Pharmacotherapy in Primary Care

Pharmacotherapy in Primary Care

William D. Linn, PharmD

Associate Professor
Feik School of Pharmacy
University of the Incarnate Word
San Antonio, Texas

Marion R. Wofford, MD, MPH

Professor of Medicine
Director of General Internal Medicine
Hypertension Division
University of Mississippi Medical Center
Jackson, Mississippi

Mary Elizabeth O'Keefe, MD

Geisinger Medical Center
Danville, Pennsylvania

L. Michael Posey, BPharm

American Pharmacists Association
Washington, D.C.

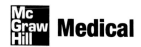 **Medical**

New York   Chicago   San Francisco   Lisbon   London   Madrid   Mexico City
New Delhi   San Juan   Seoul   Singapore   Sydney   Toronto

Pharmacotherapy in Primary Care

Copyright © 2009 by The McGraw-Hill Companies, Inc.

1 2 3 4 5 6 7 8 9 0   QPD/QPD 12 11 10 9 8

ISBN 978-0-07-145612-8
MHID 0-07-145612-0

This book was set in New Baskerville by Aptara®, Inc.
The editors were Michael Weitz and Karen Davis.
The production supervisor was Phil Galea.
Production management was provided by Samir Roy, Aptara®, Inc.
The cover designer was Elizabeth Pisacreta.
The index was prepared by Maria Coughlin.
Quebecor World Dubuque was printer and binder.

This book is printed on acid-free paper.

Library of Congress Cataloging-in-Publication Data

Pharmacotherapy in primary care / by William D. Linn . . . [et al.].
      p. ; cm.
   Includes bibliographical references.
   ISBN 978-0-07-145612-8 (softcover : alk. paper)
  1. Chemotherapy—Handbooks, manuals, etc. 2. Primary care
(Medicine)—Handbooks, manuals, etc. I. Linn, William D.
   [DNLM: 1. Drug Therapy–methods—Handbooks. 2. Primary
Health Care—methods—Handbooks. WB 39 P5358 2008]
   RM262.P473 2008
   615.5'8—dc22
                                              2008008342

CONTENTS

vi Contents

CONTRIBUTORS

Joe R. Anderson, PharmD, BCPS

Associate Professor, College of Pharmacy, University of New Mexico Health Sciences Center, Albuquerque, New Mexico
Chapter 2: Heart Failure

Michael L. Ayers, MD, FCCP

Associate, Pulmonary and Critical Care Medicine, Director of Interventional Bronchoscopy, Geisinger Medical Center, Danville, Pennsylvania
Chapter 9: Management of Chronic Obstructive Pulmonary Disease

Christina L. Barlow, MD

Assistant Professor, Division of Internal Medicine/Hypertension, University of Mississippi Medical Center, Jackson, Mississippi
Chapter 27: Thyroid Gland Disorders

Richard C. Berchou, PharmD

Department of Neurology, Psychiatry and Behavioral Neuroscience, Wayne State University School of Medicine, Detroit, Michigan, The Clinical Neuroscience Center, Southfield, Michigan
Chapter 17: Parkinson Disease

Brookie M. Best, PharmD, MAS

Assistant Clinical Professor of Pharmacy and Pediatrics, Department of Pediatrics, UCSD Skaggs School of Pharmacy and Pharmaceutical Sciences, UCSD School of Medicine, La Jolla, California
Chapter 38: Otitis Media and Sinusitis

Kendra Boell, DO

Associate, Department of Gastroenterology and Nutrition, Geisinger Medical Center, Danville, Pennsylvania
Chapter 24: Obesity

Marshall J. Bouldin, MD

Associate Professor, University of Mississippi Medical Center, Jackson, Mississippi
Chapter 25: Diabetes Mellitus Management

Julianna Burzynski, PharmD, BCPS, BCOP

Clinical Assistant Professor, University of Texas Health Science Center at San Antonio, Bone Marrow Transplant Clinical Pharmacy Specialist, Audie L. Murphy Memorial Veterans Hospital, San Antonio, Texas
Chapter 18: Persistent Pain

Lucinda M. Buys

Associate Professor, University of Iowa, College of Pharmacy, Clinical Pharmacist, Siouxland Medical Education Foundation, Inc., Sioux City, Iowa
Chapter 35: Osteoarthritis

Ann E. Canales, PharmD, BCPS

Assistant Professor, Department of Pharmacy Practice,, Texas Tech University Health Sciences Center, Abilene, Texas
Chapter 32: Urinary Incontinence

Deborah L. Cardell, MD

Clinical Assistant Professor of Medicine, Division of General Medicine, University of Texas Health Science Center at San Antonio, San Antonio, Texas
Chapter 1: Hypertension

C. Shannon Carroll, Sr., DO

Clinical Assistant Professor, Department of Obstetrics and Gynecology, University of Mississippi Medical Center, Jackson, Mississippi
Chapter 28: Contraception

Robert Chilton, DO, FACC

Professor of Medicine, Department of Medicine, Division of Cardiology, University of Texas Health Science Center, San Antonio, Texas
Chapter 4: Arrhythmias

Elizabeth C. Clark, MD, MPH

Department of Family Medicine, Robert Wood Johnson Medical School, University of Medicine and Dentistry of New Jersey, Somerset, New Jersey
Chapter 36: Gout

Michelle V. Conde, MD

Clinical Associate Professor of Medicine, University of Texas Health Science Center at San Antonio, Audie L. Murphy Division/South Texas Veterans Health Care System and Division of General Internal Medicine, San Antonio, Texas
Chapter 1: Hypertension
Chapter 23: Obstructive Sleep Apnea Hypopnea Syndrome

Elizabeth A. Coyle, PharmD

Clinical Associate Professor, University of Houston College of Pharmacy, Adjunct Clinical Assistant Professor of Medicine, Department of Infectious Diseases, Infection Control and Employee Health, UT-MD Anderson Cancer Center, Houston, Texas
Chapter 44: Urinary Tract Infections and Prostatitis

Dana Dale, MD

Assistant Professor, Division of Endocrinology, University of Mississippi Medical Center, Jackson, Mississippi
Chapter 27: Thyroid Gland Disorders

Wendy S. Dean, PharmD

*Clinical Pharmacist, HealthPark Medical Center
Fort Myers, Florida*
Chapter 28: Contraception

Leonard J. Deftos, MD, JD

Professor of Medicine, University of California, San Diego, Physician, San Diego VA Healthcare System, La Jolla, California
Chapter 33: Osteoporosis

David N. Duddleston, MD

Clinical Assistant Professor, University of Mississippi Medical Center, Jackson, Mississippi
Chapter 39: Venous Thromboembolism

Alexandria A. Dunleavy, PharmD, BCPS

School of Pharmacy, Northeastern University , Bouve College of Health Sciences, Boston, Massachusetts
Chapter 11: Peptic Ulcer Disease
Chapter 12: Inflammatory Bowel Disease

Honey East, MD

Associate Professor of Medicine, Department of Medicine, University of Mississippi Medical Center, Jackson, Mississippi
Chapter 6: Dyslipidemia

Kelly Echevarria, PharmD, BCPS

Clinical Assistant Professor, The University of Texas at Austin and the University of Texas Health Science Center at San Antonio, San Antonio, Texas
Chapter 41: Lower Respiratory Tract Infections

Mary Elizabeth Elliott, PharmD, Phd, RPh

Associate Profesor, University of Wisconsin School of Pharmacy, Clinical Pharmacist, Wm. S. Middleton VA Medical Center, Madison, Wisconsin
Chapter 35: Osteoarthritis

Michael E. Ernst, PharmD

Associate Professor, Division of Clinical and Administrative Pharmacy, College of Pharmacy and Department of Family Medicine, Roy J. and Lucille A. Carver College of Medicine, The University of Iowa, Iowa City, Iowa
Chapter 36: Gout

Susan C. Fagan, PharmD, BCPS

Professor of Pharmacy, University of Georgia, Adjunct Professor of Neurology, Medical College of Georgia, Augusta, Georgia
Chapter 16: Stroke/Transient Ischemic Attacks

Douglas N. Fish, PharmD

Professor, Department of Clinical Pharmacy, University of Colorado School of Pharmacy, Clinical Specialist in Infectious Diseases/Critical Care, University of Colorado Hospital, Denver, Colorado
Chapter 42: Skin and Soft Tissue Infections

Mark C. Granberry, PharmD

Associate Dean, Feik School of Pharmacy, University of the Incarnate Word, San Antonio, Texas
Chapter 4: Arrhythmias

Rebecca E. Greene, Pharm D, BCOP

Clinical Assistant Professsor, University of Texas at Austin College of Pharmacy, Oncology Clinical Specialist, South Texas Veterans Health Care System, San Antonio, Texas
Chapter 13: Nausea and Vomiting

R. Darryl Hamilton, MD

Assistant Professor, Division of Oncology, Department of Medicine, University of Mississippi Medical Center, Jackson, Mississippi
Chapter 40: Anemia

Michelle S. Harkins, MD

Associate Professor of Medicine, Department of Internal Medicine, Division of Pulmonary and Critical Care, University of New Mexico, Albuquerque, New Mexico
Chapter 8: Asthma Management

T. Kristopher Harrell, PharmD

Assistant Professor of Pharmacy Practice, University of Mississippi School of Pharmacy, Jackson, Mississippi
Chapter 29: Menopausal Hormone Therapy

Barbara Jean Hoeben, Maj, USAF, PharmD, MSPharm, BCPS

Clinical Pharmacy Flight Commander, Wilford Hall Medical Center, Lackland AFB, Texas
Chapter 7: Peripheral Arterial Disease

Stephen S. Im, MD

Assistant Professor, University of Texas Health Science Center at San Antonio, South Texas Veterans Health Care System, Audie L. Murphy Memorial Veterans Hospital, Division of Pulmonary and Critical Care Medicine, San Antonio, Texas
Chapter 23: Obstructive Sleep Apnea Hypopnea Syndrome

S. Rubina Inamdar, MD

Section Head, Division of Allergy and Immunology, Mercy Medical Group, Sacramento, California
Chapter 37: Allergic and Nonallergic Rhinitis
Chapter 38: Otitis Media and Sinusitis

Dena Jackson, MD

Brookhaven Internal Medicine, Brookhaven, Mississippi
Chapter 19: Headache Disorders

H. William Kelly, PharmD

Professor Emeritus of Pediatrics, Department of Pediatrics, University of New Mexico, Albuquerque, New Mexico
Chapter 8: Asthma Management

Deborah S. King, PharmD

Associate Professor, Department of General Internal Medicine, University of Mississippi Medical Center, Jackson, Mississippi
Chapter 19: Headache Disorders

Cynthia K. Kirkwood, PharmD, BCPP

Associate Professor of Pharmacy, Vice Chair for Education, Department of Pharmacy, Virginia Commonwealth University, Richmond, Virginia
Chapter 22: Anxiety Disorders

Sarah Lapey, MD

Clinical Assistant Professor of Medicine, University of Texas Health Science Center at San Antonio, Audie L. Murphy Division/South Texas Veterans Health Care System and Division of General Internal Medicine, San Antonio, Texas
Chapter 1: Hypertension

Peter A. LeWitt, MD

Professor of Neurology, Wayne State University School of Medicine, Detroit, Michigan, Editor-in-Chief, Clinical Neuropharmacology, Director, Division of Parkinson's Disease and Movement Disorders, Henry Ford Health Systems, Franklin Pointe Medical Center, Southfield, Michigan
Chapter 17: Parkinson Disease

Cara Liday, PharmD, CDE

Associate Professor, Department of Pharmacy Practice and Administrative Sciences, College of Pharmacy, Idaho State University, Pocatello, Idaho
Chapter 31: Benign Prostatic Hyperplasia

William D. Linn, PharmD

Associate Professor, Feik School of Pharmacy, University of the Incarnate Word, San Antonio, Texas
Chapter 4: Arrhythmias
Chapter 5: Hypertrophic Cardiomyopathy

Sunny A. Linnebur, PharmD, FASCP, BCPS, CGP

Assistant Professor, Department of Clinical Pharmacy, University of Colorado Denver, Denver, Colorado
Chapter 30: Erectile Dysfunction

Annette K. Low, MD

Associate Professor of Medicine, University of Mississippi Medical Center, Jackson, Mississippi
Chapter 29: Menopausal Hormone Therapy

Dalia Mack, PharmD, AE-C, CDE

School of Pharmacy, Northeastern University, Bouve College of Health Sciences, Boston, Massachusetts
Chapter 11: Peptic Ulcer Disease

Cynthia A. Mascarenas, PharmD, MSPharm, BCPP

Clinical Assistant Professor, College of Pharmacy, The University of Texas at Austin, Clinical Assistant Professor, Department of Pharmacology, The University of Texas Health Science Center at San Antonio, San Antonio, Texas
Chapter 21: Depression

Robb McIlvried, MD, MPH

Associate, Department of General Internal Medicine Geisinger Medical Center, Danville, Pennsylvania
Chapter 20: Pharmacotherapy for Alzheimer Disease

Trevor McKibbin, PharmD

Advanced Practice Masters Student, University of Texas at Austin College of Pharmacy, Oncology Pharmacy Resident, South Texas Veterans Health Care System, San Antonio, Texas
Chapter 13: Nausea and Vomiting

Nicole L. McMaster-Baxter, PharmD, MS, BCPS

Michael E. DeBakey VA Medical Center–Houston, The University of Texas at Austin College of Pharmacy, Houston, Texas
Chapter 14: Constipation and Diarrhea

Shyamal Mehta, MD, PhD

Resident in Neurology, Department of Neurology, Medical College of Georgia, Augusta, Georgia
Chapter 16: Stroke/Transient Ischemic Attacks

Deborah S. Minor, PharmD

Associate Professor of Medicine, University of Mississippi Medical Center, Jackson, Mississippi
Chapter 19: Headache Disorders

Tera D. Moore, PharmD, BCPS

Primary Care Clinical Pharmacy Specialist, South Texas Veterans Health Care System, Clinical Assistant Professor, The University of Texas at Austin College of Pharmacy, San Antonio, Texas
Chapter 2: Heart Failure

Troy A. Moore, PharmD, MSPharm, BCPP

Assistant Professor, Department of Psychiatry, Division of Schizophrenia and Related Disorders, The University of Texas Health Science Center at San Antonio, San Antonio, Texas
Chapter 21: Depression

Candis M. Morello, PharmD, CDE, FCSHP

Assistant Professor of Clinical Pharmacy, Ambulatory Care Pharmacist Specialist, Skaggs School of Pharmacy and Pharmaceutical Sciences, University of California, San Diego, La Jolla, California
Chapter 33: Osteoporosis

Laura A. Morgan, PharmD, BCPS

Assistant Professor of Pharmacy, Department of Pharmacy, Virginia Commonwealth University, Richmond, Virginia
Chapter 22: Anxiety Disorders

Nicole Murdock, PharmD, BCPS

Pocatello Family Medicine, Idaho State University, Pocatello, Idaho
Chapter 31: Benign Prostatic Hyperplasia

Rocsanna Namdar, PharmD

Assistant Professor, College of Pharmacy, University of New Mexico, Albuquerque, New Mexico
Chapter 43: Tuberculosis

Beverly D. Nixon-Lewis, DO

Assistant Professor, Department of Family and Community Medicine, Texas Tech University Health Sciences Center, Amarillo, Texas
Chapter 32: Urinary Incontinence

Robert A. O'Rourke, MD

Charles Conrad Brown Distinguished Professor in Cardiovascular Disease, Department of Medicine/Cardiology, The University of Texas Health Science Center at San Antonio, San Antonio, Texas
Chapter 3: Diagnosis and Management of Chronic Coronary Heart Disease
Chapter 5: Hypertrophic Cardiomyopathy

Charles A. Peloquin, PharmD

Director, Infectious Disease, Pharmacokinetics Laboratory, National Jewish Medical and Research Center, Denver, Colorado
Chapter 43: Tuberculosis

Randall A. Prince, PharmD, FCCP

Professor and Director, University of Houston Anti-infective Research Laboratories, Adjunct Professor of Medicine, Department of Infectious Diseases, Infection Control and Employee Health, UT-MD Anderson Cancer Center, Houston, Texas
Chapter 44: Urinary Tract Infections and Prostatitis

Susan J. Rogers, BS, PharmD, BCPS

Clinical Pharmacy Specialist, Audie L. Murphy Memorial Veterans Hospital, Assistant Clinical Professor of Pharmacology, The University of Texas Health Science Center at San Antonio, San Antonio, Texas
Chapter 15: Epilepsy

Brendan Sean Ross, MD

Clinical Associate Professor, Department of Pharmacy Practice, University of Mississippi School of Pharmacy, Staff Physician, G.V. (Sonny) Montgomery Veterans Affairs of Medical Center, Jackson, Mississippi
Chapter 6: Dyslipedemia

Leigh Ann Ross, PharmD, BCPS, CDE

Associate Professor and Chair, Department of Pharmacy Practice, University of Mississippi School of Pharmacy, Jackson, Mississippi
Chapter 6: Dyslipidemia

Rebecca A. Rottman, PharmD, BCPS, CGP

Geriatrics Clinical Pharmacy Specialist, South Texas Veterans Health Care System, Clinical Assistant Professor, University of Texas College of Pharmacy at Austin, University of Texas Health Science Center at San Antonio (UTHSCSA), San Antonio, Texas
Chapter 39: Venous Thromboembolism

Laurajo Ryan, PharmD, MSc, BCPS, CDE

Clinical Assistant Professor, University of Texas at Austin College of Pharmacy, University of Texas Health Science Center at San Antonio, San Antonio, Texas
Chapter 45: Sexually Transmitted Diseases

Kathryn Sabol, PharmD, BCPS

Infectious Diseases Clinical Pharmacy Specialist, Parkland Health and Hospital System, San Antonio, Texas
Chapter 41: Lower Respiratory Tract Infections

Robert R. Schade, MD

Professor, Department of Medicine, Chief, Section of Gastroenterology and Hepatology, Medical College of Georgia, Augusta, Georgia
Chapter 10: Gastroesophageal Reflux Disease

Arthur A. Schuna, MS, FASHP

Rheumatology Pharmacotherapist, William S. Middleton VA Medical Center, Clinical Professor, University of Wisconsin School of Pharmacy, Madison, Wisconsin
Chapter 34: Rheumatoid Arthritis

Jinna Shepherd, MD

Associate Professor, Division of General Internal Medicine/Hypertension, Department of Medicine, University of Mississippi Medical Center, Jackson, Mississippi
Chapter 40: Anemia

Renu F. Singh, PharmD

Assistant Clinical Professor, Ambulatory Care Pharmacist Specialist, Skaggs School of Pharmacy and Pharmaceutical Sciences, University of California, San Diego, La Jolla, California
Chapter 33: Osteoporosis

Ronald Solbing, MD

Idaho State University Family Medicine Residency,, Pocatello, Idaho
Chapter 31: Benign Prostatic Hyperplasia

Jimmy L. Stewart, MD

Associate Professor of Medicine and Pediatrics, Program Director, Combined Internal Medicine/Pediatrics Residency Program, University of Mississippi Medical Center, Jackson, Mississippi
Chapter 26: Metabolic Syndrome

Scott Strassels, PharmD, PhD, BCPS

Assistant Professor, Division of Pharmacy Practice, University of Texas at Austin, Austin, Texas
Chapter 18: Persistent Pain

Caryl Sumrall, FNP

Clinical Instructor, University of Mississippi Medical Center, Jackson, Mississippi
Chapter 25: Diabetes Mellitus Management

Sharon A. Jung Tschirhart, PharmD, BCPS

South Texas Veterans Healthcare System, Audie L. Murphy Division, The University of Texas at Austin College of Pharmacy, Houston, Texas
Chapter 14: Constipation and Diarrhea

Jeffrey I. Wallace, MD, MPH

Associate Professor, Department of Medicine, University of Colorado at Denver and Health Sciences Center, Denver, Colorado
Chapter 30: Erectile Dysfunction

Patrick F. Walsh, DO

Associate, Critical Care Medicine, Geisinger Medical Center, Danville, Pennsylvania
Chapter 9: Management of Chronic Obstructive Pulmonary Disease

Dianne B. Williams, PharmD, BCPS

Drug Information and Formulary Coordinator, Medical College of Georgia Health System, Clinical Associate Professor, University of Georgia College of Pharmacy, Augusta, Georgia
Chapter 10: Gastroesophageal Reflux Disease

Marion R. Wofford, MD, MPH

Professor of Medicine, Director of General Internal Medicine, Hypertension Division, University of Mississippi Medical Center, Jackson, Mississippi
Chapter 26: Metabolic Syndrome

FOREWORD

Pharmacotherapy in Primary Care is a book chock full of useful, easily accessible information and advice. Busy practitioners seeking quick overviews and practical management recommendations for many conditions seen in primary care will be pleased with its format and content. Well-laid out chapters focus on the following: Clinical Presentation, Physical Findings, Diagnostic Evaluation, and Management. Management sections comprehensively address asymptomatic and symptomatic patients, referral and consultation questions, integration of pharmacotherapy with nonpharmacologic treatment, and long-term monitoring. Particularly attractive for busy readers are the multiple tables and concise algorithms of treatment strategies, and the clearly written thumbnail summaries of key points. Unquestionably, the authors have achieved their high aim of presenting a well-reasoned and streamlined approach to therapeutic decision-making about common primary care disorders.

Cynthia Mulrow MD, MSc, MACP

Deputy Editor, Annals of Internal Medicine
Clinical Professor of Medicine
University of Texas Health Science Center at San Antonio
San Antonio, Texas

PREFACE

Clinicians are in constant need of information. It is estimated that providers need answers to two questions for every three patients seen. Unfortunately, many decisions appear to be opinion based, highly variable, and without clear justification. The difference between an outstanding clinician and an average one is the ability to quickly find high-quality evidence generalizable to their patients.

The authors of *Pharmacotherapy in Primary Care* have been carefully chosen and their clinical experience represents tens of thousands of patient visits. Their authoritative recommendations provide evidence-based information that is essential to accurate clinical decision making. This text will be a valuable resource for primary care providers of all disciplines. *Pharmacotherapy in Primary Care* is not intended to be an encyclopedic textbook. For in-depth reviews, readers should refer to texts such as *Pharmacotherapy: A Pathophysiologic Approach, Harrison's Principles of Internal Medicine,* or *The Heart.*

Pharmacotherapy in Primary Care includes the search strategy used by the authors, to allow the reader to know when the information was assessed, and to feel confident that the most relevant material is included. There are numerous tables, algorithms, and flow diagrams to facilitate finding key information. The authors include insights regarding the need for subspecialty referral or hospitalization, and each chapter closes with an evidence-based summary. *Pharmacotherapy in Primary Care* is structured so that clinicians can quickly find answers to specific questions. Readers will feel that they have consulted with a specialist after reading a chapter.

In closing, we would like to thank Karen Davis and her colleagues at McGraw-Hill for their support to *Pharmacotherapy in Primary Care.* Without their resources, dedication, and faith in us, this first edition would not have been possible.

The Editors
July 2008

INTRODUCTION

Clinicians are constantly faced with choices about how to accurately achieve a diagnosis, estimate a prognosis, choose an optimal treatment strategy, or assess the possibility of harm, in order to provide the best care to their patients. Increasingly, clinicians are turning to the principles of evidence-based medicine (EBM) to help them make these decisions. This text, *Pharmacotherapy in Primary Care*, seeks to translate the best available evidence for the most common diseases encountered daily in physician offices, ambulatory care clinics, hospitals, and pharmacies.

The practice of EBM means to (1) recognize informational need while caring for a patient, (2) identify the best existing evidence to help resolve the problem, (3) consider the evidence in light of the actual circumstances, and (4) integrate the evidence into a medical plan.

Medical information is growing incessantly—the number of citations more than doubled in the past decade. Each year, 10,000 randomized controlled trials addressing the impact of health care interventions are published. The information synthesized by the authors of this book provide a sound outline on how to care for the majority of patients clinicians see, but when presented with a patient whose clinical characteristics differ in important ways, care must be individualized. How can busy frontline clinicians sort the good from the bad and identify the best evidence to resolve their problem at the time of such patient visits?

FOCUS THE SEARCH

The search for evidence begins with identifying relevant articles in the peer-reviewed literature. To expedite and target a literature search, the clinician must phrase the problem in a clear, precise, and specific question. The acronym PICO can be helpful to clarify the question and search strategy[1]:

P = patient (including the disease, comorbidities, age, and other relevant characteristics)

I = intervention (drug therapy, diagnostic test, exposure, and other possible treatments)

C = comparison (of possible actions and interventions with other drugs, tests, procedures)

O = outcome (cure, disease avoidance, accurate diagnoses, and other clinical, humanistic, and economic measures of success or failure)

BE MORE CRITICAL

The authors of each chapter in *Pharmacotherapy in Primary Care* have carefully searched and critically appraised for the best available evidence to provide their recommendations for patients with 45 common diseases listed in the Table of Contents. Asking an expert or a colleague may be the quickest way to get advice on how to proceed with these patients, but be cautious, as these people may be just as overwhelmed by the volume and complexity of medical information as you are or their advice may be out of date. Searching PubMed or MEDLINE may simply be too labor intensive for point-of-care decisions.

In such cases, consider evidence-based resources that have conducted the search, filtered the high

---

[1]Ghosh AK, Ghosh K. Enhance your practice with evidence-based medicine. *Patient Care*. February 2000:32–56.

quality, relevant evidence, and summarized the results for the busy clinician. Reputable evidence-based databases—including the Cochrane Library, Up-to-Date, National Guideline Clearinghouse, and PIER (Physicians' Information and Education Resource from the American College of Physicians)—provide evidence-based discussions of hundreds of specific clinical situations. For example, the Cochrane Collaboration, available online at www.cochrane.org, listed the following top 10 accessed reviews when this foreword was written in September 2007:

- Membrane sweeping for induction of labor
- Vitamin C for preventing and treating the common cold
- Ear drops for the removal of ear wax
- Low glycemic index or low glycemic load diets for overweight and obesity
- Glucosamine therapy for treating osteoarthritis
- Surgery for thumb (trapeziometacarpal joint) osteoarthritis
- Surgery for degenerative lumbar spondylosis
- Effects of low sodium diet versus high sodium diet on blood pressure, renin, aldosterone, catecholamines, cholesterols, and triglyceride
- Diacerein for osteoarthritis
- Hypotonic versus isotonic saline solutions for intravenous fluid management of acute infections

Accessing these resources is like having your own personal librarian to conduct searches and an on-staff group of world-renowned experts to assess the literature for you.

INTEGRATE INTO PRACTICE

Integrating evidence into practice requires combining the best evidence with knowledge of disease and patient management. The usefulness of an intervention depends not only on its efficacy but also on whether the magnitude of the benefit outweighs the risks, costs, benefits of existing alternative and whether the intervention is realistic and acceptable considering the patient's values and health care delivery context.

The needed skills for practicing EBM may appear daunting, but once acquired, they can help the health professionals to better use available resources and time by knowing how to focus a search and be more critical of what research studies and information to integrate in their knowledge base.

Pharmacotherapy in Primary Care fulfills the four attributes to make it useful in daily clinical practice: it is relevant to everyday practice, evidence-based, concise, and reader friendly. It is intended to be the first-line resource clinicians can turn to when faced with clinical management options. For more in-depth review and discussion of disease management, the reader may refer to textbooks such as *Harrison's Principles of Internal Medicine* or the *Pharmacotherapy: A Pathophysiologic Approach* on which this primary care resource was based.

Although the chapters in this textbook vary in their content, they use a similar outline to help the reader access quickly the information they need:

- Clinical presentation
- Physical findings
- Diagnostic evaluation
- Risk stratification
- Management
- Evidence-based summary

The chapters use flow charts, figures, and tables to simplify the description of investigations and treatments recommended for the various common conditions in primary care.

Pharmacotherapy in Primary Care will help frontline clinicians identify the array of potential decisions and provide them with the evidence that, when used in conjunction with the clinicians' individual clinical judgment and their patients' values and expectations, will assist greatly in the millions of patient-care decisions that must be made daily in primary care settings.

Elaine Chiquette, PharmD
San Antonio, Texas

L. Michael Posey, BPharm
Athens, Georgia

PART 1

Cardiovascular Disorders

CHAPTERS

Chapter 1

Hypertension

Deborah L. Cardell, Sarah Lapey, and Michelle V. Conde

SEARCH STRATEGY

A comprehensive search of the medical literature was performed in January 2008. The search, limited to human subjects and English language journals, included MEDLINE®, PubMed, the Cochrane Database of Systematic Reviews, and UpToDate®. The current Seventh Report of the Joint National Committee on Prevention, Detection, Evaluation, and Treatment of High Blood Pressure (JNC VII) can be found at http://www.nhlbi.nih.gov/guidelines/hypertension/

PREVALENCE AND DISEASE BURDEN

Hypertension (HTN) is both the most common reason for office visits in the United States as well as the most common indication for prescription medicines. Twenty-four percent of the adult population, or approximately 50 million people, have HTN. Although 53% of hypertensive patients are receiving pharmacotherapy, only a disappointing 14% to 25% of these patients succeed in meeting blood pressure (BP) treatment goals.[1] Elevated BP is associated with a continuum of increasing risk for cardiovascular disease, stroke, and kidney disease. Each incremental rise in BP above 115/75 translates into an elevated risk of end-organ damage.[2] Reduction in BP decreases the risk of stroke by 35% to 40%, myocardial infarction (MI) by 20% to 25%, and heart failure by greater than 50%.[3] The successful control of BP could therefore potentially reduce the deleterious effects of three of the most common medical conditions affecting Americans.

SCREENING

The treatment of HTN is impossible without an awareness of the diagnosis. National Health and Nutrition Examination Survey (NHANES) III found that only 70% of patients meeting diagnostic criteria for HTN were in fact cognizant of their condition. Currently, the U.S. Preventive Services Task Force recommends screening all adults more than 18 years of age annually for HTN (grade A recommendation).[4]

MEASUREMENT OF BP

PROPER TECHNIQUE

The diagnosis of HTN requires accurate measurements of BP. The JNC VII includes recommendations for proper BP measurement based on expert guidelines.[2] First, an appropriate cuff size must be selected so as to avoid falsely elevated (from very small size) or falsely decreased (from very large size) BP readings. The bladder, which is the rubber, inflatable portion of the cuff, should encircle at least 75% to 80% of the upper arm, and the width of the cuff should span at least 40% of the length of the upper arm.[5] Ideally, the patient should be seated in a chair for 5 minutes prior to the measurement of BP. Ingestion of caffeine, tobacco products, or medications potentially raising the BP should be avoided for 30 to 60 minutes prior to measuring the BP. Talking during BP measurement can falsely elevate the BP, as can excessively cold temperatures or improper patient positioning. The patient's arm should be supported at the level of the heart, and the sphygmomanometer, within 3 feet of the examiner and preferably at the eye level. With its lower edge positioned 2 to 3 cm above the brachial artery, the cuff is then inflated to approximately 30 mm Hg higher than the point at which the brachial artery can no longer be palpated. This value is determined prior to the actual BP measurement by inflating the cuff while palpating the radial artery and noting the mm Hg at which the pulse disappears; this is the number above which the sphygmomanometer must be inflated. The stethoscope is then held lightly over the brachial artery while the cuff is slowly deflated at a rate of 2 to 3 mm Hg per heartbeat or per second. Deflating the cuff any faster results in an underestimation of systolic and overestimation of diastolic pressures.[5] The diagnosis of HTN can be established when there are two to three elevated readings from separate office visits at least a week apart.

Although the mercury sphygmomanometer has been the "gold standard" for decades, its use is being phased out and replaced by aneroid and electronic devices, because of the environmental concerns of potential mercury leakage. Health care personnel must ensure that their BP equipment is kept in the best possible working order by regular inspection and validation for accuracy. Tubing should be checked for leaks, hook and eye closures must be strong enough to remain fastened during inflation, and aneroid sphygmomanometers must be calibrated at least every 6 months. Over time, with repeated jostling and movement, aneroid devices become less and less accurate, causing an underestimation in the true BP.

HOME BP MONITORING

Home BP monitoring, or self-monitoring of BP by the patient outside of the clinic, represents an area of increased recent interest in the literature. An agreed-upon application includes the evaluation of patients with suspected white coat HTN.[6] White-coat HTN is defined as an elevated BP (>140/90 mm Hg) in the clinic setting, with a concomitant normal BP reading (<135/85 mm Hg) at home. As would be expected, further assessment of these patients fails to demonstrate evidence of end-organ damage.

The literature on ambulatory BP monitoring (ABPM) has uncovered a trend in which home BP readings are consistently lower than office measurements. Consequently, BP goals for home readings have been adjusted, with home BP <135/85 mm Hg corresponding to an office BP goal of <140/90 mm Hg.[7] The same factors affecting the accuracy of the office-based BP measurement also impact home BP measurement, and home BP devices often do not perform as well in the community as compared with the laboratory set-

ting.[8] In light of the above barriers, home BP monitoring should be limited to certain special circumstances, including the assessment of response to therapy, efforts to improve patient compliance, and the evaluation of suspected white-coat HTN. Its use has not been universally recommended for the regular care of all hypertensive patients.[2]

AMBULATORY BP MONITORING

ABPM refers to an outpatient-evaluation technique in which multiple-automated BP readings are obtained at specific intervals over the span of 24 to 72 hours. ABPM provides additional data that potentially provides insight into BP control during a patient's everyday activities. Similar to home BP monitoring, there is a recent and growing interest in ABPM in the medical community and literature. Prospective studies have suggested that ambulatory BP data may more accurately reflect a patient's BP and better correlate with target-organ injury (such as left ventricular hypertrophy) than office-based BP measurements;[9,10] however, long-term outcomes are lacking. In general, the research assessing long-term outcomes on the use of clinic-based BP monitoring far exceeds the corresponding studies for ABPM. Therefore, in-office BP readings still remain the gold standard for decision-making in BP management. While admittedly the literature on ABPM is newer, there is a general consensus that there are select groups of patients, including those with suspected white-coat HTN, refractory HTN with apparent drug resistance, and patients in whom efficacy of their antihypertensive regimen is under evaluation, for whom ABPM may be beneficial. Medicare has recently approved reimbursement for ABPM in patients with suspected white-coat HTN.

Advocates for ABPM point to the money that is wasted on 20% to 25% of the hypertensive patients who have white-coat HTN and are unnecessarily treated with medications. Some experts, however, argue that patients with white-coat HTN are not completely free of cardiovascular risk and have a risk that is more than normotensive patients and yet less than that of patients with sustained HTN.[11,12] Still other studies have found no increased risk for cardiovascular outcomes for patients determined to have only white-coat HTN.[13] Patients determined to have white-coat HTN need close follow-up as the incidence of stroke rises after 6 years.[7] A recent review article suggests that ABPM is best suited for more accurate assessment of risk in hypertensive patients, for evaluating nighttime BPs when clinically relevant and for evaluating the effectiveness of various antihypertensive drugs when they are being compared in clinical studies.[14]

Table 1-1. JNC VII Classification of BP for Adults[2]

BP Classification	SBP (mm Hg)	DBP (mm Hg)	Follow-up (Without Compelling Indications for Treatment)
Normal	<120	and <80	2 years
Pre-HTN	120–139	or 80–89	Recheck in 1 year
Stage 1 HTN	140–159	or 90–99	Confirm within 2 months
Stage 2 HTN	≥160	or ≥100	<180/110—Evaluate and treat within 1 month
			≥180/110—Evaluate and treat immediately or within 1 week (depending upon the clinical situation)

Source: Chobanian et al: Natl Hi BP. Hypertension 2003;42:1206

DEFINITION AND CLASSIFICATION OF BP

JNC VII introduced a new classification of "pre-HTN," corresponding to a systolic BP (SBP) of 120 to 139 mm Hg and/or a diastolic blood pressure (DBP) of 80 to 89 mm Hg. This is not a disease category but rather a designation, aiming to identify individuals at high risk for the development of HTN. Prehypertensive patients are ideal targets for early intervention through lifestyle modifications, so as to prevent the progressive increase in BP leading to HTN. Clinicians can educate these patients regarding their risk and encourage them to make lifestyle modifications. Those patients with pre-HTN who also have underlying renal insufficiency or diabetes, on the other hand, are candidates for pharmacotherapy, if their BP remains above 130/80, despite lifestyle modifications. In all other patients without compelling indications for treatment, a BP can be rechecked within 1 year (see Table 1-1).

INITIAL EVALUATION

The diagnosis of HTN requires two to three separate BP readings, higher than 140/90 mm Hg, at least a week apart. The initial approach in assessing a hypertensive patient consists of a global cardiovascular disease risk assessment, evaluation for the presence of end-organ damage, and a search for secondary causes of HTN, if indicated (Fig. 1-1 and Tables 1-2 and 1-5).

MANAGEMENT

LIFESTYLE MODIFICATIONS

Lifestyle modifications represent a crucial part of a multidisciplinary BP management approach and offer the added benefit of decreasing cardiovascular risk independent of BP changes. Health care providers should encourage all prehypertensive (SBP 120 to 139 mm Hg or DBP 80 to 89 mm Hg) and hypertensive (BP ≥ 140/90 mm Hg) patients regarding the importance of weight reduction; dietary modifications, as exemplified by the Dietary Approaches to Stop Hypertension (DASH)

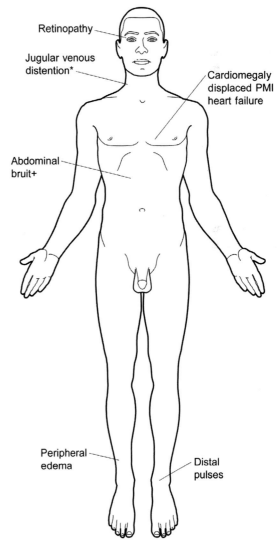

Figure 1-1. Selected physical examination findings. *Jugular venous distention: 85–100% probability of increased filling pressures[67]; +Abdominal bruit: sensitivity 39% and specificity 99% for a systolic-diastolic bruit for detecting true renal atherosclerotic disease.[68]

Table 1-2. Routine Laboratory Studies

Hematocrit	Electrolytes
Urinalysis	Fasting lipid profile
Glucose	Electrocardiogram
Creatinine	

eating plan (diet rich in fruits, vegetables, and low-fat dairy products) and dietary sodium restriction, regular physical activity, and moderation of alcohol consumption. These lifestyle changes can lower BP, and also enhance the efficacy of antihypertensive medications. The most effective nonpharmacological lifestyle modification is weight loss. The DASH diet, recommending four servings of fruit, four servings of vegetables, and three servings of low-fat dairy products per day, also has significant BP lowering effects independent of weight loss. In some individuals, this dietary plan approaches the impact of a single antihypertensive medication.[2] Exercise recommendations consist of 30 minutes of brisk, aerobic activity most days of the week. Alcohol moderation refers to limiting intake to no more than two drinks for men and one drink for women each day (Table 1-3). Additionally, given that the overall goal is reduction in cardiovascular-related disease and not simply BP reduction, health care providers should also assist patients in tobacco cessation.

INITIAL PHARMACOLOGIC THERAPY

The JNC VII recommends initial drug therapy with a thiazide-type diuretic in the absence of a compelling indication for another antihypertensive drug class.[2] This recommendation supports the findings of The Antihypertensive and Lipid Lowering Treatment to Prevent Heart Attack Trial (ALLHAT), which prospectively randomized 42 418 hypertensive patients with one addi-

tional risk factor for coronary artery disease to low-dose chlorthalidone or one of the following newer antihypertensive agents: lisinopril, amlodipine, and doxazosin.[15] The doxazosin arm was terminated prematurely as a result of the increased incidence of heart failure relative to chlorthalidone. The primary outcomes were fatal coronary heart disease and nonfatal MI, and the incidences were similar across the chlorthalidone, amlodipine, and lisinopril groups, consistent with results from other trials.[16,17] Additionally, the chlorthalidone group showed superiority in several secondary endpoints, including improved heart failure protection compared to both amlodipine and lisinopril and improved stroke protection compared with lisinopril.

The results of the ALLHAT trial have sparked controversy. First, open-label agents or "step-up agents" were used for additional BP control and included atenolol, reserpine, clonidine, and hydralazine, combinations which, in general, do not mirror clinical practice. Approximately 40% of patients required these additional agents for BP control. Additionally, increased fasting glucose levels ≥126 mg/dL in nondiabetic patients assigned to chlorthalidone were noted. Although this change did not increase cardiovascular morbidity and mortality relative to the other groups during the mean follow-up of 4.9 years, experts raised the concern that significant deleterious changes in cardiovascular morbidity and mortality might become apparent after 5 years.[18,19]

The ALLHAT trial also found that lisinopril had higher rates of stroke, heart failure, and combined cardiovascular outcomes than chlorthalidone, which was a surprising finding given reports of improved cardiovascular outcomes with angiotensin converting enzyme (ACE) inhibitors independent of its BP lowering effects.[20] Several authors highlight that the chlorthalidone arm achieved tighter BP control relative to the lisinopril arm, potentially accounting for the cardiovascular differences.[21–24]

Table 1-3. JNC VII Lifestyle Modification Recommendations[2]

Modification	Recommendation	Average SBP Reduction Range (mm Hg)
Weight reduction	Maintain normal BMI (18.5–24.9 kg/m^2)	5–20 (per 10 kg)
DASH eating plan	Eat a diet rich in fruits, vegetables, and low-fat dairy products with reduced content of saturated and total fat.	8–14
Dietary sodium reduction	Reduce dietary sodium intake to ≤100 mmol/d (2.4 g sodium or 6 g sodium chloride).	2–8
Aerobic physical activity	Regular aerobic physical activity at least 30 min/d, most days of the week.	4–9
Moderation of alcohol consumption	Men: Limit to ≤2 drinks/d; women: Limit to ≤1 drink/d; 1 drink ~12 oz beer, 5 oz wine, or 1.5 oz 80-proof whiskey.	2–4

Source: Chobanian et al: Natl Hi BP. Hypertension 2003;42:1206

The Anglo-Scandinavian Cardiac Outcomes Trial: Blood Pressure Lowering Arm (ASCOT-BPLA), which prospectively randomized 19 257 hypertensive patients, mean age of 63 years with three cardiovascular risk factors, to an amlodipine-based strategy or an atenolol-based strategy, has added another layer of complexity.[25] This trial found that an antihypertensive strategy based on amlodipine, with perindopril (an ACE inhibitor) added as required, reduced all-cause mortality, fatal and nonfatal stroke, and total cardiovascular events and procedures compared to an atenolol-based strategy, with bendroflumethiazide added as required. The trial was prematurely terminated after 5.5 years median follow-up because of an 11% risk reduction in all-cause mortality in the amlodipine/perindopril group compared with the atenolol/bendroflumethiazide group. The majority of patients (78%) were taking at least two antihypertensive agents by the end of the trial.

The results of the ALLHAT and ASCOT trials are seemingly contradictory. One explanation is that atenolol may not be a suitable first-line antihypertensive drug compared to other classes. A systematic review found no difference in cardiovascular morbidity and mortality in patients with primary HTN between placebo and atenolol, despite a lower BP achieved with atenolol relative to placebo.[26] When compared to other antihypertensive agents (thiazide diuretics, calcium-channel antagonists, ACE inhibitors, angiotensin II receptor blockers [ARBs]), mortality was higher with atenolol than with other agents (relative risk [RR] 1.13; 95% confidence interval [CI] 1.02–1.25). Other studies have also questioned the efficacy of β-blockers as first-line drug agents for HTN in the older adults.[27,28] potentially accounting for the differences in the two treatment arms of the ASCOT trial. A meta-analysis evaluated 13 randomized controlled trials comparing treatment with different β-blockers (not limited to atenolol) with other antihypertensive classes. The meta-analysis concluded that β-blocker treatment was associated with a 16% higher RR of stroke (95% CI 4–30%; $p = 0.009$) compared with other classes.[29] Thus, the results of the ASCOT trial do not negate ALLHAT's finding that thiazide diuretics are useful first-line antihypertensive drugs in patients with uncomplicated HTN.

A systematic review by the Blood Pressure Lowering Treatment Trialists' Collaboration evaluated the effects of different antihypertensive regimens on reducing major cardiovascular events and concluded that ACE inhibitors, calcium-channel blockers, and diuretics and/or β-blocker-based regimens similarly reduced the risk of total major cardiovascular events.[30] BP lowering itself reduced the risk of total major cardiovascular events regardless of the specific regimen used. In fact, the strongest determinant in reducing total major cardiovascular events was the level of BP achieved. There were differences in specific outcomes, most notably heart failure prevention: ACE inhibitors and diuretics and/or β-blocker-based regimens were associated with a decreased risk of heart failure compared with calcium-channel blocker regimens. This review, which included the ALLHAT trial but not the ASCOT trial, did not separate diuretic treatment from β-blocker treatment results and combined studies with diuretics and/or β-blockers into one category.

In summary, evidence still remains that thiazide diuretics are effective as first-line agents in the treatment of uncomplicated HTN. Despite chlorthalidone's use as the thiazide-like diuretic evaluated in most studies, hydrochlorothiazide, which is widely available in the United States, can also be considered as a rational diuretic choice.[31] ACE-inhibitor therapy and calcium-channel blockers are also reasonable antihypertensive drug agents. β-Blockers are less efficacious as a first-line agent for HTN in the older adults; however, they remain strongly indicated in patients with chronic congestive heart failure, asymptomatic left ventricular dysfunction, a history of MI or angina.[32,33] Numerous trials show that a significant number of patients will require at least two drugs to achieve adequate BP control. ARBs are also promising antihypertensive agents and, compared with atenolol, are associated with a significant reduction in cardiovascular morbidity and mortality in hypertensive patients with ECG evidence of left ventricular hypertrophy.[34] ARBs are particularly indicated in patients who develop cough with an ACE inhibitor.

SPECIAL POPULATIONS

African Americans

Non-Hispanic black ethnicity is independently associated with increased rates of HTN.[1] Furthermore, in addition to the increased likelihood of developing HTN, African American patients with HTN have the highest morbidity and mortality from HTN of any population group in the United States.[35] The reasons for the higher associated morbidity and mortality are multifactorial and require further elucidation. Contributing factors, as cited by the Hypertension in African Americans Working Group of the International Society on Hypertension in Blacks, include medical providers' nonaggressive and inconsistent efforts in diagnosing and treating HTN.[36] Additionally, African Americans consume less potassium than white Americans and this dietary characteristic may also be a contributing factor.

Drugs that inhibit the renin system, including ACE inhibitors, ARBs, and β-blockers, reportedly have a decreased BP lowering effect as compared with thiazide diuretics and calcium-channel blockers when used as monotherapy in African American hypertensive patients.[36–38] The hypothesis is that African Americans more commonly exhibit a "low renin" phenotype.[19] African American patients have a lower baseline plasma renin activity, thus, drugs that lower BP by decreasing the plasma renin activity and, henceforth, angiotensin effects may not be effective monotherapy in patients with a relatively low baseline plasma renin activity.[39] In a systematic review of antihypertensive drug monotherapy in black patients, β-blockers did not significantly differ from that of placebo in reducing SBP (−3.53 mm Hg; 95% CI −7.51–0.45 mm Hg).[40] Additionally, ACE inhibitors did not significantly differ from that of placebo in achieving a DBP goal ≤90 mm Hg or reduction in DBP β>10 mm Hg (or 10% decrease) (RR 1.35; 95% CI 0.81–2.26). Interestingly, ARBs were found to lower both SBP and DBP. Calcium-channel blockers, diuretics, central sympatholytics, α-blockers, and again, ARBs were effective in lowering BP compared to placebo. This systematic review only evaluated efficacy of monotherapy versus placebo. Frequently, patients will not be controlled on monotherapy and will require at least two drugs. Combining drugs that inhibit the renin system along with a diuretic is a synergistic, effective combination. Indeed, β-blockers, ACE inhibitors, and ARBs should not be withheld from use in the African American population (in the absence of known adverse reactions), especially in patients with an underlying compelling indication.

The African American Study of Kidney Disease and Hypertension trial and the ALLHAT trial yielded important observations on morbidity and mortality outcomes in black hypertensive patients.[35,41] In the African American Study of Kidney Disease and Hypertension trial, which included 1 094 black hypertensive patients with hypertensive renal disease (Glomerular Filtration Rate [GFR] 20–65 mL/min/1.73 m^2) ages 18 to 70 years, patients were randomly assigned to three agents: ACE inhibitor, dihydropyridine calcium-channel blocker (amlodipine), or β-blocker.[41] The primary end point was a reduction in both the chronic GFR slope after 3 months and the mean total GFR slope from baseline to the end of the study. The secondary end point was a composite of GFR decline, end-stage renal disease (ESRD), and death. The trial did not evaluate event rates for cardiovascular outcomes. Follow-up was more than 3 to 6 years. Patients assigned to each arm were on a total of 2.75 drugs, with open-labeled medications (furosemide, doxazosin, clonidine, and hydralazine or minoxidil) added in a stepwise fashion until goal BP was achieved, consistent with previous observations that most patients require more than one antihypertensive agent.

The amlodipine arm was terminated early because of the safety concerns fueled by an interim analysis showing a slower decline in GFR and a composite reduced rate of decline in renal function, ESRD, or death in the ramipril and metoprolol groups versus the amlodipine group.[42]

This was most pronounced in those hypertensive patients with baseline proteinuria >300 mg/dL. In general, ACE inhibitors were more efficacious than β-blockers or dihydropyridine calcium-channel blockers in reducing the composite endpoint of decline in GFR by ≥50% from baseline, ESRD, or death.

In the ALLHAT trial, 35% (11 792) of enrolled patients were black.[35] The trial showed that chlorthalidone, amlodipine, and lisinopril were associated with equivalent rates for coronary heart disease. Diuretic-based treatment was associated with the lowest rate of heart failure. ACE-inhibitor-based therapy was associated with an increased incidence of stroke and heart failure, although this may have been caused by the better BP control with the diuretic versus ACE-inhibitor-based therapy. ACE-inhibitor-based therapy was also associated with a higher incidence of angioedema relative to chlorthalidone-based treatment. The authors recommended that thiazide diuretics be considered as initial therapy for black hypertensive patients with normal renal function. Furthermore, the authors made the recommendation that in African American hypertensive patients who could not tolerate a diuretic, a calcium-channel blocker would be a reasonable choice.

In summary, in African American hypertensive patients without renal disease, diuretic-based therapy is reasonable as an initial first-line agent. In black hypertensive patients with proteinuric renal disease (or other compelling indications, such as decreased systolic function), ACE-inhibitor-based therapy is warranted, although multiple agents will be needed to achieve BP goal. β-blockers as monotherapy may not achieve target BP goal but should not be withheld from patients with a previous history of angina, MI, or congestive heart failure. Rational combinations include combining ACE inhibitors, ARBs, or β-blockers with a low-dose diuretic and/or a calcium-channel blocker.

Diabetes Mellitus

Patients with diabetes mellitus are at increased risk for the development of both microvascular (retinopathy, nephropathy, and neuropathy) and macrovascular complications (stroke, coronary heart disease, peripheral vascular disease, and congestive heart failure). ACE inhibitors and ARBs are first-line agents in diabetic patients with established microalbuminuria (urine albumin to creatinine ratio ≥ 30 mg/mg), regardless of BP.[43] In the absence of microalbuminuria, thiazide diuretics are also reasonable agents.[2,15] Certain β-blockers may be more efficacious than others. In the Glycemic Effects in Diabetes Mellitus: Carvedilol-Metoprolol Comparison in Hypertensives trial, carvedilol was found to decrease albumin excretion and not affect Hgb A1C, compared to metoprolol, which increased Hgb A1C by a mean of 0.15%.[44] Clinical outcomes were not evaluated in this trial.

Goal BP should be lower than 130/80 mm Hg in all diabetics.[2,45,46] Intensive BP control significantly contributes to the reduction in both microvascular and macrovascular diabetic complications.[47,48]

Nondiabetic Chronic Kidney Disease

ACE inhibitors (and ARBs in patients unable to take ACE inhibitors) are indicated in patients with nondiabetic chronic kidney disease, particularly in patients with spot urine total protein to creatinine ratio >200 mg/g. These agents slow the progression of kidney disease.[46] Examples of nondiabetic kidney disease include glomerular, hypertensive nephrosclerosis, and tubulointerstitial diseases. There is some uncertainty on the optimal BP goal; however, guidelines recommend a goal <130/80 mm Hg.[2,42] Goal SBP 110 to 129 mm Hg in patients with urinary total protein excretion >1 g/d may be even more beneficial in retarding renal decline.[49]

Upon initiation of an ACE inhibitor or ARB, patients should be monitored closely for a creatinine increase. A 20% to 30% initial increase in creatinine is acceptable upon initiation of an ACE inhibitor or ARB in hypertensive patients with chronic kidney disease.[50] This increase in creatinine reflects renal hemodynamic adjustments; the creatinine will then stabilize or improve. ACE inhibitors and ARBs should be discontinued if there is an increase of 30% in creatinine. ACE inhibitors and ARBs, in general, are contraindicated in patients with bilateral renal artery stenosis and polycystic kidney disease. The compression of the large cysts on the renal vasculature can physiologically mimic renal artery stenosis.[50] The ACE-inhibitor- (or ARB-) induced efferent arteriole vasodilatation in the presence of a reduced effective arterial blood volume in these settings can result in a deleterious decline in GFR.

Older Adults

Most elderly hypertensive patients are afflicted with systolic HTN, defined as a SBP, ≥140 mm Hg and a DBP lower than or equal to 90 mm Hg.[2] Systolic HTN is now recognized as an important risk factor for cardiovascular disease, even more so than diastolic HTN. Randomized clinical trials have shown that treatment of SBP ≥160 mm Hg reduces the risk of stroke[51,52] and incidence of cardiovascular disease.[51–53] The evidence for treating SBPs <160 mm Hg in the older adults is less

established by large-scale clinical trials;[54] however, the overall recommendation of JNC VII remains to initiate antihypertensive therapy for BP ≥140/90 mm Hg (or ≥130/80 mm Hg in the presence of coexisting diabetes mellitus or chronic kidney disease with proteinuria) if lifestyle modifications or treatment of reversible causes of HTN are not successful, irrespective of age.[2] Individual patient preferences and values and shared decision making between the practitioner and patient should guide the decision to lower BP in older patients, particularly in the BP range of 140 to 159 mm Hg.[54]

The primary drug agents used in the large-scale clinical trials evaluating the clinical management of systolic HTN in the older adults were a thiazide-like diuretic,[51] chlorthalidone, and a long-acting dihydropyridine calcium-channel blocker, nitrendipine.[52,53] Thus, these agents are often recommended as first-line agents in the treatment of uncomplicated HTN in the older adults.[54] ACE inhibitors are also reasonable first-line agents in hypertensive elderly patients. The Second Australian National Blood Pressure Trial found that enalapril provided superior cardiovascular outcomes compared to hydrochlorothiazide in white, elderly men,[55] which is in contrast to the ALLHAT findings; however, the two trials are sufficiently different in design to obviate the need for any definitive changes in JNC VII recommendations.

In a systematic review of mostly randomized trials evaluating the efficacy of diuretics (versus placebo) and β-blockers (versus placebo) in elderly hypertensive patients, thiazide diuretics were found to be superior to β-blockers in preventing cerebrovascular events, coronary heart disease, cardiovascular mortality, and all-cause mortality.[27] A meta-analysis showed an increased incidence of stroke with β-blockers compared to other classes;[29] thus, β-blockers are not standard first-line agents in the treatment of uncomplicated HTN in the older adults.

TREATMENT SUMMARY AND GLOBAL CARDIOVASCULAR RISK REDUCTION

The overall goal in HTN treatment is reduction in cardiovascular-related disease, not simply BP reduction. Health care providers should assist with lifestyle modifications, including smoking cessation, identification and treatment of dyslipidemia, and identification of high cardiovascular risk patients who would benefit from aspirin chemoprophylaxis. β-blockers and ACE inhibitors (or ARBs in patients intolerant of ACE inhibitors) are strongly indicated in all patients with: (1) established coronary artery disease or (2) heart failure from systolic dysfunction[32,33] The level of BP achieved remains a powerful determinant in reducing total cardiovascular events.[30] A significant number of

Table 1-4. Pharmacologic Management Strategies

Uncomplicated HTN	Initial Therapy Thiazide Diuretic[2,15]	Comments BP goal <140/90 mm Hg[2,33,57,59]
Coronary artery disease; LV dysfunction;	β-Blockers and ACE inhibitors (or ARBs)[32,33]	BP goal < 140/90 mm Hg[2] or BP goal < 130/80 mm Hg[33,59] Consider BP goal < 120/80 (LV dysfunction)[33] No increased risk of depression with β-blockers and only small increases in fatigue and sexual dysfunction[69]
Chronic kidney disease GFR < 60 mL/min/1.73 m² or > 300 mg urinary albumin/d[2]	ACE inhibitors (or ARBs)[2,36,41] ACE inhibitor (plus usually a second agent, e.g., a diuretic) in African Americans[36,41,42,46]	BP goal < 130/80 mm Hg[2,33,46,57,59] SBP 110–129 mm Hg may be beneficial with urinary total protein excretion >1.0 g/d[49] Avoid amlodipine as initial first-line agent[42]
African Americans (without proteinuria)	Thiazide diuretic[35]; calcium-channel blocker reasonable alternative[35]	ACE inhibitors[35] and β-blockers as monotherapy unlikely to achieve goal BP[40] Increased incidence (~0.7%) of angioedema with ACE inhibitors[32]
Diabetics (without proteinuria)	Thiazide diuretic[2,15]; ACE inhibitors[20]	BP goal < 130/80 mm Hg[2,33,57,59]
Diabetics (with proteinuria)	ACE inhibitors (or ARBs)[2,43,46]	BP goal < 130/80 mm Hg[2,33,57,59]
Older adults	Thiazide diuretic[2,15,51,54] or long-acting dihydropyridine calcium-channel blocker[52–54]; ACE inhibitors in white elderly men[55]	β-Blockers less efficacious compared to other drug classes as initial agent[26,27,29]

patients will require two or more agents. Large-scale studies and guidelines endorse thiazide diuretics as first-line therapy in uncomplicated HTN.[2,15] Table 1-4 summarizes indications for pharmacotherapy.

CLINICAL PRACTICE GUIDELINES

Several HTN clinical practice guidelines are available to aid clinicians and patients in decision making. In addition to JNC VII,[2] other guidelines include the British Hypertension Society guideline,[56] the Canadian Hypertension Education Program guideline,[57] the American Heart Association Treatment of Hypertension guideline,[33] the Scottish Intercollegiate Guidelines Network guideline,[58] and the European Society of Hypertension and European Society of Cardiology guideline.[59] Most of these guidelines have similar recommendations for first-line therapeutic agents and treating patients with specific comorbid conditions, for example, diabetes mellitus. The guidelines do have different recommendations, however, on the SBP and DBP levels that require drug therapy and target systolic and DBP goals for other comorbid conditions. As an example, in patients with established cardiovascular disease, the American Heart Association[33] and European Society of Hypertension and European Society of Cardiology[59] guidelines recommend a target BP goal of <130/80 mm Hg, while JNC VII recommends a target BP goal of <140/90.[2]

BARRIERS TO OPTIMAL CONTROL OF HTN

Data from the NHANES has highlighted the sub-optimal control of HTN in the United States, with 70% of hypertensive individuals not attaining their goal of <140/90.[1] The most commonly recognized factors contributing to the low control rate include lack of access to health care, with a disturbingly large percentage of uncontrolled HTN found in ethnic and racial minorities, and poor patient compliance.[60]

The NHANES III identified the following factors associated with improved HTN control rates: The state of being married with social support, access to private health insurance, continuity in care, regular BP measurements (at least within the past 6 to 11 months), and the adherence to lifestyle modifications.[61]

RESISTANT OR REFRACTORY HTN

Resistant HTN is most commonly defined as a BP that is not controlled despite a combination of lifestyle modifications and the use of full therapeutic doses of three medications, one of which is a diuretic appropriate for the level of renal function.[2] Difficult-to-control HTN is described as a BP that is elevated despite treatment with two to three BP medications, but not meeting formal criteria for resistant HTN. There are multiple possibilities to consider when evaluating refractory HTN, including medication nonadherence, drug-related causes such as interfering substances and inappropriate drug regimens, occult volume overload, pseudoresistance caused by office HTN or pseudohypertension, associated conditions such as obesity and obstructive sleep apnea, and the traditional causes of secondary HTN.[2,62]

Nonadherence to Therapy

Nonadherence with the medication regimen commonly contributes to poor BP control. Physicians must approach this issue in a nonjudgmental manner, first by acknowledging the difficulty in taking medications regularly and then candidly asking patients how often they miss doses.[63] Physicians can explore further by inquiring about drug costs, side effects, and complicated dosing schedules. Studies demonstrate that adherence is inversely proportional to the frequency of dose.[64] Physicians should also assess for objective signs of nonadherence, for example, the lack of expected physical examination or laboratory findings associated with the medications (such as sinus bradycardia for β-blockers or non-dihydropyridine (DHP) calcium-channel blockers and hypokalemia in patients on thiazide or loop diuretics).

Interfering Substances

There are innumerable medications, including prescription drugs, over-the-counter agents, alternative remedies, and drugs of abuse that can sabotage BP management, both by raising the BP directly as well as by interfering with the efficacy of the patient's antihypertensive medications. Common examples of interfering substances include nasal decongestants, caffeine, appetite suppressants, oral contraceptives, adrenal steroids, antidepressants, nonsteroidal anti-inflammatory drugs, sympathomimetics, and nicotine. Other notorious examples include cyclosporine, tacrolimus, adrenal steroids, erythropoietin, and licorice. Drugs of abuse such as alcohol and cocaine also negatively impact BP control, both with respect to their impact physiologically as well as in their secondary effect of potentially blunting patients' overall motivational state for adhering to the medication regimen.[60]

Occult Volume Overload

Inadequate control of extracellular volume is an extremely common cause of resistant HTN. It has been recognized that extracellular volume expansion is a compensatory response to the lowering of BP. It may also be a result of antihypertensive drugs such as direct vasodilators. Volume overload can occur in other settings such as with excessive salt intake and progressive renal insufficiency. For these reasons, a diuretic acts as a crucial component of an antihypertensive regimen. The diuretic chosen should be appropriate for the level of renal function. Thiazide diuretics act as antihypertensive agents in patients with preserved renal function but become less efficacious as GFR falls (typically once, creatinine >2.0 mg/dL or GFR <30 mL/min/1.73 m^2). In cases of end stage renal disease, combinations of diuretics are often required for volume control.

Pseudoresistance

In some cases, refractory HTN may be erroneous, in that the patient has white-coat HTN. Office HTN or white-coat HTN occurs when the office measurements overestimate the patient's true BP. When suspected, this condition can be investigated through ABPM, which would reveal normal BPs when the patient is away from the doctor's office. Patients with white-coat HTN should not have evidence of target-organ damage. Another cause of mistakenly resistant HTN arises from faulty BP measurements. A very common error involves the use of an inappropriately small BP cuff for an obese patient, leading to an incorrectly elevated reading.

Pseudohypertension is a condition to consider in elderly patients with vascular disease. An increased stiffness within the vessel walls requires higher than normal pressures to compress and occlude the vascular wall. Patients typically complain of symptoms of hypotension, such as lightheadedness and presyncope, as the BP medications are increased. In addition, they may not have the target-organ injury that would be expected for such degrees of BP elevation. The definitive diagnosis is made through an intra-arterial BP measurement.

Causes of Secondary HTN

Ninety-five percent of patients have essential HTN. Secondary HTN is more commonly seen in patients with refractory HTN. It is important to identify since treating the underlying condition may avert the need for treating the elevated BP. Some clinical clues suggesting secondary causes include the following: Onset at age <30 or >50 (except for isolated systolic HTN which is commonly seen in the older adults), refractory HTN or an acute, marked rise in BP. In contrast to essential HTN, family history is often negative in cases of secondary HTN.

Causes of secondary HTN include both associated conditions such as obesity and obstructive sleep apnea, as well as the classical secondary causes including renovascular disease, intrinsic renal disease, primary aldosteronism, pheochromocytoma, Cushing's syndrome, aortic coarctation, thyroid disorders, and hyperparathyroidism. The clinical presentations vary according to the etiology, but certain features of the history and physical examination will often suggest the specific diagnosis, allowing for a focused approach to evaluation. See Table 1-5 for causes and clinical findings of secondary HTN.

Table 1-5. Etiologies and Clinical Findings of Secondary Causes of HTN

Etiology	Physical Findings	Laboratory Findings
Cushing's syndrome	Moon facies, buffalo hump, abdominal stria, central deposition of body fat	Elevated 24-hour urinary cortisol
Renovascular	Systolic/diastolic abdominal bruit (sensitivity 39% and specificity 99% for detecting true renal atherosclerotic disease)[68] or flank bruit; onset of C in a young woman,	Rise in creatinine after ACE I or ARB; evidence of atherosclerosis elsewhere
Pheochromocytoma	Episodes of HTN, flushing, sweating, headache	Elevated urinary metanephrines or VMA
Renal disease	Late-fluid overload, uremic frost, nausea, vomiting	Elevated creatinine; abnormal urinalysis
Oral contraceptives	Rise in BP related to the initiation of contraceptive	
Obstructive sleep apnea	Nighttime snoring with episodes of apnea, daytime somnolence, large neck circumference	Apnea on sleep study
Coarctation of the aorta	Diminished BP in legs as compared with upper arm BP	Abnormalities on echo and/or cardiac catheterization
Hypothyroidism	Cold intolerance, constipation, fatigue, bradycardia, delayed deep tendon reflexes	Elevated TSH
Hyperthyroidism	Heat intolerance, hyperdefecation, lid lag, normochromic, normocytic anemia, tachycardia	Suppressed TSH
Primary hyperparathyroidism	Often none	Elevated serum calcium
Obesity	BMI >30	NA
Hyperaldosteronism	Resistant HTN	Low K off diuretics, serum aldosterone/ renin >20:1

VMA, vanillyl mandelic acid; TSH, thyroid stimulating hormone; NA, not applicable.
Adapted from Ref. 2.

Overview of Evaluation and Management of Resistant HTN

A suggested approach to the evaluation and management of resistant HTN is outlined in Fig. 1-2. Several pharmacologic strategies can be employed for HTN that persists following a comprehensive evaluation of the causes of resistant HTN. The overriding principle is to select antihypertensive agents with complementary physiologic actions in BP regulation. Medications targeted to decrease sympathetic activity are combined with agents which block peripheral vascular resistance, reverse volume overload, and promote smooth muscle relaxation. Common combinations include a diuretic, ACE inhibitor (or ARB), β-blocker, and DHP calcium-channel blocker. When BP remains elevated, subsequent potential adjustments can include a titration of the dose and frequency of diuretic (loop diuretics require at least twice a day dosing for HTN), the addition of another diuretic (aldosterone antagonist), the use of both an ACE inhibitor and an ARB (if potassium allows), the use of both DHP and non-DHP calcium-channel blockers, the use of combined α- and β-blockers (like labetalol), and finally, centrally-acting agents and direct vasodilators. Referral to a HTN specialist is warranted in cases of ongoing HTN, following evaluation and attempted management as above.[62]

Special Situations: Hypertensive Urgencies and Emergencies

In special cases, the elevation in BP is extreme enough to warrant immediate or rapid BP reduction. Hypertensive urgencies (see Table 1-6 for definitions) are defined as severe elevations in BP (typically, >180/120) without symptoms or evidence of acute end-organ damage. Hypertensive emergencies are classified as severe elevations in BP that are associated with acute injury to target organs such as the brain, heart, kidneys, retina, and other vasculature. Examples include hypertensive encephalopathy, intracerebral hemorrhage, acute MI, acute coronary syndromes, acute left ventricular failure with pulmonary edema, dissecting aortic aneurysm, and acute renal failure.[2]

The etiologies of hypertensive crises[65] include essential HTN, renal parenchymal disease (vasculitis, acute glomerulonephritis), renovascular disease, eclampsia, drug-related causes (including the withdrawal of antihypertensive agents), endocrinological causes (pheochromocytoma, Cushing's syndrome, renin-secreting tumors), and central nervous system disorders (traumatic head injury, CVA, brain tumors). Clinical evaluation focuses on assessing target-organ damage and determining possible causes.

Management of hypertensive urgencies consists of BP lowering with oral agents, over a time course of hours to

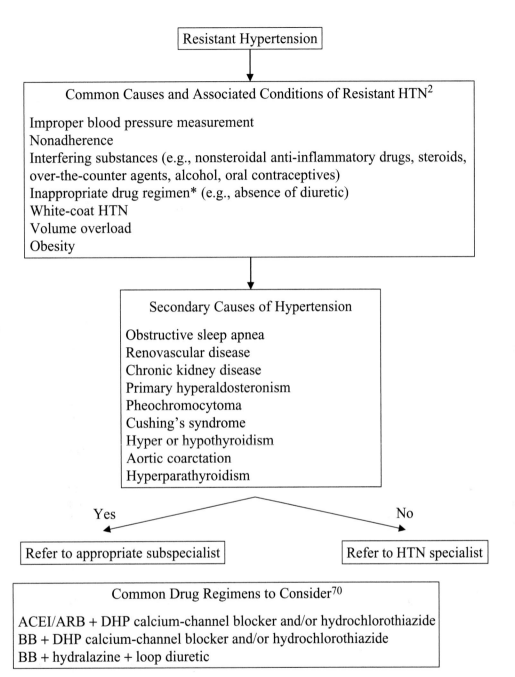

Figure 1-2. Approach to evaluation and management of resistant HTN.

Table 1-6. Definition: Hypertensive Urgency and Emergency

Definition	End-Organ Damage	Treatment
Hypertensive urgency-elevated BP without evidence of end-organ damage	No	Lower BP in 24–48 hours with combination oral therapy Follow-up appointment within 1–2 days
Hypertensive emergency-elevated BP with evidence of end-organ damage. i.e., encephalopathy, unstable angina, MI, pulmonary edema, eclampsia, stroke, dissecting aortic aneurysm	Yes	Admission to Intensive Care Unit for parenteral drug therapy

Table 1-7. Parenteral Drugs for Treatment of Hypertensive Emergencies[2]

Drug	Dose	Onset of Action	Duration of Action	Adverse Effects	Special Indications
Vasodilators					
Sodium nitroprusside	0.25–10 μg/kg/min as IV infusion	Immediate	1–2 min	Nausea, vomiting, muscle twitching, sweating, thiocyanate and cyanide intoxication	Most hypertensive emergencies; caution with high intracranial pressure or azotemia
Nicardipine hydrochloride	5–15 mg/h IV	5–10 min	15–30 min, may exceed 4 h	Tachycardia, headache, flushing, local phlebitis	Most hypertensive emergencies except acute heart failure; caution with coronary ischemia
Fenoldopam mesylate	0.1–0.3 μg/kg per min IV infusion	<5 min	30 min	Tachycardia, headache, nausea, flushing	Most hypertensive emergencies; caution with glaucoma
Nitroglycerin	5–100 μg/min as IV infusion	2–5 min	5–10 min	Headache, vomiting, methemo-globinemia, tolerance with prolonged use	Coronary ischemia
Enalaprilat	1.24–5 mg q 6 h IV	15–30 min	6–12 h	Precipitous fall in pressure in high-renin states; variable response	Acute left ventricular failure; avoid in acute MI
Hydralazine hydrochloride	10–20 mg IV, 10–40 mg IM	10–20 min IV 20–30 min IM	1–4 h IV 4–6 h IM	Tachycardia, flushing, headache, vomiting, aggravation of angina	Eclampsia
Adrenergic inhibitors					
Labetalol hydrochloride	20–80 mg IV bolus q 10 m 0.5–2.0 mg/min IV infusion	5–10 min	3–6 h	Vomiting, scalp tingling, bronchoconstric-tion, dizziness, nausea, heart block, orthostatic hypotension	Most hypertensive emergencies, except acute heart failure
Esmolol hydrochloride	250–500 μg/kg/min IV bolus, then 50–100 μg/kg/min by infusion; may repeat bolus after 5 min or increase infusion to 300 μg/min	1–2 min	10–30 min	Hypotension, nausea, asthma, first-degree heart block, heart failure	Aortic dissection, perioperative
Phentolamine	5–15 mg IV bolus	1–2 min	10–30 min	Tachycardia, flushing, headache	Catecholamine excess

Source: Chobanian et al: Natl Hi BP. Hypertension 2003;42:1206

days, ideally within 24 to 48 hours. Possible choices of medications include short-acting antihypertensive agents such as captopril, labetalol, or clonidine. Medications which rapidly lower the BP such as sublingual nifedipine should be avoided because of an associated increased morbidity and mortality likely related to the excessively rapid fall in BP.[2,66] In hypertensive emergencies, in contrast to hypertensive urgencies, BP must be lowered immediately but cautiously by parenteral therapy. Excessive falls in BP should be avoided because of the potential for precipitating renal, cerebral, or coronary ischemia. The exact rate of BP lowering depends on the clinical condition, with more rapid BP control (generally to SBP <100 mm Hg) indicated in aortic dissection. In cases involving cerebrovascular symptoms, an excessive decline in BP can be dangerous, triggering ischemia. Clinical practice guidelines advise aiming for a reduction in mean arterial BP of 25% within minutes to 1 hour, and to 160/100 mm Hg by 6 hours.[2] Pharmacotherapy for hypertensive emergencies is summarized in Table 1-7.

CONCLUSION

There is ample evidence proving the beneficial effects of lowering BP. NHANES data reveal the need for improvement, both in the number of patients treated and in the percent of patients who are treated to goal. Through doctor–patient communication, patient education, lifestyle modification, frequent follow-up, appropriate medication regimens, and timely medication adjustment, more hypertensive patients can be identified, treated, and attain their target BPs (see Evidence-Based Summary below).

EVIDENCE-BASED SUMMARY

Screen
- All adults >21 years annually[4]

Diagnosis
- BP >140/90 mm Hg on 2–3 separate readings 1 week apart[2]
- BP >130/80 mm Hg in patients with chronic kidney disease or diabetes mellitus[2]

Initial evaluation
- Global cardiovascular risk assessment
- Evaluate for end-organ damage
- Evaluate for secondary causes, if clinically indicated
- Recognize hypertensive urgency/emergency

Management
- Lifestyle modifications
- Pharmacotherapy
- Thiazide-based therapy for uncomplicated HTN[2,15,30]
- Identify high cardiovascular risk patients who would benefit from other drug classes[2]

Follow-up
- Continued patient education
- Continued lifestyle modification
- Appropriate medication adjustment(s)

REFERENCES

1. Hajjar I, Kotchen TA. Trends in prevalence, awareness, treatment, and control of hypertension in the United states, 1988–2000. *JAMA*. 2003;290:199–206.
2. Chobanian AV, Bakris GL, Black HR, et al, National High Blood Pressure Education Program Coordinating Committee. Seventh Report of the Joint National Committee on Prevention, Detection, Evaluation, and Treatment of High Blood Pressure. *Hypertension*. 2003;42:1206–1252.
3. Neal B, MacMahon S, Chapman N. Blood pressure lowering treatment Trialists C. Effects of ace inhibitors, calcium antagonists, and other blood-pressure-lowering drugs: Results of prospectively designed overviews of randomised trials. blood pressure lowering treatment trialists' collaboration. *Lancet*. 2000;356:1955–1964.
4. Calonge N, Petitti DB, DeWitt TG, et al. Screening for High Blood Presure: United States Preventive Services Task Force Reaffirmation Recommendation Statement. *Ann Intern Med*. 2007;147:783–786.
5. Beevers G, Lip GY, O'Brien E. ABC of hypertension: Blood pressure measurement. Part II-conventional sphygmomanometry: Technique of auscultatory blood pressure measurement. *BMJ*. 2001;322:1043–1047.
6. Staessen JA, Den Hond E, Celis H, et al. Treatment of hypertension based on home or office blood pressure Trial I: Antihypertensive treatment based on blood pressure measurement at home or in the physician's office: A randomized controlled trial. *JAMA*. 2004;291:955–964.
7. Yarows SA, Julius S, Pickering TG. Home blood pressure monitoring. *Arch Intern Med*. 2000;160:1251–1257.
8. Lewis JE, Boyle E, Magharious L, et al. Evaluation of a community-based automated blood pressure measuring device. *Can Med Assoc J*. 2002;166:1145–1148.
9. Staessen JA, Thijs L, Fagard R, et al. Predicting cardiovascular risk using conventional vs. ambulatory blood pressure in older patients with systolic hypertension. Systolic Hypertension in Europe Trial Investigators. *JAMA*. 1999;282:539–546.
10. Verdecchia P, Porcellati C, Schillaci G, et al. Ambulatory blood pressure. An independent predictor of prognosis in essential hypertension. *Hypertension*. 1994;24:793–801.
11. Verdecchia P, Reboldi GP, Angeli F, et al. Short- and long-term incidence of stroke in white-coat hypertension. *Hypertension*. 2005;45:203–208.
12. Karter Y, Curgunlu A, Altinisik S, et al. Target organ damage and changes in arterial compliance in white coat hypertension. Is white coat innocent? *Blood Press*. 2003;12:307–313.
13. Celis H, Staessen JA, Thijs L, et al. Ambulatory blood pressure and treatment of hypertension Trial I: Cardiovascular risk in white-coat and sustained hypertensive patients. *Blood Press*. 2002;11:352–356.
14. Pickering TG, Shimbo D, Haas D. Ambulatory blood-pressure monitoring. *N Engl J Med*. 2006;354:2368–2374.
15. The ALLHAT Officers and Coordinators for the ALLHAT Collaborative Research Group. Major outcomes in

high-risk hypertensive patients randomized to angiotensin-converting enzyme inhibitor or calcium channel blocker vs. diuretic: The Antihypertensive and Lipid-Lowering Treatment to Prevent Heart Attack Trial (ALLHAT). *JAMA.* 2002;288:2981–2997.

16. Brown MJ, Palmer CR, Castaigne A, et al. Morbidity and mortality in patients randomised to double-blind treatment with a long-acting calcium-channel blocker or diuretic in the International Nifedipine GITS study: Intervention as a goal in hypertension treatment (INSIGHT). *Lancet.* 2000;356:366–372.

17. Hansson L, Lindholm LH, Ekbom T, et al. Randomised trial of old and new antihypertensive drugs in elderly patients: Cardiovascular mortality and morbidity the swedish trial in old patients with hypertension-2 study. *Lancet.* 1999;354:1751–1756.

18. Pepine CJ, Cooper-Dehoff RM. Cardiovascular therapies and risk for development of diabetes. *J Am Coll Cardiol.* 2004;44:509–512.

19. Williams B. Recent hypertension trials: Implications and controversies. *J Am Coll Cardiol.* 2005;45:813–827.

20. The Heart Outcomes Prevention Evaluation Study Investigators. Effects of an angiotensin-converting-enzyme inhibitor, ramipril, on cardiovascular events in high-risk patients. *N Engl J Med.* 2000;342:145–153.

21. Davis BR, Furberg CD, Wright JT, et al. ALLHAT: Setting the record straight. *Ann Intern Med.* 2004;141:39–46.

22. Furberg CD, Psaty BM, Pahor M, et al. Clinical implications of recent findings from the antihypertensive and lipid-lowering treatment to prevent heart attack trial (ALLHAT) and other studies of hypertension. *Ann Intern Med.* 2001;135:1074–1078.

23. Houston MC. ALLHAT debate: Diuretics are not preferred, first-line initial therapy for hypertension. *Arch Intern Med.* 2004;164:570–571.

24. Moser M. Results of ALLHAT: Is this the final answer regarding initial antihypertensive drug therapy? *Arch Intern Med.* 2003;163:1269–1273.

25. Dahlof B, Sever PS, Poulter NR, et al. Prevention of cardiovascular events with an antihypertensive regimen of amlodipine adding perindopril as required versus atenolol adding bendroflumethiazide as required, in the Anglo-Scandinavian cardiac outcomes trial-blood pressure lowering arm (ASCOT-BPLA): A multicentre randomised controlled trial. *Lancet.* 2005;366:895.

26. Carlberg B, Samuelsson O, Lindholm LH. Atenolol in hypertension: Is it a wise choice? *Lancet.* 2004;364:1684–1689.

27. Messerli FH, Grossman E, Goldbourt U. Are beta-blockers efficacious as first-line therapy for hypertension in the elderly? A systematic review. *JAMA.* 1998;279:1903–1907.

28. Wright JM. Choosing a first-line drug in the management of elevated blood pressure: What is the evidence? Part 2: Beta-blockers. *CMAJ.* 2000;163:188–192.

29. Lindholm LH, Carlberg B, Samuelsson O. Should beta-blockers remain first choice in the treatment of primary hypertension? A meta-analysis. *Lancet.* 2005;366(9496):1545–1553.

30. Blood Pressure Lowering Treatment Trialists' Collaboration. Effects of different blood-pressure-lowering regimens on major cardiovascular events: Results of prospectively-designed overviews of randomised trials. *Lancet.* 2003;362:1527–1535.

31. Carter BL, Ernst ME, Cohen JD. Hydrochlorothiazide versus chlorthalidone: Evidence supporting their interchangeability. *Hypertension.* 2004;43:4–9.

32. Hunt SA, Abraham WT, Chin MH, et al. ACC/AHA 2005 Guideline Update for the Diagnosis and Management of Chronic Heart Failure in the Adult: A Report of the American College of Cardiology(American Heart Association Task Force on Practice Guidelines (Writing Committee to Update the 2001 Guidelines for the Evaluation and Management of Heart Failure). *Circulation.* 2005;112:e154–235.

33. Rosendorff C, Black HR, Cannon CP, et al. American Heart Association Council for High Blood Pressure Research. American Heart Association Council on Clinical Cardiology. American Heart Association Council on Epidemiology and Prevention. Treatment of hypertension in the prevention and management of ischemic heart disease: a scientific statement from the American Heart Association Council for High Blood Pressure Research and the Councils on Clinical Cardiology and Epidemiology and Prevention. *Circulation.* 2007;115(21):2761–88.

34. Dahlof B, Devereux RB, Kjeldsen SE, et al. Cardiovascular morbidity and mortality in the Losartan Intervention for endpoint reduction in hypertension study (LIFE): A randomised trial against atenolol. *Lancet.* 2002;359:995–1003.

35. Wright JT, Jr., Dunn JK, Cutler JA, et al. Outcomes in hypertensive black and nonblack patients treated with chlorthalidone, amlodipine, and lisinopril. *JAMA.* 2005;293:1595–1608.

36. Douglas JG, Bakris GL, Epstein M, et al. Management of high blood pressure in African Americans: Consensus statement of the hypertension in African Americans Working Group of the International Society on Hypertension in Blacks. *Arch Intern Med.* 2003;163:525–541.

37. Cushman WC, Reda DJ, Perry HM, et al. Regional and racial differences in response to antihypertensive medication use in a randomized controlled trial of men with hypertension in the united states. Department of veterans affairs cooperative study group on antihypertensive agents. *Arch Intern Med.* 2000;160:825–831.

38. Richardson AD, Piepho RW. Effect of race on hypertension and antihypertensive therapy. *Int J Clin Pharmacol Ther.* 2000;38:75–79.

39. Weir MR, Gray JM, Paster R, et al. Differing mechanisms of action of angiotensin-converting enzyme inhibition in black and white hypertensive patients. The trandolapril multicenter study group. *Hypertension.* 1995;26:124–130.

40. Brewster LM, van Montfrans GA, Kleijnen J. Systematic review: Antihypertensive drug therapy in black patients. *Ann Intern Med.* 2004;141:614–627.

41. Wright JT, Jr., Bakris G, Greene T, et al. Effect of blood pressure lowering and antihypertensive drug class on progression of hypertensive kidney disease: Results from the AASK trial. *JAMA.* 2002;288:2421–2431.

42. Agodoa LY, Appel L, Bakris GL, et al. Effect of ramipril vs amlodipine on renal outcomes in hypertensive nephrosclerosis: A randomized controlled trial. *JAMA*. 2001;285:2719–2728.

43. Lovell HG. Angiotensin converting enzyme inhibitors in normotensive diabetic patients with microalbuminuria. *Cochrane Database Syst Rev.* 2001;(1):CD002183.

44. Bakris GL, Fonseca V, Katholi RE, et al. Metabolic effects of carvedilol vs. metoprolol in patients with type 2 diabetes mellitus and hypertension: A randomized controlled trial. *JAMA*. 2004;292:2227–2236.

45. Bakris GL, Williams M, Dworkin L, et al. Preserving renal function in adults with hypertension and diabetes: A consensus approach. national kidney foundation hypertension and diabetes executive committees working group. *Am J Kidney Dis*. 2000;36:646–661.

46. Kidney Disease Outcomes Quality I. K/DOQI clinical practice guidelines on hypertension and antihypertensive agents in chronic kidney disease. *Am J Kidney Dis*. 2004;43:S1–290.

47. Group UKPDS. Tight blood pressure control and risk of macrovascular and microvascular complications in type 2 diabetes: UKPDS 38. *BMJ*. 1998;317:703–713.

48. Hansson L, Zanchetti A, Carruthers SG, et al. Effects of intensive blood-pressure lowering and low-dose aspirin in patients with hypertension: Principal results of the hypertension optimal treatment (hot) randomised trial. *Lancet*. 1998;351:1755.

49. Jafar TH, Stark PC, Schmid CH, et al. Progression of chronic kidney disease: The role of blood pressure control, proteinuria, and angiotensin-converting enzyme inhibition: A patient-level meta-analysis. *Ann Intern Med*. 2003;139:244–252.

50. Palmer BF. Renal dysfunction complicating the treatment of hypertension. *N Engl J Med*. 2002;347:1256–1261.

51. SHEP Cooperative Research Group. Prevention of stroke by antihypertensive drug treatment in older persons with isolated systolic hypertension. Final results of the systolic hypertension in the elderly program (SHEP): *JAMA*. 1991;265:3255–3264.

52. Staessen JA, Fagard R, Thijs L, et al. Randomised double-blind comparison of placebo and active treatment for older patients with isolated systolic hypertension. The Systolic Hypertension in Europe (Syst-Eur) Trial Investigators. *Lancet*. 1997;350:757–764.

53. Liu L, Wang JG, Gong L, et al. Comparison of active treatment and placebo in older Chinese patients with isolated systolic hypertension. Systolic Hypertension in China (Syst-China) Collaborative Group. *J Hypertens*. 1998;16:1823–1829.

54. Chaudhry SI, Krumholz HM, Foody JM. Systolic hypertension in older persons. *JAMA*. 2004;292:1074–1080.

55. Wing LM, Reid CM, Ryan P, et al. A comparison of outcomes with angiotensin-converting-enzyme inhibitors and diuretics for hypertension in the elderly. *N Engl J Med*. 2003;348:583–592.

56. Williams B, Poulter NR, Brown MJ, et al. British Hypertension Society Guidelines for hypertension management 2004 (BHS-IV): Summary. *BMJ*. 2004;328:634–640.

57. Canadian Hypertension Education Program. The 2007 Canadian Hypertension Education Program recommendations: the scientific summary–an annual update. *Canad J Cardiol*. 2007;23(7):521–527.

58. Scottish Intercollegiate Guidelines Network. Hypertension in Older People. A national clinical guideline. Edinburgh, Scotland. 2001:1–50. http://www.sign.ac.uk/guidelines/fulltext/49/index.html/. Accessed January 15, 2008.

59. The Task Force for the Management of Arterial Hypertension of the European Society of Cardiology. 2007 Guidelines for the Management of Arterial Hypertension: The Task Force for the Management of Arterial Hypertension of the European Society of Hypertension (ESH) and of the European Society of Cardiology (ESC). *European Heart Journal*. 2007; 28(12): 1462–536.

60. Schwartz GL, Sheps SG , Hypertension. In: Dale DC, Federman DD, eds. *ACP Medicine*. New York, NY: WebMD Inc. 2006. http://www.acpmedicine.com

61. He J, Muntner P, Chen J, et al. Factors associated with hypertension control in the general population of the united states. *Arch Intern Med*. 2002;162:1051–1058.

62. Kaplan NM, Rose BD Resistant hypertension. http://www.uptodate.com/. Accessed January 13, 2007.

63. Osterberg L, Blaschke T. Adherence to medication. *N Engl J Med*. 2005;353:487–497.

64. Claxton AJ, Cramer J, Pierce C. A systematic review of the associations between dose regimens and medication compliance. *Clin Ther*. 2001;23:1296–1310.

65. Vaughan CJ, Delanty N. Hypertensive emergencies. *Lancet*. 2000;356:411–417.

66. Cherney D, Straus S. Management of patients with hypertensive urgencies and emergencies: A systematic review of the literature. *J Gen Intern Med*. 2002;17:937–945.

67. Badgett RG, Lucey CR, Mulrow CD. Can the clinical examination diagnose left-sided heart failure in adults? *JAMA*. 1997;277:1712–1719.

68. Turnbull JM. The rational clinical examination. Is listening for abdominal bruits useful in the evaluation of hypertension? *JAMA*. 1995;274:1299–1301.

69. Ko DT, Hebert PR, Coffey CS, et al. Beta-blocker therapy and symptoms of depression, fatigue, and sexual dysfunction. *JAMA*. 2002;288:351–357.

70. Moser M, Setaro JF. Clinical practice. Resistant or difficult-to-control hypertension. *N Engl J Med*. 2006;355:385–392.

Chapter 2
Heart Failure

Tera D. Moore and Joe R. Anderson

SEARCH STRATEGY

A systematic search of the medical literature was performed on January 11, 2008. The search, limited to human subjects and English language journals, included National Guideline Clearinghouse, the Cochrane database, PubMed, pier® and UpToDate®. The current American College of Cardiology/ American Heart Association Chronic Heart Failure Guidelines can be found at www.acc.org. The European Society of Cardiology Acute Heart Failure and Chronic Heart Failure Guidelines can be found at www.escardio.org and the HFSA 2006 Heart Failure Practice Guideline can be found at www.onlinejcf.com

INTRODUCTION

Heart failure (HF) is a serious and growing health problem affecting approximately 5 million persons in the United States with an additional 550,000 individuals diagnosed yearly. HF contributes to approximately 300,000 deaths each year. The estimated direct and indirect costs attribute to HF for 2006 is $29.6 billion.[1]

HF was once described as "a condition in which the heart fails to discharge its contents adequately" (Thomas Lewis 1933); however, the simplistic model of pump failure has evolved into a complex disorder that affects the cardiovascular, musculoskeletal, renal, and neuroendocrine systems.

CLINICAL PRESENTATION

The cardinal manifestations of HF include dyspnea, fatigue, and fluid retention. The development of symptoms characteristic in HF result from pulmonary and systemic congestion. The presence of signs and symptoms of HF (Table 2-1) may vary considerably over time in a given patient. The mechanism of fatigue in HF is complex and originates from low cardiac output, peripheral hypoperfusion, and skeletal muscle deconditioning. As left ventricular function deteriorates and the ability to accept and eject the increased blood volume is impaired, pulmonary venous and capillary pressures elevate, leading to interstitial and bronchial edema, increased airway resistance, and dyspnea. In early HF, dyspnea may occur only with exertion. As HF progresses, the degree of exertion necessary to induce dyspnea decreases and eventually leads to dyspnea at rest.[2] Associated symptoms include orthopnea and paroxysmal nocturnal dyspnea (PND). Orthopnea, that is, dyspnea in the supine position, results from redistribution of fluid from the abdomen and lower extremities into the chest, which increases the pulmonary capillary pressure, combined with elevation of the diaphragm. Orthopnea is relieved by sitting upright and typically is prevented by elevating the head with pillows. PND is a result of severe pulmonary and bronchial congestion and refers to severe shortness of breath and coughing that generally occurs after 2 to 4 hours of sleep; patients awaken with a sense of suffocation.[3] The period between the initiation of ventricular dysfunction and the onset of symptoms may occur very quickly after a myocardial infarction (MI) or extend for a long period of time. With more chronic processes, such as hypertension or idiopathic cardiomyopathies, this interval may extend for months to years. There is a discordance between the degree of ventricular dysfunction and the degree of functional impairment in HF; therefore, the severity of symptoms does not directly correlate with the amount of left-ventricular (LV) dysfunction.[4]

Table 2-1. Clinical Presentation of HF

Symptoms
  Dyspnea
  Orthopnea
  PND
  Exercise intolerance
  Tachypnea
  Cough
  Fatigue
  Abdominal pain
  Anorexia
  Nausea
  Bloating
  Ascites
  Mental status changes
Signs
Vitals
  Pulse rate, rhythm, quality
  Pulse pressure
  Positional blood pressure
  Respiratory rate, depth, periodicity
  Temperature
Cardiovascular
  Elevated jugular venous pressure
  Abdominal jugular reflux
  Displaced LV maximal impulse
  S_3 gallop
  Heart murmurs
  Diminished S_1 or S_2
  Prominent P_2
  Friction rub
  Peripheral pulses
  Temperature of extremities
Neurologic
  Mental status changes
Pulmonary
  Rales
  Rhonchi
  Pleural effusion
Abdominal
  Ascites
  Hepatosplenomegaly
  Pulsatile liver
  Decreased bowel sounds
Systemic
  Edema
  Cachexia

Adapted from: Goswami NJ, O'Rourke RA, Shaver JA, et al. The History, Physical Examination and Parker RB. Heart Failure. In: DiPiro JT, Talbert RL, Yee GC (eds). *Pharmacotherapy: A Pathophysiologic Approach*, 6th ed. New York, NY: McGraw Hill; 2005:219–260.

PHYSICAL FINDINGS

Important information concerning the patient with HF is obtained by a careful and deliberate physical examination. In the first stages of HF, the patient typically has no symptoms at rest except for discomfort when lying flat for more than a few minutes. The venous pressure may be normal at rest but may become elevated with sustained pressure on the abdomen (positive abdomi-

nal jugular reflux). In acutely decompensated HF, systolic hypotension may be present, with cool, diaphoretic extremities, and Cheyne-Stokes respiration (breathing with rhythmic waxing and waning of depth of breaths and regularly recurring apneic periods). Central venous pressure is often elevated which is reflected by distention of the jugular veins. Third and fourth heart sounds are often audible with auscultation but are not specific for HF. In severe HF, the pulse pressure may be increased because of generalized vasoconstriction.[3]

The thorough cardiovascular examination should initially include an assessment of the vital signs. The arterial pulse which begins with aortic valve opening and the onset of LV ejection is inspected for rhythm, intensity, and pulsus alternans. Pulsus alternans, a pattern of regular alteration of the pressure pulse amplitude despite a regular rhythm, indicates severe impairment of LV function and often occurs in patients with a loud third heart sound.[5]

Examination of the neck veins include inspection of waveforms and estimation of central venous pressure which is best estimated by evaluation of the jugular venous pulse (JVP) in the right internal jugular vein. Assessment of the JVP is optimal when the trunk is inclined less than 30 degrees; however, patients with elevated venous pressure or jugular venous distention may require further elevation of the trunk. Palpation of the left carotid artery may aid in distinguishing venous pulses. The vertical distance from the top of the oscillating venous column to the level of the sternal angle is generally less than 3 cm if the patient is euvolemic.[3] In those patients with normal resting venous pressure, but suspected right ventricular failure, the abdominal jugular reflux test may be useful.

Auscultation of the lungs is used to determine the presence of rales, rhonchi, wheezes, or pleural effusion. The rate and depth of respiration should also be noted. Cardiac auscultation is important for the evaluation of the patient with HF to identify the presence of third or fourth heart sounds and to rule out underlying or precipitating causes of HF. Peripheral edema typically is not observed until a fluid weight gain of 10 pounds occurs. Edema typically is located in dependent parts of the body, such as the feet and ankles in ambulatory patients and sacrum in patients who are bedridden.[2] Other physical findings include hepatomegaly (liver more than 12 cm upon percussion at the midclavicular line) and cardiac cachexia.

EVALUATON

INITIAL

The initial evaluation of the patient presenting with signs and symptoms of HF should include an electrocardiogram

Table 2-2. Potential Contributing Factors of HF

Hypertension
Diabetes
Coronary artery disease
Valvular disease
Rheumatic fever
Collagen vascular disease
Hypothyroidism or hyperthyroidism
Exposure to cardiotoxic agents
Excessive alcohol use
Illicit drug use

(ECG) and a CXR. A B-type natriuretic peptide (BNP) level should also be evaluated. A normal ECG or low to normal BNP concentrations have high negative predictive values so that LV dysfunction can be ruled out. Point-of-care testing is available for BNP which increases its utility as a screening tool in primary care and emergency department settings. If any of these tests are abnormal, a transthoracic Doppler echocardiogram should be obtained. The echocardiogram provides a measurement of the left ventricular ejection fraction (LVEF). Additionally, the echocardiogram provides assessment of cardiac dimensions and geometry, wall motion and thickness, and valvular function. Individuals with an ejection fraction (EF) of less than 40% are considered to have systolic dysfunction.

A careful evaluation for potential causative factors should be initiated with onset of signs and symptoms of HF (Table 2-2). An inquiry of past history of hypertension, diabetes, coronary artery disease (CAD), valvular disease, rheumatic fever, collagen vascular disease, hypo- or hyperthyroidism, exposure to cardiotoxic agents (e.g., anthracyclines), alcohol use, and illicit drug use should be assessed. Laboratory testing should include a complete blood count, serum electrolytes (including magnesium), serum blood urea nitrogen and creatinine, hepatic transaminases, and thyroid-stimulating hormone. Patients with systolic dysfunction, CAD, and angina should be referred for coronary angiography to evaluate if they are candidates for revascularization. Although there is no evidence that revascularization improves morbidity or mortality in patients without angina, many experts believe coronary angiography should be performed in all patients with newly diagnosed congestive HF.[4,6]

ONGOING

At every visit the clinician should make a full inquiry into the patient's symptoms (type, severity, and duration) and perform an assessment of volume status. When assessing symptoms, the patient should be questioned about their ability to accomplish several activities such as activities of daily living (bathing, dressing, climbing stairs, and household chores) or exercise routine. Additionally, an inquiry should be made into whether the patient is experiencing chest pain, orthopnea, or PND. The evaluation of symptoms should include an assessment of the patient's functional capacity. This is accomplished through the use of the New York Heart Association Functional Classification (NYHA-FC). Patients are categorized as NYHA-FC I–IV based on the presence or absence and severity of symptoms (Table 2-3).

The assessment of volume status is critical for the determination of HF treatment and should be performed at every visit. This is accomplished through monitoring of patient weight and several physical examination procedures. The simplest assessment is patient weight. Patients should be encouraged to measure and record daily weights and the provider must determine the patient's dry weight to guide diuretic therapy. Abrupt changes in weight, for example an increase of ≥3 to 5 lbs in a period of 24 to 48 hours, signal fluid retention. Measurement of JVP is one of the most accurate physical signs of volume status. In addition to JVP, clinicians should assess for the presence of peripheral edema, hepatomegaly, ascites, and pulmonary rales or crackles. The absence of these signs does not always indicate an absence of fluid retention. For instance, the majority of patients with advanced HF and elevated LV filling pressure do not exhibit pulmonary rales. Therefore, patient history, weight, and physical examination all need to be considered when determining volume status.

In addition to history and physical examination, laboratory analyses for serum electrolytes and renal function should be performed periodically. Serum potassium, blood urea nitrogen (BUN), and serum creatinine (SCr) are particularly important to monitor for patients treated with diuretics, digoxin, angiotensin-converting enzyme (ACE) inhibitors, angiotensin II receptor blockers (ARBs), or aldosterone antagonists. Hypokalemia as a result of diuresis may increase the risk of digoxin toxicity, therefore, potassium levels of between 4 and 5 mEq/dL represent a reasonable target range. Renal function should also be monitored closely when diuresing a patient or when adding an ACE inhibitor, ARB, or aldosterone antagonist. Increases in

Table 2-3. NYHA-FC

NYHA-FC I	Ordinary exercise/activity does not cause symptoms (fatigue and dyspnea)
NYHA-FC II	Slight limitation in activity. Ordinary exercise/activity results in symptoms.
NYHA-FC III	Marked limitation in activity. Less than ordinary activity results in symptoms.
NYHA-FC IV	Any physical activity results in symptoms. Symptoms occur at rest.

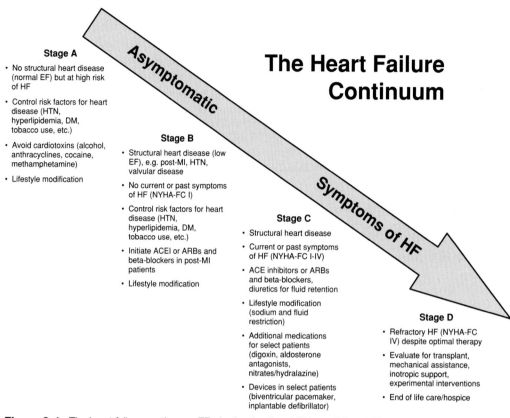

The Heart Failure Continuum

Asymptomatic

Symptoms of HF

Stage A
- No structural heart disease (normal EF) but at high risk of HF
- Control risk factors for heart disease (HTN, hyperlipidemia, DM, tobacco use, etc.)
- Avoid cardiotoxins (alcohol, anthracyclines, cocaine, methamphetamine)
- Lifestyle modification

Stage B
- Structural heart disease (low EF), e.g. post-MI, HTN, valvular disease
- No current or past symptoms of HF (NYHA-FC I)
- Control risk factors for heart disease (HTN, hyperlipidemia, DM, tobacco use, etc.)
- Initiate ACEI or ARBs and beta-blockers in post-MI patients
- Lifestyle modification

Stage C
- Structural heart disease
- Current or past symptoms of HF (NYHA-FC I-IV)
- ACE inhibitors or ARBs and beta-blockers, diuretics for fluid retention
- Lifestyle modification (sodium and fluid restriction)
- Additional medications for select patients (digoxin, aldosterone antagonists, nitrates/hydralazine)
- Devices in select patients (biventricular pacemaker, inplantable defibrillator)

Stage D
- Refractory HF (NYHA-FC IV) despite optimal therapy
- Evaluate for transplant, mechanical assistance, inotropic support, experimental interventions
- End of life care/hospice

Figure 2-1. The heart failure continuum. EF, ejection fraction; HF, heart failure; HTN, hypertension; DM, diabetes mellitus; MI, myocardial infarction; NYHA-FC, new york heart association functional classification; ACEI, angiotensin-converting enzyme inhibitors; ARBs, angiotensin II receptor blockers. Adapted from Hunt SA, Abraham WT, Chin MH, Feldman et al. ACC/AHA 2005 Guideline Update for the Diagnosis and Management of Chronic Heart Failure in the Adult: A Report of the American College of Cardiology/American Heart Association task Force on Practice Guidelines (Writing Committee to Update the 2001 Guidelines for the Evaluation and Management of Heart Failure). Available at: http://www.acc.org/clinical/guidelines/failure//index.pdf.

the BUN/SCr ratio (more than 20:1) may indicate central vascular volume depletion. BNP levels may be helpful in monitoring patients when symptoms of HF do not correlate with the physical examination. However, BNP levels need to be interpreted with caution as they may be elevated in females, older patients, and patients with renal disease. Routine measurement of ventricular function is not recommended unless there is a substantial change in clinical status.[4,6,7]

CLASSIFICATION OF HF

The American College of Cardiology and the American Heart Association developed four stages of HF (Stages A–D).[6] These stages were developed in an attempt to describe the development and progression of HF along a continuum (Fig. 2-1). It was hoped that the creation of these stages along with treatment recommendations for each would prompt earlier recognition and treatment. The ultimate goal would be to decrease the development of HF in susceptible patients and decrease the

progression in patients with HF. Stages A and B represent populations at risk for the development of HF. Stage C represents patients who have either current or past symptoms of HF and Stage D represents patients with end-stage HF. The NYHA-FC applies to patients in Stages C and D. Current evidence for HF medication therapy was derived using the NYHA-FC.

MANAGEMENT

PATIENTS AT HIGH RISK FOR DEVELOPING HF

Stage A represents the importance of early recognition and modification of risk factors associated with an increased risk of structural heart disease. The goal of therapy is to prevent development of LV remodeling, cardiac dysfunction, and HF. Risk factors include hypertension, hyperlipidemia, atherosclerosis, diabetes mellitus, obesity, physical inactivity, excessive alcohol intake, and smoking. Management of these risk factors is vital to decrease the risk of developing HF (Table 2-4).

Table 2-4. Treatment Goals of Risk Factors for the Development of HF

Risk Factor	Treatment Goal
Hypertension	<140/90 mm Hg
	Diabetes and/or coronary artery
	$\quad$ disease: <130/80 mm Hg
	Renal insufficiency
	$\quad$ >1g/d proteinuria: <130/85 mm Hg
	$\quad$ ≤1g/d proteinuria: <125/75 mm Hg
Diabetes	American Diabetes
	$\quad$ Association Guideline
	HgbA1c < 7%
Hyperlipidemia	National Cholesterol Education
	$\quad$ Program Guideline
Sedentary lifestyle	Sustained aerobic activity 20–30 min,
	$\quad$ 3–5 times weekly
Obesity	Weight reduction BMI < 30
Alcohol intake	Men
	$\quad$ Limit 1–2 drink equivalents/d
	Women
	$\quad$ Limit 1 drink equivalent/d
Smoking	Cessation
Dietary sodium	Maximum 2–3 g/d

Adapted from: Adams KF, Lindenfeld J, Arnold JMO, et al. Executive Summary: HFSA 2006 Comprehensive Heart Failure Practice Guidelines. *J Cardiac Failure.* 2006;12:10–38.

Specific medication management includes an ACE inhibitor for patients with CAD, peripheral vascular disease, stroke, or diabetes. Individuals with a prior MI should receive a β-blocker to reduce mortality, recurrent MI, and development of HF.[6]

ASYMPTOMATIC LV DYSFUNCTION

As a general rule, the lower the EF, the higher the risk of developing HF or sudden death. The goal of pharmacological treatment in asymptomatic patients (American College of Cardiology/American Heart Association Stage B) with documented LV systolic dysfunction is to delay or prevent the development of HF and reduce the risk of MI and sudden death by prevention, attenuation, or even reversal of LV dilatation and hypertrophy.[5] In addition to the treatment measures in Stage A, medication therapy should include an ACE inhibitor and β-blocker despite the EF; similarly, patients with a reduced LVEF should receive both medications, regardless of a history of MI. The dose of the ACE inhibitor or β-blocker should be optimized in individual patients with a goal of reaching the target dose used in large controlled trials. ARBs are recommended for those intolerant of ACE inhibitors as a result of cough or angioedema.

SYMPTOMATIC HF

Chronic HF

Stage C is defined as structural heart disease with prior or current symptoms of HF. The NYHA-FC is uti-

lized in chronic HF to classify patient's symptoms and guide pharmacologic treatment (Table 2-5). Goals for treating HF patients with LV systolic dysfunction include: (1) improving symptoms and quality of life, achieved by reduction of volume overload and maintaining a stable volume status, (2) slowing the progression of cardiac and peripheral dysfunction, and (3) reducing mortality. ACE inhibitors and β-blockers, the cornerstone of HF therapy, improve symptoms, delay progression of cardiac dysfunction, and reduce mortality.[6,7]

Patients with NYHA-FC I–IV who are euvolemic should have an ACE inhibitor initiated followed by a β-blocker. Patients with evidence of volume overload should first be treated with loop diuretics and may simultaneously have ACE-inhibitor therapy initiated. The dose of the diuretic is adjusted based on volume status (Fig. 2-2). If response is insufficient, the dose can be increased or a combination of diuretics (loop and metolazone or hydrochlorothiazide) can be given. Combination diuretic therapy should be used with caution because of the risk of severe electrolyte depletion. Once the patient is euvolemic, β-blocker therapy should be initiated and titrated to target doses (Table 2-6).

Digoxin is effective in patients with normal sinus rhythm to decrease hospitalizations and improve functional status and should be continued in those individuals who have symptomatically improved.

Aldosterone antagonists, ARBs, and hydralazine-isosorbide dinitrate may be beneficial in select patients. In addition to the treatment measures in Stage A, general measures include salt restriction, modest physical activity, daily weight measurement, immunization against influenza and pneumococcus, and avoidance of medications that can exacerbate HF (nonsteroidal anti-inflammatory drugs, calcium channel blockers, sympathomimetics, thiazolidinediones).

Acute Decompensated Heart Failure

Acute decompensated heart failure (ADHF) is diagnosed primarily on signs and symptoms. Elevated LV filling pressures and systemic vascular resistance (SVR) directly contribute to fluid redistribution, pulmonary edema, and respiratory distress. Most patients with ADHF present with significant volume overload and congestive symptoms. Clinical symptoms indicate whether the filling pressure is elevated (wet or dry) and perfusion is adequate (warm or cold), yielding four hemodynamic profiles (Fig. 2-3) that can be used to predict early and late mortality.[8] Management of ADHF is focused on reversal of acute hemodynamic abnormalities, relief of congestion and volume overload, identification of precipitating factors, and initiation of treatments that will decrease disease progression and improve survival. After evaluation and stabilization in

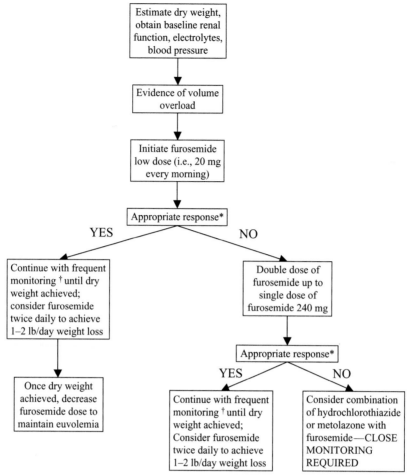

Figure 2-2. Diuretic algorithm (*Appropriate response defined by urination within 30–40 min of initial furosemide dose, then 4–6 repeat urination over 4–6 h; †Renal function, electrolytes, blood pressure [use potassium supplementation to maintain serum potassium 4.5 mEq per liter; if BUN/SCr >20, indication of intravascular volume depletion, evaluate rate of diuresis).

the emergency department, most patients will require hospital admission. Renal function and blood pressure are powerful predictors of in-hospital mortality among patients with ADHF and may be extended to patients in clinic to guide the primary care clinician to determine if hospitalization is required (Table 2-7).[9] An analysis of 32,229 patients in the Acute Decompensated Heart Failure (ADHERE) National Registry found that a baseline BUN level ≥43 mg/dL was the most useful predictor of in-hospital mortality, followed by a systolic blood pressure of less than 115 mm Hg and creatinine level of ≥2.75 mg/dL.

Advanced HF

Despite recent treatment advances, some patients progress to Stage D, refractory end-stage HF. Patients with Stage D HF have symptoms at rest (NYHA FC IV) or with minimal exertion (such as with activities of

daily living) and require frequent hospitalizations and/or emergency department visits for management. As patients frequently fluctuate in their NYHA FC, clinicians should make certain that the patient is receiving optimal medical therapy and that no exacerbating factors are contributing to the current symptoms before the patient is categorized as end-stage. Potential exacerbating factors include dietary sodium indiscretion, contraindicated medications (nonsteroidal anti-inflammatory drugs, calcium channel blockers, sympathomimetics, thiazolidinediones), substance abuse, arrhythmias, uncontrolled hypertension, myocardial ischemia, or anemia. Once the patient is classified as Stage D, they should be considered for the following: treatment with a mechanical assist device, intravenous inotropic support, referral for cardiac transplantation, or hospice care. In addition, if they have not already been, the patient should be referred to a HF disease

Table 2-5. Pharmacological Therapy of HF

	Survival/Morbidity	**Symptom Treatment**
NYHA I	ACE inhibitor/ARB if ACE inhibitor intolerant Aldosterone antagonist if post-MI β-Blocker if post-MI	Decrease/discontinue diuretic
NYHA II	ACE inhibitor/ARB if ACE inhibitor intolerant β-Blocker Aldosterone antagonist if post-MI	Diuretic if evidence of fluid retention
NYHA III	ACE inhibitor/ARB if ACE inhibitor intolerant β-Blocker Aldosterone antagonist	Diuretic Digoxin continued symptoms
NYHA IV	ACE inhibitor β-Blocker Aldosterone antagonist	Diuretic Digoxin ± Inotropic support

Adapted from: Swedberg K, Cleland J, Dargie H, et al. *Guidelines for the Diagnosis and Treatment of Chronic Heart Failure: Executive Summary* (update 2005): The Task Force for the Diagnosis and Treatment of Chronic Heart Failure of the European Society of Cardiology. *Eur Heart J.* 2005;26:1115–1140.

management program and advance directives should be discussed with the patient and their family. A recently validated tool, the Seattle Heart Failure Model, can be helpful to discuss prognosis as well as to demonstrate the potential benefit of various HF treatments (β-blockers, ACE inhibitors, etc).[10] Stage D HF treatment decisions, including end-of-life care, should be made by HF specialists in conversation with the primary care provider.

Heart transplantation represents the most accepted form of surgical intervention for end-stage HF patients; however, it is not readily available because of the shortage

Table 2-6. Cardiovascular Medications for HF Treatment

Medication	**Initial Dose (mg)**	**Maximum Dose (mg)**
ACE inhibitors		
Captopril	6.25 tid	50 tid
Enalapril	2.5 bid	20 bid
Lisinopril	2.5–5 qd	40 qd
Perindopril	2 qd	8–16 qd
Quinapril	5 bid	20 bid
Ramipril	1.25–2.5 qd	10 qd
Trandolapril	1 qd	4 qd
β-Blockers		
Bisoprolol	1.25 qd	10 qd
Carvedilol	3.125 bid	25 bid; 50 bid if >85 kg
Metoprolol succinate	12.5–25 qd	200 qd
Loop diuretics		
Bumetanide	1	4-8
Furosemide	40	160–200
Torsemide	10	100–200
Thiazide diuretics		
Hydrochlorothiazide	25 qd	50 mg qd
Chlorthalidone	25 qd	50 mg qd
Thiazide-related diuretics		
Metolazone	1.25–2.5	10 bid
Digoxin	0.125 qod–0.25 qd	
Isosorbide dinitrate	10 tid	80 tid
Hydralazine	25 tid	150 qid
Angiotensin receptor blockers		
Candesartan	4–8 qd	32 qd
Losartan	25–50 qd	50–100 qd
Valsartan	20–40 bid	160 bid
Aldosterone antagonists		
Spironolactone	12.5–25 qd	25 qd
Eplerenone	25 qd	50 qd

Congestion at Rest

		No	Yes
Adequate Perfusion at Rest	Yes	**Warm & Dry** PCWP normal CI normal	**Warm & Wet** PCWP elevated CI normal
	No	**Cold & Dry** PCWP low/normal CI decreased	**Cold & Wet** PCWP elevated CI decreased Normal/high SVR

Figure 2-3. Hemodynamic profile.

of donor hearts. Indications for heart transplantation are provided in Table 2-8. Common contraindications to transplantation include but are not limited to the following: current alcohol or substance abuse, uncontrolled mental illness, severe pulmonary hypertension, and systemic disease with multiorgan involvement.[4] Left-ventricular assist devices (LVADs) or intra-aortic balloon pumps have been used to maintain hemodynamic support for those awaiting transplant. Recently, LVADs have been used as "destination" therapy for patients with an estimated 1-year mortality of more than 50% and who are not transplant candidates.[6] Intermittent intravenous positive inotropic infusions, such as, dobutamine or milrinone, have been used to alleviate symptoms and help bridge patients to transplant. Every attempt should be made to wean the patient from the inotropic infusions as they may hasten mortality. How-

Table 2-8. Indications for Heart Transplantation[6]

Absolute indications in appropriate patients
For hemodynamic compromise to HF
Refractory cardiogenic shock
Documented dependence on IV inotropic support to maintain organ perfusion
Peak VO$_2$ < 10 mL/kg per minute with achievement of anaerobic metabolism
Severe symptoms of ischemia that consistently limit routine activity and are not candidates for surgical or percutaneous intervention
Recurrent symptomatic refractory ventricular arrhythmias
Relative indications
Peak VO$_2$ 11–14 mL/kg per minute and major limitation in patient's ADLs
Recurrent unstable angina not amenable to surgery
Recurrent instability of fluid and renal function
Insufficient indications
Low LV function
History of NYHA FC III or IV symptoms of HF
Peak VO$_2$ > 15 mL/kg per minute

HF, heart failure; ADLs, activities of daily living; IV, intravenous; VO$_2$ oxygen consumption per unit time; NYHA FC, New York Heart Association functional classification.
Source: Lippincott W&W web page

ever, in some instances, intravenous infusions may be used as part of palliative care to allow the patient to die in comfort. For Stage D patients with implantable cardioverter-defibrillators (ICDs) who are entering end-of-life care, the decision to inactivate the ICD should be discussed with the patient and their family.[6]

HF WITH PRESERVED SYSTOLIC FUNCTION

It is now recognized that approximately 50% of patients with HF have normal or near normal systolic function (EF > 40%). These patients can present with the same signs and symptoms as patients with impaired systolic function (dyspnea, fatigue, fluid retention). In addition, BNP levels will typically be elevated in symptomatic patients and cannot be used to differentiate the two types of HF. Diagnosis of HF with preserved systolic dysfunction (HFPSF) is typically made based on the presence of symptoms and normal or near normal EF without evidence of valvular abnormalities. Previously, HFPSF was termed diastolic dysfunction, and while diastolic dysfunction is the underlying pathology of HFPSF, it is estimated that as many as 50% of patients with HF and systolic dysfunction have a component of diastolic dysfunction. Diastolic dysfunction is characterized by decreased ventricular compliance and altered relaxation. The decrease in compliance and relaxation is generally caused by hypertension and LV hypertrophy and can be exacerbated by tachyarrhythmias such as atrial fibrillation. The epidemiology of HFPSF is still being characterized; however; the mortality in patients may be similar to those with reduced LVEF.[11,12]

Table 2-7. Consideration for Hospitalization for ADHF

Recommendation	Clinical Circumstances
Recommend hospitalization	Evidence of severely decompensated HF: Hypotension (SBP < 115 mm Hg) Worsening renal function (BUN ≥ 43 mg/dL, SCr ≥ 2.75 mg/dL) Altered mentation Dyspnea at rest Hemodynamically significant arrhythmia Acute coronary syndrome
Consider hospitalization	Worsened congestion Weight gain ≥ 5 kilograms Signs and symptoms of pulmonary or systemic congestion Major electrolyte disturbance Associated comorbid conditions Pneumonia Pulmonary embolus Symptoms suggestive of TIA or stroke Repeated ICD firings Previously undiagnosed HF with signs and symptoms of systemic or pulmonary congestion

Adapted from: Adams KF, Lindenfeld J, Arnold JMO, et al. Executive Summary: HFSA 2006 Comprehensive Heart Failure Practice Guidelines. *J Cardiac Failure.* 2006;12:10–38.

Treatment recommendations for HFPSF are based largely on the presence of comorbid conditions, such as, hypertension, arrhythmia, CAD, as only a few clinical trials exist in this population. However, a recently completed large clinical trial with the ARB, candesartan, demonstrated the feasibility of clinical studies in patients with HFPSF.[13] However, the results were underwhelming because candesartan was demonstrated to have nonsignificant reductions in HF hospitalizations and no effect on mortality (cardiovascular or all-cause). Current HF guidelines recommend control of blood pressure, heart rate, and volume status in patients with HFPSF. Agents to control blood pressure should be selected based on the presence of comorbid conditions. In the absence of comorbid conditions, ACE inhibitors or ARBs are preferred agents. ACE inhibitors are preferred for patients with diabetes or atherosclerotic cardiovascular disease. β-Blockers are recommended for patients requiring control of heart rate or for those with CAD. Calcium channel blockers, such as, verapamil or diltiazem, are alternatives for rate control in patients either unresponsive or intolerant to β-blockers. Diuretics (thiazide and/or loop) should be used to control volume. Patients with myocardial ischemia should be evaluated for coronary revascularization. Finally, patients with symptomatic atrial fibrillation should be considered for cardioversion and maintenance of sinus rhythm.

MEDICATIONS

DIURETICS

Diuretics inhibit the reabsorption of sodium and chloride at specific sites in the renal tubules and are necessary adjuncts for symptomatic treatment of HF. The cause of edema in HF is complex and includes renal vasoconstriction, elevated aldosterone and vasopressin, and/or elevated venous pressures.[5] HF leads to increased sympathetic tone and an activation of the renin–angiotensin–aldosterone system that results in sodium retention and potassium loss. Accumulation of sodium and water lead to an expanded extravascular volume, peripheral edema, and pulmonary congestion. The goal of diuretic therapy is to reduce fluid retention and pulmonary congestion, improve quality of life, and reduce hospitalizations from HF.[6] Furosemide, torsemide, and bumetanide act at the loop of Henle, whereas thiazides, metolazone, and potassium-sparing diuretics act in the distal portion of the renal tubule. Furosemide is the most commonly used loop diuretic. With evidence of volume overload, furosemide is initiated at low doses and increased until urine output increases with a desired weight loss of approximately 1 to 2 lbs daily (Figure 2-2). Multiple adjustments of diuretic therapy may be required over days or weeks to restore normal volume status. After

the desired diuresis is attained with once daily administration of furosemide, which is evident by urination within 30 to 60 minutes of first morning dose, the frequency of administration may be increased to twice daily until euvolemia is achieved. Generally, patients requiring diuretic therapy require chronic treatment, although often at lower doses than those required for initial diuresis. Close monitoring is required to prevent adverse effects, including electrolyte abnormalities, renal dysfunction, and symptomatic hypotension.[7]

Torsemide, which has better oral absorption and a longer duration of action than furosemide, may be considered in patients with poor absorption of oral medication or erratic diuresis. Concomitant therapy with thiazides or metolazone and loop diuretics may be considered in patients with persistent fluid retention despite high-dose loop diuretic therapy. However, patients must be monitored closely because of the potential for profound electrolyte and volume depletion. Electrolyte and renal function should be monitored every 2 to 3 days with combination therapy. Potassium-sparing diuretics may be added if hypokalemia persists after ACE inhibition, but requires close monitoring.

ACE INHIBITORS

ACE inhibitors decrease circulating levels of angiotensin II and have many beneficial effects in HF including reduction in sodium and water retention by inhibiting angiotensin II stimulation of aldosterone release and decreasing sympathetic nervous system (SNS) activity. ACE inhibitors decrease both afterload and preload resulting in reduced SVR, arterial pressure, LV and right ventricular end-diastolic pressures, myocardial oxygen consumption, and increased cardiac output. ACE inhibitors improve symptoms, quality of life, exercise tolerance, and survival. They are recommended for all patients with asymptomatic or symptomatic HF and LV systolic dysfunction (Stage B through D) and for the prevention of HF in patients with a history of vascular disease, diabetes mellitus, or hypertension (Stage A).[6,14]

Low doses should be used initially and then doubled as tolerated to the target doses that have been shown to reduce the risk of cardiovascular events in clinical trials (Table 2-5). Blood pressure, renal function, and potassium should be reassessed within 1 to 2 weeks after initiation and followed closely after changes in dose. Although a 30% increase in SCr from baseline is acceptable, doubling of the SCr should warrant consideration of renal dysfunction related to ACE inhibitor use, a need to reduce the dose of the diuretic, or exacerbation of HF.

Contraindications for ACE inhibitor use include history of angioedema, anuric renal failure, or bilateral renal artery stenosis. They should be used with caution for patients with hypotension (systolic blood pressure less than 80 mmHg), elevated levels of SCr (more than 3mg/dL), or elevated levels of serum potassium (more than 5.5 mEq/L).[4,6]

ANGIOTENSIN II RECEPTOR BLOCKERS

ARBs inhibit the angiotensin II receptor subtype AT_1, which diminishes the detrimental effects of the renin-angiotensin system. The clinical evidence for ARBs in HF is considerably less than with ACE inhibitors; however, several placebo-controlled studies with long-term therapy of ARBs in HF produced hemodynamic, neurohormonal, and clinical effects consistent with ACE inhibition.[6,15,16] For patients unable to tolerate ACE inhibitors due to cough or angioedema, valsartan and candesartan have shown benefit by reducing hospitalizations and mortality.[6,15]

ACE inhibitors remain the first choice for inhibition of the renin-angiotensin system in chronic HF. ARBs should be used for patients in stages A through D who are intolerant to ACE inhibitors due to cough or angioedema.[4,6]

Low doses should be used initially and then doubled as tolerated to the target dose (Table 2-5). Blood pressure, renal function, and potassium should be reassessed within 1 to 2 weeks after initiation and followed closely after changes in dose. Particular caution is warranted in patients with a systolic blood pressure below 80 mmHg, low serum sodium, diabetes mellitus, or impaired renal function. The risks of treatment with ARBs include renal dysfunction, hypotension, and hyperkalemia and are greater in combination with ACE inhibitors or aldosterone antagonists. Although the incidence of angioedema is less frequent with ARBs, there are case reports of patients who developed angioedema to ACE inhibitors and later to ARBs.[6,15]

β-ADRENERGIC RECEPTOR ANTAGONISTS

β-Blockers inhibit the cardio-stimulatory effects of SNS activation. Activation of the SNS occurs in response to a decrease in cardiac output. However, in chronic HF, SNS activation has the following undesirable effects: increased myocardial oxygen demand, production of ventricular arrhythmias, ventricular remodeling, myocyte apoptosis, and increases in preload and afterload. β-Blockers antagonize these detrimental effects and have been demonstrated to reduce total mortality, cardiovascular mortality, sudden death, and all-cause hospitalizations. In addition, β-blockers have been demonstrated to improve NYHA-FC and patient quality of life.

β-Blockers should be used for patients in stages B through D. Stage B would include patients with a history of MI either with or without evidence of LV dys-

function. In addition, patients in stage B who do not have a history of MI nor symptoms of HF but with evidence of LV dysfunction should receive a β-blocker. All stable stage C patients should receive a β-blocker with demonstrated mortality benefits (Table 2-5).[6]

Prior to initiation of β-blocker therapy, patients should be stable without signs of moderate to severe fluid retention. Low doses should be used initially and then doubled, as tolerated, at biweekly intervals to the target dose (see Table 2-6). Patients should be instructed to weigh themselves each morning and record weights. They should also be instructed to call for worsening symptoms or increased weight. If symptoms worsen, diuretics should be increased and β-blocker dose should be held at the same dose or decreased if no response to diuretics. For patients experiencing symptoms of hypotension, the diuretic or the ACE inhibitor should be decreased and the administration times of the ACE inhibitor and β-blocker should be separated. Every attempt should be made to continue the β-blocker. If a patient receiving chronic β-blocker therapy requires inotropic support, a phosphodiesterase inhibitor, such as milrinone, would be preferred as their activity would not be diminished by the β-blockade. Absolute contraindications to β-blockade are few and include the following: documented reactive airway disease, severe obstructive pulmonary disease, symptomatic bradycardia, and greater than first-degree heart block (not treated with a pacemaker).

ALDOSTERONE ANTAGONISTS

Aldosterone has many deleterious effects on the renal-cardiovascular system in patients with HF. In the kidneys, increased aldosterone levels result in sodium and water retention, potassium and magnesium loss, and renal fibrosis. Aldosterone also causes vascular inflammation and fibrosis, modulation of the vasculature to vasoconstrictors such as angiotensin II, and endothelial dysfunction. The cardiac implications of increased aldosterone levels include: catecholamine potentiation, decreased coronary blood flow, inflammation, myocardial fibrosis, ventricular hypertrophy, and ventricular arrhythmias.[17–20] While short-term therapy with ACE inhibitors and ARBs can lower levels of aldosterone, this suppression may not persist during long-term treatment.[21]

The introduction of aldosterone antagonists to HF therapy was implemented following the Randomized Aldactone Evaluation Study (RALES) trial, which studied 1600 class III or class IV HF patients receiving standard HF therapy, randomized to spironolactone 25 mg daily or placebo.[22] The risk of death was reduced from 46% to 35% (30% relative risk reduction) over 2 years, with a 35% reduction in hospitalizations due to HF and an improvement in functional class. The novel selective aldosterone receptor antagonist, eplerenone, was compared with placebo in 6642 patients with LV dysfunction after MI receiving usual therapy (ACE inhibitor, β-blocker, aspirin, and diuretics).[23] Mortality was decreased by 13.6% at 1-year and HF hospitalizations were reduced by 23%. The benefits of aldosterone antagonists in HF appear to be due largely to their neurohormonal inhibition, more specifically, inhibition of aldosterone-mediated cardiac fibrosis and ventricular remodeling.

While aldosterone antagonists have been demonstrated to reduce mortality, HF hospitalizations, and improve functional class when added to standard HF therapy, spironolactone and eplerenone were studied in two specific subgroups of HF patients. Therefore, the initiation of an aldosterone antagonist should be considered in select patients with moderate to severe HF symptoms (NYHA-FC III and IV) and recent decompensation or LV dysfunction early after a MI. Although patients with NYHA-FC II and stable class III have yet to be studied, it might be reasonable to consider initiation of an aldosterone antagonist if the patient requires potassium supplementation. Patients would be excluded from this therapy with a recent history of renal dysfunction or hyperkalemia. In addition, the benefit of decreased mortality and hospitalization from HF must be weighed against the potential risk of hyperkalemia. Upon initiation of an aldosterone antagonist, the SCr should be less than 2.0 to 2.5 mg/dL without recent worsening and serum potassium should be less than 5.0 mEq/dL without a history of hyperkalemia.[6] Aldosterone antagonists should not be given to patients with a creatinine clearance less than 30 mL/min.

The recommended initial doses of the available aldosterone antagonists are spironolactone 12.5 mg or eplerenone 25 mg daily and if tolerated may be increased to 25 mg and 50 mg, respectively. Renal function and serum potassium should be evaluated within 3 days and again in one week after initiation. Routine monitoring of renal function and serum potassium is recommended monthly for the first 3 months, then every 3 months thereafter. Close monitoring would be necessary with any change in spironolactone or eplerenone, ACE inhibitor or ARB therapy. It is recommended to avoid the combination of an aldosterone antagonist, ACE inhibitor, and ARB. If the serum potassium exceeds 5.5 mEq/L, the aldosterone antagonist should be discontinued or the dose reduced. Additionally, prior to the initiation of aldosterone antagonists, potassium supplementation should be discontinued.

The use of aldosterone antagonists requires patient education. Patients should be instructed to avoid foods that are high in potassium. Patients should also be advised against using nonsteroidal anti-inflammatory agents and cyclo-oxygenase-2 inhibitors, and to discontinue the aldosterone antagonist if loop diuretic therapy is interrupted or during an episode of diarrhea.

The most significant adverse effect with aldosterone antagonists is the risk of hyperkalemia. Recent data from clinical practice suggests that the minimal risk of hyperkalemia and renal dysfunction evident from clinical trials poses a larger problem than originally apparent.[22–25] Therefore, therapy with either aldosterone antagonist requires close monitoring.[24,25]

DIGITALIS GLYCOSIDES

Digitalis glycosides exert their effects in HF by inhibition of the enzyme sodium-potassium (Na^+-K^+) adenosine triphosphatase (ATPase) in cardiac and noncardiac tissues. Inhibition of this enzyme on the surface membrane of myocardial cells results in an increase in the amount of intracellular calcium, thereby increasing cardiac contractility. The noncardiac effects of digitalis glycosides in HF are primarily through the attenuation of neurohormonal activation. These include sensitization of cardiac baroreceptors, which reduces sympathetic outflow from the central nervous system, and decreased renal tubular reabsorption of sodium in the kidney, which leads to suppression of renin secretion from the kidneys. Collectively, the effects augment myocardial performance while reducing peripheral resistance.

Of the digitalis glycosides, digoxin has a relatively rapid onset and intermediate duration of action and is the only glycoside that has been evaluated in placebo-controlled trials. Digoxin has greater hemodynamic effects with decreased ventricular function and has been shown to improve symptoms, quality of life, and exercise tolerance in patients with mild to moderate HF, regardless of the underlying rhythm (normal sinus rhythm or atrial fibrillation), cause of HF (ischemic or nonischemic cardiomyopathy), or associated therapy (with or without ACE inhibitor).[6] Digoxin is indicated in patients with LV dysfunction (LVEF < 40%) who continue to have NYHA-FC II, III, and IV symptoms despite appropriate therapy. As demonstrated in the Digitalis Investigation Group (DIG) trial,[26] digoxin therapy was associated with a significant reduction in hospitalization for HF, but had no mortality benefit.

The recommended daily dose of digoxin is 0.125 to 0.25 mg if the SCr is within normal limits. A digoxin serum level of 0.5 to 0.8 ng/mL is therapeutic. Lower doses, such as 0.125 mg every other day, should be initiated if patients are greater than 70 years of age, have impaired renal function, low lean body mass, or receiving interacting drugs, such as amiodarone. Digoxin should not be initiated in an acutely decompensated patient, but is indicated in chronic HF patients who are receiving appropriate HF therapy and still experiencing symptoms. The major adverse effects associated with digoxin are somewhat dependent on serum levels. When digoxin is dosed appropriately it is well tolerated by most HF patients. The major adverse effects include cardiac arrhythmias, especially ectopic and re-entrant cardiac rhythms and heart block and central nervous symptoms such as anorexia, nausea, vomiting, visual disturbances, and disorientation. Contraindications to digoxin therapy include bradycardia, second and third-degree atrioventricular block, sick sinus syndrome, carotid sinus syndrome, Wolff-Parkinson-White syndrome, hypertrophic cardiomyopathy, and hypo- or hyperkalemia.[6] Routine measurement of renal function and electrolytes is necessary due to the risk of increased toxicity with hypokalemia, hypomagnesemia, and worsening renal function.

Prior to initiation of medications that can increase serum digoxin concentrations and increase the risk of digoxin toxicity (e.g., clarithromycin, erythromycin, amiodarone, itraconazole, cyclosporine, verapamil, or quinidine), the dose of digoxin should be decreased.

VASODILATORS

A number of direct vasodilators have been studied for use in HF. The only one to demonstrate reductions in morbidity and mortality is the combination of isosorbide dinitrate and hydralazine. Alpha-antagonists should not be used as individual agents as they were demonstrated to be no better than placebo in patients with chronic HF and their use for the treatment of hypertension was shown to increase the incidence of HF as compared to other classes of antihypertensive medication.[27,28] Calcium channel blockers should also be avoided in patients with systolic dysfunction.[6] The exceptions are the dihyropyridines, amlodipine and felodipine, which have neutral effects on mortality and morbidity.[27,28] However, their use should be limited to patients with hypertension or angina refractory to treatment with ACE inhibitors, β-blockers, and nitrates.

Nitrates are primarily venodilators which act to reduce preload and hydralazine is an arterial vasodilator that acts to reduce SVR (afterload). The combination of isosorbide dinitrate and hydralazine has proven mortality benefits versus placebo in patients with HF and LV dysfunction.[29] These agents have been demonstrated to improve survival, decrease hospitalizations, and improve quality of life in African American patients with NYHA-FC III/IV HF already receiving treatment with ACE inhibitors and β-blockers.[30] Therefore, the combination should be strongly considered for use in this select population. It would be reasonable to consider the addition of the combination for all patients with systolic dysfunction and progressive symptoms despite therapy with ACE inhibitors and β-blockers.

Additionally, patients unable to tolerate ACE inhibitors and ARBs should be considered for treatment with the combination of nitrates and hydralazine.[6,7]

The target daily doses of isosorbide dinitrate and hydralazine are 160 mg and 300 mg, respectively. Side effects such as headache and symptomatic hypotension are often dose-limiting. The initial doses of each drug should be low and titrated toward the target dose. Recently, a combination tablet of isosorbide dinitrate and hydralazine (BiDil®) was approved for use in African American patients for the treatment of HF. The formulation consists of isosorbide dinitrate 20 mg and hydralazine 37.5 mg administered as 1 to 2 tablets three times daily.

NESIRITIDE

Nesiritide (Natrecor®) is a synthetic form of BNP and is indicated for use in patients with ADHF who have dyspnea at rest or minimal activity. Nesiritide is a vasodilator that dilates both the venous and arterial systems thereby decreasing preload and afterload. In addition, nesiritide increases sodium excretion (natriuresis) without activating the renin-angiotensin-aldosterone system. Nesiritide is administered by continuous intravenous infusion for a period no longer than 48 hours. Due to the risk of hypotension, patients receiving nesiritide should have frequent monitoring of their blood pressure and patients having a systolic blood pressure of <90 mm Hg should not receive nesiritide.

Two recent analyses of data provided to the US Food and Drug Administration by the drug's sponsor Scios during the initial review revealed a potential worsening of renal function and a potential increase in mortality.[31,32] As a result of these findings, as well as increasing pressure from healthcare professionals, Scios convened an expert panel of HF specialists to review all nesiritide data. The panel recommended that nesiritide use be limited to patients presenting to the hospital with ADHF and dyspnea at rest and that nesiritide use in this situation should be balanced against the possible risks and against alternative therapies.[33] In addition, the panel stated that nesiritide should not be used as a diuretic or for intermittent outpatient infusions. Until such time that prospective, randomized trials demonstrate that nesiritide decreases morbidity and mortality associated with HF, its use in the treatment of HF should be extremely limited.

INOTROPES

Routine use of positive inotropic agents should be avoided as they are associated with increased mortality.[4,6,7,34] Their use should be reserved for patients with

ADHF who have evidence of systemic hypoperfusion unresponsive to vasodilators and diuretics.[7,34]

The agents commonly used are the β_1-receptor agonists, dopamine and dobutamine, and the type III phosphodiesterase inhibitors, milrinone and enoximone. All inotropes have the net result of increasing intracellular calcium resulting in enhanced contractility. Unfortunately, inotropes are associated with an increased risk of arrhythmias and increased risk of myocardial ischemia due to increased myocardial oxygen demand. When inotropic therapy is necessary, it should be accompanied by continuous hemodynamic and electrophysiologic monitoring, and frequent serum electrolyte (potassium and magnesium) determination.[7,35]

When selecting between the inotropic agents, consideration should be given to whether or not the patient is being treated with a β-blocker as these patients would be expected to have a diminished response to typical doses of the β_1-receptor agonists. These patients should preferentially be treated with the type III phosphodiesterase inhibitors as their pharmacologic effect is not dependent on β-receptors.

ANTIARRHYTHMICS

Although sudden cardiac death (SCD), presumably as a result of arrhythmia, is one of the leading causes of death in HF patients, studies of antiarrhythmic agents have not demonstrated reductions in mortality and in fact may worsen LV dysfunction and increase sudden death. It is recommended that Class I and III antiarrhythmics be avoided in patients with LV systolic dysfunction for the primary and secondary prevention of sudden death.[4,6,7] Instead efforts should focus on placing patients on agents that are associated with decreasing disease progression such as β-blockers (class II antiarrhythmic) and aldosterone antagonists since these agents have been demonstrated to decrease both sudden death and all-cause mortality in patients with LV dysfunction post-MI as well as with chronic HF.

The lone exception is amiodarone (class III) which has been demonstrated to have a neutral effect on all-cause mortality. Therefore, the use of amiodarone may be considered for management of patients with supraventricular arrhythmias or to reduce the recurrence of ICD discharge for ventricular arrhythmias.[6] Chronic amiodarone therapy is associated with several toxicities such as hyper- and hypothyroidism, pulmonary fibrosis, hepatitis, and neuropathy (optic and peripheral). Therefore, it is imperative to consistently monitor for potential toxicities through patient history and laboratory analysis. Baseline monitoring parameters should include thyroid studies, hepatic transaminase levels, chest radiograph (or chest X-ray) (CXR),

pulmonary function tests with diffusion capacity and eye examination. Thyroid studies and hepatic transaminase levels should be repeated every 6 months. Symptoms of pulmonary fibrosis are nonspecific and often confused with symptoms of HF; however, any patient that develops a nonproductive cough and dyspnea while on amiodarone should be considered for a CXR and pulmonary function tests with diffusion capacity. Patients reporting any changes in visual acuity should be referred for ophthalmologic examination. Maintenance doses of 100 to 200 mg per day are associated with a lower incidence of toxicity and are therefore preferred.

In addition to potential toxicities, amiodarone is associated with several clinically important drug interactions. Amiodarone inhibits the cytochrome P450 isoenzymes 2C9 (warfarin), 2D6 (β-blockers), and 3A4 (calcium channel blockers and HMG Co-A reductase inhibitors) and can therefore increase plasma concentrations of P450 substrates. Amiodarone inhibits the renal clearance of digoxin by 50%; therefore, the dose of digoxin should be decreased by half in patients on concomitant therapy.

DEVICES

Sudden cardiac death (SCD) is a leading cause of death worldwide accounting for more than 3 million deaths each year. LVEF< 40% and signs and symptoms of congestive HF are important predictors of SCD. As previously mentioned, antiarrhythmic agents (with the exception of β-blockers) are ineffective at preventing SCD and are associated with significant risks. Recent research has focused on cardiac device therapy, such as implantable cardioverter defibrillators (ICDs). ICDs have two main parts, the pulse generator which is implanted in a subcutaneous pectoral pocket, and the lead electrodes. Current ICDs are typically dual chamber electrode systems, with leads in the right atria and ventricle. There are several functions of ICDs, including sensing atrial and ventricular electrical signals and detection of the rhythm. If a ventricular tachycardia (VT) or fibrillation (VF) rhythm is detected, the ICD delivers appropriate treatment in the form of either a shock or antitachycardia pacing (ATP).[35] ATP can terminate VT without delivering a shock by pacing at a faster rate than the detected VT which interrupts the re-entrant circuit. Additionally, ICDs can provide pacing for bradycardia and for cardiac resynchronization therapy (CRT).

ICD therapy has been demonstrated in recent years to decrease total mortality by virtue of decreasing SCD in several distinct groups of patients with HF and impaired systolic function. Current guidelines recommend ICD therapy as secondary prevention to prolong survival in patients with current or past symptoms of HF and reduced LVEF who have a history of either cardiac arrest, VF, or hemodynamically unstable sustained VT.[4,6,7] The exception to this recommendation is for patients with refractory HF (Stage D) who are not considered candidates for cardiac transplantation because survival would be expected to be short regardless of ICD therapy. Guidelines recommend ICD therapy for primary prevention to decrease total mortality as a result of a decrease in SCD in patients with or without a history of ischemic cardiomyopathy (≥40 days post-MI) who have an LVEF of ≤30% and NYHA FC II or III symptoms despite optimal chronic HF therapy (ACE inhibitors or ARBs and β-blockers).[4,6,7] Primary prevention patients meeting the above criteria with the exception of an LVEF of 30% to 35% should be considered for ICD therapy; however, patients with either refractory HF symptoms or a life expectancy of less than a year should not receive ICD therapy regardless of LVEF.[4,6]

Another important innovation in device therapy is the development of biventricular CRT. Intraventricular conduction delays (such as left bundle branch block) result in dyssynchronous ventricular contraction and a reduction in cardiac output. CRT capability involves a third electrode lead that is placed into the left ventricle. Biventricular CRT stimulates both ventricles to contract in a more simultaneous or synchronous fashion. When added to optimal medical therapy, CRT has been demonstrated to improve symptoms, exercise tolerance, quality of life, EF and lead to reductions in hospitalizations and overall mortality. Current guidelines recommend CRT therapy for patients with an LVEF ≤ 35%, normal sinus rhythm, NYHA FC III or IV symptoms on optimal medical therapy, and a QRS duration >120 ms.[4,6,7]

Patients with cardiac devices should receive frequent follow-up by a cardiology device specialist, such as an electrophysiologist, every 1 to 6 months for device testing and interrogation and determination of battery longevity (typically, 4–7 years).[35,36] Patients reporting a single shock without a change in symptoms do not require immediate evaluation; however, the decision of whether or not the patient needs to be seen should be made in consultation with the patient's electrophysiologist. Patients experiencing a single shock but not feeling well or those having multiple shocks (>1) within a relatively brief time frame (hours) need immediate evaluation and the patient should be instructed to contact emergency medical services. Such patients need evaluation to determine if the arrhythmia is ongoing, determine secondary causes of arrhythmia (acute MI, hypokalemia), or determine the possibility of ICD malfunction. If the arrhythmia is ongoing upon evaluation, treatment should be according to appropriate advanced cardiac life support guidelines. However, electrodes for external defibrillation should not be placed over the area of the ICD to reduce risk of damage to the device. ICD therapy can be interrupted through the placement of a magnet directly over the pulse generator. This will terminate arrhythmia detection as well as therapy; therefore, external ECG monitoring should be in place.

PATIENT EDUCATION

Education is essential for both patients and their caregivers to improve quality of life, decrease hospitalizations, and delay progression of HF.

WEIGHT MONITORING

Weight monitoring enables the patient and the clinician to objectively evaluate changes in volume status. Patients should weigh themselves in the morning, after voiding, as part of a daily routine and record the results. An action plan can be developed to contact their provider or use a sliding scale diuretic regimen if patient exceeds their "dry" weight.

SODIUM AND FLUID RESTRICTION

Sodium should be restricted to less than two grams per day. Noncompliance with sodium restrictions can lead to volume retention, marked elevations in LV end-diastolic pressures, and increased hospitalizations. Fluid restriction to 1.5 to 2 liters per day is needed in more advanced HF. Alcohol consumption should be restricted to no more than one alcoholic beverage per day and patients with alcoholic cardiomyopathy must abstain completely. Education regarding sodium and fluid restriction must be strongly emphasized and reinforced at each appointment.[6,37]

PHYSICAL ACTIVITY

To prevent exercise intolerance and improve skeletal muscle function and overall functional capacity, patients should be given recommendations for daily physical and leisure activities and specifically instructed to cease exercise if worsening symptoms of HF occur. Exercise should be done at least four days a week; common recommendations include walking outdoors or in an enclosed fitness center or mall. Patients should be instructed to avoid physical activity in excessive heat or cold.[4,6]

MEDICATION REGIMENS

HF medication regimens are complex and they usually require a large number of pharmacologic agents. Ensure that patients and their caregivers understand when and how to take the medications. This can be accomplished by: providing them with a detailed medication list with drug name, dose, and frequency of administration along with common side effects; plan of diuretic adjustment for weight increase with subsequent electrolyte management; and instructions not to discontinue any medication without notifying their provider. Compliance with medications should be assessed and their importance reinforced at each appointment.

INSTRUCTIONS FOR PROVIDER CONTACT

Patients and caregivers must be educated when to contact their provider. Some examples include weight gain ($\geq$3 lbs/24–48 h), uncertainty about increasing diuretics, onset of edema of the feet or abdomen, decreased exercise tolerance, inability to lie flat in bed or awakening from sleep due to dyspnea, worsening cough, nausea and vomiting, decreased appetite, signs or symptoms of postural hypotension, or prolonged palpitations. Although not all inclusive, early intervention by the provider may prevent a hospital admission. If the patient experiences a sudden onset of symptoms including chest pain, severe dyspnea, loss of consciousness, visual changes, or impairment in speech or strength in an extremity, the patient or caregiver should be instructed to call emergency medical services.[4]

EVIDENCE-BASED SUMMARY

Screen
- Early recognition and modification of risk factors associated with an increased risk of HF
- Includes hypertension, hyperlipidemia, atherosclerosis, diabetes mellitus, obesity

Patient evaluation
- Assess symptoms
- Assess physical findings and determine volume status

Diagnostic evaluation
- ECG, CXR,
- CBC, SCr, TSH, BNP
- Transthoracic Doppler echocardiogram
- Patients with LV dysfunction and CAD should be referred for coronary angiography

Management
- All HF patients in Stages B, C (current or past HF symptoms), or D (refractory HF) should be treated with ACE inhibitors or ARBs and β-blockers

- Prior to initiation of β-blockers, the patient should be stable and euvolemic. Diuretics (loop or thiazide) are used to manage volume and helpful in enabling initiation and titration of β-blockers.
- Patients who remain symptomatic despite treatment with ACE inhibitors and β-blockers can be considered for treatment with additional agents such as aldosterone antagonists (spironolactone and eplerenone), ARBs, digoxin or nitrates/hydralazine
- Digoxin has neutral effects on mortality but does decrease morbidity (hospitalizations). If used for the treatment of HF, low doses should be used to achieve serum concentrations between 0.5 and 0.8 ng/mL.
- SCD, presumably due to arrhythmia, is the leading cause of death in HF. Device therapy, with ICDs, has been shown to decrease the incidence of SCD in certain populations of patients with systolic dysfunction
- Individuals with intraventricular conduction delays and subsequent ventricular dyssynchrony as well as significant systolic dysfunction (EF $\leq$ 35%) despite optimal medical therapy, should be considered for biventricular CRT.
- Noncompliance with both diet and medications is the leading cause of rehospitalization in HF patients. Therefore, patient education is an integral component of HF management

Follow-up
- Symptoms, volume status
- BUN, SCr, serum electrolytes

REFERENCES

1. American Heart Association. Heart Disease and Stroke Statistics—2006 Update. Dallas, TX: American Heart Association; 2006.
2. Braunwald E. Heart failure and cor pulmonale, In: Kasper DL, Braunwald E, Fauci AS (eds.). *Harrison's Principles of Internal Medicine*, 16th ed. New York, NY: McGraw-Hill; 2005:1370–1371.
3. Goswami NJ, O'Rourke RA, Shaver JA, Silverman ME. The history, physical examination, and cardiac auscultation. In: O'Rourke RA, Fuster V, Alexander RW (eds). *Hurst's The Heart Manual of Cardiology*, 11th ed. New York, NY: McGraw-Hill; 2005:1–12.
4. Swedberg K, Cleland J, Dargie H, et al. Guidelines for the diagnosis and treatment of chronic heart failure: Executive summary (update 2005): The task force for the diagnosis and treatment of chronic heart failure of the european society of cardiology. *Eur Heart J.* 2005;26: 1115–1140.

5. LeJemtel TH, Sonnenblick EH, Frishman WH. Diagnosis and management of heart failure. In: Fuster V, Alexander RW, O'Rourke RA (eds). *Hurst's The Heart*, 11th ed. New York, NY: McGraw-Hill; 2005:723–729.

6. Hunt SA, Abraham WT, Chin MH, Feldman et al. ACC/AHA 2005 Guideline Update for the Diagnosis and Management of Chronic Heart Failure in the Adult: A Report of the American College of Cardiology/American Heart Association task Force on Practice Guidelines (Writing Committee to Update the 2001 Guidelines for the Evaluation and Management of Heart Failure). Available at: http://www.acc.org/clinical/guidelines/failure//index.pdf. Accessed January 11, 2008.

7. Adams KF, Lindenfeld J, Arnold JMO, et al. Executive summary: HFSA 2006 comprehensive heart failure practice guidelines. *J Card Fail.* 2006;12:10–38.

8. Nohria A, Tsang SW, Fang JC, et al. Clinical assessment identifies hemodynamic profiles that predict outcomes in patients admitted with heart failure. *J Am Coll Cardiol.* 2003;41:1797–1804.

9. Fonarow GC, Adams KF, Abraham WT, et al. Risk stratification for in-hospital mortality in acutely decompensated heart failure. *JAMA.* 2005;293:572–580.

10. Levy WC, Mozaffarian D, Linker DT, et al. The seattle heart failure model: Prediction of survival in heart failure. *Circulation.* 2006;113:1424–1433.

11. Owan TE, Hodge DO, Herges RM, et al. Trends in prevalence and outcome of heart failure with preserved ejection fraction. *N Engl J Med.* 2006;355;251–259.

12. Bursi F, Weston SA, Redfield MM, et al. Systolic and diastolic heart failure in the community. *JAMA.* 2006;296;2209–2216.

13. Yusuf S, Pfeffer MA, Swedberg K, et al. Effects of candesartan in patients with chronic heart failure and preserved left-ventricular ejection fraction: The CHARM-preserved trial. *Lancet.* 2003;362:777–781.

14. Garg R. Yusuf, for the collaboration group on ace inhibitor trials. Overview of randomized trials of angiotensin-converting enzyme inhibitors on mortality and morbidity in patients with heart failure. *JAMA.* 1995;273:1450–1456.

15. Granger CB, McMurray JJ, Yusuf S, et al. Effects of candesartan in patients with chronic heart failure and reduced left-ventricular systolic function intolerant to angiotensin-converting-enzyme inhibitors: The CHARM-Alternative trial. *Lancet.* 2003;362:772–776.

16. Cohn JN, Tognoni G. A randomized trial of the angiotensin-receptor blocker valsartan in chronic heart failure. *N Engl J Med.* 2001;345:1667–1675.

17. Rocha R, Williams GH. Rationale for the use of aldosterone antagonists in congestive heart failure. *Drugs.* 2002;62:723–731.

18. Christ M, Douwes K, Eisen C, et al. Rapid effects of aldosterone on sodium transport in vascular smooth muscle cells. *Hypertension.* 1995;25:117–123.

19. Alzamora R, Michea L, Marusic ET. Role of 11 beta-hydroxysteroid dehydrogenase in nongenomic aldosterone effects in human arteries. *Hypertension.* 2000;35:1099–1104.

20. Rajagopalan S, Pitt B. Aldosterone as a target in congestive heart failure. *Med Clin North Am.* 2003;87:441–457.

21. McKelvie RS, Yusuf S, Pericak D, et al. Comparison of candesartan, enalapril, and their combination in congestive heart failure: Randomized evaluation strategies for left ventricular dysfunction (RESOLVD) pilot study. The RESOLVD pilot study investigators. *Circulation.* 1999;100:1056–1064.

22. Pitt B, Zannad F, Remme WJ, et al. The effect of spironolactone on morbidity and mortality in patients with severe heart failure. *N Engl J Med.* 1999;341:709–717.

23. Pitt B, Remme W, Zannad F, et al. Eplerenone, a selective aldosterone blocker, in patients with left ventricular dysfunction after myocardial infarction. *N Engl J Med.* 2003;348:1309–1321.

24. Bozkurt B, Agoston I, Knowlton AA. Complications of inappropriate use of spironolactone in heart failure: When an old medicine spirals out of new guidelines. *J Am Coll Cardiol.* 2003;41:211–214.

25. Svensson M, Gustafsson F, Galatius S, et al. Hyperkalaemia and impaired renal function in patients taking spironolactone for congestive heart failure: Retrospective study. *Br Med J.* 2003;327:1141–1142.

26. The Digitalis Investigation Group. The effect of digoxin on mortality and morbidity in patients with heart failure. *N Engl J Med.* 1997;336:525–533.

27. Packer M, O'Connor CM, Ghali JK, et al. Effect of amlodipine on morbidity and mortality in severe chronic heart failure. *N Engl J Med.* 1996;335:1107–1114.

28. Cohn JN, Ziesche S, Smith R, et al. Effect of the calcium antagonist felodipine as supplementary vasodilatory therapy in patients with chronic heart failure treated with enalapril: VHeFT III. *Circulation.* 1997;96:856–863.

28. Cohn JN, Archibald DG, Ziesche S, et al. Effect of vasodilator therapy on mortality in chronic congestive heart failure. Results of a veterans administration cooperative study. *N Engl J Med.* 1986;314:1547–1552.

29. ALLHAT Research Group. Major cardiovascular events in hypertensive patients randomized to doxazosin vs chorthalidone. *JAMA.* 2000;283:1967–1975.

30. Taylor AL, Ziesche S, Yancy C, et al. Combination of isosorbide dinitrate and hydralazine in blacks with heart failure. *N Engl J Med.* 2004;351:2049–2057.

31. Sackner-Bernstein JD, Kowalski M, Fox M, Anderson K. Short-term risk of death after treatment with nesiritide for decompensated heart failure. *JAMA.* 2005;293:1900–1905.

32. Sackner-Bernstein JD, Skopiki HA, Aaronson KD. Risk of worsening renal function with nesiritide in patients with acutely decompensated heart failure. *Circulation.* 2005;111:1487–1491.

33. Scios Inc. Press Release: Panel of Cardiology Experts Provides Recommendations to Scios Regarding Natrecor®. June 13, 2005. Available at http://www.sciosinc.com/scios/pr_1118721302. Accessed April 22, 2006.

34. Nieminen MS, Bohm M, Cowie MR, et al. Guidelines on the diagnosis and treatment of acute heart failure: Executive summary (update 2005): The task force on acute

heart failure of the european society of cardiology. *Eur Heart J.* 2005;26:384–416.

35. Stevenson WG, Chaitman BR, Ellenbogen KA, et al for the Subcommittee on electrocardiography and arrhythmias of the american heart association council on clinical cardiology, in collaboration with the heart rhythm society. Clinical assessment and management of patients with implanted cardioverter-defibrillators pre-senting to nonelectrophysiologists. *Circulation.* 2004;110:3866–3869.

36. Schoenfeld MH. Contemporary pacemaker and defibrillator device therapy: Challenges confronting the general cardiologist. *Circulation.* 2007;115;638–653.

37. Goldberg LR, Eisen H. Heart Failure. Physicians' Information and Education Resource (PIER). July 2005; http://pier.acponline.org. Accessed January 11, 2008.

Chapter 3

Diagnosis and Management of Chronic Coronary Heart Disease

Robert A. O'Rourke

SEARCH STRATEGY

A systematic search of the medical literature was performed in January 2008. The search, limited to human subjects and English language journals, included the National Guideline Clearinghouse, the Cochrane database, PubMed, UpToDate®, and PIER. The current American College of Cardiology (ACC)/American Heart Association (AHA) 2007 Chronic Angina Focused Update of the 2002 Guidelines for the Management of Patients with Chronic Stable Angina can be found at www.acc.org.

INTRODUCTION

Ischemic heart disease remains a major health problem. Chronic stable angina is the first manifestation of ischemic heart disease in approximately 50% of patients.[1–3] The reported yearly incidence of angina is 213 per 100 000, in the population that comprise more than 30 years of age.[4] The prevalence of angina can also be determined by extrapolating from the number of myocardial infarctions (MIs) in the United States.[5] Thus, the number of patients with stable angina can be calculated as 30 × 550 000 or 16.5 million.[2,3] This approximation does not include patients who fail to seek medical attention for their chest pain, or who are shown to have a noncardiac cause of chest discomfort.[2,3]

Despite a recent reduction in cardiovascular deaths, ischemic heart disease is still the leading cause of mortality in the United States and causes one of every 4.8 deaths.[6] Many patients are hospitalized for the assessment and treatment of stable chest pain syndromes and many patients with chronic stable angina are unable to perform normal activities for varying periods of hours or days, and thus have a diminished quality of life. The economic costs of chronic coronary heart disease (CHD) are enormous with direct costs of hospitalization exceeding $15 billion a year.[7]

The main objective of this chapter is to discuss the usefulness of noninvasive tests for the cost-effective diagnosis and risk stratification of patients with suspected or definite CHD, emphasizing the role of various imaging modalities for both diagnosis and risk stratification, the difference between the two often being arbitrary.

It must be emphasized *that not every patient needs every test* and that a markedly positive low-level electrocardiogram (ECG) exercise test precludes the need for additional more costly imaging studies prior to coronary angiography and likely myocardial revascularization. The use of additional noninvasive imaging tests in this situation is usually financially driven. The management of patients with symptomatic and asymptomatic CHD will be discussed in detail. In general, when myocardial ischemia is produced, an ischemic cascade occurs. Regional diastolic and systolic dysfunction precede global diastolic and then systolic dysfunction, which in turn often occurs prior to changes in ECG and before the symptoms of angina pectoris (Fig. 3-1). Noninvasive testing is often useful in detecting ischemia. The detection of left-ventricular (LV) diastolic dysfunction by Doppler mitral valve recording or by diastolic filling curves using radionuclide ventriculography has many limitations. The prevalence of MI, unstable angina, variant

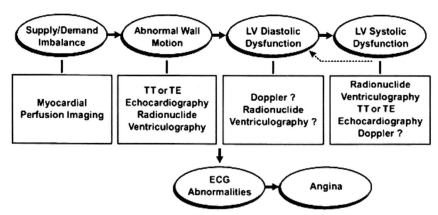

Figure 3-1. Sequence of events in the ischemic cascade plus noninvasive tests for detecting its presence. (TT, transthoracic; TE, transesophageal.)

angina, and silent ischemia is greatest in the morning during the first 2 hours, after awakening, and the threshold for precipitating angina attacks in patients with stable angina also appears to be lowest in the morning (Fig. 3-2).

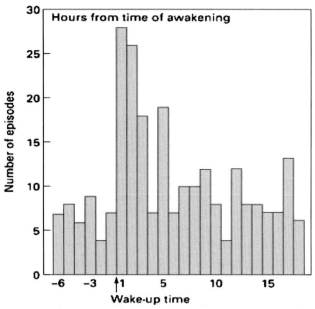

Figure 3-2. When the frequency of episodes is displayed hourly from the time of awakening, the peak activity occurs in the first and second hour after arising. (Adapted from Rocco MB, Barry J, Campbell S, et al. Circadian variation of transient myocardial ischemia in patients with coronary artery disease. *Circulation.* 1987;75:395–400.)

DIAGNOSIS

Angina is a clinical syndrome that consists of discomfort or pain in the chest, jaw, shoulder, back, or arm. It is typically precipitated or aggravated by exertion or emotional stress and relieved by nitroglycerin. Angina usually occurs in patients with CHD affecting one or more large epicardial arteries. However, angina often is present in individuals with valvular heart disease, hypertrophic cardiomyopathy, and uncontrolled hypertension.[2,3] It also occurs in patients with normal coronaries and myocardial ischemia caused by coronary artery spasm or endothelial dysfunction. The symptom of angina is often observed in patients with noncardiac disorders affecting the esophagus, chest wall, or lungs.

HISTORY AND PHYSICAL EXAMINATION

The first step is to obtain a detailed description of the *symptom complex* that is used by the clinician to characterize the chest pain or chest discomfort. *Five descriptors* are typically considered: (1) location, (2) quality, (3) duration of the discomfort, and the factors that (4) induce and (5) relieve the pain.

After the description of the chest discomfort is obtained, the physician makes an integrated assessment of the symptom complex. The most commonly used classification scheme for chest pain divides patients into three groups: Typical angina, atypical angina, or noncardiac chest pain (Table 3-1).[8]

Following a comprehensive interview concerning the chest pain, the *presence of risk factors* for CHD should be determined. Smoking, hyperlipidemia, diabetes,

Table 3-1. Clinical Classification of Chest Pain

Typical angina (definite)
  Substernal chest discomfort with a characteristic quality and
    duration that is
  Provoked by exertion or emotional stress and
  Relieved by rest or nitroglycerin.
Atypical angina (probable)
  Meets two of the above characteristics.
Noncardiac chest pain
  Meets one or none of the typical anginal characteristics.

Adapted from: Diamond GA, Staniloff HM, Forrester JS, Pollock BH, Swan HJ. Computer-assisted diagnosis in the noninvasive evaluation of patients with suspected coronary disease. *J Am Coll Cardiol.* 1983;1:444–455.

hypertension and a family history of premature CHD increase the likelihood of CHD. A past history of cerebrovascular or peripheral vascular disease also increases the probability of CHD.

The physical examination is often normal in patients with stable angina. However, an examination performed during an episode of pain can be useful. A third or fourth heart sound, a mitral regurgitant systolic murmur, a paradoxically split S_2, bibasilar pulmonary rales, or palpable precordial impulses that disappear when the pain subsides are all predictive of CHD. Evidence of noncoronary atherosclerotic disease such as a carotid bruit, diminished pedal pulse, or abdominal aneurysm increases the likelihood of CHD. An elevated blood pressure, xanthomas, and retinal exudates indicate the presence of CHD risk factors.[2,3]

CLINICAL ASSESSMENT OF THE LIKELIHOOD OF CHD

The clinicopathological study performed by Diamond and Forrester demonstrated that it is possible to predict the probability of CHD after the history and the physical examination.[8] By combining data from a series of angiography studies performed in the 1960s and the 1970s, they showed that simple clinical observations of pain type, age, and sex were powerful predictors of the probability of CHD.

The utility of the Diamond and Forrester approach was confirmed subsequently in prospective studies at Duke and Stanford.[9–13] In both men and women referred to cardiology clinics for cardiac catheterization or for cardiac stress testing, the initial clinical characteristics most helpful in predicting CHD were determined. In these studies, age, sex, and pain type were the most powerful predictors[8,9] (Tables 3-2 and 3-3). Smoking Q-waves or ST-T changes on ECG, hyperlipidemia, and diabetes strengthened the predictive abilities of these models.

ECG AND CHEST ROENTGENOGRAM

A resting 12-lead ECG should be recorded in all patients with symptoms suggestive of angina; but will be normal in up to 50% of patients with chronic stable angina.[2,3] ECG evidence of LV hypertrophy or ST-T wave changes consistent with myocardial ischemia favor the diagnosis of angina pectoris. Evidence of prior Q-wave MI on the ECG makes CHD very likely.

The presence of arrhythmias (e.g., atrial fibrillation or ventricular tachyarrhythmias) on the ECG in patients with chest pain also increase the probability of underlying CHD,[2,3] however, these arrhythmias are frequently caused by other types of cardiac disease. Various degrees of AV block occur in patients with chronic CHD, but have a very low specificity for the diagnosis. Left anterior fascicular block, right bundle branch block, and left bundle branch block (LBBB) often are present in patients with CHD and frequently indicate multivessel CHD. However, these findings

Table 3-2. Pretest Likelihood of CAD in Symptomatic Patients According to Age and Sex* (Combined Diamond/Forrester and Cass Data)*,†

Age (y)	Nonanginal Chest Pain		Atypical Angina		Typical Angina	
	Men	Women	Men	Women	Men	Women
30–39	4	2	34	12	76	26
40–49	13	3	51	22	87	55
50–59	20	7	65	31	93	73
60–69	27	14	72	51	94	86

*Each value represents the percent with significant CAD on catheterization.
†Diamond GA, Staniloff HM, Fonester JS, et al: Computer-assisted diagnosis in the noninvasive evaluation of patients with suspected coronary disease. *J Am Coll Cardiol.* 1983;1:444–455; Chaitman BR, Bourassa MG, David K, et al. Angiographic prevalence of high-risk coronary artery disease in patient subsets (CASS). *Circulation.* 1981;64:360–367; Lange RA, Cigarroa RG, Yancy CWJ, et al. Cocaine-induced coronary-artery vasoconstriction. *N Engl J Med.* 1989;321:1557–1562.
Source: Gibbons RJ, Chatterjee K, Daley J, et al. ACC/AHA/ACP guidelines for the management of chronic stable angina: A Report of the American College of Cardiology/American Heart Association/American College of Physicians Task Force on Practice Guidelines (Committee on the Management of Patients with Chronic Stable Angina). *J Am Coll Cardiol.* 1999;33:2097–2197; Gibbons RJ, Abrams J, Chatterjee K, et al. ACC/AHA 2002 guideline update for the management of patients with chronic stable angina. *J Am Coll Cardiol.* 2003;41:159–168.

Table 3-3. Comparing Pretest Likelihoods of CAD in Low-Risk Symptomatic Patients with High-Risk Symptomatic Patients*—Duke Database

Age (y)	Nonanginal Chest Pain		Atypical Angina		Typical Angina	
	Men	Women	Men	Women	Men	Women
35	3–35	1–19	8–59	2–39	30–88	10–78
45	9–47	2–22	21–70	5–43	51–92	20–79
55	23–59	4–25	45–79	10–47	80–95	38–82
65	49–69	9–29	71–86	20–51	93–97	56–84

*Each value represents the percent with significant CHD. The first is the percentage for a low-risk, mid-decade patient without diabetes, smoking, or hyperlipidemia. The second is that of the same age patient with diabetes, smoking, and hyperlipidemia. Both high- and low-risk patients have normal resting ECGs. If ST-T wave changes or Q waves would have been present, the likelihood of CAD would be higher in each entry of the table.
Source: Pryor et al. CAD. Ann Intern Med. 1993;118:81–90. Value of the history and physical in identifying patients at increased risk for coronary artery disease. *Ann Intern Med.* 1993;118:81–90.

also lack specificity for the diagnosis of chronic stable angina.

An ECG obtained *during chest pain* is abnormal in approximately 50% of patients with angina and a normal resting ECG. Sinus tachycardia occurs commonly; bradyarrhythmias are less common. ST-segment elevation or depression establishes a high likelihood of angina and indicates ischemia at a low workload, portending an unfavorable prognosis. Many *high-risk* patients with severe episodes of angina need *no further noninvasive testing.* Coronary arteriography usually defines the severity of coronary artery stenoses and defines the necessity and feasibility of myocardial revascularization. In patients with ST-T wave depression or inversion on the resting ECG, a pseudo-normalization of these abnormalities *during pain* is another indicator that CHD is likely.[2,3] The occurrence of tachyarrhythmias, AV block, left anterior fascicular block, or bundle branch block during chest pain also increases the probability of CHD and often leads to coronary arteriography.

The *chest roentgenogram* is often normal in patients with stable angina pectoris. Its usefulness as a routine test is *not* well established. It is more likely to be abnormal in patients with previous or acute MI, those with a noncoronary artery cause of chest pan, and those with noncardiac chest discomfort.

Coronary artery calcification increases the likelihood of symptomatic CHD. *Fluoroscopically detectable* coronary calcification is correlated with major vessel occlusion in 94% of patients with chest pain[2,3]; however, the sensitivity of the test is only 40%.

Electron beam computed tomography (EBCT) and *multislice computed tomography* are being used with increased frequency for the detection and quantification of coronary artery calcification.[14–16] In studies of selected patients, the sensitivity of a positive EBCT detection of calcium for the presence of CHD varied from 85% to 100%; the specificity ranged from only 41% to 76%; the positive predictive value varied considerably from 55% to 84% and the negative predictive value from 84% to 100%.[16] The role of EBCT has been controversial. The current report of an American College of Cardiology/American Heart Association (ACC/AHA) expert consensus writing group does not recommend EBCT for screening of asymptomatic patients for CHD or for its use in most patients with chest pain.[16] However, when the coronary artery calcium score is high (≥400 units), it is useful for further risk stratification of patients at intermediate risk by conventional Framingham risk factors.

EXERCISE ECG STRESS TESTING

Exercise (ECG) testing is a well-established procedure that has been in widespread clinical use for many decades.[17] Although usually safe, both MI and death occur at a rate of up to one per 2500 tests. Absolute contraindications to exercise testing include acute MI within 2 days, cardiac arrhythmias causing symptoms or hemodynamic compromise, symptomatic and severe aortic stenosis, symptomatic heart failure, acute pulmonary embolus or infarction, acute myocarditis or pericarditis, and acute aortic dissection. Relative contraindications include left main coronary artery stenosis, moderate aortic stenosis, electrolyte abnormalities, systolic hypertension >200 mm Hg, diastolic blood pressure >100 mm Hg, tachyarrhythmias or bradyarrhythmias, hypertrophic cardiomyopathy and other forms of outflow tract obstruction, and high-degree AV block.

For optimizing the information obtained, the protocol should be tailored to the individual patient with exercise lasting at least 6 minutes. Exercise capacity should be reported in estimated METs of exercise (*one MET is the standard basal oxygen uptake of 3.5 mL/kg per minute*), and also the duration of exercise in minutes.

The ECG, heart rate, and blood pressure should be carefully monitored and recorded during each stage of exercise, as well as during ST-segment abnormalities and chest pain. The patient should be monitored continuously for transient rhythm disturbances, ST-segment changes, and other ECG manifestations of myocardial ischemia. Although exercise testing often is stopped when subjects reach a standard percentage of predicted maximum heart rate, there is great variability in maximum heart rates among individuals, and predicted values may be suboptimal for some patients. *Absolute indications* for termination of the test include a decline in systolic blood pressure of >10 mmHg from baseline despite an increase in workload when accompanied by other evidence of ischemia; moderate to severe angina; increasing ataxia, dizziness, or near syncope; signs of poor perfusion such as cyanosis or pallor; technical difficulties monitoring the ECG or systolic blood pressure; subjects desire to stop; sustained ventricular tachycardia; or ST elevation more than or equal to 1.0 mm in leads without diagnostic Q waves.

The interpretation of the exercise test should include symptomatic response, exercise capacity, hemodynamic response, and ECG changes. The occurrence of ischemic chest pain consistent with angina is important, particularly if it necessitates termination of the test. Abnormalities in exercise capacity, the systolic blood pressure, or the heart rate response to exercise are important findings. The most important ECG findings are ST depression and ST elevation. The most commonly used definition for a positive exercise test is more than or equal to 1 mm of horizontal or downsloping ST-segment depression or elevation for at least 60 to 80 milliseconds after the end of the QRS complex.

A meta-analysis of 147 published reports describing 24074 patients who underwent both coronary angiography and exercise testing found wide variation in sensitivity and specificity.[17] The mean sensitivity was 68% and the mean specificity was 77%. When the analysis considered only studies that excluded patients with a prior MI, the mean sensitivity was 67% and the mean specificity was 72%. When the analysis was restricted to the few studies that avoided work-up bias by including only patients who agreed in advance to have both exercise testing and coronary angiography, the sensitivity was 50% and the specificity was 90%.[18] Therefore, the true diagnosis value of the exercise ECG relates to its relatively high specificity when positive.

Diagnostic testing is most valuable when the pretest probability of obstructive CHD is *intermediate*. In these conditions, the test result has the largest effect on the posttest probability of disease and thus on clinical decisions. Intermediate probability has been arbitrarily defined as between 10% and 90%[19]; this definition has been utilized in several studies[20,21] including ACC/AHA exercise test guidelines.[17]

SPECIAL ISSUES IN ECG EXERCISE TESTING

Digoxin produces abnormal exercise-induced ST-depression in 25% to 40% of apparently healthy normals.[22] Whenever possible, it is recommended that β-*blockers* (and other anti-ischemic drugs) be withheld for 48 to 72 hours prior to exercise stress testing when used for the *diagnosis* of patients with suspected CHD. When β-blockers cannot be stopped, ECG exercise testing usually will still be positive in patients at very high risk.

Exercise-induced ST-depression usually occurs with *LBBB* and has no association with ischemia.[23] In right bundle branch block, ST-depression in the left chest leads (V_{5-6}) or inferior leads (II, AVF), has the same significance as it does when the resting ECG is normal.

Left-ventricular hypertrophy (LVH) with repolarization abnormalities on the resting ECG is associated with more false-positive test results as a result of decreased specificity. Even in hypertensive patients with LV hypertrophy on echo but not on ECG, false-positive ST-segment changes often occur with exercise (Mercado M and O'Rourke RA, 1992).

Resting ST-segment depression is a marker for adverse cardiac events in patients with and without known CHD.[17] Additional exercise-induced ST-segment depression in the patient with ≤1 mm resting ST-segment depression is a reasonably sensitive indicator of CHD.

The difficulties of using exercise testing for diagnosing obstructive CHD in *women* have led to speculation that stress imaging may be preferred instead of standard stress testing. However, there is insufficient data to justify replacing standard exercise testing with stress imaging *routinely* when evaluating women for CHD. In many women with a low pretest likelihood of disease, a negative exercise test will be sufficient, and imaging procedures will not be required.[17,24]

RESTING ECHOCARDIOGRAPHY

Echocardiography can be useful for establishing a diagnosis of CHD and in defining the consequences of CHD in select patients with chronic chest pain presumed to be chronic stable angina. However, most patients undergoing a *diagnostic* evaluation for angina *do not need* a resting *echocardiogram*.

Chronic ischemic heart disease, whether or not associated with angina, can result in impaired systolic and/or ventricular function. The extent and severity of regional and global abnormalities are important considerations in choosing appropriate medical or surgical therapy.

Echocardiographic findings, which may help establish the diagnosis of chronic ischemic heart disease, include regional systolic wall motion abnormalities such as hypokinesis, akinesis, dyskinesis, and failure of a wall segment to thicken normally during systole.[25] Care must be taken to distinguish chronic CHD as a cause of ventricular septal wall motion abnormalities from other conditions such as LBBB, presence of an intraventricular pacemaker, right ventricular volume overload, or prior cardiac surgery.

Mitral regurgitation demonstrated by Doppler echocardiography may result from global LV systolic dysfunction, regional papillary muscle dysfunction, scarring and shortening of the chordae tendineae, papillary muscle rupture, or other causes.[25]

STRESS IMAGING

Patients who are good candidates for cardiac stress testing *with imaging* for the diagnosis of CHD as opposed to exercise ECG alone, include those in the following categories: (1) complete LBBB, electronically paced ventricular rhythm, preexcitation syndromes, and other similar ECG conduction abnormalities, (2) patients who have more than 1 mm of resting ST-segment depression including those with LVH or taking drugs such as digitalis, (3) patients who are unable to exercise sufficiently to give meaningful results on routine stress ECG (these patients should be considered for pharmacologic stress imaging test), and (4) patients with angina who have undergone prior revascularization, in whom localization of ischemia, establishing the functional significance of lesions, and demonstrating myocardial viability are important considerations.

Several methods can be used to induce stress: (1) exercise (treadmill or bicycle) and (2) pharmacological techniques (dobutamine or vasodilator drugs). When the patient can exercise to develop an appropriate level of cardiovascular stress of 6 to 12 minutes, exercise stress (usually treadmill), is preferred to pharmacologic stress. However, when the patient cannot exercise to the appropriate level, or in other specified circumstances (the assessment of myocardial viability), pharmacologic stress may be preferable. Three drugs are commonly used as substitutes for exercise stress testing. Dipyridamole and adenosine are vasodilators that are commonly used in conjunction with myocardial perfusion scintigraphy, whereas dobutamine is a positive inotropic (and chronotropic) agent commonly used in conjunction with echocardiography.

MYOCARDIAL PERFUSION IMAGING

In patients with suspected or known chronic stable angina, the largest accumulated experience in myocardial perfusion imaging has been with the isotope thallium-201; however, the available evidence suggests that the newer isotopes technetium Tc-99m sestamibi and technetium-99m tetrofosmin provide similar diagnostic accuracy.[26–34] Thus, for the most part, thallium-201, Tc-99m sestamibi, or Tc-99m tetrofosmin can be used interchangeably, with a similar diagnostic accuracy for CHD.[35]

Myocardial perfusion imaging may use either planar or single photon emission computed tomographic (SPECT) techniques and visual analyses[36] or quantitative techniques. Quantification using horizontal[37] or circumferential[38] profiles may improve the test's sensitivity, especially in patients with single-vessel disease. For thallium-201 planar scintigraphy, average reported values of sensitivity and specificity (not corrected for posttest referral bias) have been in the range of 83% to 88%, respectively, by visual analysis, and 90% to 80%, respectively, for quantitative analyses.[2,3] Thallium-201 SPECT is generally more sensitive than planar imaging for diagnosing CHD, localizing hypoperfused vascular segments, identifying left anterior descending and left circumflex coronary artery stenoses, and correctly predicting multivessel CHD.[2,3] The average sensitivity and specificity of exercise thallium-201 SPECT imaging (uncorrected for referral bias) is in the range of 89% to 76%, respectively, for qualitative analyses and 90% to 70%, respectively, for quantitative analyses.[2,3]

Since the introduction of dipyridamole- or adenosine-induced coronary vasodilatation as an adjunct to thallium-201 myocardial perfusion imaging,[39] pharmacologic stress has become an alternative to exercise in the noninvasive diagnosis of CHD.[40] Dipyridamole planar scintigraphy has a high sensitivity (90% average) and acceptable specificity (70% average) for detection of CHD.[41] Dipyridamole SPECT imaging with thallium-201 or Tc-99m sestamibi appears to be at least as accurate as planar imaging.[42] Results of myocardial perfusion imaging during adenosine infusion are similar to those obtained with dipyridamole and exercise imaging.[41] Evidence of CHD is demonstrated by redistribution defects comparing stress and resting scintigrams (ischemia); fixed defects at rest and during stress (so called "scar"), and by LV dilation or lung uptake of isotope during stress.[43]

STRESS ECHOCARDIOGRAPHY

Stress echocardiography relies on imaging LV segmental wall motion and thickening during stress compared with baseline. Echocardiographic findings suggestive of myocardial ischemia include: (1) decrease in wall motion in one or more LV segments with stress, (2) decrease in wall thickening in one or more LV segments with stress, and (3) compensatory hyperkinesis in complementary (nonischemic) wall segments. The advent of digital acquisition and storage, as well as side-by-side (or quad screen) display of cine loops of LV images acquired at different levels of (rest or) stress, have facilitated efficiency and accuracy in interpretation of stress echocardiograms.[41,44]

Stress echocardiography has been reported to have sensitivity and specificity for detecting CHD similar to stress myocardial imaging. In 36 studies reviewed, including 3210 patients, the range of reported overall sensitivities (uncorrected for posttest referral bias) ranged from 70% to 97%. The average figure was 85% for overall sensitivity for exercise echocardiography and 82% for dobutamine stress echocardiography.[25] As expected, the reported sensitivity of exercise echocardiography for multivessel disease was higher (average approximately 90%) than the sensitivity for single-vessel disease (average approximately 79%).[25] In this series of studies, specificity ranged from 72% to 100%, with an average of approximately 86% for exercise echocardiography and 85% for dobutamine echocardiography.

Pharmacologic stress echocardiography is best accomplished using dobutamine since it enhances myocardial contractile performance and wall motion, which can be evaluated directly by echocardiography.[45] *Dobutamine stress echocardiography* has substantially higher sensitivity than *vasodilator stress echocardiography* for detecting coronary artery stenoses.[46] In a recent review of 36 studies, average sensitivity and specificity (uncorrected for referral bias) of dobutamine stress echocardiography in the detection of CHD were in the range of 82% to 85%, respectively.[2,3]

Most special tests in patients with suspected stable angina are performed either to establish a diagnosis and/or to determine the risk for coronary events. In Fig. 3-3, the probability of coronary artery disease is depicted, comparing the pretest and posttest likelihood of CAD using ECG exercise testing, myocardial perfusion imaging, and radionuclide cineangiography.

SPECIAL ISSUES IN STRESS IMAGING

The sensitivity of the exercise imaging study for the *diagnosis* of CHD appears to be lower in patients taking β-blockers for the treatment of ischemia.[47] Nevertheless, in patients who exercise to a submaximal level, perfusion or echocardiographic imaging still affords higher sensitivity than the exercise ECG alone.[25]

Several studies have observed an increased prevalence of myocardial perfusion defects in the interventricular septum during exercise imaging, in the absence of angiographic coronary disease, in patients with *LBBB*.[48] Multiple studies indicate that perfusion imaging with pharmacologic vasodilatation is more accurate for identifying CHD in patients with LBBB.[49] In contrast, only a single small study has reported on the diagnostic utility of stress echocardiography in the presence of LBBB.[50]

Myocardial perfusion imaging or echocardiography could be a logical addition to treadmill testing in women who have a lower pretest likelihood of CHD than men. Photon attenuation artifacts because of breast attenuation, usually manifest in the anterior wall, can be an important caveat in the interpretation of women's perfusion scans, especially when thallium-201 is used as a tracer. Similar artifacts involving the inferior wall diaphragmatic are common in very obese patients. This is a less common problem with ECG-gated technetium 99m sestamibi SPECT.[51]

COMPARISON OF MYOCARDIAL PERFUSION IMAGING AND ECHOCARDIOGRAPHY

In an analysis of 11 studies[52] involving 808 patients who had contemporaneous treadmill (or pharmacologic) stress echocardiography and myocardial perfusion scintigraphy, the overall sensitivity was 83% for stress perfusion imaging versus 78% for stress echocardiography (*p* = NS). On the other hand, overall specificity tended to favor stress echocardiography (86% vs. 77%, *p* = NS).

More recently, Fleishmann et al.[53] performed a meta-analysis on 44 articles that examined the diagnostic accuracy of exercise tomographic myocardial perfusion imaging or exercise echocardiography. The overall sensitivity and specificity, respectively, were 85% to 77% for exercise echocardiography; 87% to 64% for exercise myocardial perfusion imaging; and 52% to 71% for exercise ECG.

SPECT has afforded diagnostic improvement over planar imaging for more precise localization of the

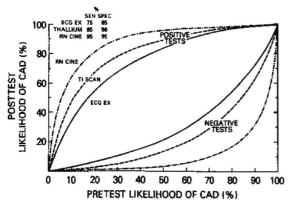

Figure 3-3. Probability of CAD. Comparison of ECG exercise testing (ECG Ex), thallium perfusion imaging (TI Scan), and radionuclide cineangiography (RN CINE). Sensitivity (SEN) and specificity (SPEC) values are approximations derived from published series. (Adapted from Epstein et al. *Am J Cardiol.* 1980;46:491.)

vascular territories involved, particularly for identifying left circumflex coronary artery stenoses and predicting multivessel CHD.[41] For localization of disease to the circumflex coronary artery, the radionuclide method conferred a significant advantage in sensitivity (72% vs. 33%, $p < 0.001$).

Echocardiographic and radionuclide stress imaging have complementary roles and both add value to routine stress ECG under circumstances outlined above. A summary of the comparative advantages of stress myocardial perfusion imaging and stress echocardiography is provided in Table 3-4.

CORONARY ANGIOGRAPHY

Recommendations for coronary angiography to establish a diagnosis of CHD are listed in Table 3-5 according to the ACC/AHA/American College of Physicians (ACC/AHA/ACP) Guidelines on Chronic Stable Angina.[2,3]

RISK STRATIFICATION

The prognosis for the patient with chronic coronary artery disease is usually related to four patient factors. *LV function is the strongest predictor* of long-term survival in patients with CHD and the ejection fraction is the

Table 3-4. Comparative Advantages of Stress Echocardiography in Diagnosis and Stress Radionuclide Perfusion Imaging in Diagnosis of CAD

Advantages of stress echocardiography
  Higher specificity
  Versatility. More extensive evaluations of cardiac anatomy and function
  Greater convenience/efficacy/availability
  Lower cost
Advantages of stress perfusion imaging
  Higher technical success rate
  Higher sensitivity, especially for single-vessel coronary diease involving the left circumflex
  Better accuracy in evaluating possible ischemia when multiple resting LV wall motion abnormalities are present
  More extensive published data base, especially in evaluation of prognosis

Source: Gibbons RJ, Chatterjee K, Daley J, et al. ACC/AHA/ACP guidelines for the management of chronic stable angina: A Report of the American College of Cardiology/American Heart Association/American College of Physicians Task Force on Practice Guidelines (Committee on the Management of Patients with Chronic Stable Angina). *J Am Coll Cardiol.* 1999;33:2097–2197; Gibbons RJ, Abrams J, Chatterjee K, et al. ACC/AHA 2002 guideline update for the management of patients with chronic stable angina. *J Am Coll Cardiol.* 2003;41:159–168.

most commonly used measure of the presence and the degree of LV dysfunction. The anatomic *extent and severity of atherosclerotic* involvement of the coronary arteries is the *second predictive factor.* The number of stenosed coronary arteries is the most common measure of this

Table 3-5. Invasive Testing: Coronary Angiography (Recommendations for Coronary Angiography to Establish a Diagnosis in Patients with Suspected Angina, Including Patients with Known CAD Who Have a Significant Change in Anginal Symptoms)

Class I*
  Patients with known or possible angina pectoris who have survived sudden cardiac death

Class II†
  IIa
    Patients with an uncertain diagnosis after noninvasive testing in whom the benefit of a more certain diagnosis outweighs the risk and cost of coronary angiography
    Patients who cannot undergo noninvasive testing because of disability, illness, or morbid obesity
    Patients with an occupational requirement for a definitive diagnosis
    Patients who by virtue of young age at onset of symptoms, noninvasive imaging, or other clinical parameters are suspected of having a nonatherosclerotic cause of myocardial ischemia (coronary artery anomaly, Kawasaki disease, primary coronary artery dissection, radiation-induced vasculoplasty)
    Patients in whom coronary artery spasm is suspected and provocative testing may be necessary
    Patients with a high pretest probability of left main or three-vessel CAD
  IIb
    Patients with recurrent hospitalization for chest pain in whom a definite diagnosis is judged necessary
    Patients with an overriding desire for a definitive diagnosis and a greater than low probability of CAD

Class III‡
  Patients with significant comorbidity in whom the risk of coronary arteriography outweighs the benefit of the procedure
  Patients with an overriding personal desire for a definitive diagnosis and a low probability of CAD

*Class I: Conditions for which there is evidence and/or general agreement that a given procedure or treatment useful and effective.
†Class II: Conditions for which there is conflicting evidence and/or a divergence of opinion about the usefulness/efficacy of a procedure or treatment; IIa: Weight of evidence/opinion is in favor of usefulness/efficacy; IIb: Usefulness/efficacy is less well established by evidence/opinion.
‡Class III: Conditions for which there is evidence and/or general agreement that the procedure/treatment is not useful/effective and in some cases may be harmful.
Source: Gibbons RJ, Chatterjee K, Daley J, et al. ACC/AHA/ACP guidelines for the management of chronic stable angina: A Report of the American College of Cardiology/American Heart Association/American College of Physicians Task Force on Practice Guidelines (Committee on the Management of Patients with Chronic Stable Angina). *J Am Coll Cardiol.* 1999;33:2097–2197; Gibbons RJ, Abrams J, Chatterjee K, et al. ACC/AHA 2002 guideline update for the management of patients with chronic stable angina. *J Am Coll Cardiol.* 2003;41:159–168.

characteristic. A *third patient factor* influencing prognosis is *evidence of a recent coronary plaque rupture*, indicating a substantially greater short-term risk for cardiac death or nonfatal MI. Worsening clinical symptoms with unstable features is the major clinical marker of a complicated plaque. The *fourth prognostic factor is general health and noncoronary comorbidity.*

STEPS IN DETERMINING PROGNOSIS PRIOR TO NONINVASIVE TESTING

History and Physical Examination

Very useful information relevant to prognosis can be obtained from the history. This includes demographics such as age and gender, as well as medical history focusing on hypertension, diabetes, hypercholesterolemia, smoking, peripheral arterial disease, and previous MI.[2,3] As discussed under the Section "Diagnosis," the description of the patient's chest discomfort can usually be readily assigned to one of three categories: (1) typical angina, (2) atypical angina, and (3) nonanginal chest pain.

The physical examination may be useful in risk stratification by defining the presence or absence of signs that might alter the probability of *severe* CHD. Useful findings include those suggesting vascular disease (abnormal fundi, decreased peripheral pulses, bruits), long-standing hypertension (blood pressure, abnormal fundi); aortic valve stenosis or hypertrophic obstructive cardiomyopathy (systolic murmur, abnormal carotid pulse, abnormal apical pulse); left heart failure (third heart sound, displaced apical impulse, bibasilar rales), or right heart failure (jugular venous distension, hepatomegaly, ascites, pedal edema).

Hubbard et al.[54] identified five clinical parameters that were independently predictive of severe three vessel or left main CHD including age, typical angina, diabetes, gender and prior MI and developed a 5-point cardiac risk score.

ECG and Chest Roentgenogram

Patients with chronic stable angina who have resting ECG abnormalities are at greater risk than those with normal ECGs.[2,3] Evidence of one or more prior MIs on ECG indicates an increased risk for cardiac events. In fact, the presence of Q waves in multiple ECG leads, often accompanied by a R-wave in lead V_1 (posterior infarction), often is associated with a markedly reduced LV ejection fraction, an important determinant of the natural history of patients with CHD.

The aggregation of certain historical and ECG variables in an angina score offers prognostic information that is independent of, and incremental to, that detected by catheterization.[55] The angina score comprised three differentially weighted variables: (1) the anginal course, (2) anginal frequency, (3) resting ECG ST-T wave abnormalities. On the chest roentgenogram, the presence of cardiomegaly, an LV aneurysm, or pulmonary venous congestion is associated with a poorer long-term prognosis than occurs in patients with a normal chest X-ray.

The presence of calcium in the coronary arteries on chest X-ray or fluoroscopy in patients with symptomatic CHD suggests an increased risk of cardiac events.[2,3] Although the presence and amount of coronary artery calcification by *electron beam or multislice computed tomography* correlate to some extent with the severity of CHD; there is considerable patient variation.[16]

NONINVASIVE TESTING FOR RISK STRATIFICATION

Assessment of LV Function

LV global systolic function and volumes are important predictors of prognosis. In patients with chronic ischemic heart disease, LV ejection fraction measured at rest by either echocardiography or radionuclide angiography is predictive of long-term prognosis; as LV ejection fraction declines subsequent mortality increases. A resting ejection fraction of <35% is associated with an annual mortality rate of >3% per year.[2,3]

Radionuclide LV ejection fraction may be measured at rest using a gamma camera, a technetium-99m tracer, and first pass or gated equilibrium blood pool angiography[41] or by gated SPECT perfusion imaging using a technetium-based isotope.[56,57] LV diastolic function can also be estimated by radionuclide ventriculography.[41] LV systolic function can also be measured by quantitative 2D echocardiography[41] and LV diastolic function assessed by transmitral valve Doppler recordings.[25]

In patients with chronic stable angina and a history of previous MI, segmental wall motion abnormalities can be seen not only in the zone(s) of prior infarction, but also in areas with ischemic stunning or hibernation of myocardium that are nonfunctional but still viable.[2,3,58] In patients with chronic ischemic heart disease the presence, severity, and mechanism of mitral regurgitation can be detected reliably using transthoracic 2D echocardiography (TTE) and Doppler echocardiographic techniques.[25]

Echocardiography is the definition for detecting intracardiac thrombi.[25] LV thrombi are most common in stable angina pectoris patients who have significant LV wall motion abnormalities. In patients with anterior and apical infarctions, the presence of LV thrombi denotes an increased risk of both embolism and death.[59]

ECG Exercise Testing

Unless cardiac catheterization is clearly indicated, symptomatic patients with suspected or known CHD should usually undergo exercise testing to assess the risk of future cardiac events, unless they have confounding features on their resting ECG or are unable to exercise. Also, *documentation of exercise-induced ischemia* is desirable for most patients who are being evaluated for revascularization.[2,3]

Several studies have shown that risk assessment in patients with a normal ECG who are not taking digoxin and are physically capable *usually* should start with the exercise test.[2,3,60–63] In contrast, a stress-imaging technique should be used for patients with ECG evidence of LVH, widespread resting ST-depression (>1 mm), complete LBBB, ventricular paced rhythm, or preexcitation. One of the strongest and most consistent prognostic markers is the maximum exercise capacity.[64,65]

A second group of prognostic markers relates to exercise-induced ischemia. ST-segment depression and ST-segment elevation (in leads without pathologic Q-waves and not in AVR) best summarize the prognostic information related to ischemia.[63] Other variables are less powerful, including angina, the number of leads with ST-segment depression, the configuration of the ST-depression (downsloping, horizontal, or upsloping), and the duration of the ST deviation into the recovery phase.

The Duke Treadmill Score combines this information and provides a way to calculate risk.[17,63,64,66,67] The Duke Treadmill Score equals the exercise time in minutes minus 5 times the ST-segment deviation during or after exercise in mm minus 4 times the angina index that has a value of 0 if there is no angina, 1 if angina occurs, and 2 if angina is the reason for stopping the test. Among outpatients with suspected CHD, the two-thirds of patients with scores indicating low risk had a 4-year survival of 99% (average annual mortality of 0.25%), and the 4% who had scores indicating high risk had a 4-year survival of 79% (average annual mortality rate of 5%) (see Table 3-6). Recent studies[66–68] indicate that this approach is equally applicable in men and women.

Stress Imaging

Stress imaging studies using radionuclide myocardial perfusion imaging techniques or 2D echocardiography at rest and during stress are useful for risk stratification and determining the most beneficial management strategy for patients with chronic stable angina.[2,3] Whenever possible, treadmill or bicycle exercise should be used as the most appropriate form of stress since it provides the most information concerning patient's symptoms, cardiovascular function, and

Table 3-6. Survival According to Risk Groups Based on Duke Treadmill Scores*

Risk Group (Score)	Percentage of Total	Four-Year Survival	Annual Mortality (%)
Low (≥+5)	62	0.99	0.25
Moderate (−10 to +4)	34	0.95	1.25
High (< −10)	4	0.79	5.0

*Patients with a predicted average annual cardiac mortality of less than or equal to 1% per year (low-risk score) can be managed medically without need for cardiac catheterization. Patients with a predicted average annual cardiac mortality of greater than or equal to 3% per year (high-risk score) should be referred for cardiac catheterization.
Source: Gibbons RJ, Chatterjee K, Daley J, et al. ACC/AHA/ACP guidelines for the management of chronic stable angina: A Report of the American College of Cardiology/American Heart Association/American College of Physicians Task Force on Practice Guidelines (Committee on the Management of Patients with Chronic Stable Angina). *J Am Coll Cardiol.* 1999;33:2097–2197; Gibbons RJ, Abrams J, Chatterjee K, et al. ACC/AHA 2002 guideline update for the management of patients with chronic stable angina. *J Am Coll Cardiol.* 2003;41:159–168.

hemodynamic response during usual forms of activity.[17] In fact, the inability to perform a bicycle or exercise treadmill test is in itself a negative prognostic factor for patients with chronic CHD.

In patients who cannot perform an adequate amount of bicycle or treadmill exercise, various types of pharmacologic stress are useful for *risk stratification.*[25,41] The selection of the type of pharmacologic stress will depend on specific patient factors such as the patient's heart rate and blood pressure, the presence or absence of bronchospastic disease, the presence of LBBB or a pacemaker, and the likelihood of ventricular arrhythmias.

Myocardial perfusion imaging has played a major role in the risk stratification of patients with CHD. Either planar or single photon emission computed tomography (SPECT) imaging utilizing thallium-201 or technetium-99m-perfusion tracers with images obtained at stress and during rest, provide important information concerning the severity of functionally significant CHD.[2,3,41,69]

Stress echocardiography has been used more recently for assessing patients with chronic stable angina; thus, the amount of prognostic data obtained with this approach is somewhat limited. Nevertheless, the presence or absence of inducible myocardial wall motion abnormalities has useful predictive value in patients undergoing exercise or pharmacologic stress echocardiography. A negative stress echocardiography study denotes a low cardiovascular event rate during follow-up.[2,3,25,70,71]

Myocardial Perfusion Imaging

Normal poststress thallium scan results are highly predictive of a benign prognosis even in patients with known coronary disease.[41] A collation of 16 studies involving 3594 patients followed for a mean of 29 months indicated a rate per year of cardiac death and MI of 0.9%, almost no different from that of the general population. In a recent prospective study of 5183 consecutive patients who underwent myocardial perfusion studies during stress and later at rest, patients with normal scans were at low risk (0.5/year) for cardiac death and MI during 642 ± 226 days of mean follow-up and rates of both outcomes increased significantly with worsening scan abnormalities.[72]

The number, extent, and site of abnormalities on stress myocardial perfusion scintigrams reflect the location and severity of functionally significant coronary artery stenoses. Lung uptake of thallium-201 on postexercise or pharmacologic stress images is an indicator of stress-induced global LV dysfunction and is associated with pulmonary venous hypertension in the presence of multivessel CHD.[73] Transient poststress ischemic LV dilatation also correlates with severe two or three vessel CHD. Several studies have suggested that SPECT may be more accurate than planar imaging for determining the size of defects, for detecting CHD and particularly left circumflex disease, and for localizing abnormalities in the distribution of individual coronary arteries.[2,3,41] However, more false-positive results are likely to result from photon attenuation during SPECT imaging.[41]

Information concerning both myocardial perfusion and ventricular function at rest may be helpful in determining the extent and severity of coronary disease.[2,3,41] This combined information can be obtained by performing two separate exercise tests (e.g., stress perfusion scintigraphy and stress radionuclide ventriculography) or by combining the studies after a single exercise test (e.g., first pass radionuclide angiography with technetium-99-based agents followed by perfusion imaging or perfusion imaging utilizing ECG gating). The use of ECG gated technetium sestamibi SPECT imaging provides important prognostic information concerning LV EF as well as the extent of reversible ischemia.

The treadmill ECG test is less accurate for the diagnosis of CHD in women who have a lower pretest likelihood than men.[17] However, the sensitivity of thallium perfusion scans may be lower in women than in men.[2,3,41] As mentioned previously, Tc-99m sestamibi may be preferable to thallium-201 scintigraphy in women with large breasts and those with breast implants for determining prognosis as well for diagnosing CHD.[41]

Pharmacologic stress perfusion imaging is preferable to exercise perfusion imaging in patients with LBBB. Recently, 245 patients with LBBB underwent SPECT imaging with thallium-201 ($n = 173$) or technetium 99m sestamibi ($n = 72$) during dipyridamole ($n = 153$) or adenosine ($n = 92$) stress.[74] The 3-year survival was 57% in the high-risk group compared to 87% in the low-risk group ($p = 0.001$).

Stress Echocardiography

Stress echocardiography is both sensitive and specific for detecting inducible myocardial ischemia in patients with chronic stable angina.[25] Compared with standard exercise treadmill testing, stress echocardiography provides an additional clinical value for detecting and localizing myocardial ischemia. The results of stress echocardiography may provide important *prognostic value*. Several studies indicate that patients at low, intermediate, and high risk for cardiac events can be stratified by the presence or absence of inducible wall motion abnormalities on stress echocardiography testing.

The presence of ischemia on the exercise echocardiogram is independent and incremental to clinical and exercise data in predicting cardiac events both in men and women.[75,76]

The prognosis is not benign in patients with a positive stress echocardiographic study. In this subset, morbid or fatal cardiovascular events are more likely, but the overall event rates are rather variable. Hence, the cost-effectiveness of using routine stress echocardiographic testing to establish prognosis is uncertain.

Coronary Angiography

The availability of powerful but expensive strategies to reduce the long-term morbidity and mortality of CHD mandate that the patients most likely to benefit because of increased risk, be determined. The prevalence of 0 to 3-vessel CHD on coronary angiography in men and women related to severity of angina is shown in Fig. 3-4.

Assessment of cardiac risk and decisions regarding further testing usually begin with simple, repeatable and inexpensive assessments of history and physical examination and extend to noninvasive or invasive testing depending on outcome. Clinical risk factors are in general additive, and a crude estimate of 1-year mortality can be obtained from these variables.

Risk stratification of patients with chronic stable angina by stress testing with exercise or pharmacologic agents has been shown to permit identification of groups of patients with low, intermediate, or high risk for subsequent cardiac events.[6,19,41] The objective is to identify patients in whom coronary angiography and subsequent revascularization might improve survival. Such an approach can only be effective if the patient's prognosis on medical therapy is sufficiently poor that it can be improved.

Previous experience in the randomized trials of coronary artery bypass grafting (CABG) demonstrated that

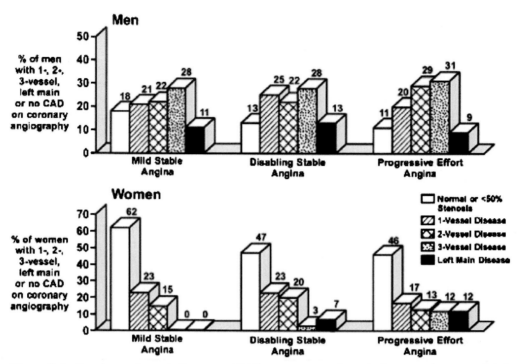

Figure 3-4. Prevalence of zero- to three-vessel CAD on coronary angiography in men and women related to severity of angina. (Adapted from Douglas JS Jr., Hurst JW. Limitation of symptoms in the recognition of coronary atherosclerotic heart disease. In: Hurst JW, ed. *Update I: The Heart*. New York, NY: McGraw-Hill; 1979:3.)

patients randomized to initial CABG had a lower mortality than those treated with medical therapy only if they were at sustained risk.[77] Low-risk patients, who did not have a lower mortality with CABG, were those who had a 5-year survival with medical therapy of approximately 95%. This is equivalent to an annual mortality of 1%. As a result, coronary angiography to identify patients whose prognosis can be improved is inappropriate when the patient's estimated annual mortality is less than 1%. In contrast, patients with a survival advantage with CABG such as those with three-vessel disease, have an annual mortality of more than or equal to 3%. Coronary angiography is appropriate for patients whose mortality risk is in this range.

Noninvasive test findings that identify high-risk patients are listed in Table 3-7. Patients identified as high-risk are generally referred for coronary arteriography independent of their symptomatic status. Noninvasive tests when appropriately utilized are less costly than coronary angiography and have an acceptable predictive value for adverse events. This is most true when the pretest probability of severe CHD is low. When the pretest probability of severe CHD is high, direct referral for coronary angiography without noninvasive testing has been shown to be most cost-effective as the total number of tests is reduced.[78]

OTHER NONINVASIVE TESTS

Certain other noninvasive tests have been utilized in some patients with chronic stable angina. These include ambulatory ECG recordings, magnetic resonance imaging, and positron emission tomography.

AMBULATORY ECG RECORDINGS

Ambulatory ECG recordings have been utilized to detect symptomatic and asymptomatic episodes of myocardial ischemia in individuals during their normal activities. This is a relatively insensitive technique for detecting coronary artery disease even when there is 0.08 seconds of ST-segment depression for 60 seconds or greater, the usual definition for a positive test. It should be emphasized that this test is *not a reliable diagnostic test* for determining the presence of myocardial ischemia[17] and its role in monitoring therapy in patients with known ischemic heart disease is still under investigation.

MAGNETIC RESONANCE IMAGING

Magnetic resonance imaging is an excellent technique for defining LV systolic function, wall motion, and the presence of valvular regurgitation. Because of its

Table 3-7. Noninvasive Risk Stratification

High-Risk (>3% annual mortality rate)
  Severe resting LV dysfunction (LVEF < 35%)
  High-risk treadmill score (score ≤ −11)
  Severe exercise LV dysfunction (exercise LVEF < 35%)
  Stress-induced large perfusion defect (particularly if anterior)
  Stress-induced multiple perfusion defects of moderate size
  Large, fixed perfusion defect with LV dilatation or increased
    lung uptake (thallium-201)
  Stress-induced moderate perfusion defect with LV dilatation or
    increased lung uptake (thallium-201)
  Echocardiographic wall motion abnormality (involving >two
    segments developing at low dose of dobutamine (≤10 mg/kg
    per minute) or at a low heart rate (It; 120 beats/min)
  Stress echocardiographic evidence of extensive ischemia
Intermediate-Risk (1% to 3% annual mortality rate)
  Mild/moderate resting LV dysfunction (LVEF = 35–49%)
  Intermediate-risk Duke treadmill score* (score of −10 to +4)
  Stress-induced moderate perfusion defect without LV
    dilatation or increased lung uptake (thallium-201)
  Limited stress echocardiographic ischemia with a wall motion
    abnormality only at higher doses of dobutamine involving
    ≤ two segments
Low-Risk (<1% annual mortality rate)
  Low-risk treadmill score (score = or >5)
  Normal or small myocardial perfusion defect at rest or with
    stress†
  Normal stress echocardiographic wall motion or no change of
    limited resting wall motion abnormalities during stress†

*Duke treadmill score, see text.
†Although the published data are limited, patients with these findings will probably not be at low risk in the presence of either a high-risk treadmill score or severe LV dysfunction (LVEF 35%).
Source: Gibbons RJ, Chatterjee K, Daley J, et al. ACC/AHA/ACP guidelines for the management of chronic stable angina: A Report of the American College of Cardiology/American Heart Association/American College of Physicians Task Force on Practice Guidelines (Committee on the Management of Patients with Chronic Stable Angina). *J Am Coll Cardiol.* 1999;33:2097–2197; Gibbons RJ, Abrams J, Chatterjee K, et al. ACC/AHA 2002 guideline update for the management of patients with chronic stable angina. *J Am Coll Cardiol.* 2003;41:159–168.

expense and its applicability primarily to patients at rest, this technique is not commonly used for the assessment of patients with chronic stable angina.[79]

POSITRON EMISSION TOMOGRAPHY

This technique is extremely useful for defining areas of myocardial tissue that are active metabolically, in the presence of normal or markedly diminished myocardial perfusion. When available, this technique is applicable to many patients who have severely diminished LV function and a decision must be made as to whether or not improved coronary blood flow to these regions will result in the perfusion of contracting myocardium.

TREATMENT OF CHRONIC STABLE ANGINA

There are two major purposes in the treatment of stable angina. The first is to prevent MI and death and *thereby*

increase the quantity of life. The second is to reduce symptoms of angina and the frequency and severity of ischemia, which should *improve the quality of life.* Therapy directed toward preventing death has the highest priority. The choice of therapy often depends on the clinical response to initial medical therapy, although some patients (and many physicians) prefer coronary revascularization in situations where either may be successful. It must be stressed that the pharmacologic treatment of chronic CHD has greatly improved and may even be superior to revascularization therapy for many patients.[80,81] Patient education, cost-effectiveness, and patient preference are important components in this decision-making process.

PHARMACOTHERAPY TO PREVENT MI

Antiplatelet Agents

Aspirin exerts an antithrombotic effect by inhibiting cyclooxygenase and synthesis of platelet thromboxane A_2. In the Physician's Health Study, aspirin given on alternate days to asymptomatic individuals was associated with a decreased incidence on MI.[82] In the Swedish Angina Pectoris Aspirin Trial in patients with stable angina, the addition of 75 mg of aspirin to sotalol resulted in a 34% reduction in primary outcome events of MI and sudden death and a 32% decrease in secondary vascular events.[83] A recent meta-analysis of 200 000 patients showed similar benefits of aspirin doses from 75 to 325 mg.[84]

Ticlopidine is a thienopyridine derivative that inhibits platelet aggregation induced by adenosine diphosphate and low concentrations of thrombin, collagen, thromboxane A_2, and platelet-activating factors.[85] It has *not* been shown to decrease adverse cardiovascular events and may induce neutropenia and often-thrombotic thrombocytopenic purpura.

Clopidogrel, also a thienopyridine derivative, is chemically related to ticlopidine, but it appears to possess a greater antithrombotic effect than ticlopidine. In a randomized trial that compared clopidogrel with aspirin in patients with previous MIs, stroke, or peripheral vascular disease, clopidogrel was slightly more effective than aspirin in decreasing the combined risk of MI, vascular death, and ischemic stroke.[88]

The greater reduction in event rates with clopidogrel in the CURE, PCI CURE, and CREDO studies cannot yet be applied to patients not undergoing revascularization.[87,88]

Aspirin, 75 to 325 mg per day, should be used routinely in all patients with acute and chronic ischemic heart disease and with and without clinical symptoms in the absence of contraindications. In those unable to take aspirin, clopidogrel may be used instead. Warfarin is the third choice.[89]

Antithrombotic Therapy

Disturbed fibrinolytic function after exercise appears to be associated with an increased risk of subsequent cardiovascular death in patients with chronic stable angina, providing the rationale for long-term antithrombotic therapy. In small placebo-controlled trials among patients with chronic stable angina, daily subcutaneous administration of low-molecular-weight heparin decreased the fibrinogen level and improved the exercise time to ST-segment depression[90] The clinical experience of such therapy, however, is extremely limited. The efficacy of newer antiplatelet and antithrombotic agents such as glycoprotein IIIb/IIa inhibitors and recombinant hirudin in the management of patients with chronic stable angina has not been established. Low-intensity oral anticoagulation with warfarin decreased the risk of ischemic events in a randomized trial of patients with risk factors for atherosclerosis but without symptoms of angina.[91]

Lipid-Lowering Agents

Recent clinical studies have convincingly demonstrated that low-density lipoprotein (LDL)-lowering agents can decrease the risk of adverse ischemic events in patients with established CHD (see Chapter 6). In the 4S trial,[92,93] treatment with an HMG-CoA reductase inhibitor in patients with documented CHD (including stable angina) and a baseline total cholesterol concentration between 212 and 308 mg/dL was associated with a 30% to 35% reduction in both mortality rate and major coronary events. In the Cholesterol and Recurrent Events (CARE) study,[94] in men, and women with previous MI and total cholesterol levels of less than 240 mg/dL and LDL-cholesterol levels of 115 to 174 mg/dL, treatment with an HMG-CoA reductase inhibitor (statin) was associated with a 24% reduction in risk for nonfatal MI. The Cholesterol Treatment Trialists' Collaborators performed a meta-analysis of data from 90056 participants in 14 randomized trials of statin therapy.[95] These data emphasize that statin therapy can safely reduce the 5-year incidence of CHD mortality, total mortality, major coronary events, coronary revascularization, and stroke. The mean baseline LDL-cholesterol in the meta-analysis was 148 mg/dL and at follow-up, 105 mg/dL representing a 29% reduction.

Angiotensin-Converting Enzyme Inhibitors

The potential cardiovascular protective effects of angiotensin-converting enzyme (ACE) inhibitors have been suspected for some time. As early as 1990, several randomized clinical trials showed that ACE inhibitors reduced the incidence of recurrent MI and that this effect could not be attributed to the effect on blood pressure alone.

The results of the Heart Outcomes Prevention Evaluation (HOPE) trial now confirm that use of the ACE inhibitor ramipril[96] (10 mg/d) reduces the rate of cardiovascular death, MI, and stroke in patients who are at high risk or have vascular disease in the absence of heart failure.[97,97a]

More than 90% of ACE is tissue-bound, whereas only 10% of ACE is present in soluble form in the plasma. In nonatherosclerotic arteries, the majority of tissue ACE is bound to the cell membranes of endothelial cells on the luminal surface of the vessel walls, and there is a large concentration of ACE within the adventitial vasa vasorum endothelium. It is now well appreciated that atherosclerosis represents different stages of a process that is in large part mediated by the endothelial cell. Thus, in the early stage, ACE, with its predominant location for the endothelial cells, would be an important mediator of local angiotensin II and bradykinin levels that could have an important impact on endothelial function.

ACE inhibition shifts the balance of ongoing vascular mechanisms in favor of those promoting vasodilatory, antiaggregatory, antiproliferative, and antithrombotic effects.

The HOPE study was unique in that of the 9541 patients in this study, 3577 (37.5%) had diabetes.[97] There was a significant reduction in diabetic complications, a composite for the development of diabetic nephropathy, need for renal dialysis, and laser therapy for diabetic retinopathy in those patients receiving ramipril. The Microalbuminuria, Cardiovascular, and Renal Outcomes-HOPE, a substudy of the HOPE study,[98] provided new clinical data on the cardiorenal therapeutic benefits of ACE inhibitor intervention in a broad range of middle-aged patients with diabetes mellitus who are at high risk for cardiovascular events.

ACE inhibitors should be used as routine secondary prevention for patients with known CHD,[99] particularly in diabetics without severe renal disease and in CHD patients with depressed LV systolic function.[98]

Antianginal and Anti-Ischemic Therapy

The major relevant determinate of myocardial oxygen consumption are heart rate, contractility, and systolic wall stress (Fig. 3-5). Heart rate is one of the most important determinates of MVO_2 and can be altered easily by medical therapy.

Systolic wall stress is directly related to the LV systolic pressure (P) and the radius (r) and inversely related to wall thickness decreasing preload by venodilation and thus reducing LV size and is an important mechanism for nitrate therapy in angina.

Antianginal and anti-ischemic drug therapy consists of β-adrenoreceptor blocking agents (β-blockers), calcium

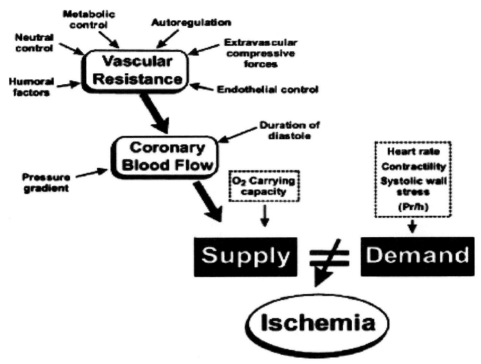

Figure 3-5. Factors controlling myocardial oxygen demand. (P, systolic pressure; r, radius; h, wall thickness.) (Adapted from Ardehali A, Ports TA. Myocardial oxygen supply and demand. *Chest.* 1990;98:699–705.)

antagonists, and nitrates. There is a tendency for physicians to give *lower doses* of antianginal medications than those proven to be effective in clinical trials; higher doses and combined therapy are often not utilized in patients who could be "angina-free" if treated more appropriately; this is particularly true with β-blocker therapy. For example, the usual dose for angina is 50 to 200 mg of metoprolol XL twice daily or a dose that produces an equivalent attenuation of heart rate (50–60 bpm). Other β-blockers should be given with the dose adjusted to maintain a bradycardia throughout the day (Fig. 3-5).

β-Blockers

The decrease in heart rate, contractility, arterial pressure, and usually LV wall stress with β-blockers is associated with decreased MVO$_2$ (Fig. 3-5). A reduction in heart rate also increases diastolic coronary artery perfusion time, which may enhance LV perfusion. Although β-blockers have the potential to increase coronary vascular resistance by the formation of cyclic AMP, the clinical relevance of this pharmacodynamic effect remains to be demonstrated.

All β-blockers without intrinsic sympathetic activity appear to be equally effective in angina pectoris. In patients with chronic stable exertional angina, these agents decrease the heart rate–blood pressure product during exercise, and the onset of angina or the ischemic threshold during exercise is delayed or avoided[1] (Fig. 3-5). In treating stable angina, it is essential that the dose of β-blockers be adjusted to lower the resting heart rate to 60 beats or less per minute. In patients with severe angina, the heart rate can be reduced to less than 50 beats per minute if there are no symptoms associated with bradycardia and AV block does not develop. In patients with exertional angina, β-blockers attenuate the increase in heart rate during exercise, which ideally should not exceed 75% of the heart rate response associated with the onset of ischemia. It is often useful for the patient to perform exercise (sit-ups, running in place) before and after the institution of β-blocker therapy. If the heart rate increase with exercise is not significantly reduced by therapy, the dose of the β-blocker is inadequate. β-Blockers are definitely effective in reducing exercise-induced angina. Three controlled studies comparing β-blockers with calcium antagonists[100–102] report equal efficacy in the treatment of chronic stable angina.

In the International Multicenter Angina Exercise study,[103] both metoprolol and nifedipine were effective as monotherapy in increasing exercise time, although metoprolol was more effective than nifedipine. The combination therapy also significantly increased the exercise time to ischemia compared with either drug alone. The absolute contraindications to the use of β-blockers are severe bradycardia, preexisting high-degree AV block, sick sinus syndrome, and severe, unstable LV failure. Asthma and bronchospastic disease, severe depression, and peripheral vascular disease are relative contraindications. Fatigue, inability to perform exercise, lethargy, insomnia, nightmares, worsening claudication, and impotence are frequently experienced side effects. Most patients with chronic CHD and diabetes can be treated with β-blockers. However, the heart rate may not be attenuated in diabetics with autonomic nervous system involvement.

In patients with postinfarction stable angina and those who require antianginal therapy after revascularization, treatment with β-blockers appears to be effective in controlling symptomatic and asymptomatic ischemic episodes. β-Blockers are still the anti-ischemic drugs of choice in elderly patients with stable angina.[104]

β-Blockers are frequently combined with nitrates for treating chronic stable angina. This combination of therapy appeared to be more effective in several studies than nitrates or β-blockers alone.[105–107] β-Blockers may also be combined with calcium antagonists. For combination therapy, slow-release dihydropyridine derivatives or new-generation long-acting dihydropyridine derivatives are the calcium antagonists of choice.[106]

Calcium Antagonists

These agents reduce the transmembrane flux of calcium by the calcium channels. There are three types of voltage-dependent calcium channels: L type, T type, and N type.

All calcium antagonists exert a negative inotropic effect, depending on dosage. In smooth muscle, calcium ions also regulate the contractile mechanism, and calcium antagonists reduce smooth muscle tension in the peripheral vascular bed, thus causing vasodilation. All the calcium antagonists cause dilatation of the epicardial conduit vessels and the arterial resistance vessels, the former being the primary mechanism for the beneficial effect of calcium antagonists for relieving vasospastic angina. Calcium antagonists also decrease MVO_2 demand, primarily by reducing the systemic vascular resistance and arterial pressure. The negative inotropic effect of calcium antagonists also decreases the MVO_2 (Fig. 3-5).

Randomized clinical trials comparing calcium antagonists and β-blockers have demonstrated that calcium antagonists are equally effective as β-blockers in relieving angina and improving exercise time to onset of angina or ischemia.[1] The calcium antagonists are effective in reducing the incidence of angina in patients with vasospastic angina.[108,109]

In a retrospective case-controlled study reported in patients with hypertension, treatment with immediate-acting nifedipine, diltiazem, or verapamil was associated with an increased risk of MI of 31% to 61%.[110] Although a subsequent meta-analysis of immediate release and short-acting nifedipine in patients with MI and unstable angina reported a dose-related influence on excess mortality,[111] further analysis of the published reports failed to confirm an increased risk of adverse cardiac events with calcium antagonists.[112,113] Importantly, long-acting calcium antagonists, including slow-release and long-acting dihydropyridine and nondihydropyridine derivatives, are effective in relieving symptoms in patients with chronic stable angina. They should be used in combination with β-blockers when initial treatment with β-blockers is not successful or as a substitute for β-blockers when initial treatment leads to unacceptable side effects. The use of calcium blockers may decrease the incidence of coronary artery spasms, which β-blockers do not. Many patients with two or three-vessel CHD are asymptomatic on combined β-blocker and calcium antagonist therapy. Some have further improvement on triple therapy (combined β-blocker, calcium antagonist, and long-acting nitrates). Further information concerning the potential side effects of the calcium antagonists is given elsewhere (Chapter 30).

Nitroglycerin and Nitrates

Nitrates are endothelium-independent vasodilators that produce beneficial effects by both reducing the MVO_2 and improving CBF perfusion. The decreased MVO_2 results from the reduction of LV volume and arterial pressure, primarily because of the reduced preload. Nitroglycerin also exerts antithrombotic and antiplatelet effects in patients with stable angina[1] (Fig. 3-5).

Nitrates dilate large epicardial arteries and collateral vessels. The vasodilating effect on epicardial coronary arteries with or without atherosclerotic CHD is beneficial in relieving coronary vasospasm in patients with vasospastic angina.

In patients with exertional stable angina, nitrates improve exercise tolerance, time to onset of angina, and time to ST-segment depression during treadmill exercise testing. In combination with β-blockers or calcium antagonists, nitrates produce greater antianginal and anti-ischemic effects in patients with stable angina.[114–117] The interaction between nitrates and sildenafil (Viagra®) is discussed in detail elsewhere.[118] The coadministration of nitrates and sildenafil greatly increases the risk of potentially life-threatening hypotension.

The major problem with long-term use of nitroglycerin and long-acting nitrates is development of nitrate tolerance.[119] Tolerance develops not only to antianginal and hemodynamic effects but also to platelet anti-aggregatory effects.[120] The mechanism for development of nitrate tolerance remains unclear. For practical purposes, the administration of nitrates with an adequate nitrate-free interval (8–12 h) appears to be the most effective method of preventing nitrate tolerance. Unfortunately, this means that patients with unpredictable episodes of myocardial ischemia should not be treated with *nitrate therapy alone* because they will be "unprotected" for part of each 24-hour day.

The primary consideration in the choice of pharmacologic agents for treatment of angina should be to improve prognosis. Aspirin and lipid-lowering therapies have been shown to reduce the risk of death and nonfatal MI in both primary and secondary prevention trials. β-Blockers also reduce the cardiac events, when used as secondary prevention in post infarction patients and reduce mortality and morbidity among patients with hypertension. Nitrates have not been shown to reduce mortality with acute infarction or in patients with chronic CHD.

Recommended drug therapy using calcium antagonists versus β-blockers in patients with angina-associated conditions are listed in Table 3-8.

Table 3-8. Recommended Drug Therapy (Calcium Antagonist vs. β-Blocker) in Patients with Angina and Associated Conditions

Condition	Recommended Treatment and Alternative	Avoid
Medical conditions		
Systemic hypertension	β-Blockers (calcium antagonists)	
Migrane or vascular headaches	β-Blockers (verapamil or diltiaziem)	
Asthma or chronic obstructive pulmonary disease with bronchospasm	Verapamil or diltiazem	β-Blockers
Hyperthyroidism	β-Blockers	
Raynaud's syndrome	Long-acting slow-release calcium antagonists	β-Blockers
Insulin-dependent diabetes mellitus	β-Blockers (particularly if prior MI) or long-acting slow-release calcium antagonists	
Noninsulin-dependent diabetes mellitus	β-Blockers or long-acting slow-release calcium antagonists	
Depression	Long-acting slow-release calcium antagonists	β-Blockers
Mild peripheral vascular disease with rest ischemia	β-Blockers or calcium antagonists	
Severe peripheral vascular disease with rest ischemia	Calcium antagonists	β-Blockers
Cardiac arrhythmias and conduction abnormalities		
Sinus bradycardia	Long-acting slow-release calcium antagonists that do not decrease heart rate	β-Blockers, diltiazem, verapamil
Sinus tachycardia (not because of heart failure)	β-Blockers	
Supraventricular tachycardia	Verapamil, diltiazem, or β-blockers	
Atrioventricular block	Long-acting slow-release calcium antagonists that do not slow AV conduction	β-blockers, verapamil, diltiazem
Rapid atrial fibrillation (with digitalis)	Verapamil, diltiazem, or β-blockers	
Venticular arrhythmias	β-Blockers	
LV dysfunction		
Congestive heart failure		
Mild (LVEF ≤40%)	β-Blockers	
Moderate to severe (LVEF <40%)	Amlodipine or felodipine (nitrates)	Verapamil, diltiazem
Left-sided valvular heart disease		
Mild aortic stenosis	β-Blockers	
Aortic insufficiency	Long-acting slow-release dihydropyridines	
Mitral regurgitation	Long-acting slow-release dihydropyridines	
Mitral stenosis	β-Blockers	
Hypertrophic cardiomyopathy	β-Blockers, nondihydropyridine calcium antagonist	Nitrates, dihydropyridine calcium antagonists

Source: Gibbons RJ, Chatterjee K, Daley J, et al. ACC/AHA/ACP guidelines for the management of chronic stable angina: A Report of the American College of Cardiology/American Heart Association/American College of Physicians Task Force on Practice Guidelines (Committee on the Management of Patients with Chronic Stable Angina). *J Am Coll Cardiol.* 1999;33:2097–2197; Gibbons RJ, Abrams J, Chatterjee K, et al. ACC/AHA 2002 guideline update for the management of patients with chronic stable angina. *J Am Coll Cardiol.* 2003;41:159–168.

A NEW CLASS OF ANTIANGINA DRUGS, pFOX INHIBITORS

Antianginal drugs currently being studied includes the partial fatty acid oxidation (pFOX) inhibitor class of drugs, which partially inhibit fatty acid oxidation and improve cardiac efficiency. Clearly, the development of drugs that modulate myocardial metabolism, have the potential to reduce extent of myocardial ischemia and angina symptoms, yet have no clinically significant effects on heart rate, blood pressure, or coronary blood flow, are of considerable interest. Ranolazine has recently obtained U.S. Food and Drug Administration's approval for patient use as *adjuvant therapy for patients with angina on optimal medical trial.* The biochemical rationale, and progress in development of pFOX inhibitors is the result of approximately two decades of research.

The pFOX inhibitor drugs partially relieve the inhibition of pyruvate dehydrogenase through an inhibition of the enzyme sequence necessary for β-oxidation of plasma free fatty acids in mitochondria (when there is sufficient residual oxygen supply to the myocardium to allow pyruvate oxidation). The sustained release formulation of ranolazine was tested for chronic angina in both the MARISA and CARISA trials.[121]

The MARISA and CARISA studies indicate that ranolazine (Ranexa) is a potentially effective drug to alleviate chronic angina in patients with moderately severe symptoms. The increase in exercise time with monotherapy or when combined with other antianginal drugs averaged approximately 30 s with more marked improvements in individual patients. The average increase of 30 s over placebo approximates the magnitude of increase seen with β-blockers or calcium channel antagonists when time-dependent placebo controls were used.

Treatment of Risk Factors

The recommendations of the AHA for the treatment of risk factors are detailed elsewhere.[122] Interventions that have been shown to reduce the incidence of CHD events include those that lead to declines in (1) cigarette smoking, (2) LDL cholesterol, (3) systemic hypertension, (4) LV hypertrophy, and (5) thrombogenic factors.

The causal role of LDL cholesterol in the pathogenesis of atherosclerotic CHD has been affirmed by recent randomized, controlled clinical trials of lipid-lowering therapy. Several primary and secondary prevention trials have shown that the lowering of LDL cholesterol is associated with a reduced risk of CHD events. Angiographic trials provide firm evidence linking cholesterol reduction to favorable trends in coronary anatomy.[123–126]

Data from numerous observational studies indicate a continuous and graded relation between blood pressure and cardiovascular disease risk.[127] Hypertension predisposes patients to coronary events both as a result of the direct vascular injury caused by increases in blood pressure and by its effects on the myocardium (Fig. 3-5), including increased wall stress and MVO_2.

CHD, diabetes, LV hypertrophy, heart failure, retinopathy, and nephropathy are indicators of increased cardiovascular disease risk in hypertensive patients. The target of therapy is a reduction in blood pressure to less than 130 mm Hg systolic and less than 85 mm Hg diastolic in patients with CHD and coexisting diabetes, heart failure, or renal failure.[128] In diabetics, an even lower systolic blood pressure (<120 mm Hg) appears to be of greater benefit.

Treatment of hypertension begins with nonpharmacologic means. When lifestyle modifications and dietary alterations adequately reduce blood pressure, pharmacologic intervention may be unnecessary (see Chapter 1).

When pharmacologic treatment is necessary (as is usually the case), β-blockers or calcium antagonists may be especially useful in patients with hypertension and angina pectoris; however, short-acting calcium antagonists should not be used.[129]

Epidemiologic studies have implicated LV hypertrophy as a risk factor for the development of MI, congestive heart failure, and sudden death.[130] LV hypertrophy has also been shown to predict a poorer prognosis in patients with definite CHD.[131] In the Framingham Heart Study,[132] the subjects who demonstrated ECG evidence of LV hypertrophy regression on follow-up were at a substantially reduced risk for cardiovascular events.

Coronary artery thrombosis is a trigger of acute MI. Aspirin has been documented to reduce the risk for CHD in both primary and secondary prevention studies.[11] Elevated plasma fibrinogen levels predict CHD risk in prospective observational studies.[133]

Interventions that are likely to reduce the incidence of CHD events include those that lead to declines in diabetes mellitus, LDL cholesterol, obesity, physical inactivity, and possibly postmenopausal status.

Diabetes mellitus, which is defined as a fasting blood sugar level of more than 126 mg/dL.[134] is present in a significant minority of adult Americans (see Chapter 25). Data supporting an important role of diabetes mellitus as a risk factor for cardiovascular disease comes from a number of observational settings. This is true for both type 1 and type 2 diabetes. Atherosclerosis accounts for 80% of all diabetic mortality.[135,136] The goal is to maintain blood glucose HbA_1c level of less than 7% and a blood glucose level of less than

140 mg/dL. In diabetic patients with hypertension, microalbuminuria, or decreased LV systolic function, ACE inhibitors appear indicated. This may apply to most diabetics with CHD.[1,137] Observational studies and clinical trials have demonstrated a strong inverse association between high-density lipoprotein (HDL) cholesterol and CHD risk. This inverse relation is observed in both men and women and among asymptomatic persons as well as patients with established CHD.[1] The National Cholesterol Adult Treatment Panel III has defined a low HDL–cholesterol level as less than 40 mg/dL.[137]

Obesity is a common condition associated with increased risk for CHD and mortality. New AHA guidelines for weight control have recently been published[138] (see Chapter 47).

Multiple randomized, controlled trials comparing exercise training with a "no exercise" control group have demonstrated a statistically significant improvement in exercise tolerance for the exercise group versus the control group. The threshold for ischemia is likely to increase with exercise training, because training reduces the heart rate–blood pressure product at a given submaximal exercise workload.[1]

Postmenopausal Hormonal Replacement Therapy

Both estrogenic and androgenic hormones produced by the ovary have appeared to be protective against the development of atherosclerotic cardiovascular disease. When hormonal production decreases in the perimenopausal period over several years, the risk of CHD rises in postmenopausal women. By 75 years of age, the risk of atherosclerotic cardiovascular disease among men and women is equal. Women have an accelerated risk of developing CHD if they experience an early menopause or abrupt onset of menopause through surgical removal or chemotherapeutic ablation of the ovaries. Loss of estrogen and onset of menopause result in an increase in LDL cholesterol, a small decrease in HDL cholesterol, and therefore an increased ratio of total cholesterol to HDL cholesterol. Numerous epidemiologic studies have suggested a favorable influence of estrogen replacement therapy on the primary prevention of CHD in postmenopausal women.

Based on the above, postmenopausal estrogen replacement has previously been advocated for both primary and secondary prevention of CHD in women (see Chapter 29). However, the first published randomized trial of estrogen plus progestin therapy in postmenopausal women with known CHD did not show any reduction in cardiovascular events over 4 years of follow-up[139] despite an 11% lower LDL cholesterol level and a 10% higher HDL-cholesterol level

in those women receiving hormone replacement therapy.

The Women's Health Initiative, a randomized controlled primary prevention trial of estrogen plus progestin, found that the overall health risks of this therapy exceeded its benefits.[140] Thus, current information suggests that *hormone replacement therapy in postmenopausal women does not reduce risk for major vascular events* or coronary deaths in secondary prevention. Women who are taking hormone replacement therapy and who have vascular disease can continue this therapy if it is being prescribed for other well-established indications (e.g., osteoporosis) and no better alternative therapies are appropriate. There is, however, at the present time no basis for adding or continuing estrogens in postmenopausal women with clinically evident CHD or cerebrovascular disease in an effort to prevent or retard progression of their underlying disease.

Other randomized trials of hormone replacement therapy in primary and secondary prevention of CHD in postmenopausal women are being conducted.[141] As their results become available over the next several years, this recommendation may require modification.

Interventions that may reduce the incidence of CHD events include those that lead to declines in psychosocial factors, triglycerides, lipoprotein(a), homocysteine, oxidative stress, and consumption of alcohol.

Triglyceride levels are predictive of CHD in a variety of observational studies and clinical settings.[142] However, much of the association of triglycerides with CHD risk is related to other factors, including diabetes, obesity, hypertension, high LDL cholesterol, and low HDL cholesterol.[143]

Lipoprotein(a) is a lipoprotein particle that has been linked to CHD risk in observational studies. Elevated levels of lipoprotein(a) are largely genetically determined.

MYOCARDIAL REVASCULARIZATION

There are currently two well-established revascularization approaches to treatment of chronic stable angina caused by coronary atherosclerosis. One is coronary artery bypass graft surgery, in which segments of autologous arteries or veins are used to reroute blood around relatively stenotic segments of the proximal coronary artery. The other is percutaneous coronary intervention (PCI) using catheter-borne or laser techniques to open usually short areas of stenosis from within the coronary artery. Revascularization is also potentially feasible with transthoracic (laser) myocardial revascularization in patients in whom neither CABG nor PCI is feasible. The recommendations of the

ACC/AHA/ACP-American Society of Internal Medicine (ACC/AHA/ACP-ASIM) for revascularization with PCI or CABG in patients with stable angina are listed in Table 3-9.

Patients with stable angina pectoris may be appropriate candidates for revascularization either by CABG surgery or PCI. In general, this is an individual decision to be made by the patient with knowledge of the advantages and disadvantages either of medical therapy alone or revascularization with either CABG or PCI.

There are two general indications for revascularization procedures: The presence of symptoms that are not acceptable to the patient either because of (1) restriction of physical activity and lifestyle as a result of limitations or side effects from medications or (2) the presence of findings that indicate clearly that the patient would have a better prognosis with revascularization than with medical therapy. Considerations regarding revascularization are based on an assessment of the grade or class of angina experienced by the

Table 3-9. Revascularization for Chronic Stable Angina* (Recommendations for Revascularization with PTCA or Other Catheter-Based Techniques and CABG in Patients with Stable Angina)

Class I

CABG for patients with significant left main coronary disease.

CABG for patients with three-vessel disease. The survival benefit is greater in patients with abnormal LV function (ejection fraction <50%),

CABG for patients with two-vessel disease with significant proximal left anterior descending CAD and either abnormal LV function (ejection fraction < 50%) or demonstrable ischemia on noninvasive testing.

PCI for patients with two- or three-vessel disease with significant proximal left anterior descending CAD, who have anatomy suitable for catheter-based therapy, normal LV function, and no treated diabetes.

PCI or CABG for patients with one- or two-vessel CAD without significant proximal left anterior descending CAD but with a large area of viable myocardium and high-risk criteria on noninvasive testing.

CABG for patients with one- or two-vessel CAD without significant proximal left anterior descending CAD who have survived sudden cardiac death or sustained ventricular tachycardia.

In patients with prior PCI, CABG, or PCI for recurrent stenosis associated with a large area of viable myocardium or high-risk criteria on noninvasive testing.

PTCA[†] or CABG for patients who have not been treated successfully by medical therapy and can undergo revascularization with acceptable risk.

Class IIa

Repeat CABG for patients with multiple saphenous vein graft stenoses, especially when there is significant stenosis of a graft supplying the LAD. It may be appropriate to use PTCA for focal saphenous vein graft lesions or multiple stenoses in poor candidates for reoperative surgery.

Use of PCI or CABG for patients with one- or two-vessel CAD without significant proximal LAD disease but with a moderate area of viable myocardium and demonstrable ischemia on noninvasive testing.

Use of PCI or CABG for patients with on-vessel disease with significant proximal LAD disease.

Class IIb

Compared with CABG, PCI for patients with two- or three-vessel disease with significant proximal left anterior descending CAD, who have anatomy suitable for catheter-based therapy, and who have treated diabetes or abnormal LV function.

Use of PCI for patients with significant left main coronary disease who are not candidates for CABG.

PCI for patients with one- or two-vessel CAD without significant proximal left anterior descending CAD who have survived sudden cardiac death or sustained ventricular tachycardia.

Class III

Use of PCI or CABG for patients with one- or two-vessel CAD without significant proximal left anterior descending CAD, who have mild symptoms that are unlikely because of myocardial ischemia or who have not received an adequate trial of medical therapy and

Have only a small area of viable myocardium or

Have no demonstrable ischemia on noninvasive testing.

Use of PCI or CABG for patients with borderline coronary stenoses (50–60% diameter in locations other than the left main coronary artery) and no demonstrable ischemia on noninvasive testing.

Use of PCI or CABG for patients with borderline coronary stenoses (<50% diameter).

Use of PCI in patients with significant left main coronary disease who are candidates for CABG.

*Recommendations for revascularization with PTCA (or other catheter-based techniques) and CA BG in patients with stable angina.
[†]PTCA is used in these recommendations to indicate PTCA or other catheter-based techniques, such as stents, atherectomy, and laser therapy. See Notes classes I to III as described at the bottom of Table 3-5.
CABG, coronary artery bypass graft; CAD, coronary artery disease; LAD, left anterior descending (coronary artery); LV, left ventricular; PCI, percataneous coronary intervention; PTCA, percataneous transluminal coronary angioplasty.
Source: Gibbons RJ, Chatterjee K, Daley J, et al. ACC/AHA/ACP guidelines for the management of chronic stable angina: A Report of the American College of Cardiology/American Heart Association/American College of Physicians Task Force on Practice Guidelines (Committee on the Management of Patients with Chronic Stable Angina). *J Am Coll Cardiol.* 1999;33:2097–2197. Gibbons RJ, Abrams J, Chatterjee K, et al. ACC/AHA 2002 guideline update for the management of patients with chronic stable angina. *J Am Coll Cardiol.* 2003;41:159–168.

patient, the presence and severity of myocardial ischemia or noninvasive testing, the degree of LV function, and the distribution and severity of coronary artery stenoses.

A recent meta-analysis of three major large, multicenter, randomized trials of initial surgery versus medical management (performed in the 1970s) as well as other smaller trials has confirmed the surgical benefits achieved by surgery at 10 postoperative years for patients with three-vessel disease, two-vessel disease, or even one-vessel disease that included a severe stenosis of the proximal left anterior descending coronary artery.[144–146]

The advantages of PCI for the treatment of CHD include a low level of procedure-related morbidity, a low procedure-related mortality rate in properly selected patients, a short hospital stay, early return to activity, and the feasibility of multiple procedures. However, PCI is not feasible in all patients; it remains accompanied by a significant incidence of restenosis, and there is an occasional need for emergency CABG surgery.

Three randomized studies have compared PCI with medical management alone for the treatment of chronic stable angina[147–150] All these randomized studies of PCI versus medical management have involved patients at a low risk of mortality even with medical management and did not assess patients with moderate to severe CHD. Multiple trials have compared the strategy of an initial PCI with initial CABG surgery for treatment of multivessel CHD. The results of all these trials have shown that early and late survival rates have been equivalent for the PCI and CABG surgery groups.[150] In the BARI trial, the subgroups of patients with treated diabetes had a significantly better survival rate with CABG surgery.[151] This was true, however, on post hoc analysis of the clinical variables, including diabetes, which was not a prerandomization-blocking variable.

The randomized studies on invasive therapy for chronic angina have all excluded patients who developed recurrent angina after previous CABG surgery. Few existing data define outcomes for risk-stratified groups of patients who develop recurrent angina after bypass surgery. Those that do indicate that patients with ischemia produced by late atherosclerotic stenoses in vein grafts are at a higher risk with medical management alone than are patients with ischemia produced by native-vessel disease.

OTHER THERAPIES IN PATIENTS WITH REFRACTORY ANGINA

Recent evidence has emerged regarding the relative efficacy, or lack thereof, of a number of techniques for the management of refractory chronic angina pectoris. These techniques should only be used in patients who cannot be managed adequately by medical therapy and who are not candidates for revascularization (interventional and/or surgical). Data are reviewed regarding three techniques: spinal cord stimulation (SCS), enhanced external counterpulsation, and laser transmyocardial revascularization (TMR).[1]

SPINAL CORD STIMULATION

The efficacy of SCS depends on the accurate placement of the stimulating electrode in the dorsal epidural space, usually at the C7-T1 level. A review of the literature has revealed two small-randomized clinical trials involving implanted spinal stimulators, one of which directly tested its efficacy. The authors concluded that SCS was effective in the treatment of chronic intractable angina pectoris and that its effect was exerted through an anti-ischemic action.[1]

ENHANCED EXTERNAL COUNTERPULSATION

This technique uses a series of cuffs that are wrapped around both of the patient's legs. Using compressed air, pressure is applied via the cuffs to the patient's lower extremities in a sequence synchronized with the cardiac cycle. Specifically, in early diastole, pressure is applied sequentially from the lower legs to the lower and upper thighs, to propel blood back to the heart. The procedure results in an increase in arterial blood pressure and retrograde aortic blood flow during diastole (diastolic augmentation). Treatment was relatively well tolerated and free of limiting side effects in most patients. However, the sample size in this study was relatively small.[1] (Two multicenter registry studies found the treatment to be generally well tolerated and efficacious; anginal symptoms were improved in approximately 75% to 80% of patients. However, additional clinical trial data is necessary before this technology can be recommended definitively.)

LASER TMR

Another emerging technique for the treatment of more severe chronic stable angina refractory to medical or other therapies is laser TMR. This technique has either been performed in the operating room (using a carbon dioxide or holmium: YAG laser) or by a percutaneous approach with a specialized (holmium: YAG laser) catheter. Eight prospective randomized clinical trials have been performed, two using the percutaneous technique and the other six using an epicardial surgical technique.[1]

PERCUTANEOUS TMR

The two randomized percutaneous TMR trials assessed parameters such as angina class, freedom from angina, exercise tolerance, and quality of life score. In general, these studies have shown improvements in severity of angina class, exercise tolerance, and quality of life, as well as increased freedom from angina.[1] However, percutaneous TMR technology has not been approved by the Food and Drug Administration; therefore, percutaneous TMR should still be considered an experimental therapy.

SURGICAL TMR

The surgical TMR technique has also generally been associated with improvement in symptoms in patients with chronic stable angina. The mechanism for improvement in angina symptoms is still controversial.[1] Three studies also assessed myocardial perfusion using thallium scans. Only one of these studies demonstrated an improvement in myocardial perfusion in patients who underwent TMR versus those continuing to receive only medical therapy. Despite the apparent benefit in decreasing angina symptoms, no definite benefit has been demonstrated in terms of increasing myocardial perfusion.[1]

FOLLOW-UP OF PATIENTS WITH CHRONIC STABLE ANGINA

Published evidence of the efficacy of specific strategies for the follow-up of patients with chronic stable angina on patient outcome is nonexistent. The ACC/AHA/

Table 3-10. Recommendations for Echocardiography, Treadmill Exercise Testing, Stress Imaging Studies, and Coronary Angiography during Patient Follow-Up

Class I

Chest X-ray for patients with evidence of new or worsening congestive heart failure.

Assessment of LV ejection fraction and segmental wall motion in patients with new or worsening congestive heart failure evidence of intervening MI by history or ECG.

Echocardiography for evidence of new or worsening valvular heart disease.

Treadmill exercise test for patients without prior revascularization who have a significant change in clinical status, are able to exercise, and do not have nay of the ECG abnormalities listed below.

Stress imaging procedures for patients without prior revascularization who have a significant change in clinical status and are unable to exercise or have one of the following ECG abnormalities:

    Preexcitation (Wolff-Parkinson-White) syndrome.

    Electronically paced ventricular rhythm.

    More than 1 mm of rest ST-segment depression.

    Complete LBBB.

Stress imaging procedures for patients who have a significant change in clinical status and required a stress imaging procedure on their initial evaluation because of equivocal or intermediate-risk treadmill results.

Stress imaging procedures for patients with prior revascularization who have a significant change in clinical status.

Coronary angiography in patients with marked limitation of ordinary activity. (CCS class III despite maximal medical therapy.)

Class IIb

Annual treadmill exercise testing in patients who have no change to clinical status, can exercise, have none of the ECG abnormalities listed in number 5 above, and have an estimated annual mortality of >1%.

Class III

Echocardiography or radionuclide imaging for assessment of LV ejection fraction and segmental wall motion in patients with a normal ECG, no history of MI, and no evidence of congestive heart failure.

Repeat treadmill exercise testing in <3 years in patients who have no change in clinical status and an estimated annual mortality ≥1% on their initial evaluation as demonstrated sby one of the following:

    Low-risk Duke treadmill score without imaging.

    Low-risk Duke treadmill score with negative imaging.

    Normal LV function and a normal coronary angiogram.

    Normal LV function and insignificant CAD.

Stress imaging procedures for patients who have no change in clinical status and a normal rest ECG, are not taking digoxin, are able to exercise, and did not require a stress imaging procedure on their initial evaluation because of equivocal or intermediate-risk treadmill results.

Repeat coronary angiography in patients with no change in clinical status, no change on repeat exercise testing or stress imaging, and insignificant CAD on initial evaluation.

Note: See footnotes of Table 3-5 for classes I–III.

Source: Gibbons RJ, Chatterjee K, Daley J, et al. ACC/AHA/ACP guidelines for the management of chronic stable angina: A Report of the American College of Cardiology/American Heart Association/American College of Physicians Task Force on Practice Guidelines (Committee on the Management of Patients with Chronic Stable Angina). *J Am Coll Cardiol.* 1999;33:2097–2197;Gibbons RJ, Abrams J, Chatterjee K, et al. ACC/AHA 2002 guideline update for the management of patients with chronic stable angina. *J Am Coll Cardiol.* 2003;41:159–168.

ACP-ASIM guidelines[1] for the monitoring of symptoms and antianginal therapy during patient follow-up are as follows:

For the patient with successfully treated chronic stable angina, a follow-up evaluation every 4 to 12 months is appropriate. During the first year of therapy, evaluations every 4 to 6 months are recommended. After the first year of therapy, annual evaluations are recommended if the patient is stable and reliable enough to return for evaluation when anginal symptoms become worse or other symptoms occur.[1] At the time of follow-up, a general assessment of the patient's functional and health status and quality of life may reveal additional issues that affect angina. Symptoms that have worsened should follow reevaluation as outlined above. A detailed history of the patient's daily activity is critical because anginal symptoms may remain stable only because stressful activities have been eliminated.

A careful history of the characteristics of the patient's angina, including provoking and alleviating factors, must be repeated at each visit. Detailed questions should be asked about common drug side effects. The patient's adherence to the treatment program must be assessed.

The physical examination should be focused by the patient's history. Every patient should have his or her weight, blood pressure, and pulse noted. The jugular venous pressure, carotid pulse magnitude and upstroke, and presence or absence of carotid bruits should be noted. Pulmonary examination with special attention to rales, rhonchi, wheezing, and decreased breath sounds is required. A cardiac examination should note the presence of fourth and third heart sounds, a new or changed systolic murmur, the location of the LV impulse, and any change from previous examinations. Clearly, the vascular examination should identify any change in peripheral pulses and new bruits; the abdominal examination should identify hepatomegaly and the presence of any pulsatile mass suggesting an abdominal aortic aneurysm. The presence of new or worsening peripheral edema should be noted.

The American Diabetes Association recommends that patients not known to have diabetes should have a fasting blood glucose measured every 3 years and an annual measurement of glycosylated hemoglobin for individuals with established diabetes. Fasting blood work, 6 to 8 weeks after initiating lipid-lowering drug therapy, should include liver function testing and assessment of the cholesterol profile. This should be repeated every 8 to 12 weeks during the first year of therapy and at 4 to 6-month intervals thereafter.

An ECG should be repeated when medications affecting cardiac conduction are initiated or changed. A repeat ECG is indicated for a change in the anginal pattern, symptoms or finding suggestive of an arrhythmia or conduction abnormality, and near or frank syncope. There is no clear evidence showing that routine, periodic ECGs are useful in the absence of a change in history or physical examination.

In the absence of a change in clinical status, low-risk patients with an estimated annual mortality rate of less than 1% over each year of the interval do not require repeat stress testing for 3 years after the initial evaluation.[1] Annual follow-up for noninvasive testing in the absence of a change in symptoms has not been studied adequately; it may be useful in high-risk patients with an estimated annual mortality rate of greater than 5%. Follow-up testing should be performed in a stable high-risk patient only if the initial decision not to proceed with revascularization may change if the patient's estimated risk worsens. Patients with an immediate-risk (>1 and $<3\%$) annual mortality rate are more problematic because of limited data. They may need testing at an interval of 1 to 3 years depending on the individual circumstances. The ACC/AHA/ACP-ASIM recommendations for echocardiography, treadmill exercise testing, stress imaging studies, and coronary angiography during patient follow-up are also listed in Table 3-10.

EVIDENCE-BASED SUMMARY

- Ischemic heart disease is the leading cause of mortality in the United States
- Diagnostic testing is most valuable when the pretest probability of obstructive CHD is intermediate
- Resting ST-segment depression is a marker for adverse cardiac events in patients with and without known CHD
- LV function is the strongest predictor of long-term survival in patients with CHD
- Aspirin 75 to 325 mg per day should be used routinely in all patients with acute and chronic ischemic heart disease. In those unable to take aspirin, clopidogrel may be used instead
- Evidence supports that lowering LDL-cholesterol by 30% using a statin reduces total and cardiac mortality
- Heart rate is one of the most important determinates of MVO_2 and can be altered easily by medical therapy.

REFERENCES

1. Kannel WB, Feinleib M. Natural history of angina pectoris in the Framingham study. Prognosis and survival. *Am J Cardiol.* 1972;29:154–163.
2. Gibbons RJ, Chatterjee K, Daley J, et al. ACC/AHA/ACP guidelines for the management of chronic stable angina: A Report of the American College of Cardiology/American Heart Association/American College of Physicians Task Force on Practice Guidelines (Committee on the Management of Patients with Chronic Stable Angina). *J Am Coll Cardiol.* 1999;33:2097–2197.
3. Gibbons RJ, Abrams J, Chatterjee K, et al. ACC/AHA 2002 guideline update for the management of patients with chronic stable angina. *J Am Coll Cardiol.* 2003;41:159–168.
4. Elveback LR, Connolly DC, Melton LJ 3rd. Coronary heart disease in residents of rochester, minnesota. VII. Incidence, 1950 through 1982. *Mayo Clin Proc.* 1986;61:896–900.
5. Ryan TJ, Anderson JL, Antman EM, et al. ACC/AHA guidelines for the management of patients with acute myocardial infarction. A Report of the American College of Cardiology/American Heart Association Task Force on Practice Guidelines (Committee on Management of Acute Myocardial Infarction). *J Am Coll Cardiol.* 1996;28:1328–1428.
6. The American Heart Association. Biostatistical Fact Sheets. Dallas, TX: 1997.
7. O'Rourke RA, O'Gara P, Douglas JS Jr. Diagnosis and management of patients with chronic ischemic heart disease. In: Fuster V, Alexander FW, O'Rourke RA, et al (eds). *Hurst's the Heart,* 11th ed. New York, NY: Mc-Graw-Hill; 2004:1465–1493.
8. Diamond GA, Staniloff HM, Forrester JS, Pollock BH, Swan HJ. Computer-assisted diagnosis in the noninvasive evaluation of patients with suspected coronary disease. *J Am Coll Cardiol.* 1983;1:444–455.
9. Diamond GA, Forrester JS. Analysis of probability as an aid in the clinical diagnosis of coronary-artery disease. *N Engl J Med.* 1979;300:1350–1358.
10. Pryor DB, Harrell FE, Lee KL, Califf RM, Rosati RA. Estimating the likelihood of significant coronary artery disease. *Am J Med.* 1983;75:771–780.
11. Sox HC, Hickam DH, Marton KI, et al. Using the patient's history to estimate the probability of coronary artery disease: A comparison of primary care and referral practices. *Am J Med.* 1990;89;7–14; Erratum. *Am J Med.* 1990;89(4)550.
12. Pryor DB, Shaw L, McCants CB, et al. Value of the history and physical in identifying patients at increased risk for coronary artery disease. *Ann Intern Med.* 1993;118: 81–90.
13. Chaitman BR, Bourassa MG, Davis K, et al. Angiographic prevalence of high-risk coronary artery disease in patient subsets (CASS). *Circulation.* 1981;64:360–367.
14. Wexler L, Brundage B, Crouse J, et al. Coronary artery calcification: Pathophysiology, epidemiology, imaging methods, and clinical implications. A statement for health professionals from the American Heart Association Writing Group. *Circulation.* 1996;94:1175–1192.
15. Mautner SL, Mautner GC, Froehlich J, et al. Coronary artery disease: Predication with in vitro electron beam CT. *Radiology.* 1994;192:625–630.
16. O'Rourke RA, Froelicher VF, Greenland P, et al. ACC/AHA expert consensus document on electron beam computed tomography for the diagnosis of coronary artery disease. *J Am Coll Cardiol.* 2000;36:326–341.
17. Gibbons RJ, Balady GJ, Beasley JW, et al. ACC/AHA guidelines for exercise testing: Executive summary. A Report of the Americans College of Cardiology/American Heart Association Task Force on Practice Guidelines (Committee on Exercise Testing). *J Am Coll Cardiol.* 1999; 30:260–311.
18. Froelicher VF, Lehmann KG, Thomas R, et al. The electrocardiographic exercise test in a population with reduced workup bias: Diagnostic performance, computerized interpretation, and multivariable prediction. Veterans affairs cooperative study in health services #016 (QUEXTA) study group. Quantitative exercise testing and angiography. *Ann Intern Med.* 1998;128:965–974.
19. Diamond GA, Forrester JS, Hirsch M, et al. Application of conditional probability analysis to the clinical diagnosis of coronary artery disease. *J Clin Invest.* 1980;65:1210–1221.
20. Goldman L, Cook EF, Mitchell N, et al. Incremental value of the exercise test for diagnosing the presence or absence of coronary artery disease. *Circulation.* 1982;66:945–953.
21. Melin JA, Wijns W, Vanbutsele RJ, et al. Alternative diagnostic strategies for coronary artery disease in women: Demonstration of the usefulness and efficiency of probability analysis. *Circulation.* 1985;71:535–542.
22. LeWinter MM, Crawford MH, O'Rourke RA, Karliner JS. The effects of oral propranolol, digoxin, and combination therapy on the resting and exercise electrocardiogram. *Am Heart J.* 1977;93:202–209.
23. Whinnery JE, Froelicher VF, Stuart AJ. The electrocardiographic response to maximal treadmill exercise in asymptomatic men with left bundle branch block. *Am Heart J.* 1977;94:316–324.
24. Pennel DJ, Sechtem U, Higgins C, et al. European Society of Cardiology and Society of Cardiovascular Magnetic Resonance-Clinical indications for cardiovascular magnetic resonance: Consensus Panel Report. *Eur Heart J.* 2004;25:1940–1965.
25. Cheitlin MD, Alpert JS, Armstrong WF, et al. ACC/AHA Guidelines for the clinical application of echocardiography. A Report of the American College of Cardiology/American Heart Association Task Force on Practice Guidelines (Committee on Clinical Application of Echocardiography). Developed in collaboration with the American Society of Echocardiography. *Circulation.* 1997;95:1686–1744.
26. Kiat H, Berman DS, Maddahi J. Comparison of planar and tomographic exercise thallium-201 imaging methods for the evaluation of coronary artery disease. *J Am Coll Cardiol.* 1989;13:613–616.
27. Iskandrian AS, Heo J, Kong B, Lyons E, Marsch S. Use of technetium-99m isonitrile (RP-30A) in assessing left ventricular perfusion and function at rest and during

exercise in coronary artery disease, and comparison with coronary arteriography and exercise thallium-201 SPECT imaging. *Am J Cardiol.* 1989;64:270–275.

28. Taillefer R, Laflamme L, Dupras G, Picard M, Phaneuf DC, Leveille J. Myocardial perfusion imaging with 99mTc-methoxy-isobutyl-isonitrile (MIBI): Comparison of short and long time intervals between rest and stress injections. Preliminary results. *Eur J Nucl Med.* 1988;13: 515–522.

29. Maddahi J, Kiat H, Van Train FK, et al. Myocardial perfusion imaging with technetium-99m sestamibi SPECT in the evaluation of coronary artery disease. *Am J Cardiol.* 1990;66:55E–62E.

30. Kahn JK, McGhie I, Akers MS, et al. Quantitative rotational tomography with 201T and 99mTc 2-methoxy-isobutyl-isonitrile. A direct comparison in normal individuals and patients with coronary artery disease. *Circulation.* 1989;79:1282–1293.

31. Wackers FJ, Berman DS, Maddahi J, et al. Technetium-99m hexakis 2-methoxyisobutyl isonitrile: Human biodistribution, dosimetry, safety, and preliminary comparison to thallium-201 for myocardial perfusion imaging. *J Nucl Med.* 1989;30:301–311.

32. Maisey MN, Mistry R, Sowton E. Planar imaging techniques used with technetium-99m sestamibi to evaluate chronic myocardial ischemia. *Am J Cardiol.* 1990;66: 47E–54E.

33. Maddahi J, Kiat H, Friedman JD, Berman DS, Van Train KK, Garcia EV. Technetium-99m-sestamibi myocardial perfusion imaging for evaluation of coronary artery disease. In: Zaret BL, Beller GA. (eds). *Nuclear Cardiology: State of the Art and Future Directions.* St. Louis, MO: Mosby;1993:191–200.

34. Zaret BL, Rigo P, Wackers FJ, et al. Myocardial perfusion imaging with 99m TC-tetrofosmin. Comparison to 201-T1 imaging and coronary angiography in a Phase III Multicenter trial. *Circulation.* 1995;91:313–319.

35. Klocke FJ, Barid MG, Lorell BH, et al. ACC/AHA/ASNC guidelines for the clinical use of cardiac radionuclide imaging-executive summary: A Report of the American College of Cardiology/American Heart Association Task Force on Practice Guidelines. *J Am Coll Cardiol.* 2003; 42(7):1318–1333.

36. Detrano R, Janosi A, Lyons KP, Marcondes G, Abbassi N, Froelicher VF. Factors affecting sensitivity and specificity of a diagnostic test: The exercise thallium scintigram. *Am J Med.* 1988;84:699–710.

37. Watson DD, Campbell NP, Read EK, Gibson RS, Teates CD, Beller GA. Spatial and temporal quantitation of plane thallium myocardial images. *J Nucl Med.* 1981;22: 577–584.

38. Garcia E, Maddahi J, Berman D, Waxman A. Space/time quantitation of thallium-201 myocardial scintigraphy. *J Nucl Med.* 1981;22:309–317.

39. Gould KL. Noninvasive assessment of coronary stenoses by myocardial perfusion imaging during pharmacologic coronary vasodilatation. I. Physiologic basis and experimental validation. *Am J Cardiol.* 1978;41: 267–278.

40. Verani MS. Pharmacologic stress myocardial perfusion imaging. *Curr Probl Cardiol.* 1993;18:481–525.

41. Ritchie JL, Bateman TM, Bonow RO, et al. Guidelines for clinical use of cardiac radionuclide imaging. Report of the American College of Cardiology/American Heart Association Task Force on Assessment of Diagnostic and Therapeutic Cardiovascular Procedures (Committee on Radionuclide Imaging). Developed in collaboration with the American Society of Nuclear Cardiology. *J Am Coll Cardiol.* 1995;25:521–547.

42. Parodi O, Marcassa C, Casucci R, et al. Accuracy and safety of technetium-99m hexakis 2-methoxy-2-isobutylisonitrile (Sestamibi) myocardial scintigraphy with high dose dipyridamole test in patients with effort angina pectoris: A multicenter study. Italian group of nuclear cardiology. *J Am Coll Cardiol.* 1991;18:1439–1444.

43. Berman DS, Hachamovitch R, Shaw LJ, et al. Nuclear cardiology. In: Fuster V, Alexander RW, O'Rourke RA, et al. (eds). *Hurst's the Heart,* 11th ed. New York, NY: McGraw-Hill; 2004:563–598.

44. Marwick TH. *Stress Echocardiography.* Boston, MS: Kluwer Academic Publishers; 1994.

45. C, Kwok YS, Heagerty P, Redberg R. Pharmacologic stress testing for coronary disease diagnosis. *Am Heart J.* 2001;142(6):934–944.

46. Dagianti A, Penco M, Agati L, Sciomer S, Rosanio S, Fedele F. Stress echocardiography: Comparison of exercise, dipyridamole and dobutamine in detecting and predicting the extent of coronary artery disease. *J Am Coll Cardiol.* 1995;26:18–25; Erratum. *J Am Coll Cardiol.* 1995;26(4):1114.

47. Hockings B, Saltissi S, Croft DN, Webb-Peploe MM. Effect of beta adrenergic blockade on thallium-201 myocardial perfusion imaging. *Br Heart J.* 1983;49:83–89.

48. DePuey EG, Guertler-Krawczynska E, Robbins WL. Thallium-201 SPECT in coronary artery disease patients with left bundle branch block. *J Nucl Med.* 1988;29: 1479–1485.

49. O'Keefe JH Jr., Bateman TM, Barnhart CS. Adenosine thallium-201 is superior to exercise thallium-201 for detecting coronary artery disease in patients with left bundle branch block. *J Am Coll Cardiol.* 1993;21:1332–1338.

50. Mairesse GH, Marwick TH, Arnese M, et al. Improved identification of coronary artery disease in patients with left bundle branch block by use of dobutamine stress echocardiography in comparison with myocardial perfusion tomography. *Am J Cardiol.* 1995;76:321–325.

51. Smanio PE, Watson DD, Segalla DL, Vinson EL, Smith WH, Beller GA. Value of gating of technetium-99m sestamibi single-photon emission computed tomographic imaging. *J Am Coll Cardiol.* 1997;30:1687–1692.

52. O'Keefe JH, Barnhart CS, Bateman TM. Comparison of stress echocardiography and stress myocardial perfusion scintigraphy for diagnosing coronary artery disease and assessing its severity. *Am J Cardiol.* 1995;75:25D–34D.

53. Fleischmann KE, Hunink MGM, Kuntz KM, Douglas PS. Exercise echocardiography or exercise SPECT imaging: A meta-analysis of diagnostic test performance. *JAMA.* 1998; 280: 913–920.

54. Hubbard BL, Gibbons JR, Lapeyre AC III, Zinsmeister AR, and Clements IP. Prospective evaluation of a clinical and exercise-test model for the prediction of left main coronary artery disease. *Archives Intern Med.* 1992; 152: 309–312.

55. Califf RM, Mark DB, Harrell FE, et al. Importance of clinical measures of ischemia in the prognosis of patients with documented coronary artery disease. *J Am Coll Cardiol.* 1998;11:20–26.

56. Germano G, Erel J, Lewin H, Kavanagh PB, Berman DS. Automatic quantitation of regional myocardial wall motion and thickening from gated technetium-99m sestamibi myocardial perfusion single-photon emission computed tomography. *Circulation.* 1996;93:463–473.

57. Shaw LJ, Iskandrian AE. Prognostic value of gated myocardial perfusion SPECT. *J Nucl Cardiol.* 2004;11(2): 171–185.

58. Oh JK, Gibbons RJ, Christina TF, et al. Correlation of regional wall motion abnormalities detected by two-dimensional echocardiography with perfusion defect determined by technetium 99m sestamibi imaging in patients treated with reperfusion therapy during acute myocardial infarction. *Am Heart J.* 1996;131:32–37.

59. Spirito P, Bellotti P, Chiarella F, Domenicucci S, Sementa A, Vecchio C. Prognostic significance and natural history of left ventricular thrombi in patients with acute anterior myocardial infarction: A two-dimensional echocardiographic study. *Circulation.* 1985;72:774–780.

60. Gibbons RJ, Zinsmeister AR, Miller TD, Clements IP. Supine exercise electrocardiography compared with exercise radionuclide angiography in noninvasive identification of severe coronary artery disease. *Ann Intern Med.* 1990;112:743–749.

61. Ladenheim ML, Kotler TS, Pollock BH, Berman DS, Diamond GA. Incremental prognostic power of clinical history, exercise electrocardiography and myocardial perfusion scintigraphy in suspected coronary artery disease. *Am J Cardiol.* 1987;59:270–277.

62. Mattera JA, Arain SA, Sinusas AJ, Finta L, Wackers FJ, 3rd. Exercise testing with myocardial perfusion imaging in patients with normal baseline electrocardiograms: Cost savings with a stepwise diagnostic strategy. *J Nucl Cardiol.* 1998;5:498–506.

63. Mark DB, Hlatky MA, Harrell FE, Lee KL, Califf RM, Pryor DB. Exercise treadmill score for predicting prognosis in coronary artery disease. *Ann Intern Med.* 1987;106:793–800.

64. Morrow K, Morris CK, Froelicher VF, et al. Prediction of cardiovascular death in men undergoing noninvasive evaluation for coronary artery disease. *Ann Intern Med.* 1993;118:689–695.

65. Brunelli C, Cristofani R, L'Abbate A. Long-term survival in medically treated patients with ischaemic heart disease and prognostic importance of clinical and electrocardiographic data (the Italian CNR multicentre prospective study OD1). *Eur Heart J.* 1989;10:292–303.

66. Shaw LS, Peterson ED, Shaw LK, et al. Use of prognostic treadmill score in identifying diagnostic coronary disease subgroups. *Circulation.* 1998;98:1622–1630.

67. Alexander KP, Shaw LJ, Delong ER, Mark DB, Peterson ED. Value of exercise treadmill testing in women. *J Am Coll Cardiol.* 1998;32:1657–1664.

68. Alexander KP, Shaw LJ, Shaw LK, et al. Value of exercise treadmill testing in women. *J Am Coll Cardiol.* 1998; 32(6):1657–1664.

69. Boyne TS, Koplan BA, Parsons WJ, Smith WH, Watson DD, Beller GA. Predicting adverse outcome with exercise SPECT technetium-99m sestamibi imaging in patients with suspected or known coronary artery disease. *Am J Cardiol.* 1997;79:270–274.

70. Williams MJ, Odabashian J, Lauer MS, Thomas JD, Marwick TH. Prognostic value of dobutamine echocardiography in patients with left ventricular dysfunction. *J Am Coll Cardiol.* 1996;27:132–139.

71. Afridi I, Quinones MA, Zoghbi WA, Cheirif J. Dobutamine stress echocardiography: Sensitivity, specificity, and predictive value for future cardiac events. *Am Heart J.* 1994;127:1510–1515.

72. Hachamovitch R, Berman DS, Shaw JF, et al. Incremental prognostic value of myocardial perfusion single photon emission computed tomography (SPECT) for the prediction of cardiac death: Differential stratification for risk of cardiac death and myocardial infarction. *Circulation.* 1998;97(6)533–543; Erratum. *Circulation.* 1998; 98(2):190.

73. Cox JL, Wright LM, Burns RJ. Prognostic significance of increased thallium-201 lung uptake during dipyridamole myocardial scintigraphy: Comparison with exercise scintigraphy. *Can J Cardiol.* 1995;11:689–694.

74. Wagdy HM, Hodge D, Christian TF, Miller TD, Gibbons RJ. Prognostic value of vasodilator myocardial perfusion imaging in patients with left bundle branch block. *Circulation.* 1998; 97:1563–1570.

75. Marwick TH, D'Hondt AM, Baudhuin T, et al. Optimal use of dobutamine stress for the detection and evaluation of coronary artery disease: Combination with echocardiography or scintigraphy, or both? *J Am Coll Cardiol.* 1993;22:159–167.

76. Marwick TH. Use of stress echocardiography for the prognostic assessment of patients wtih stable chronic coronary artery disease. *Eur Heart J.* 1997;18(Suppl D): D97–D101.

77. Califf RM, Armstrong PW, Carver JR, D'Agostino RB, Strauss WE. Stratification of patients into high, medium and low risk subgroups for purposes of risk factor management. *J Am Coll Cardiol.* 1996;27:1007–1019.

78. Patterson RE, Eisner RL, Horowitz SF. Comparison of cost-effectiveness and utility of exercise ECG, single photon emission tomography, positron tomography and coronary angiography for diagnosis of coronary artery disease. *Circulation.* 1995;91:51–68.

79. Gibbons RJ, Balady GJ, Bricker JT, et al. ACC/AHA 2002 guideline update for exercise testing-summary article. *J Am Coll Cardiol.* 2002;106:1883–1892.

80. O'Rourke RA, Boden W, Weintraub W, et al. Medical therapy versus percutaneous coronary intervention: Implications of the Avert Study and Courage Trial. *Curr Pract Med.* 1999;2(11):225–227.

81. O'Rourke RA. Optimal medical management of patients with chronic ischemic heart disease. *Curr Probl Cardiol.* 2001;26:195–244.

82. Final Report on the aspirin component of the ongoing Physicians' Health Study. Steering Committee of the Physicians' Health Study Research Group. *N Engl J Med.* 1989;321:129–135.

83. Juul-Moller S, Edvardsson N, Jahnmatz B, et al. Double-blind trial of aspirin in primary prevention of myocardial infarction in patients with stable chronic angina pectoris: The Swedish Angina Pectoris Aspirin Trial (SAPAT) group. *Lancet.* 1992;340:1421–1425.

84. O'Rourke RA. Hurst's Online-Meta-Analysis of 200,000 patients with low/high doses of aspirin. www.accessmedicine.com. Accessed January, 2008.

85. McTavish D, Faulds D, Goa KL. Ticlopidine: An updated review of its pharmacology and therapeutic use in platelet-dependent disorders. *Drugs.* 1990;40(2):238–259.

86. Yusuf S, Zhao R, Mehta SR, et al. Effects of Clopidogrel in addition to aspirin in patients with acute coronary syndromes without ST-segment-elevation. *N Engl J Med.* 2001;345(7):494–502.

87. O'Rourke RA, Hurst's Online Editorial. Are the One Year Results of the CREDO Trial Compelling? http://www.cardiology.accessmedicine.com. Accessed January, 2008.

88. Khot UN, Nissen SE. Is CURE a cure for acute coronary syndromes? Statistical versus clinical significance. *J Am Coll Cardiol.* 2002;40:218–219.

89. CAPRIE Steering Committee. A randomized, blinded trial of clopidogrel versus aspirin in patients at risk of ischemic events (CAPRIE). *Lancet.* 1996;348(9038):1329–1339.

90. Melandri G, Semprini F, Cervi V, et al. Benefit of adding low molecular weight heparin to the conventional treatment of stable angina pectoris: A double-blind, randomized, placebo-controlled trial. *Circulation.* 1993;88(6):2517–2523.

91. Thrombosis prevention trial: Randomized trial of low-intensity oral anticoagulation with warfarin and low-dose aspirin in the primary prevention of ischaemic heart disease in men at increased risk. The medical research council's general practice research framework. *Lancet.* 1998;351:233–241.

92. Randomized trial of cholesterol lowering in 4444 patients with coronary heart disease: The Scandinavian Simvastatin Survival Study (4S). *Lancet.* 1994;344:1383–1389.

93. Pedersen T, Olsson A, Faergeman O, et al. Lipoprotein changes and reduction in the incidence of major coronary heart disease events in the Scandinavian Simvastatin Survival Study (4S). *Circulation.* 1998;97:1453–1460.

94. Sacks FM, Pfeffer MA, Moye LA, et al. The effect of pravastatin on coronary events after myocardial infarction in patients with average cholesterol levels: Cholesterol and recurrent events trial investigators. *N Engl J Med.* 1996;335(14):1001–1009.

95. Cholesterol Treatment Trialists' (CTT) Collaborators. Efficacy and safety of cholesterol-lowering treatment: prospective meta-analysis of data from 90056 participants in 14 randomized trials of statins. *Lancet.* 2005;366:1267–1278.

96. Yusef S, Sleight P, Pogue J, et al. Effects of an angiotensin-converting-enzyme inhibitor, ramipril, on cardiovascular events in high-risk patients. The heart outcomes prevention evaluation study investigators. *N Engl J Med.* 2000;342:145–153.

97. Braunwald E, Domanski, MJ, Fowler SE, et al. Angiotensin converting enzyme inhibition in stable coronary artery disease. *N Engl J Med.* 2004;38:2058–2060.

97a. Heart Outcomes Prevention Evaluation Study Investigators. Effects of ramipril on cardiovascular outcomes in people with diabetes mellitus: Results of the HOPE study and MICRO-HOPE sub-study. *Lancet.* 2000;355:253–259.

98. HOPE/HOPE-TOO study investigators. Long-term effects of ramipril on cardiovascular events and on diabetes. Results of the HOPE study extension. *Circulation.* 2005;112:1339–1346.

99. Al-Mallah MH, Tleyjeh IM, Abdel-Latif AA, Weaver WD. Angiotensin-converting enzyme inhibitors in coronary artery disease and preserved left ventricular systolic function. A systematic review and meta-analysis of randomized controlled trials. *J Am Coll Cardiol.* 2006;47:1576–1583.

100. Wallace WA, Wellington KL, Chess MA, Liang CS. Comparison of nifedipine gastrointestinal therapeutic system and atenolol on antianginal efficacies and exercise hemodynamic responses in stable angina pectoris. *Am J Cardiol.* 1994;73(1):23–28.

101. de Vries RJ, van den Heuvel AF, Lok DJ, et al. Nifedipine gastrointestinal therapeutic system versus atenolol in stable angina pectoris: The Netherlands Working Group on Cardiovascular Research (WCN). *Int J Cardiol.* 1996;57:143–150.

102. Fox KM, Mulcahy D, Findlay I, et al. The total ischaemic burden European trial (TIBET): Effects of atenolol, nifedipine SR and their combination on the exercise test and the total ischaemic burden in 608 patients with stable angina. The TIBET study group. *Eur Heart J.* 1996;17(1):96–103.

103. Gibbons RJ, Chatterjee K, Daley J, et al. American College of Cardiology/American Heart Association, American College of Physicians-American Society of Internal Medicine (ACC/AHA/ACP-ASIM) guidelines for the management of patients with chronic stable angina: A Report of the ACC/AHA Task Force on Practice Guidelines (Committee on the Management of Patients with Chronic Stable Angina). *J Am Coll Cardiol.* 2002;41:160–168.

104. Savonitto S, Ardissiono D, Egstrup K, et al. Combination therapy with metoprolol and nifedipine versus monotherapy in patients with stable angina pectoris: Results of the international multicenter angina exercise (IMAGE) study. *J Am Coll Cardiol.* 1996;27(2):311–316.

105. van de Ven LL, Vermeulen A, Tana JG, et al. Which drug to choose for stable angina pectoris: A comparative study between bisoprolol and nitrates. *Int J Cardiol.* 1995;47(3):217–223.

106. Waysbort J, Meshulam N, Brunner D. Isosorbide-t-mononitrate and atenolol in the treatment of stable exertional angina. *Cardiology.* 1991;79(Suppl 2):19–26.

107. Krepp HP. Evaluation of the antianginal and anti-ischemic efficacy of slow release isosorbide-5-monitrate capsules,

bupranolol and their combination, in patients with chronic stable angina pectoris. *Cardiology.* 1991;79(Suppl 2):14–18.

108. Pepine CJ, Feldman RL, Whittle J, et al. Effect of diltiazem in patients with variant angina: A randomized double-blind trial. *Am Heart J.* 1981;101(6):719–725.

109. Antman E, Muller J, Goldberg S, et al. Nifedipine therapy for coronary-artery spasm: Experience in 127 patients. *N Engl J Med.* 1980;302(23):1269–1273.

110. Psaty BM, Heckbert SR, Koepsell TD, et al. The risk of myocardial infarction associated with antihypertensive drug therapies. *JAMA.* 1995;92(5):1326–1331.

111. Furberg CD, Psaty BM, Meyer JV. Nifedipine: Dose-related increase in mortality in patients with coronary heart disease. *Circulation.* 1995;92(5):1326–1331.

112. Opie LH, Messerli FH. Nifedipine and mortality: Grave defects in the dossier. *Circulation.* 1995;92(5):1068–1073.

113. Ad Hoc Subcommittee of the Liaison Committee of the world health organization and the international society of hypertension. Effects of calcium antagonists on the risks of coronary heart disease, cancer and bleeding. *J Hypertens.* 1997;15:105–115.

114. Schneider W, Maul FD, Bussmann WD, et al. Comparison of the antianginal efficacy of isosorbide dinitrate (ISDN) 40 mg and verapamil 120 mg three times daily in the acute trial and following two-week treatment. *Eur Heart J.* 1998;9:149–158.

115. Ankier SI, Fay L, Warrington SJ, Woodings DF. A multicentre open comparison of isosorbide-5-mononitrate and nifedipine given prophylactically to general practice patients with chronic stable angina pectoris. *J Int Med Res.* 1989;17(2):172–178.

116. Emanuelsson H, Ake H, Kristi M, Arina R. Effects of diltiazem and isosorbide-5-mononitrate, alone and in combination, on patients with stable angina pectoris. *Eur J Clin Pharmacol.* 1989;36:561–566.

117. Akhras F, Jackson G. Efficacy of nifedipine and isosorbide mononitrate in combination with atenolol in stable angina. *Lancet.* 1991;338(8774):1036–1039.

118. Cheitlin MD, Hutter AM, Jr., Brindis RG, et al. ACC/AHA expert consensus documents: Use of sildenafil (Viagra) in patients with cardiovascular disease. *J Am Coll Cardiol.* 1999;33:273–282.

119. Fung HL, Bauer JA. Mechanisms of nitrate tolerance. *Cardiovasc Drugs Ther.* 1994;8(3):489–499.

120. Chirkov YY, Chirkova LP, Horowitz JD. Nitroglycerin tolerance at the platelet level in patients with angina pectoris. *Am J Cardiol.* 1997;80(2):128–131.

121. Chaitman BR, Skettino S, DeQuattro V. Improved exercise performance on ranolazine in patients with chronic angina and a history of heart failure: The MARISA trial. *J Am Coll Cardiol.* 2001;37(Suppl A):149A.

122. Maron DJ, Grundy SM, Ridker PM, Pearson TA. Dyslipidemia, other risk factors, and the prevention of coronary heart disease. In: Fuster V, O'Rourke RA, Alexander RW, et al. (eds). *Hurst's the Heart,* 11th ed. New York, NY: Mc Graw-Hill; 2004:1093–1122.

123. Pearson TA, Blari SN, Daniels SR, et al. AHA guidelines for primary prevention of cardiovascular disease and stroke: 2002 update: Consensus panel guide to comprehensive risk reduction for adult patients without coronary or other atherosclerotic vascular diseases. *Circulation.* 2002;106:388–391.

124. Smith SC, Blair SN, Bonow RO, et al: AHA/ACC Guidelines for preventing heart attach and death in patients with atherosclerotic cardiovascular disease: 2001 Update: A Statement for Healthcare Professionals from the American Heart Association and the American College of Cardiology. *Circulation.* 2001;104:5177–1579.

125. Third Report of the National Cholesterol Education Program (NCEP) Expert Panel on Detection, Evaluation, and Treatment of High Blood Cholesterol in Adults (Adult Treatment Panel III). Final Report. *Circulation.* 2002;106:3143–3421.

126. Third Report of the National Cholesterol Education Program (NCEP) Expert Panel on Detection, Evaluation, and Treatment of High Blood Cholesterol in Adults (Adult Treatment Panel III). Final Report. National Heart, Lung, and Blood Institute, National Institutes of Health, Bethesda, MD. NIH publication No. 02–5215. September 2002. Available at: http://www.nhlbi.nih.gov/guidelines/cholesterol/atp3_rpt.htm. Accessed April 6, 2004.

127. Stamler J, Neaton J, Wentworth DN. Blood pressure (systolic and diastolic) and risk of fatal coronary heart disease. *Hypertension.* 1989;13(Suppl 5):I2–I12.

128. The Sixth Report of the Joint National Committee on Prevention, Detection, Evaluation, and Treatment of High Blood Pressure. *Arch Intern Med.* 1997;157(21):2413–2446.

129. Alderman MH, Cohen H, Roque R, Madhavan S. Effect of long-acting and short-acting calcium antagonist on cardiovascular outcomes in hypertensive patients. *Lancet.* 1997;349(9052):594–598.

130. Kannel WB, Gordon T, Castelli WP, Margolis JR. Electrocardiographic left ventricular hypertrophy and risk of coronary heart disease: The framingham study. *Ann Intern Med.* 1970;72(6):813–822.

131. Ghali JK, Liao Y, Simmons B, et al. The prognostic role of left ventricular hypertrophy in patients with or without coronary artery disease. *Ann Intern Med.* 1992;117(10):831–836.

132. Levy D, Salomon M, D'Agostino RB, et al. Prognostic implications of baseline electrocardiographic features and their serial changes in subjects with left ventricular hypertrophy. *Circulation.* 1994;90(4):1786–1793.

133. Ernst E, Resch KL. Fibrinogen as a cardiovascular risk factor: A meta-analysis and review of the literature. *Ann Intern Med.* 1993;118(12):956–963.

134. American Diabetes Association. Clinical Practice Recommendations 1998: Screening for type 2 diabetes. *Diabetes Care.* 1998;21(Suppl 1):1–98.

135. The effect of intensive treatment of diabetes on the development and progression of long-term complications in insulin-dependent diabetes mellitus: The diabetes control and complications trial research group. *N Engl J Med.* 1993;329:977–986.

136. Getz GS. Report on the Workshop on Diabetes and Mechanisms of Atherogenesis, September 17 and 18, 1992, Bethesda, MD. *Arterioscler Thromb.* 1993;13:459–464.

137. National Cholesterol Education Program. Third Report of the Expert Panel on Detection, Evaluation, and Treatment of High Blood Cholesterol in Adults (Adult Treatment Panel III). *Circulation.* 2002;106:3143–3421.

138. Eckel RH. Obesity and heart disease: A statement for healthcare professionals from the Nutrition Committee, American Heart Association. *Circulation.* 1997;96(9): 3248–3250.

139. Hulley S, Grady D, Bush T, et al. Randomized trial of estrogen plus progestin for secondary prevention of coronary heart disease in postmenopausal women: Heart and Estrogen/Progestin Replacement Study (HERS) Research Group. *JAMA.* 1998;280(7):605–613.

140. Curb JD, McTiernan A, Heckbert SR, et al. Outcomes ascertainment and adjudication methods in the women's health initiative. *Ann Epidemiol.* 2003;95: S122–S128.

141. Barrett-Connor E, Ensrud KE, Harper K, et al. Post hoc analysis of data from the multiple outcomes of raloxifene evaluation (MORE) trial on the effects of 3 years of raloxifene treatment on glycemic control and cardiovascular disease risk factors in women with and without type 2 diabetes. *Clin Ther.* 2003;25(3):919–930.

142. Jeppesen J, Hein HO, Suadicani P, Gyntelberg F. Triglyceride concentration and ischemic heart disease: An 8-year follow-up in the Copenhagen Male Study. *Circulation.* 1998;97(11):1029–1036; Erratum. *Circulation.* 1999;98(2):190.

143. Reaven GM. Insulin resistance and compensatory hyperinsulinemia: Role in hypertension, dyslipidemia, and coronary heart disease. *Am Heart J.* 1991;121(4 pt 2): 1283–1288.

144. The VA Coronary Artery Bypass Surgery Cooperative Study Group. 18-year follow-up in the Veterans Affairs Cooperative Study of Coronary Artery Bypass Surgery for Stable Angina. *Circulation.* 1992;86:121–130.

145. Varnauskas E. 12-year follow-up of survival in the randomized European Coronary Surgery Study. *N Engl J Med.* 1988;319:332–337.

146. Passamani E, Davis KB, Gillespie MJ, Killip T. A randomized trial of coronary artery bypass surgery. Survival of patients with a low ejection fraction. *N Engl J Med.* 1985;312:1665–1671.

147. Coronary Heart Disease. Triglyceride, high-density lipoprotein, and coronary heart disease. *JAMA.* 1993;269: 505–510.

148. Genest JJ, Jenner JL, McNamara JR, et al. Prevalence of lipoprotein (a) [Lp(a)] excess in coronary artery disease. *Am J Cardiol.* 1991;67(13):1039–1045.

149. Clarke R, Daly L, Robinson K, et al. Hyperhomocysteinemia: An independent risk factor for vascular disease. *N Engl J Med.* 1991;324(17):1149–1155.

150. Stampfer MJ, Malinow MR, Willett WC, et al. A prospective study of plasma homocysteine and risk of myocardial infarction in US physicians. *JAMA.* 1992;268(7):877–881.

151. Bypass Angioplasty Revascularization Investigation (BARI) Investigators. Comparison of coronary artery bypass surgery with angioplasty in patients with multivessel disease. *N Engl J Med.* 1996;335(4):217–225; Erratum. *N Engl J Med.* 1997;336(2):147.

Chapter 4

Arrhythmias

Mark C. Granberry, William D. Linn, and Robert Chilton

SEARCH STRATEGY

A systematic search of the medical literature was performed on January 9, 2008. The search, limited to human subjects and English language journals, included the National Guideline Clearinghouse, the Cochrane database, PubMed, UpToDate®, and PIER. The current American College of Cardiology (ACC)/American Heart Association (AHA)/European Society of Cardiology 2006 Guidelines for Management of Patients with Ventricular Arrhythmias and the Prevention of Sudden Cardiac Death, and the Management of Patients with Supraventricular Arrhythmias can be found at www.acc.org.

OFFICE EVALUATION

HISTORY

Cardiac arrhythmia is an abnormality of impulse generation, impulse propagation, or a combination of both. Although arrhythmias can occur in all age groups, significant rhythm disturbances are relatively uncommon in young, healthy individuals. The primary purposes of the history in evaluating a cardiac arrhythmia are to determine the underlying etiology, anatomic abnormalities, physiologic disturbances, cardiac status, and prognosis.

PHYSICAL FINDINGS

The symptoms associated with cardiac arrhythmias vary widely. They may be very minor such as an awareness of the heartbeat (palpitations). More serious symptoms usually reflect a decrease in cardiac output resulting from reduced ventricular filling during the tachycardia. Patients may describe a rapid, sustained heartbeat that may be regular or irregular, or may describe intermittent accelerations or decelerations of the heartbeat. Some patients are able to detect even slight variations in the heart rate or rhythm while others may have no awareness of any arrhythmia—even ventricular tachycardia (VT). Patients will commonly seek medical attention because of palpitations, presyncope, syncope, or symptoms of angina or heart failure.

INTERPRETATION OF THE ELECTROCARDIOGRAM

WIDE-COMPLEX RHYTHM

Wide QRS complexes result from impulses that have at least some conduction outside the normal conduction system. By definition, wide-complex tachycardias have a rate greater than 100 beats per minute and have a QRS duration greater than or equal to 120 ms. VT is one form of a wide-QRS-complex tachycardia, but a wide QRS complex may also occur in supraventricular tachycardia (SVT) when there is a conduction delay in the His–Purkinje system or there is conduction over a parallel route from the atria to the ventricle, that is, an accessory pathway. In general, the wider the QRS complex, the more likely the rhythm is to be ventricular in origin, especially when the complexes are greater than 160 ms in duration.[1] The patient's age and risk factors play a significant role in general as to the potential etiology of a wide complex rhythm. Other evidences to support the diagnosis of VT include the independent P-wave activity, fusion beats, AV dissociation, and concordance throughout the precordial leads. The absence of an RS complex in all precordial leads, or an RS interval of more than 100 ms, is indicative of VT.[2] If the origin of the wide-complex tachycardia cannot be determined, the safest option is to treat it as VT.

NARROW-COMPLEX RHYTHM

Narrow-complex tachyarrhythmias almost always have a supraventricular origin. The most common causes of a narrow-QRS-complex tachycardia are sinus tachycardia, atrial tachycardia, atrial fibrillation, atrial flutter, atrioventricular node reentrant tachycardia (AVNRT), and atrioventricular reentrant tachycardia (AVRT).

SPECIFIC ARRHYTHMIAS

SUPRAVENTRICULAR ARRHYTHMIAS

Atrial Fibrillation

Patients with atrial fibrillation often present with symptoms of palpitations, fatigue, dyspnea, or systemic emboli. However, many patients with atrial fibrillation are asymptomatic. A serious consequence of atrial fibrillation is a stroke due to thromboembolism with the embolic origin most commonly being from the left atrial appendage. If left untreated, the yearly risk for ischemic stroke averages 4.5%, but varies from greater than 1% to over 20% and is dependent upon associated disease states but not upon the duration of the arrhythmic episodes.[3] Atrial fibrillation is usually associated with hypertension, advanced age, heart failure, valvular (primarily mitral) or ischemic heart diseases, and coronary artery bypass surgery. Hyperthyroidism, pulmonary emboli, excessive alcohol intake, myocarditis, or pericarditis must also be considered. It commonly occurs after a cardiac surgery. Patients may present without heart disease or other systemic illness; a condition that has been called "lone atrial fibrillation." Recurrent atrial fibrillation can be classified as paroxysmal, persistent, and permanent. By definition, paroxysmal atrial fibrillation terminates without any intervention, persistent atrial fibrillation requires an intervention for termination, while permanent atrial fibrillation does not terminate.[4]

Diagnosis. The electrocardiogram (ECG) recording is characterized by an absence of P waves and instead shows a flat or slightly undulating baseline reflecting chaotic atrial activity. Ventricular response is irregularly irregular, most often ranging between 120 and 180 QRS complexes per minute (see Fig. 4-1A). With atrioventricular (AV) nodal blocking therapy or when intrinsic disease of the AV node is present, the ventricular rate will frequently be lower and more regular. The QRS morphology is normal unless a concomitant condition affecting the QRS exists.

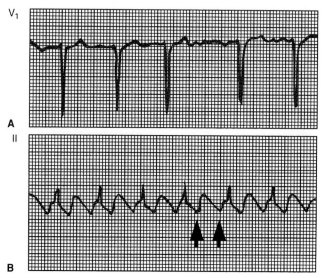

Figure 4-1. Atrial fibrillation and atrial flutter. (A) Lead V_1 demonstrates an irregularly irregular ventricular rhythm with chaotic atrial activity associated with atrial fibrillation. (B) Lead II demonstrates atrial flutter as identified by regular ventricular activity and a "saw-tooth-like" pattern (arrows) of atrial activity at an atrial rate of 300 beats per minute with a 2:1 ventricular response. (Reproduced with permission from Kasper DL et al. Harrison's Principles of Internal Medicine. NY, McGraw-Hill;2005:1345.)

Management. Atrial fibrillation is the most common arrhythmia that requires treatment. Immediate direct-current, synchronized cardioversion under mild sedation, initially at 200 J, is recommended for patients who are highly symptomatic due to the arrhythmia. Optimal chronic management is directed at stroke prevention and reduction or elimination of symptoms through either ventricular rate control or cardioversion to sinus rhythm. In addition, ECG, chest radiograph, echocardiogram, and thyroid function should be evaluated.

Both the American College of Chest Physicians (ACCP)[3] and the ACC/AHA/European Society of Cardiology have guidelines for the prevention of stroke in patients with atrial fibrillation.[5] These guidelines are centered on risk stratification to determine which patients should be treated with adjusted-dose warfarin alone, with aspirin alone, or with a combination of both. See Table 4-1 for specific recommendations from each organization. For patients who are being considered for elective cardioversion, it is important to consider the duration of the atrial fibrillation when determining the need for antithrombotic therapy. For those patients known to have had atrial fibrillation for more than 48 hours or for an unknown duration, anticoagulation with warfarin, target international normalized ratio (INR) 2.5 (range 2–3), is recommended for 3 weeks prior to elective cardioversion and for at

Table 4-1. Antithrombotic Therapy for Patients with Atrial Fibrillation

ACCP	Recommendation	ACC–AHA–ESC	Recommendation
		Age >75 y, primary prevention, considered at increased risk of bleeding	Warfarin INR 2; range 1.6–2.5
Age >75 y or presence of any risk factor*	Warfarin target INR 2.5; range 2–3	Patients at high risk of stroke[†]	Warfarin target INR 2–3
Age 65–75 y in the absence of other risk factors*	Warfarin target INR, 2.5; range 2–3 or aspirin 325 mg daily		
Age <65 y in the absence of risk factors*	Aspirin 325 mg daily	Age <60 y, no heart disease	Aspirin 325 mg daily or no therapy
		Age <60 y with heart disease but no risk factors[†]	Aspirin 325 mg daily
		Age 60–75 y, no risk factors	Aspirin 325 mg daily
		Patients with CAD	Aspirin <100 mg daily or clopidogrel 75 mg daily may be given with warfarin INR, 2–3

*Prior ischemic stroke/TIA/systemic embolism, diabetes mellitus or history of hypertension, impaired LV systolic function or heart failure.
[†]Heart failure, LV EF ≤0.35, or history of hypertension.
ACCP, American College of Chest Physicians; ACC–AHA–ESC, American College of Cardiology–American Heart Association–European Society of Cardiology; CAD, coronary artery disease; DM, diabetes mellitus; EF, ejection fraction; INR, international normalized ratio; LV, left ventricular; TIA, transient ischemic attack.

least 4 weeks afterward.[3] The P wave on the ECG may return but the mechanical contraction may not become functional for many weeks. The need for anticoagulant drug therapy for paroxysmal atrial fibrillation is controversial and should be based on the risk for thromboembolism.

The management of symptoms is best viewed in context of the pattern of atrial fibrillation (paroxysmal, persistent, or permanent). For patients with a first episode of paroxysmal atrial fibrillation, antiarrhythmic drug therapy may or may not be necessary, depending on the severity of the associated symptoms. Ventricular rate control with drug therapy can be used if symptoms warrant their use. The goals for the ventricular rate during episodes of atrial fibrillation are 60 to 80 beats per minute at rest and 90 to 115 beats per minute during exercise. The pharmacologic agents available to control the ventricular rate response include the β-adrenergic antagonists, non-dihydropyridine calcium-channel blockers (non-DHP CCBs), and digoxin. Because of its inability to control the ventricular rate during exercise, digoxin is best used in combination with other agents; but may be used alone when these other agents are not tolerated.

Recurrent paroxysmal atrial fibrillation, with minimal or no symptoms, can be managed with ventricular rate control using drugs as described at the end of this chapter. Patients who display debilitating symptoms, conversion to sinus rhythm can be attempted with the antiarrhythmic drugs such as amiodarone, propafenone, ibutilide, dofetilide, or flecainide. These drugs vary in

effectiveness and the optimal choice should be based on their safety profile in the presence of the conditions listed. Their use has diminished due to their risk for adverse drug reactions. Antithrombotic therapy should be used in patients with recurrent paroxysmal atrial fibrillation who are at high risk for stroke, that is, patients having any of the following: prior ischemic stroke, transient ischemic attach or systemic embolism, age greater than 75 years, moderately or severely impaired left ventricular (LV) systolic function and/or heart failure, history of hypertension, or diabetes mellitus.[3]

For persistent atrial fibrillation, two strategies have been developed that are targeted at either ventricular rate control or rhythm control. Occasionally, when AV nodal blocking drugs are used, the patient's heart rate is reduced to unacceptably low values. However, when therapy is withdrawn, unacceptably high ventricular rates may result. It may then be necessary to insert a ventricular pacemaker before reinitiating AV nodal blocking therapy.

Restoration of sinus rhythm (a rhythm-control strategy) can be made with electrical cardioversion alone, drug therapy alone, or a combination of both. Drugs effectively used for the conversion of atrial fibrillation to sinus rhythm include flecainide, propafenone, moricizine, procainamide, dofetilide, amiodarone, and sotalol. Therapy should be chosen based on the presence of underlying cardiac conditions. Three studies have compared the rate-control versus the rhythm-control strategies on cardiovascular events, mortality, and safety endpoints. The Atrial Fibrillation Follow-up Investigation of Rhythm Management trial found no significant difference in mortality between the two strategies after 5 years of therapy.[6] The Rate Control Versus Electrical Cardioversion for Persistent Atrial Fibrillation trial compared the rate-control strategy to the rhythm-control strategy on the primary composite endpoint of deaths from cardiovascular causes, heart failure, thromboembolic complications, bleeding, implantation of a pacemaker, and severe adverse effects of drugs.[7] There was no significant difference between the two groups after approximately 2 years, neither in the primary composite endpoint, which showed the percentages as 17.2% versus 22.6%, an absolute difference of −5.4% (90% confidence interval, −11.0–0.4), nor in any of the individual components of the composite. Pharmacological Intervention in Atrial Fibrillation study similarly found no significant difference in the percentage of patients who had an improvement in symptoms because of a rhythm-control strategy and because of a rate-control strategy.[8] Therefore, treatment of permanent atrial fibrillation should be directed at ventricular rate control and appropriate antithrombotic drug therapy.

Atrial Flutter

Atrial flutter is often due to a reentry tract around the tricuspid valve; although less common than atrial fibrillation, it has a similar presentation. The arrhythmia may be paroxysmal, persistent, or rarely permanent. If it lasts for more than 1 week, it often converts to atrial fibrillation.

Diagnosis. The ECG shows discrete P waves at a rate of 250 to 350 per minute without a flat baseline between waves; these represent the so-called flutter waves. The P waves are quite prominent in leads II and III and are often described in a sawtooth pattern. AV blocks of 2:1 (2 flutter waves:1 QRS) are most common; however, 3:1 and 4:1 blocks can also be seen, especially when drugs that block the AV node are administered (Fig. 4-1B). Changing a 2:1 block to a 3:1 or 4:1 block may make it easier to identify the sawtooth pattern. Carotid massage or AV nodal blocking drugs can accomplish this.

Management. For patients with atrial flutter, the ACCP and ACC/AHA recommend that antithrombotic therapy decisions should follow the guidelines established for atrial fibrillation.[3] For immediate conversion, direct-current, synchronized cardioversion at 25 to 50 J under mild sedation is very effective. If immediate conversion to sinus rhythm is not indicated, AV nodal blocking drugs such as digoxin, β-adrenergic antagonists, or the non-DHP calcium-channel antagonists may

be used to control the ventricular response. Once ventricular rate control has been accomplished, attempts to convert to sinus rhythm with antiarrhythmic drugs should be considered. Additionally, ablation of the reentry tract responsible for the arrhythmia is a highly effective treatment and can cure more than 85% of patients.

Paroxysmal Supraventricular Tachycardia

While atrial fibrillation and atrial flutter can be considered supraventricular arrhythmias, the term paroxysmal supraventricular tachycardia (PSVT) generally refers to AVNRT and AVRT. PSVT can present at any time of life, and recurrences are common. Patients with PSVT often present with fatigue, chest pain, palpitations, dizziness, and neck pulsations. Heart rates are usually between 150 and 250 per minute during the arrhythmia, usually with an abrupt onset and termination. Termination by vagal maneuvers suggests a bypass tract involving AV nodal tissue. Supraventricular tachyarrhythmias almost always involve one or more bypass tracts and require either atrial or AV junctional tissues for either the initiation or the maintenance of the arrhythmia. The key features of these arrhythmias are differences in conduction and refractoriness between the AV node and a bypass tract. One pathway has relatively slow conduction velocity (slow pathway) with a short refractory period and the other pathway (fast pathway) has relatively rapid conduction velocity with a long refractory period (Fig. 4-2).

AVNRT is the more common form of PSVT. It results from two or more functionally distinct conduction pathways, either within or adjacent to the AV node. During sinus rhythm, conduction from the atria to the ventricles occurs over the fast pathway that results in a normal PR interval. A requirement for arrhythmia initiation is a critically timed atrial premature depolarization that is blocked in the fast accessory pathway secondary to its long refractory period. Anterograde conduction down the slow pathway allows time for repolarization of the fast pathway, facilitating retrograde conduction. Depending upon a critical balance of conduction velocity and refractoriness of the pathways, the arrhythmia may be sustained or may be spontaneously terminated. The near-simultaneous depolarization of the atria and the ventricles results in P waves that are inscribed upon the QRS and are therefore not usually visible on the ECG. A less-common initiating mechanism occurs when a critically timed ventricular premature depolarization results in retrograde conduction over the slow pathway and anterograde conduction over the fast pathway. When this reentry circuit is sustained, clearly visible inverted P waves are evident.

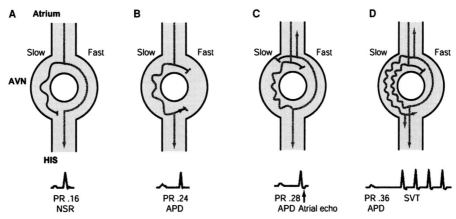

Figure 4-2. Mechanism of AV nodal reentry: The atrium, AV node (AVN), and His bundle are shown schematically. The AV node is longitudinally dissociated into two pathways, slow and fast, with different functional properties. In each, red lines denote excitation in the AV node, which is manifest on the surface electrocardiogram (ECG), while black lines denote conduction that is concealed and not apparent on the surface ECG. (A) During sinus rhythm (NSR), the impulse from the atrium conducts down both pathways. However, only conduction over the fast pathway is manifest on the surface ECG, producing a normal PR interval of 0.16 s. (B) An atrial premature depolarization (APD) blocks the fast pathway. The impulse conducts over the slow pathway to the His bundle and the ventricles, producing a PR interval of 0.24 s. Because the impulse is premature, conduction over the slow pathway occurs more slowly than it would during sinus rhythm. (C) A more premature atrial impulse blocks the fast pathway, conducting with increased delay in the slow pathway, producing a PR interval of 0.28 s. The impulse conducts retrogradely up the fast pathway producing a single atrial echo. Sustained reentry is prevented by subsequent block in the slow pathway. (D) A still more premature atrial impulse blocks initially the fast pathway, conducting over the slow pathway with increasing delay, producing a PR interval of 0.36 s. Retrograde conduction occurs over the fast pathway and reentry occurs, producing a sustained ventricular tachycardia (SVT). (Reproduced with permission from Josephson ME: *Clinical Cardiac Electrophysiology*, 2nd ed. Philadelphia, Lea & Febiger, 2002.)

AVRT occurs when one or more accessory pathways exist that are distinct from the AV node. The accessory pathway often has relatively fast conduction velocity together with a long refractory period while the AV node provides the slow pathway with a short refractory period. During sinus rhythm, conduction to the ventricles occurs through the AV node, but there is early activation of ventricular tissue through the fast accessory pathway. This condition is called preexcitation. Initiation of the arrhythmia may occur similar to the mechanism described for AVNRT except that the accessory pathway is outside of the AV node. Similar to AVNRT, conduction may travel in the opposite direction where there is anterograde conduction from the atria to ventricle over the accessory pathway and retrogradely up the bundle branches, bundle of His, and AV node back to the atria.

Diagnosis

AVNRT. The history and physical examination typically reveal few clues to aid in the diagnosis of PSVT. However, rapid jugular venous pulsations, referred to as frog sign, can occur in AVNRT due to the simultaneous activation of the atria and ventricles, which results in atrial contraction against closed AV valves. The typical slow or fast AVNRT uses the slow pathway for anterograde conduction and the fast pathway for retrograde conduction. Usually, the P wave is obscured by the QRS complex. Carotid sinus massage or a Valsalva maneuver may terminate the rhythm.

AVRT. During sinus rhythm, a delta wave and a short PR interval due to preexcitation of ventricular tissue may be seen and is called Wolff-Parkinson-White (WPW) syndrome. During the episodes of AVRT, if the reentry circuit results in conduction down the slow pathway and up the fast pathway, the QRS complex will appear normal and there will be inverted P waves following the QRS. This more common form of the arrhythmia is called orthodromic AVRT. Antidromic AVRT occurs when the impulse travels from the atria to the ventricle by the accessory pathway and from the ventricles to the atria through the bundle branches, bundle of His, and the AV node. In this situation, the

QRS complex will be wide, and inverted P waves will again be seen following the QRS.

Management. Referral to an arrhythmia specialist is recommended for patients with a wide-complex tachycardia of unknown origin, WPW syndrome, patients desiring no drug treatment, and those with severe symptoms such as syncope or dyspnea during palpitations.[9] Synchronized direct-current cardioversion, initially at 100 J, should be administered to patients with hemodynamic instability or severe symptoms related to the arrhythmia.

AVNRT

ACUTE MANAGEMENT.   Acute management of AVNRT involves vagal maneuvers such as carotid massage, Valsalva maneuver, cold-water facial immersion, or intravenous (IV) administration of adenosine, a non-DHP, calcium-channel blocker, or a β-adrenergic antagonist. Adenosine has the advantage of a very rapid onset and short duration of action and is the preferred drug therapy except in patients with asthma. Longer acting calcium-channel blocker and β-adrenergic antagonists have the benefit of suppression of atrial and ventricular depolarizations and may be preferred as means to suppress recurrences of PSVT. Similar to the treatment of other supraventricular tachyarrhythmias, synchronized direct-current cardioversion should be used to manage patients with hemodynamic instability related to the arrhythmia.

CHRONIC MANAGEMENT.   Chronic management of AVNRT can involve no therapy, catheter ablation, or drug therapy. Indications for ablation therapy depend on clinical judgment and patient preference. Ablation targeting the slow pathway has been shown to be more than 95% effective with a very low incidence of significant complications (second- or third-degree AV block) when performed in centers of excellence.[5] AV nodal blocking drugs (non-DHP, calcium-channel antagonists, β-blockers, digoxin, etc.), although less effective than ablation, are equally effective among themselves and are considered first-line drug therapy. Therapy decisions are therefore dependent on patient tolerance. For patients who do not respond to AV nodal blocking drugs and who do not have structural heart disease, flecainide or propafenone are options. These drugs can be combined with β-adrenergic antagonists to increase efficacy and to reduce the risk of one-to-one conduction over the AV node if atrial flutter occurs.[5] Sotalol, amiodarone, and dofetilide, while effective, are rarely used due to the risk of proarrhythmia and other toxicities.

For patients with infrequent episodes of PSVT, no therapy, and vagal maneuvers alone or in combination with single-dose oral-drug therapy, may be considered.

Single-dose drug therapy, the so-called "pill-in-the-pocket" therapy, may reduce the need for emergency department visits. Options shown to be effective include flecainide and diltiazem plus propranolol. In this situation, immediate release preparations should be used.

AVRT

ACUTE MANAGEMENT.   Immediate direct-current cardioversion is recommended for the treatment of hemodynamically unstable tachyarrhythmias. For the acute management of suspected AVRT in stable patients, it should be noted that if the QRS is wide (>120 ms) it is important to differentiate SVT from VT. If no definitive diagnosis can be made, then the arrhythmia should be treated as VT.

CHRONIC MANAGEMENT.   Similar to AVNRT, options for the chronic management of AVRT include no therapy, catheter ablation, or drug therapy. While catheter ablation may be used in most patients, it is first-line therapy for those with WPW syndrome and those who experience hemodynamic instability during the arrhythmia. In patients with AVRT that is poorly tolerated but is without preexcitation, catheter ablation is preferred. If drug therapy is preferred, flecainide, propafenone, sotalol, or amiodarone may be used. Verapamil and diltiazem should not be used as monotherapy for patients with an accessory pathway capable of rapid conduction during atrial fibrillation or atrial flutter. For patients without preexcitation and who have minimal symptoms during the arrhythmia, vagal maneuvers with or without drug therapy may be preferred. AV nodal blocking drugs, flecainide, propafenone, "pill-in-the-pocket," and possibly amiodarone, or sotalol are options for drug therapy. In general, the use of drugs other than β-blockers or calcium channel blockers should be directed by experts in arrhythmia management because of important side effects.

VENTRICULAR ARRHYTHMIAS

It is important to distinguish between SVT with aberrant ventricular conduction and VT. Table 4-2 outlines the specific criteria for each. Treatments for SVT such as adenosine, verapamil, and β-adrenergic antagonists are ineffective in patients with VT and rapid deterioration could occur.

Ventricular Premature Complexes and Nonsustained VT

Ventricular premature complexes (VPCs) may occur as single isolated events, in pairs (couplets), or in patterns with a sinus beat in which the VPC occurs at every second (bigeminy) or third (trigeminy) beat. VT occurs

Table 4-2. Diagnostic Criteria for the Differential Diagnosis of Ventricular Tachycardia and Wide-QRS-Complex Supraventricular Tachycardia

Factors that predict VT:
Absence of RS complex in all precordial leads
If RS complex present in one or more leads, RS interval >100 ms
    as measured from the onset of the R wave to the deepest part
    of the S wave
If RS complex present in one or more leads, RS interval <100 ms,
    evidence of AV dissociation
RS interval <100 ms, AV dissociation not clearly demonstrated
    (P waves not associated with QRS complexes, QRS
    morphology criteria)

when three or more VPCs occur consecutively at a rate greater than 100 beats per minute. Non-sustained VT is defined as the one lasting for less than 30 s. Both the rates and consequences of VT vary. The severity of the symptoms is related to the duration of the arrhythmia and underlying cardiac abnormalities. Patients with VPCs and nonsustained VTs are frequently asymptomatic while patients with sustained VTs almost always have symptoms related to reduced cardiac output.

Diagnosis. VPCs occur early in relation to the expected beat of the basic rhythm. The QRS complexes are abnormal in duration and configuration. There is usually a full compensatory pause following the VPC. The morphology of the complexes may vary in the same patient.

Management. Patients with VPCs or nonsustained VTs without organic heart disease have a relatively low risk of adverse outcomes. The risk of treatment with antiarrhythmic agents outweighs the benefit because the proarrhythmic effects of these drugs often increase the risk of sudden cardiac death. The Cardiac Arrhythmia Suppression Trial evaluated postmyocardial infarction patients who had frequent asymptomatic VPCs without significant VT.[10] Patients received flecainide, encainide (no longer available), or placebo. They were followed for an average of 10 months. These drugs were highly effective at reducing the number of VPCs. However, the relative risk of death or cardiac arrest due to arrhythmia was over 2.5 times greater in the treatment group as compared to the placebo group. Another arm of this study was stopped early because of increased mortality in patients receiving moricizine therapy.[11] Thus, eliminating asymptomatic or minimally symptomatic VPCs with antiarrhythmic therapy is not recommended.

Sustained VT

Sustained VT has a duration greater than 30 s. Usually the ventricular rate is between 140 and 200 beats per minute. Impaired LV function is a risk factor for sudden death and an assessment of sustained VT should include an evaluation of LV function. Symptoms are related to the rate of the VT and the degree of LV impairment. Sustained VT can be classified as monomorphic or polymorphic based on the shape of the QRS complexes. This has important prognostic implications.

Monomorphic VT

Diagnosis. The diagnosis of monomorphic VT can be made when three or more wide QRS complexes occur at a rate of over 100 beats per minute without a change in the morphology. Although a QRS duration of more than 140 ms favors VT, in patients with a preexisting bundle branch block, SVT can also have prolonged QRS complexes. The presence of fusion beats also favor the diagnosis of VT. The RR interval in monomorphic VT is generally constant.

Management. Immediate cardioversion of VT to sinus rhythm can be achieved through direct-current cardioversion for patients who are hemodynamically unstable and should be delivered in a series of synchronized shocks beginning at 100 J. Chronic management may include the use of an implantable cardioverter defibrillator (ICD); a summary of these indications is provided later in this chapter. The options for the treatment of sustained monomorphic VT include drug therapy, cardioversion, and pacing. The treatment should also consist of the optimal management of impaired LV function, if present, with angiotensin-converting-enzyme inhibitors, aldosterone antagonists, and β-adrenergic antagonists. Overdrive right ventricular pacing at a rate 10% to 30% in excess of the tachycardia rate can be effective. Pacing is generally reserved for patients who remain hemodynamically stable during the arrhythmia and who do not tolerate or respond to antiarrhythmic drug therapy. Drug therapy should take into consideration any impairment of LV function.[12] For patients with monomorphic VT and normal ventricular function, procainamide or sotalol are preferred; other acceptable options are amiodarone or lidocaine. For patients with impaired LV function, amiodarone or lidocaine is preferred. Only one agent should be used in order to minimize the potential proarrhythmic effect of these drugs.

Polymorphic VT

Diagnosis. VT with a continuously varying QRS morphology is called polymorphic VT. Polymorphic VT includes a specific syndrome referred to as torsades de pointes, which is characterized by QRS peaks that "twist" around the baseline. A prolonged baseline QT interval (usually greater than 500 ms) suggests torsades de pointes.[13] Torsades de pointes can be caused by drugs that prolong refractoriness of ventricular tissue (antiarrhythmics such as quinidine and procainamide, tricyclic antidepressants, phenothiazines, and some antibiotics), hypokalemia, hypomagnesemia, and congenital prolongation of the QT interval.[14]

Management. Polymorphic VT is often associated with acute myocardial ischemia and tends to be more electrically unstable than monomorphic VT. Hemodynamic collapse is common. As with other tachyarrhythmias, VT causing hemodynamic collapse or severe symptoms should be treated immediately with direct-current cardioversion. For stable patients with polymorphic VT, a primary consideration is the baseline QT interval. For patients with a normal baseline QT interval, treatment should be directed towards correction of ischemia or any electrolyte abnormality. Drug therapy may include β-adrenergic antagonists, lidocaine, amiodarone, procainamide, or sotalol.[5] For those patients with impaired LV function, amiodarone is preferred.

Treatment of torsade de pointes consists of discontinuing an offending agent, correction of electrolyte abnormalities, and administration of magnesium, even in the face of a normal serum magnesium level. Long-term management of congenital forms of torsades de pointes may include ventricular pacing. Additional treatment options include overdrive pacing, use of isoproterenol as a chronotrope prior to pacing, or use of lidocaine.[5]

BRADYARRHYTHMIAS

Sinus Node

Sinus bradycardia is a sinus rhythm with a rate of less than 60 beats per minute. It can occur as a result of conditions such as sick sinus syndrome, inferior-wall myocardial infarction (Bezold–Jarisch reflex), hypothyroidism, or from the use of β-adrenergic antagonists.[15] Bradycardia may occur normally in persons with good physical conditioning or during sleep. Treatment should be considered for persons with symptoms caused by decreased cardiac output related to the bradycardia. Sinus node dysfunction may present as either impaired automaticity of the sinus node or impaired conduction from the sinus node to the atria.[16] Sick sinus syndrome is one form of sinus node dysfunction and can lead to sinus bradycardia, sinoatrial (SA) block, or sinus arrest. Any of these conditions can be interspersed with periods of normal sinus rhythm. When sinus arrest occurs or the bradycardia becomes severe, the subsidiary pacemaker activity is shifted to tis-

sues with lower levels of automaticity such as the atria, AV node, or His–Purkinje system. Sinus node dysfunction can also result in bradycardia–tachycardia syndrome in which sinus node automaticity is depressed by atrial fibrillation, flutter, or tachycardia such that sinus bradycardia or sinus arrest follows the tachycardia.

AV Node

Conduction blocks at the AV node are frequent and important causes of bradyarrhythmias. These blocks are classified by whether the impulses are delayed, intermittently blocked, or completely blocked.

First-degree AV block consists of an impulse conduction delay at the AV node. This results in a prolongation of the PR interval, which becomes greater than 200 ms, where each P wave is followed by a QRS complex. The ventricles are activated in a normal manner and the QRS complex is narrow. First-degree AV block alone does not result in symptoms, but it may progress to higher grades of AV block. High vagal tone, as well as drugs that slow AV conduction, can cause first-degree AV block.

Second-degree AV block results from intermittent block of the AV node. Because of this blockage, some impulses from the atria are not conducted to the ventricles. As a result, some P waves are not followed by a QRS complex and the ratio of P waves to QRS complexes varies greatly. Two forms of second-degree AV block exist: Mobitz type I (also called Wenckebach) (Fig. 4-3) and Mobitz type II (Fig. 4-4). In Mobitz type I, the block usually occurs at the level of the AV node. There is a progressive delay in conduction through the AV node so that the PR interval increases over several successive beats until an impulse is not conducted to the ventricles. After the nonconducted P wave, the cycle repeats. In Mobitz type II, intermittent atrial impulses are not conducted to the ventricles. The PR interval of the conducted beats remains constant. This impaired conduction is located in the bundle of His or the bundle branches; thus, wide QRS complexes are frequently observed. Mobitz type I is usually associated with a heart rate that is adequate to maintain a sufficient cardiac output so that the patient remains asymptomatic. However, this arrhythmia can progress to the more severe heart blocks. In Mobitz type II, the heart rate is often low enough to cause symptoms.

Third-degree AV block occurs when no impulse from the atria is conducted to the ventricle. On the ECG, the P waves have no relationship to the QRS complexes and are usually more frequent than QRS complexes. The heart rate and the configuration of the QRS complex will depend upon the site of the ventricular pacemaker. If the pacemaker is within the AV node, the heart rate

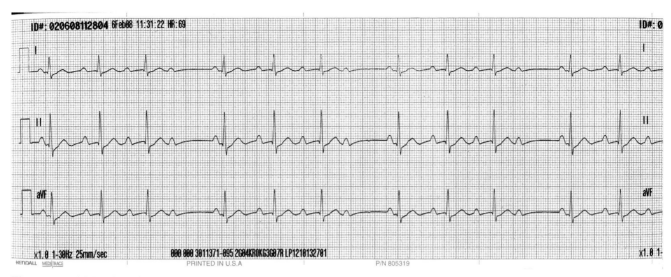

Figure 4-3. Mobitz Type I.

will usually be 40 to 60 beats per minute. Heart rates will be lower if the pacemaker is within the bundle of His, 40 to 50 beats per minute, or within the ventricle, 15 to 40 beats per minute. When the pacemaker is located below the bifurcation of the common bundle, the QRS duration will be prolonged.

CARDIAC PACING

The indications for the placement of a permanent pacemaker can be divided into the following categories: bradyarrhythmias and nonbradyarrhythmias. Recommendations for permanent pacing in bradyarrhythmias can be categorized into those indicated for AV block, AV block associated with myocardial infarction, chronic bifascicular or trifascicular block, and sinus node dysfunction.[17] See Table 4-3 for specific indications.

While the majority of indications are related to bradyarrhythmias, pacing can also be used to prevent or terminate tachyarrhythmias and also for hemodynamic improvement. Pacing can prevent the pause-dependent tachycardia in patients with torsades de pointes associated with the long QT syndrome. In addition, several studies also suggest that pacing can prevent recurrences

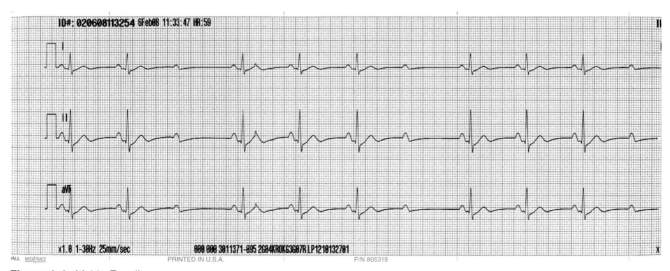

Figure 4-4. Mobitz Type II.

Table 4-3. Major Indications for Permanent Pacing*

Acquired AV Block in Adults
- Third-degree and advanced second-degree AV block associated with one of the following:
  - bradycardia with symptoms
  - documented asystole of ≥3 s
  - arrhythmias and other medical conditions that require drugs that result in symptomatic bradyarrhythmia
  - catheter ablation of the AV junction
  - postoperative AV block that is not expected to resolve after cardiac surgery
  - neuromuscular diseases with AV block
- Second-degree AV block associated with symptomatic bradycardia
- Asymptomatic third-degree block with average awake ventricular rates of 40 bpm (especially if cardiomegaly or left ventricular dysfunction is present)

Chronic Bifascicular and Trifascicular Block
- Intermittent third-degree AV block
- Type II second-degree AV block
- Alternating bundle–branch block

Atrioventricular Block Associated with Acute Myocardial Infarction
- Persistent second-degree AV block in the His–Purkinje system with bilateral bundle block or third-degree AV block within or below the His–Purkinje system
- Transient advanced (second- or third-degree) infranodal AV block and associated bundle–branch block
- Persistent and symptomatic second- or third-degree AV block
- Persistent second- or third-degree AV block

Sinus Node Dysfunction
- Sinus node dysfunction with documented symptomatic bradycardia, including frequent sinus pauses that produce symptoms
- Symptomatic chronotropic incompetence
- Sinus node dysfunction occurring spontaneously or as a result of necessary drug therapy, with heart rate <40 bpm when a clear association between significant symptoms consistent with bradycardia and actual presence of bradycardia has not been documented

*See guidelines for complete listing.
AV, atrioventricular; bpm, beats per minutes.
Adapted from: Gehi AK, Mehta D, Gomes JA. Evaluation and management of patients after implantable cardioverter defibrillator shock. *JAMA.* 2006;296: 2839–2847.

of arrhythmias in patients with intermittent atrial fibrillation and coexisting sinus node dysfunction. Although rarely needed as a treatment, overdrive pacing may be used to control SVT in the unlikely event of failure of catheter ablation and drugs. Indications related to hemodynamic improvement are enhancement of the AV synchrony in dilated cardiomyopathy and reduction of the LV outflow gradient in hypertrophic obstructive cardiomyopathy.

MONITORING A PATIENT WITH A PACEMAKER

Patients with pacemakers should receive regular follow-up either in the clinic or by primarily transtelephonic

monitoring in addition to the clinical follow-up. In either situation, the assessment should include a collection of a nonmagnet ECG strip—an ECG strip with a magnet applied to the pacemaker—and measurement of magnet rate and pulse width (duration over which the output is delivered). The schedule of follow-up should begin with a monitoring every 2 weeks for the first month after implantation followed by monitoring every 4 to 8 weeks thereafter.

IMPLANTABLE CARDIOVERTER DEFIBRILLATORS

The indications for the use of ICDs in the prevention and treatment of ventricular arrhythmias have expanded since the first device was implanted in 1980. Currently, ICDs are indicated for patients who survive a life-threatening ventricular arrhythmia (i.e., secondary prophylaxis). ICDs are also known to benefit certain patients who are at increased risk for sudden cardiac death but have not experienced a life-threatening arrhythmia (primary prophylaxis). Such patients are those who have an ischemic, dilated cardiomyopathy, an ejection fraction (EF) of less than 0.35, New York Heart Association class II or III heart failure in addition to a prior myocardial infarction, or those with a nonischemic dilated cardiomyopathy for more than 9 months, NYHA class II or III heart failure, and an EF less than 0.35.[18] Antiarrhythmic drug therapy can be initiated in patients with ICDs in order to reduce the frequency of defibrillator shocks. One study showed that after 1 year of therapy, shock rates were 10.3% for patients treated with a combination of β-blockers and amiodarone, 24.3% in those treated with sotalol, and 38.5% for those treated with other β-blockers.[19] However, most antiarrhythmic drugs alter the fibrillation threshold and the ICD may not be able to terminate the arrhythmia. Before starting any antiarrhythmic drug, an electrophysiologist should be consulted.

HIGH-RISK ECGs

Electrocardiography is the most commonly performed procedure used in the diagnosis of heart diseases. ECG abnormalities may indicate myocardial ischemia, metabolic disturbances, or arrhythmias. Unfortunately, recent studies suggest that the overall performance in interpreting ECGs is low.[20,21] Certain ECGs represent conditions that a primary care provider may be expected to treat in an emergency situation. These include VT, complete heart block, ST-segment-elevation myocardial infarction, prolonged QT interval, and hyperkalemia (see Figures 4-5 to 4-9).

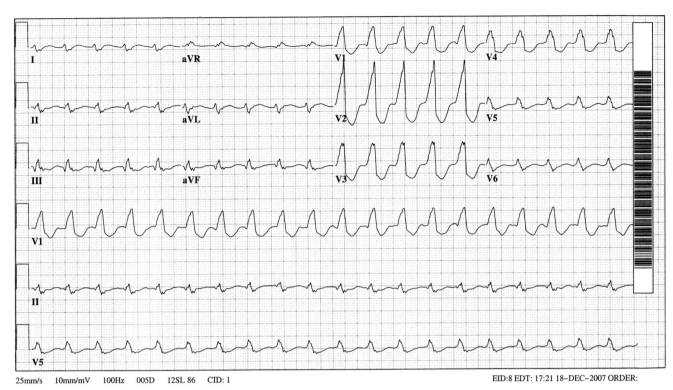

25mm/s   10mm/mV   100Hz   005D   12SL 86   CID: 1
EID:8 EDT: 17:21 18–DEC–2007 ORDER:

Figure 4-5. VT in a 71 year-old man. The patient has known coronary artery disease. He complained of palpitations and acute chest pain just prior to this ECG. The ECG shows sustained VT with a rate of 114 bpm, QRS prolongation, and AV dissociation.

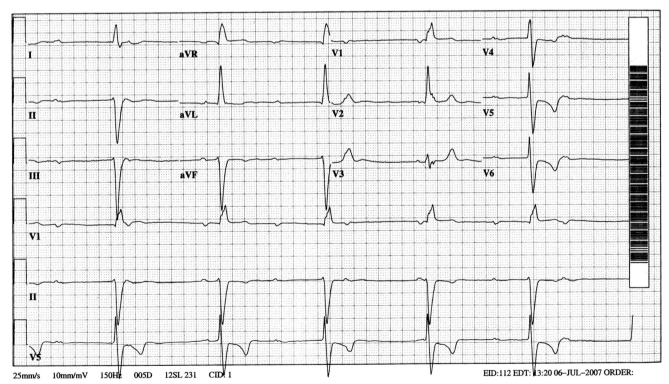

25mm/s   10mm/mV   150Hz   005D   12SL 231   CID: 1
EID:112 EDT: 13:20 06–JUL–2007 ORDER:

Figure 4-6. Complete heart block in an 84 year-old man. The patient presented with weakness, nausea, and some dyspnea. The ECG shows third-degree AV block with a wide QRS junctional escape rhythm.

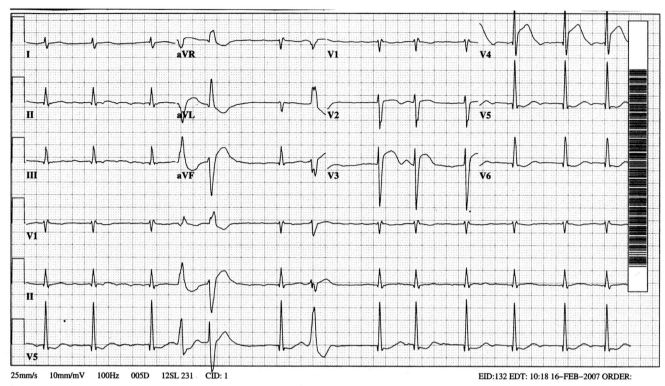

25mm/s 10mm/mV 100Hz 005D 12SL 231 CID: 1   EID:132 EDT: 10:18 16–FEB–2007 ORDER:

Figure 4-7. ST elevation MI in an 85 year-old man. The patient awoke with a crushing 10/10 midsternal chest pain radiating to both arms. The pain improved slightly with sublingual nitroglycerin. The ECG shows atrial fibrillation with premature ventricular complexes in the rightward axis with ST elevation in V3 and V4 (anterior wall) and mild ST depression in V5 and V6.

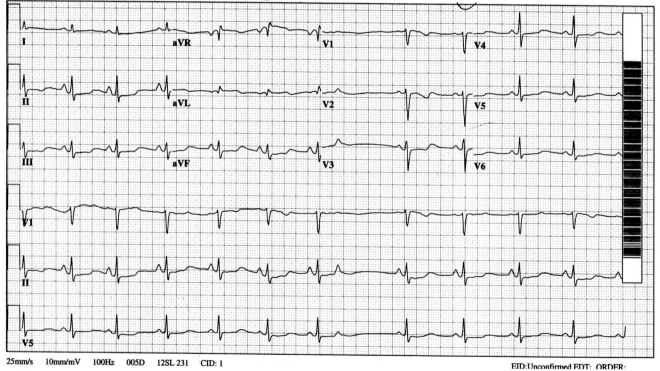

25mm/s 10mm/mV 100Hz 005D 12SL 231 CID: 1   EID:Unconfirmed EDT: ORDER:

Figure 4-8. Prolonged QT syndrome.

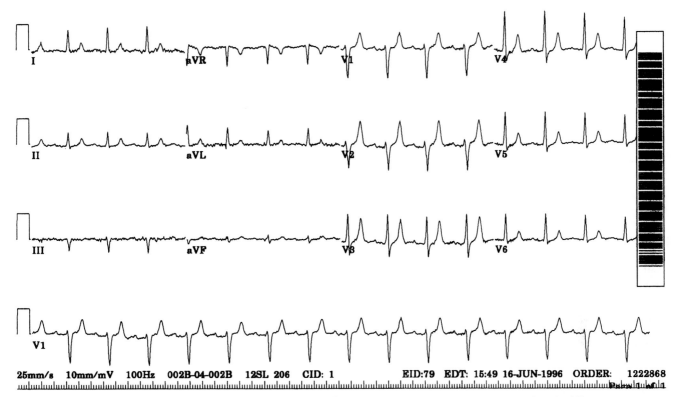

25mm/s 10mm/mV 100Hz 002B-04-002B 12SL 206 CID: 1   EID:79 EDT: 15:49 16-JUN-1996 ORDER: 1222868

Figure 4-9. T-wave changes secondary to hyperkalemia. The ECG shows sinus rhythm with tall, narrow, and peaked T-waves.

PERIOPERATIVE USE OF ANTIARRHYTHMIC AGENTS

β-adrenergic antagonists have been shown to decrease both the risk for perioperative cardiac events and the 6-month mortality rates in high-risk patients undergoing noncardiac surgery.[22] High-risk patients are those who have required β-adrenergic antagonists in the recent past to control symptoms of angina, hypertension, or symptomatic arrhythmias. β-adrenergic antagonists are also recommended for patients undergoing vascular surgery who are at high cardiac risk due to ischemia found in preoperative testing. These agents may also be beneficial for patients who are identified to have untreated hypertension, coronary artery diseases, or other major coronary risk factors. The β-adrenergic antagonist should be started several days to weeks prior to surgery and be titrated to achieve a resting heart rate between 50 and 60 beats per minute.

Arrhythmias commonly occur after cardiac surgery with rates of atrial fibrillation and atrial flutter of up to 40% after coronary artery bypass graft surgery and 60% following valve replacement.[23] The proposed mechanisms include atrial distension, atrial inflammation due to trauma, altered atrial repolarization due to elec-trolyte and volume shifts, and ischemic injury.[24] Most occurrences of atrial fibrillation after cardiac surgery are self-limiting but can often recur. Limited data are available to guide therapeutic options but recommendations have been published that suggest amiodarone for pharmacologic conversion of atrial fibrillation or atrial flutter in hemodynamically stable perioperative patients with depressed LV function.[25] For patients without heart failure, sotalol is a reasonable choice. It is recommended that therapy be continued for 4 to 6 weeks following surgery.

SPECIFIC ANTIARRHYTHMIC AGENTS

ADENOSINE

Adenosine is a naturally occurring compound in the body and is useful as an antiarrhythmic agent; it causes activation of the delayed rectifier potassium channels (I_{Kr}) channel by activating the A_1 receptor. This results in marked hyperpolarization that directly inhibits AV nodal conduction. It is highly effective (>95%) for the conversion of PSVT to sinus rhythm and is the drug of choice for this arrhythmia. Adenosine should be given as a peripheral IV bolus of 6 mg over 1 to 2 s and can be repeated with 12 mg after 1 to 2 minutes, if necessary. If given by a central line, the dose should be reduced to 3 mg. It has a very short half-life of 10 s and therefore requires a rapid bolus administration. In addition to its antiarrhythmic properties, it also produces vasodilation and may cause flushing and hypotension in approximately 20% of patients. Complete AV block often occurs but is short lived. It is contraindicated in patients with asthma. Theophylline and caffeine reduce the effects of adenosine by blocking the A_1 receptor, and dipyridamole potentiates its effects.

AMIODARONE

Amiodarone is classified as a Vaughan Williams class III antiarrhythmic agent due to its ability to prolong the action potential duration. (See Table 4-4 for Vaughan Williams classification of antiarrhythmic drugs.) Amiodarone is indicated for both ventricular and supraventricular arrhythmias and is safe for use in patients with impaired LV function and heart failure.[26] Its mechanism of action is complex and includes the blockade of calcium, sodium and I_{Kr} channels and β-adrenergic receptors. Its effects on heart rate, QT/QTc intervals, and effective refractory period are more pronounced with chronic oral administration when compared to IV administration. It is metabolized by the liver to an active metabolite, desethylamiodarone, and has a prolonged elimination half-life of approximately 35 to 110 days.[27] Amiodarone therapy is initiated with a loading dose of approximately 10 g in the first 1 to 2 weeks. For supraventricular arrhythmias, the loading dose can be given as 400 mg twice daily for 2 weeks, 400 mg once daily for 2 weeks, and then a maintenance dose of 200 mg daily. For ventricular arrhythmias, the doses are 800 to 1600 mg daily in two doses for 1 to 3 weeks, then 600 to 800 mg daily in two doses for 1 month, and then a maintenance dose of 400 mg once daily. IV therapy should start with 150-mg bolus given for over 10 minutes, followed by an infusion at 1 mg per minute for 6 hours, and then 0.5 mg per minute for 18 hours. Amiodarone interacts with other drugs metabolized by the liver and also P-glycoprotein, resulting in increased blood levels of warfarin, digoxin, and phenytoin. Adverse effects include pulmonary fibrosis, peripheral neuropathy, optic neuritis, hypo- and hyperthyroidism, hepatotoxicity, photosensitivity, blue-gray skin discoloration, nausea, and vomiting. Prior to initiation of therapy, liver, thyroid, and pulmonary functions should be measured.

β-ADRENERGIC ANTAGONISTS

β-adrenergic antagonists are Vaughan Williams class II agents that slow the rate of depolarization of the SA node and prolong AV node conduction. There are many agents in this class that have varying properties such as β-1 selectivity, intrinsic sympathomimetic activity, α-adrenergic antagonism, and membrane stabilizing effects. Examples of these agents are atenolol, carvedilol, metoprolol, and propranolol. They effectively suppress ventricular ectopic depolarizations, reduce the ventricular response rate during atrial fibrillation and flutter, and may terminate PSVT. β-adrenergic antagonists have been shown to reduce mortality rates in patients who have had a myocardial infarction or have depressed LV systolic function.

CALCIUM-CHANNEL BLOCKERS

The non-DHP CCBs, verapamil, and diltiazem are Vaughan Williams class IV antiarrhythmic agents that slow conduction, prolong the refractory period, and decrease automaticity. In atrial tachyarrhythmias, these agents can slow the ventricular response by slowing AV node conduction. During atrial fibrillation, these agents decrease the ventricular rate both at rest and during exercise. They are more effective than digoxin alone and their effects are additive.[28] IV verapamil and diltiazem are also drugs of choice for the acute management of PSVT. The recommended dose for IV verapamil is 5 mg given over 2 minutes, followed in 5 to 10 minutes by a second dose of 5 to 7.5 mg. The recommended dose for oral verapamil is 80 mg 3 times daily

Table 4-4. Vaughan Williams Classification of Antiarrhythmic Drugs

Class	Drugs	Electrophysiologic/ Pharmacologic Properties
Ia	Procainamide	Blocks sodium and potassium channel
	Disopyramide	Prolongs QRS duration and QT interval
	Quinidine	Little or no effect on SA or AV node
Ib	Lidocaine	Blocks sodium channel
		No effect on SA or AV node
Ic	Flecainide	Blocks sodium channels
		Increases QRS duration
	Propafenone	Beta-adrenergic antagonist
II	Propranolol	Beta-adrenergic antagonist
	Atenolol	Reduces SA nodal rate
	Metoprolol	Increases AV nodal refractoriness
III	Amiodarone	Blocks potassium channels
	Dofetilide	Increases QT interval
	Ibutilide	Reduces SA nodal rate (amiodarone)
		Increases AV nodal refractoriness (amiodarone)
IV	Diltiazem	Blocks calcium channels
	Verapamil	Increases AV nodal refractoriness

AV, atrioventricular; SA, sinoatrial.

up to a maximum of 480 mg in a day. Sustained-release preparations are available for once-daily dosing. Diltiazem should be given as a dose of 0.25 mg/kg IV followed by a second dose of 0.35 mg/kg, if needed.[29] A maintenance infusion may be given at 5 to 15 mg per hour. Oral diltiazem should be started at 30 mg, 4 times daily, up to a maximum of 360 mg daily. Sustained-release preparations are available for once- or twice-daily dosing. Both verapamil and diltiazem have negative inotropic properties and diltiazem is preferred in patients with depressed LV systolic function. Other common adverse effects of CCBs are hypotension, constipation, bradycardia, and peripheral edema. Verapamil and diltiazem are hepatically metabolized by the cytochrome P450 system (CYP3A4) and can inhibit the metabolism of certain 3-hydroxy-3-methylglutaryl coenzyme A reductase inhibitors, ranolazine, cyclosporine, and eplerenone among others. The DHP CCBs such as amlodipine and nifedipine do not prolong conduction or refractoriness and are not useful as antiarrhythmic agents.

DIGOXIN

Digoxin effectively converts PSVT to sinus rhythm and reduces the ventricular response in atrial fibrillation and atrial flutter.[30] It slows conduction through the AV node by augmenting vagal tone. Because sympathetic stimulation can overcome the effects of digoxin on the AV node, its usefulness is limited as monotherapy for atrial fibrillation. In addition to its effects on AV conduction, digoxin increases myocardial contractility and is useful in patients who have reduced LV systolic function in addition to a supraventricular arrhythmia. A loading dose of 0.75 to 1.25 mg over 24 hours in 3 to 4 divided doses is usually required because of its long half life of approximately 36 hours in patients with normal renal function. The maintenance dose is usually 0.125 to 0.5 mg daily. Patients with impaired renal function require a dosage reduction. Therapeutic digoxin blood levels range from 0.8 to 2 ng/mL, but major clinical practice guidelines recommend keeping the level below 1.0 ng/mL. Digoxin levels should be drawn predose. Digoxin is contraindicated in patients with hypokalemia or PSVT with an unblocked accessory pathway. Amiodarone, verapamil, and quinidine reduce digoxin's elimination, and concomitant therapy usually requires a reduction in the digoxin dose by about 50%. In about 10% of patients, oral digoxin is inactivated by colonic bacteria, and the use of tetracycline or erythromycin may result in increased digoxin blood levels. Digoxin toxicity may lead to gastrointestinal complaints, central nervous system disturbances, and arrhythmias.

DOFETILIDE

Dofetilide prolongs the cardiac action potential duration by blocking the I_{Kr} channel and is classified as a Vaughan Williams class III agent.[31] It is indicated for the conversion of atrial fibrillation and flutter to sinus rhythm. Because of its potential to increase the QT/QTc intervals and cause torsade de pointes, its use in the United States is restricted to "confirmed providers." It is primarily excreted unchanged by the kidney and dosage should be adjusted in patients with renal impairment. It is available for oral use only and should be dosed at 500 mcg every 12 hours if creatinine clearance is greater than 60 mL/min and QTc is less than 440 ms. If CrCl is between 40 and 60 mL/min and QTc is less than 440 ms, the dose should be reduced to 250 mcg every 12 hours. If CrCl is between 20 and 40 mL/min and QTc is less than 440 ms, the dose is further reduced to 125 mcg every 12 hours. Its use is not recommended if the CrCl is less than 20 mL/min or if the QTc increases to more than 500 ms after the initiation of therapy. The QTc should be monitored for 2 to 3 days after the initiation of therapy. Noncardiac adverse effects are rare.

FLECAINIDE

Flecainide depresses phase 0 of the action potential by inhibiting the inward sodium channel and the potassium channel. It is indicated for the treatment of both ventricular and atrial arrhythmias in patients without structural heart disease. The initial oral dose for sustained VT is 100 mg every 12 hours to a maximum of 200 mg every 12 hours. For PSVT and paroxysmal atrial fibrillation or flutter, the initial dose is 50 mg every 12 hours. It is contraindicated in patients with structural heart disease and a prolonged QT interval. It has potent negative inotropic effects and should not be used in patients with depressed LV systolic function. Flecainide should not be used with protease inhibitors (saquinavir, retonavir, nelfinavir, etc.), thioridazine, or ranolazine due to an increased risk of torsade de pointes.

IBUTILIDE

Ibutilide is a Vaughan Williams class III agent that increases action potential duration primarily by blocking the I_{Kr} channel.[32] It is indicated for the conversion of atrial fibrillation or flutter to sinus rhythm. It is more effective against atrial flutter than atrial fibrillation. Ibutilide is only available for IV administration; and 1 mg should be given over 10 minutes for patients weighing greater than or equal to 60 kg. A second dose of the same amount may be given 10 minutes after the conclusion of the first infusion, as necessary. For patients weighing less than 60 kg, the recommended dose is 0.01 mg/kg initially with a second dose of the same amount given 10 minutes later, if necessary. Ibutilide increases the QT/QTc interval, and nonsustained polymorphic VT has been shown to occur in approximately 5% of patients. It should not be used in patients at increased risk for arrhythmias such as those with a baseline QT of more than 500 ms, with a history of polymorphic VT, or those receiving concomitant therapy with Vaughan Williams class I or class III agents. Patients should be monitored for QT prolongation for at least 4 hours after the drug has been given.

MAGNESIUM

Magnesium has antiarrhythmic properties in patients with hypomagnesemia and normal serum magnesium levels.[33] Magnesium's antiarrhythmic mechanism of action is unknown, but it is known to activate sodium–potassium ATPase (enzyme that catalyzes adenosine triphosphate) and to affect sodium, potassium, and calcium channels. It is useful for the treatment of drug-induced torsade de pointes in patients with normal magnesium levels or for that of digoxin toxicity. It is usually given as 1-g magnesium sulfate as an IV infusion over 20 minutes and can be repeated once if necessary.

PROCAINAMIDE

Procainamide is a Vaughan Williams class Ia agent that has inhibitory properties on both the sodium and potassium channels. It prolongs the QRS duration and the QT interval on the ECG. Procainamide can cause vasodilation and hypotension. It is effective against most atrial and ventricular arrhythmias. Procainamide is available in both oral and parenteral preparations. IV use should begin with a loading dose of 15 to 17 mg/kg administered over at least 30 minutes, followed by a continuous infusion at 1 to 6 mg/min. The loading dose should be stopped if the QRS widens by greater than or equal to 50%, hypotension develops, the arrhythmia terminates, or the maximum loading dose is administered. Therapeutic blood concentrations can be monitored and should take into account an active metabolite, N-acetyl procainamide. Oral dosing is recommended at a maximum of 50 mg/kg per day in 2 to

4 divided doses. Dosage reductions are necessary for patients with impaired renal function. Adverse effects include torsade de pointes, a lupus-like syndrome, and hypotension.

PROPAFENONE

Propafenone is a Vaughan Williams class Ic agent with class II properties. It depresses phase 0 of the action potential by inhibiting the inward sodium channel. It also has weak β-adrenergic antagonistic properties. Propafenone prolongs AV conduction with little or no effect on sinus node function. It has an approved indication in the prevention of the recurrence of atrial fibrillation. Additionally, propafenone is useful in the treatment of PSVT and life-threatening ventricular arrhythmias. It should not be used in patients with atrial fibrillation and structural heart disease. It is available in both immediate-release and sustained-release preparations. The initial oral dose for immediate release is 150 mg every 8 hours and may be increased to a maximum of 300 mg every 8 hours. The sustained-release formulation should be initiated at 225 mg every 12 hours and increased to a maximum of 450 mg every 12 hours.

SOTALOL

Sotalol is marketed as a racemic mixture of d- and l-sotalol. While both isomers delay cardiac repolarization by blockade of the I_{Kr} channel, the l isomer is primarily responsible for the β-adrenergic blockade activity.[34] It is approved for use in the treatment of life-threatening ventricular arrhythmias and atrial fibrillation and flutter. Sotalol is primarily excreted (>90%) unchanged by the kidney. The initial oral dose is 80 mg every 12 hours. The dose may be increased every 3 days to a maximum of 320 mg every 12 hours. For patients with renal insufficiency, the dosing interval should be increased. If the CrCl is between 30 and 59 mL/min, the interval should be increased to every 24 hours, and if the CrCl is between 10 and 29 mL/min, the dosing interval should be 36 to 48 hours. Adverse effects are usually related to its β-adrenergic blockade properties or prolongation of the QT/QTc interval. Torsade de pointes may occur in 2% to 4% of patients receiving sotalol. It is not recommended for the treatment of atrial fibrillation and flutter in patients with structural heart disease or for patients with asthma or a prolonged QT interval (>450 ms). It does not elevate defibrillation threshold and thus may be a preferred agent for use with ICDs.[35]

EVIDENCE-BASED SUMMARY

- Supraventricular arrhythmias are rarely life-threatening while ventricular arrhythmias can be relatively benign or life-threatening.
- Atrial fibrillation is the most common arrhythmia that requires treatment.
- Treatment of atrial fibrillation should be focused on stroke prevention and symptom reduction.
- A rate-control or a rhythm-control strategy may be used in the management of recurrent atrial fibrillation.
- Treatment of asymptomatic or mildly symptomatic VPCs is not warranted.

REFERENCES

1. Edhouse J, Morris F. ABC of clinical electrocardiography: Broad complex tachycardia—Part I. *BMJ.* 2002;324:719–722.
2. Brugada P, Brugada J, Mont L, et al. A new approach to the differential diagnosis of a regular tachycardia with a wide complex. *Circulation.* 1991;83(5):1649–1659.
3. Singer DE, Albers GW, Dalen JE, et al. Antithrombotic therapy in atrial fibrillation: The Seventh ACCP Conference on antithrombotic and thrombolytic therapy. *Chest.* 2004;126:429S–456S.
4. Wyse DG, Gersh BJ. Atrial fibrillation: A perspective: Thinking inside and outside the box. *Circulation.* 2004;109: 3089–3095.
5. Fuster V, Ryden LE, Asinger RW, et al. ACC/AHA/ASC Guidelines for the Management of Patients with Atrial Fibrillation—Executive summary: A report of the American College of Cardiology/American Heart Association Task Force on Practice Guidelines and the European Society of Cardiology Committee for Practice Guidelines and Policy Conferences (Committee to develop guidelines for the management of patients with atrial fibrillation): Developed in collaboration with the North American Society of Pacing and Electrophysiology. *Circulation.* 2001;104:2118–2150.
6. Wyse DG, Waldo AL, DiMarco JP, et al. A comparison of rate control and rhythm control in patients with atrial fibrillation. *N Engl J Med.* 2002;347:1825–1833.
7. Van Gelder IC, Hagens VE, Bosker HA, et al. A comparison of rate control and rhythm control in patients with recurrent persistent atrial fibrillation. *N Engl J Med.* 2002; 347:1834–1840.
8. Hohnloser SH, Kuck KH, Lilienthal J. Rhythm or rate control in atrial fibrillation—Pharmacological intervention in atrial fibrillation (PIAF): A randomized trial. *Lancet.* 2000;356:1789–1794.
9. Blomström-Lundqvist C, Scheinman MM, Aliot EM, et al. ACC/AHA/ESC Guidelines for the Management of Patients with Supraventricular Arrhythmias—Executive Summary: A report of the American College of Cardiology/American Heart Association Task Force on Practice Guidelines and the European Society of Cardiology Committee for Practice Guidelines (writing committee to develop guidelines for the management of patients with supraventricular arrhythmias.). *J Am Coll Cardiol.* 2003;42: 1493–1531.
10. Echt DS, Liebson PR, Mitchell LB, et al. Mortality and morbidity in patients receiving encainide, flecainide, or placebo. *N Engl J Med.* 1991;324:781–788.
11. The Cardiac Arrhythmia Suppression Trial II Investigators. Effect of the antiarrhythmic agent moricizine on survival after myocardial infarction. *N Engl J Med.* 1992;327: 227–233.
12. American Heart Association. 7D: The tachycardia algorithms. *Circulation.* 2000;102(I):I158–I165.
13. Olsen KM. Pharmacologic agents associated with QT interval prolongation. *J Fam Pract.* 2005:S8–S14. Available at: http://findarticles.com/p/articles/mi_m0689/is_6_54/ai_n14732746/pg_1 Accessed March 5, 2007.
14. Edhouse J, Morris F. ABC of clinical electrocardiography: Broad complex tachycardia—Part II. *BMJ.* 2002;324: 776–779.
15. Da Costa D, Brady WJ, Edhouse J. ABC of clinical electrocardiography: Bradycardias and atrioventricular conduction block. *BMJ.* 2002;324:535–538.
16. Ufberg JW, Clark JS. Bradydysrhythmias and atrioventricular conduction blocks. *Emerg Med Clin North Am.* 2006; 24(1):1–9.
17. Gregoratos G, Abrams J, Esptein AE, et al. ACC/AHA/NASPE 2002 Guideline Update for Implantation of Cardiac Pacemakers and Antiarrhythmia Devices: Summary Article. A Report of the American College of Cardiology/American Heart Association Task Force on Practice Guidelines (ACC/AHA/NASPE Committee to Update the 1998 Pacemaker Guidelines). *Circulation.* 2002;106: 2145–2161.
18. Goldberg Z, Lampert R. Implantable cardioverter defibrillators: Expanding indications and technologies. *JAMA.* 2006;295:809–818.
19. Gehi AK, Mehta D, Gomes JA. Evaluation and management of patients after implantable cardioverter defibrillator shock. *JAMA.* 2006;296:2839–2847.
20. Berger JS, Eisen L, Nozad V, et al. Competency in electrocardiogram interpretation among internal medicine and emergency medicine residents. *Am J Med.* 2005;118: 873–880.
21. Masoudi FA, Magid DJ, Vinson DR, et al. Implications of the failure to identify high-risk electrocardiogram findings for the quality of care of patients with acute myocardial infarction. Results of the Emergency Department Quality in Myocardial Infarction (EDQMI) Study. *Circulation.* 2006;114:1565–1571.
22. Eagle KA, Berger PB, Calkins H, et al. ACC/AHA Guideline Update for Perioperative Cardiovascular Evaluation for Noncardiac Surgery—Executive Summary: A Report of the American College of Cardiology/American Heart

Association Task Force on Practice Guidelines (committee to update the 1996 Guidelines on Perioperative Cardiovascular Evaluation for Noncardiac Surgery). *Circulation.* 2002;105:1257–1267.

23. Maisel WH, Rawn JD, Stevenson WG. Atrial fibrillation after cardiac surgery. *Ann Intern Med.* 2001;135(12): 1061–1073.

24. Heintz KM, Hollenberg SM. Perioperative cardiac issues: Postoperative arrhythmias. *Surg Clin North Am.* 2005;85: 1103–1114.

25. Martinez EA, Bass EB, Zimetbaum P. Pharmacologic control of rhythm: American College of Chest Physicians Guidelines for the Prevention and Management of Postoperative Atrial Fibrillation after Cardiac Surgery. *Chest.* 2005;128:48S–55S.

26. Singh SN, Fletcher RD, Fisher SG, et al. Amiodarone in patients with congestive heart failure and asymptomatic ventricular arrhythmia. *N Engl J Med.* 1995;333:77–82.

27. Singh BN. Antiarrhythmic actions of amiodarone: A profile of a paradoxical agent. *Am J Cardiol.* 1996;78(4A):41–53.

28. McNamara RL, Tamariz LJ, Segal JB, et al. Management of atrial fibrillation: Review of the evidence for the role of pharmacologic therapy, electrical cardioversion, and echocardiography. *Ann Intern Med.* 2003;139:1018–1033.

29. Ferguson JD, DiMarco JP. Contemporary management of paroxysmal supraventricular tachycardia. *Circulation.* 2003; 107:1096–1099.

30. Gheorghiade M, Adams KF, Colucci WS. Digoxin in the management of cardiovascular disorders. *Circulation.* 2004;109:2959–2964.

31. Mounsey JP, DiMarco JP. Dofetilide. *Circulation.* 2000;102: 2665–2670.

32. Murray KT. Ibutilide. *Circulation.* 1998;97:493–497.

33. Tzivoni A, Keren A. Suppression of ventricular arrhythmias by magnesium. *Am J Cardiol.* 1990;65:1397–1399.

34. Hohnloser SH, Woosley RL. Sotalol. *N Engl J Med.* 1994; 331:31–38.

35. Anderson JL, Prystowsky EN. Sotalol: An important new antiarrhythmic. *Am Heart J.* 1999;137:388–409.

Chapter 5

Hypertrophic Cardiomyopathy

William D. Linn and Robert A. O'Rourke

SEARCH STRATEGY

A systematic search of the medical literature was performed on April 1, 2008. The search, limited to human subjects and English language journals, included the National Guideline Clearinghouse, the Cochrane database, PubMed, UpTo-Date®, and PIER. The current American College of Cardiology/European Society of Cardiology Clinical Expert Consensus Document for Hypertrophic Cardiomyopathy can be found at www.acc.org

Hypertrophic cardiomyopathy (HCM) is a complex cardiac disease that can manifest in multiple ways and can occur in patients of all ages.[1] The prevalence of HCM is much higher than what was previously thought and it occurs in *one out of 500 people*. It is now recognized that a gene mutation is responsible for HCM and that it is the most common genetic cardiovascular disease. Many people with HCM are asymptomatic and their lives are not affected by HCM. Others may experience severe limitations in their daily lives and some will have sudden cardiac death (SCD) at an early age. Therefore, it is important for primary care providers to recognize this common cardiac condition and to provide proper management options.

CLINICAL PRESENTATION

Symptoms of HCM can manifest at any phase of a person's life; many of these people have relatives with known HCM. Symptoms do not always correlate to the severity of the left ventricular (LV) outflow tract obstruction. Dyspnea on exertion occurs in almost 90% of the symptomatic patients, usually in the presence of preserved systolic function.[2] This is due to the increased stiffness of the LV wall leading to elevated LV diastolic and left atrial pressures. Other symptoms range from fatigue to near-syncope or syncope. Typical or atypical chest pain can occur in patients with a normal coronary arteriogram. This may reflect microvascular angina. Unfortunately, the first manifestation of HCM can be sudden death occurring in children or young adults after strenuous physical activity.

Atrial fibrillation (AF) occurs late in the disease process and is generally poorly tolerated. Patients with a stiff, noncompliant left ventricle need the atrial contribution for adequate ventricular filling during diastole. AF in patients with HCM increases the risk for systemic embolization.

PHYSICAL FINDINGS

In asymptomatic patients with HCM, the physical examination may be normal or may provide nonspecific findings such as a fourth heart sound (some specific recommendations are mentioned in Table 5-1). However, as the outflow obstruction increases, several characteristic abnormalities can be elicited (Fig. 5-1). High-grade obstruction creates a harsh crescendo–decrescendo systolic murmur at the lower left sternal border and apex. The murmur may radiate to the axilla and base, but usually not to the neck. It begins just after S1 and usually represents aortic outflow obstruction often with mitral regurgitation. A prominent S4 is usually present unless the patient is in AF.

Maneuvers that increase outflow obstruction, usually by decreasing LV volume, will increase the intensity of the murmur.[2,3] These include assuming an upright posture after squatting, the Valsalva maneuver, and the posture after the administration of nitroglycerin (Table 5-2). Conversely, increasing LV volume will decrease the murmur of HCM. This can be accomplished by squatting,

Table 5-1. Specific Recommendations[3]

- Evaluate the carotid pulse
- Perform cardiac auscultation for murmurs
- Determine how murmurs change with maneuvers that alter venous return Valsalva or squatting

performing a handgrip, or passively elevating the legs. The systolic murmur of aortic stenosis is generally not influenced by these maneuvers.

On physical examination, the neck veins may reveal a prominent "a" wave. In HCM, the carotid pulse (bisferiens) has a brisk upstroke, declines in midsystole secondary to a sudden deceleration of blood due to midsystolic obstruction, and then has a secondary rise. In aortic stenosis, the carotid upstroke is slow and low in amplitude (parvus and tardus).

DIAGNOSTIC EVALUATION

ECHOCARDIOGRAPHY

After a careful consideration of the cardiovascular history and physical examination, the clinical diagnosis of HCM is most readily established using two-dimensional echocardiography. The usual image seen is that of left ventricular hypertrophy (LVH) without a dilated LV chamber in the absence of other cardiac diseases such as hypertension or aortic stenosis. The clinical diagnostic criterion for HCM is a maximal LV wall thickness of greater than or equal to 15 mm. However, in patients with diagnosed HCM, the values for LV wall thickness

vary from mild (13–15 mm) to massive (=30 mm) with the normal thickness being 12 mm.

Outflow gradients are responsible for the loud, apical midsystolic murmur. The subaortic obstruction is caused by the systolic anterior motion (SAM) of the mitral valve leaflets and the midsystolic contact with the ventricular septum. Doppler echocardiography is used to determine the presence and degree of SAM and the presence of midsystolic obstruction. These hemodynamic parameters are useful for establishing the degree of outflow tract obstruction and in monitoring the progression of the disease. A subaortic gradient of 30 mm Hg is an independent predictor of HCM-related deaths.[1]

Despite being the sine qua non in the diagnosis of HCM, echocardiography has several limitations. The LV wall thickness criteria may not identify those patients with inherited disease who have not yet developed LVH. The criteria may exclude patients with HCM if they have a coexisting disease such as hypertension. Lastly, there could be false-positive results in patients with borderline increases in LV wall thickness.

ELECTROCARDIOGRAM

The 12-lead electrocardiogram (ECG) is abnormal in 75% to 95% of patients with HCM. Patients without ECG abnormalities are usually family members who have been identified as part of the pedigree screening or those who have only mild, localized LVH.[4] The ECG should be examined for LVH with repolarization abnormalities

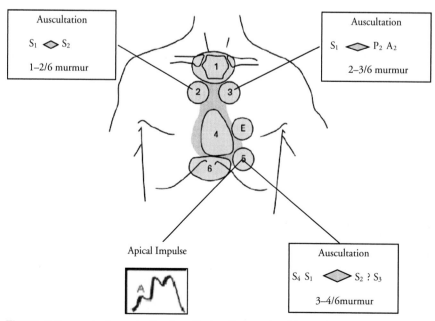

Figure 5-1. Physical examination in patients with hypertrophic cardiomyopathy.

Table 5-2. Loudness of Systolic Murmurs During Dynamic Auscultation

| Maneuver | Response of Murmur | | | |
	HCM	AS	MR	MVP
Decreased LV cavity size (Valsalva, standing)	Increased	Decreased	Decreased	Click occurs earlier and murmur increases
Increased LV cavity size (squatting, passive leg elevation)	Decreased	No change or slight increase	No change or slight increase	Click and murmur decrease or disappear

HCM, hypertrophic cardiomyopathy; LV, left ventricular; AS, aortic stenosis; MR, mitral regurgitation; MVP, mitral valve prolapse.

and for abnormal Q waves (septal hypertrophy) that mimic myocardial infarction.

CARDIOLOGY CONSULTATION[3]

Patients with HCM should be evaluated by a cardiovascular specialist to confirm the diagnosis and also for risk stratification. Physical findings and test results may be inconclusive and may require specialized diagnostic procedures. The diagnosis may be difficult in patients with coexisting conditions. The cardiovascular specialist can also assess the severity of outflow obstruction and evaluate the risk for sudden death (some considerations for hospitalization are given in Table 5-3).

RISK STRATIFICATION[1,5,6,7]

For some patients with HCM, SCD may be their first presentation of the disease. SCD frequently occurs in asymptomatic or mildly symptomatic patients and is common in adolescents and young adults. This risk does extend beyond midlife. As a result, reaching a certain age does not negate the potential of SCD. HCM patients at a high risk for SCD represent a minority of the overall population. The task is to identify this small subset of patients and focus on the prevention of SCD.

In order to create a risk profile, one must collect data from several different clinical parameters. No single diagnostic test can accurately predict SCD. Genetic typing is usually not justified. However, there is good consensus on the major risk factors for SCD in HCM (Table 5-4). These include a personal history or family history of

SCD, syncope, spontaneous sustained ventricular tachycardia, nonsustained ventricular tachycardia, abnormal blood pressure response, or extreme LVH. The strength of one risk factor alone, such as a family history of SCD or extreme LVH may warrant the prophylactic implantation of an implantable cardioverter defibrillator. The challenge remains on how to best identify HCM-related sudden death.

MANAGEMENT

ASYMPTOMATIC PATIENTS

Most patients, including those who are unaware of their disease, are asymptomatic or have only mild symptoms. Attempting to prevent or delay the onset of symptoms in this cohort of patients with HCM is unproven. Treatments should be reserved for preventing SCD in high-risk patients. The primary treatment strategies for patients with HCM are shown in Fig. 5-2.

SYMPTOMATIC PATIENTS

Pharmacologic therapy should be considered in patients experiencing dyspnea, anginal-type chest pain, or other symptoms of heart failure. These manifestations often occur in patients with preserved systolic function. The pathophysiology associated with HCM involves impaired ventricular filling due to abnormal

Table 5-3. Considerations for Hospitalization[3]

- New onset atrial fibrillation—It may cause hemodynamic compromise due to loss of atrial kick in filling a hypertrophied ventricle.
- Patients who have experienced syncope or sudden death—They may require invasive testing.
- Patients with refractory symptoms of angina or heart failure—They need a maximization of medical therapies and an evaluation for pacemaker or other surgical therapies.

Table 5-4. Risk Factors for Sudden Death in Hypertrophic Cardiomyopathy[1,7]

- Cardiac arrest (ventricular fibrillation).
- Spontaneous sustained ventricular tachycardia.
- Family history of sudden HCM-related death (especially first-degree relatives).
- Syncope (especially if recurrent or exertional or in the young).
- Nonsustained ventricular tachycardia on Holter ECG monitoring.
- Abnormal BP response with exertion (a fall in BP or a failure to rise = 20 mm Hg)
- Massive LVH (maximum LV thickness = 30 mm by echocardiography).

HCM, hypertrophic cardiomyopathy; ECG, electrocardiogram; BP, blood pressure; LVH, left ventricular hypertrophy; LV, left ventricular.

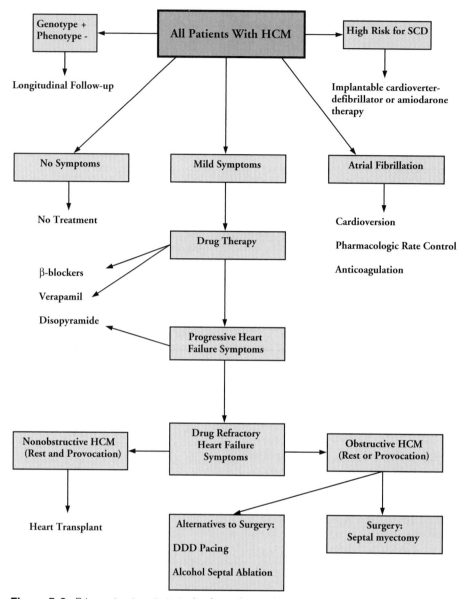

Figure 5-2. Primary treatment strategies for patients with hypertrophic cardiomyopathy. (HCM, hypertrophic cardiomyopathy; SCD, sudden cardiac death; DDD, dual-chamber.)

relaxation that leads to diastolic heart failure. These symptoms can occur in patients without significant outflow obstruction. For those with LV outflow problems and resultant elevated LV pressures, mitral regurgitation with or without AF can occur and lead to severe disabling symptoms.

Chest pain can occur without atherosclerotic disease of the epicardial arteries. The pain may be classified as typical or atypical in nature. Most of the episodes of chest pain are probably due to abnormalities in the coronary microvasculature. However, atherosclerotic coronary artery disease can occur in patients with HCM. Patients at high risk for coronary artery disease should have arteriography.

β-ADRENERGIC BLOCKING AGENTS

The negative inotropic and chronotropic properties of β-blockers are useful in patients with HCM. The symptoms of dyspnea can be relieved by β-blocker therapy due to the decrease in heart rate that allows for increased diastolic filling. Decreasing contractility decreases myocardial oxygen consumption and may help relieve outflow tract obstruction, especially with exertion.

Propranolol was the first β-blocker to be used for the relief of symptoms in patients with HCM. Doses up to 480 mg per day can be used. Currently, standard doses of longer acting agents such as metoprolol and atenolol are being used. Caution should be used if these drugs are prescribed to children or adolescents. β-blockers can impair academic performance or lead to depression.

VERAPAMIL

In patients who are not responding to β-blocker therapy or have severe asthma, the negative inotropic effects of verapamil may improve ventricular diastolic filling and relieve chest pain. Doses up to 480 mg per day in a sustained-release preparation can be used. In addition to the constipating effects of verapamil, another serious adverse effect should be considered. In HCM patients with marked outflow obstruction at rest combined with severe symptoms, verapamil has been associated with sudden death. It is postulated that the vasodilating properties of verapamil can lead to increased outflow tract obstruction, pulmonary edema, and cardiogenic shock. The combination of a β-blocker and disopyramide may be preferable in patients with significant symptoms.

DISOPYRAMIDE

Disopyramide is a type I-A antiarrhythmic agent with significant negative inotropic properties. It may provide relief from symptoms in patients with severe resting outflow tract obstruction. Disopyramide is not a first-line agent and should be reserved for those who fail treatment with a β-blocker or verapamil. Since disopyramide can increase atrioventricular conduction, low-dose β-blocker therapy should also be used in HCM patients with AF.

MANAGEMENT OPTIONS IN DRUG-FAILURE PATIENTS

SURGERY

Surgery should be considered in patients with significant outflow tract obstruction are refractory to drug therapy. This is defined as a LV outflow gradient of more than 50 mmHg. The goal of surgery is to eliminate the SAM of the mitral valve and the septal–mitral contact by widening the LV outflow tract. The ventricular septal myectomy operation (the Morrow procedure) is the gold standard for obstructive HCM and severe drug-failure symptoms. In expert hands, it is successful in approximately 70% of patients and has an annual mortality rate of 1% to 2%.

ALCOHOL SEPTAL ABLATION[8]

An alternative to surgery is a recently developed technique in which 1 to 4 mL of absolute alcohol is infused into a target septal perforator branch of the left anterior descending coronary artery. This produces an infarction in the proximal ventricular septum that would provide the same hemodynamic benefits of a septal myectomy. Data for long-term outcomes (>8 years) are lacking.

DUAL-CHAMBER PACING

A second alternative to surgery is dual-chamber pacing; its initial outcomes were based on observational or uncontrolled trial data. Subsequent randomized trial data showed only modest decreases in the outflow gradient. However, symptomatic improvement does not correlate well with gradient reduction. The mechanisms by which pacing reduces outflow tract obstruction are not fully elucidated. Pacing is not a primary therapy and it should be reserved for those patients not responding to maximum medical therapy.

ATRIAL FIBRILLATION

AF, the most common sustained arrhythmia in patients with HCM, warrants immediate attention. Episodes of AF can cause decreased diastolic filling with resultant lowered cardiac output. The hypertrophied left ventricle relies on atrial contractions for ventricular filling. The increased heart rate in AF coupled with loss of atrial contributions can lead to progressive heart failure, stroke, and death.

AF in HCM patients should be managed according to currently accepted guidelines.[9] In general, if a patient presents within 48 hours after the onset of AF, pharmacologic or direct-current cardioversion can be attempted. An attempt should be made to maintain sinus rhythm. Amiodarone is considered the most effective pharmacologic agent. Anticoagulation therapy with warfarin is indicated for chronic or paroxysmal AF.

INFECTIVE ENDOCARDITIS PROPHYLAXIS[10]

The American Heart Association no longer recommends that HCM patients with evidence of outflow obstruction receive endocarditis prophylaxis at the time of dental or other selected surgical procedures. The new guidelines state that only patients with the highest risk of adverse outcomes from infective endocarditis would benefit from antibiotic prophylaxis. These cardiac conditions include patients with prosthetic cardiac valves or prosthetic material used for valve repair, patients with previous infective endocarditis, or patients with congential heart disease (CHD) (unrepaired cyanotic CHD, repaired CHD with prosthetic material, repaired CHD with residual defects).

EVIDENCE-BASED SUMMARY

- Common symptoms for HCM include dyspnea on exertion, exertional chest pain, near-syncope or syncope.
- The systolic murmur of HCM increases with Valsalva and after assuming an upright posture and decreases with squatting.
- Risk factors for SCD include a history of cardiac arrest, sustained ventricular tachycardia, family history of HCM-related death, nonsustained ventricular tachycardia, and massive LVH.
- Echocardiography is the most useful tool in establishing the diagnosis of HCM.
- β-Blockers are the mainstay for treating the symptoms of exertional chest pain or dyspnea.

REFERENCES

1. American College of Cardiology/European Society of Cardiology Clinical Expert Consensus Document on Hypertrophic Cardiomyopathy. A Report of the American College of Cardiology Foundation Task Force on Clinical Expert Consensus Documents and the European Society of Cardiology Committee for Practice Guidelines. 2003. Available at www.acc.org. Accessed 2003.

2. Fifer MA, Vlahakes GJ. Management of Symptoms in Hypertrophic Cardiomyopathy. *Circulation.* 2008;117:429–439.

3. Bhat G. Hypertrophic Cardiomyopathy. Physicians' Information and Education Resource (PIER). http://pier.acponline.org. Accessed December, 2007.

4. Maron BJ. Hypertrophic cardiomyopathy—A systematic review. *JAMA.* 2002;287:1308–1320.

5. Spirito P, Seidman CE, McKenna WJ, Maron BJ. The management of hypertrophic cardiomyopathy. *N Engl J Med.* 1997;336:775–758.

6. Hess OM. Risk stratification in hypertrophic cardiomyopathy. *J Am Coll Cardiol.* 2003;42:880–881.

7. Maron BJ, Spirito P, Shen WK, et al. Implantable Cardioverter-Defibrillators and Prevention of Sudden Cardiac Death in Hypertrophic Cardiomyopathy. *JAMA.* 2007;298:405–412.

8. Olivotto I, Ommen SR, Maron MS, Cecchi F, Maron BJ. Surgical Myectomy Versus Alcohol Septal Ablation For Obstructive Hypertrophic Cardiomyopathy. *J Am Coll Cardiol.* 2007;50:831–840.

9. Fuster V, Ryden LE, Cannom DS, et al. ACC/AHA/ESC 2006 Guidelines for the Management of Patients with Atrial Fibrillation. A report of the American College of Cardiology/American Heart Association Task Force on Practice Guidelines and the European Society of Cardiology Committee for Practice Guidelines (Writing Committee to Revise the 2001 Guidelines for the Management of Patients with Atrial Fibrillation) Developed in Collaboration with the European Heart Rhythm Association and the Heart Rhythm Society. *J Am Coll Cardiol.* 2006;48: e149–246.

10. Wilson W, Taubert KA, Gewitz M, et al. Prevention of Infective Endocarditis. Guidelines from the American Heart Association. A Guideline From the American Heart Association Rheumatic Fever, Endocarditis, and Kawasaki Disease Committee, Council on Cardiovascular Disease in the Young, and the Council on Clinical Cardiology, Council on Cardiovascular Surgery and Anesthesia, and the Quality of Care and Outcomes Research Interdisciplinary Working Group. *Circulation.* 2007;116:1736–1754.

Chapter 6

Dyslipidemia

Leigh Ann Ross, Brendan Sean Ross, and Honey East

SEARCH STRATEGY

A formal MEDLINE review was conducted (January 1994 to March 2007) using the following terms (limited to adult humans): cholesterol *or* low-density lipoprotein cholesterol AND guidelines *or* clinical trial. The Cochrane Controlled Trials Registry, references from the American College of Physicians, American Heart Association/American College of Cardiology lipid statements, and the National Cholesterol Education Program (NCEP) 2002 final report and 2004 update were also reviewed. The NCEP recommendations can be viewed at www.nhlbi.nih.gov/guidelines/cholesterol/index.htm.

INTRODUCTION

Dyslipidemia is a prerequisite risk factor in the development of the leading cause of mortality in the United States—atherosclerotic vascular disease (ASCVD). Dyslipidemia is prevalent in the United States; some estimates place the number of affected adults at one out of every two.[1] Dyslipidemia is a modifiable ASCVD risk factor, unlike age, gender, or family predisposition, and its treatment reduces the rate of nonfatal myocardial infarction (MI), stroke, peripheral arterial disease, revascularization procedures, and all-cause mortality.[2] However, many individuals with dyslipidemia go unrecognized and most patients with lipid abnormalities fail to achieve adequate metabolic control.[3] To address these inadequacies, the National Heart, Lung, and Blood Institute of the National Institutes of Health convened an expert panel of researchers and clinicians to release a series of consensus guidelines on the detection, evaluation, and treatment of dyslipidemia. The latest NCEP recommendations were released in 2001.[4] This

Third Adult Treatment Panel (ATP-III) Report has been the focus of comment for guidelines issued from other specialty organizations.[5,6] The ATP-III authors updated the report in 2004 to account for the implications of several large prospective clinical trials of lipid interventions.[7] These clinical practice parameters emphasize the early identification of the individuals at risk and the targeted dietary, lifestyle, and pharmacologic treatment of dyslipidemia to prevent ASCVD events.

LIPOPROTEIN CLASSIFICATION

Dyslipidemia is a term encompassing a variety of abnormal lipid profiles. Dyslipidemia includes elevated levels of total cholesterol, low-density lipoprotein (LDL) cholesterol, and triglycerides, and low levels of high-density lipoprotein (HDL) cholesterol. In the past, these abnormalities were often referenced by their Fredrickson classification (Table 6-1). Dyslipidemia is now more fully described through sophisticated serum analyses to yield information on particle characteristics and their atherogenic potential. However, epidemiologic and clinical trial data continue to identify elevated LDL as the major lipid abnormality related to the development of ASCVD and recurrent adverse events.[8] Poor diet, lack of exercise, tobacco use, prescription medications, and underlying medical disorders can all contribute to alterations in lipid metabolism. It is important to exclude such secondary causes of dyslipidemia prior to initiating treatment for a presumed primary lipid abnormality (Table 6-2).

Cholesterol is a structural element in cell membranes and is a precursor in the formation of steroid hormones, vitamin D, and bile acids. It can be obtained from the diet, but the majority is synthesized in the liver and peripheral tissues. Cholesterol homeostasis is

Table 6-1. Fredrickson Classification of Lipid Disorders

Phenotype	Lipoprotein Elevation	Total Cholesterol	Triglycerides	Atherogenicity
I	chylomicrons	normal/+	+	no increase
IIa	LDL	++	normal	++
IIb	LDL and VLDL	++	+	++
III	IDL	+	+	++
IV	VLDL	normal/+	++	+
V	VLDL and chylomicrons	+	+++	+

IDL, intermediate-density lipoprotein; LDL, low-density lipoprotein; VLDL, very low density lipoprotein; +, increase.

regulated through lipid metabolism and transport. The liver is the central organ responsible for maintaining cholesterol balance. Dietary cholesterol and fats are absorbed in the intestine, assembled into chylomicrons, released into the circulation at the thoracic lymph duct, and subsequently hydrolyzed by lipoprotein lipase (LPL) into remnant particles before being removed from the plasma by the liver. Cholesterol synthesized in the liver is either secreted into bile, or released into the circulation associated with phospholipid and apopeptide macromolecules. The triglyceride content of these circulating very low-density lipoproteins (VLDL) is liberated by the enzyme LPL to be stored in adipose tissue or to be converted into energy by muscle tissue. The residual lipid particles, now known as intermediate-density lipoproteins (IDL), can be removed by the liver or undergo further conversion to LDL. The half-life of IDL can be measured in hours, while that of LDL is measured in days. At any time, LDL constitutes two-

thirds of the circulating cholesterol content. Both the liver and extrahepatic tissues can obtain the needed cholesterol by variably expressing LDL receptors. Plasma LDL can also accumulate in the arterial endothelium, incite local inflammatory processes, and promote the formation of atherosclerotic plaques. Atheromas may impede blood flow leading to downstream ischemia, or these lipid-rich lesions may rupture leading to thrombosis and tissue necrosis. Thus, elevated levels of VLDL, IDL, LDL, and triglycerides can be viewed as atherogenic. HDL is considered to be antiatherogenic, since it is able to accept free cholesterol and triglyceride-rich lipoproteins, esterify them, and then transport these cholesterol esters back to the liver in a process of reverse cholesterol transport.

Dyslipidemia is usually asymptomatic, so a screening lipoprotein analysis should be conducted in adults beginning at the age of 20 years. If the results are acceptable, testing should be repeated every 5 years. Earlier and more frequent testing may be appropriate, if indicated by genetic predisposition or medical comorbidity. No upper age limit beyond which treatment for dyslipidemia yields no benefit has been identified, thus testing should continue throughout life.[9] A complete lipid profile, consisting of total cholesterol, LDL, triglycerides, and HDL, should be drawn after an overnight, 12-hour fast, but direct measurements of random total cholesterol and HDL levels may suffice for initial screening. If the nonfasting total cholesterol value is equal to or greater than 200 mg/dL or the HDL is less than 40 mg/dL, then a complete fasting profile should be obtained. The risk relationship between dyslipidemia and ASCVD is continuous, but normal and pathologic ranges for lipoprotein values have been delineated (Table 6-3).

Most ASCVD events occur in patients with nonobstructive arterial lesions that are unstable and thus prone to ulceration and thrombus formation. Arterial plaques are rendered vulnerable to rupture due to the inflammation stimulated by the presence of oxidized lipoproteins. Cholesterol reduction can beneficially impact the progression of atheromatous disease, but more importantly, it can stabilize these vulnerable plaques. Clinical trials of drug therapy for dyslipidemia have demonstrated results that are congruent with

Table 6-2. Secondary Causes of Dyslipidemia

Secondary Cause	Lipid Changes Seen
End-stage renal disease	Increase in triglycerides, decrease in HDL
Nephrotic syndrome	Increase in VLDL and triglycerides
Hypothyroidism	Increase in LDL and triglycerides
Drugs: glucocorticoids, anabolic steroids, estrogens and progestins, tamoxifen, protease inhibitors, diuretics, β-blockers	Variable effects
Cigarette use	Decrease in HDL
Diabetes mellitus	Increase in triglycerides, decrease in HDL
Excessive alcohol consumption	Increase in triglycerides
Obstructive liver disease	Increase in LDL
Pregnancy	Increase in LDL and triglycerides
Anorexia	Increase in LDL
Caloric excess or diet high in saturated fat	Increase in LDL

HDL, high-density lipoprotein; VLDL, very low density lipoprotein; LDL, low-density lipoprotein.

Table 6-3. Classification of Dyslipidemia

	Value (mg/dL)
LDL Cholesterol	
Optimal	<100
Near or above optimal	100–129
Borderline high	130–159
High	160–189
Very high	≥190
Total Cholesterol	
Desirable	<200
Borderline high	200–239
High	≥240
HDL Cholesterol	
Low	<40
High	≥60
Triglycerides	
Normal	<150
Borderline high	150–199
High	200–499
Very high	≥500

HDL, high-density lipoprotein; LDL, low-density lipoprotein.

Table 6-4. Major Atherosclerotic Vascular Disease Risk Factors

Major Risk Factors that Modify LDL Goals*

Cigarette smoking
Blood pressure ≥140/90 mm Hg, or on antihypertensive medication
HDL cholesterol <40 mg/dL
First-degree relative with premature ASCVD with age:
  Male <55 year
  Female <65 year
Age of the individual:
  Men ≥45 year
  Women ≥55 year

*HDL cholesterol ≥60 mg/dL is a "negative" risk factor that removes one risk factor from the total count.
LDL, low-density lipoprotein; HDL, high-density lipoprotein; ASCVD, atherosclerotic vascular disease.

epidemiologic studies: Lowering total cholesterol leads to fewer ASCVD events.[10] As the evidence supporting treatment interventions is more robust for LDL lowering, the ATP-III states the primary goals of dyslipidemia therapy and the cutpoints for initiating treatment in terms of LDL. It is estimated that for every 1% decrease in LDL cholesterol, the risk for ASCVD events is reduced by 1% to 2%.[11] Recent evidence reveals that in high-risk patients, who are most prone to ASCVD events, LDL reductions of 50% or more may be needed.[12] Lipoprotein determination and classification is an essential element in ASCVD risk reduction.

ASCVD RISK ASSESSMENT

CORONARY HEART DISEASE RISK FACTORS

The intensity of dyslipidemia treatment should be in accord with a patient's ASCVD risk. In this context, cardiovascular risk must be considered globally, not simply as that conferred by dyslipidemia. The pharmacologic management of dyslipidemia is associated with significant costs and the potential for precipitating drug-related adverse effects. ASCVD risk assessment must balance cardiovascular benefits against costs and treatment-emergent risks. The ATP-III report weighs risks by utilizing a validated ASCVD risk calculator, and then sets lipid-modifying-treatment goals accordingly.[13] As adequate treatment is primarily defined by LDL goal attainment, initial risk assessment is made without reference to baseline LDL level. LDL is a major ASCVD risk factor, but ATP-III assesses risk status through accompanying risk determinants (Table 6-4).

Patients with established ASCVD are at the highest risk of an adverse event and are placed in the highest risk category (Table 6-5). ATP-III stratification states risk in terms of incident nonfatal or fatal MI in patients with coronary heart disease (CHD) over a 10-year period. As this risk is equivalent in patients with clinical forms of ASCVD other than CHD, symptomatic carotid artery disease, peripheral arterial disease, or abdominal aortic aneurysm, these manifestations of ASCVD are considered "CHD risk equivalent." Diabetes mellitus is also a CHD risk equivalent, as epidemiologic studies have

Table 6-5. ATP-III LDL Goals and Cutpoints for TLC and Drug Therapy by Risk Category

Risk Category	LDL Goal	Initiate TLC	Consider Drug Therapy
High risk: CHD, CHD risk equivalents, 10-year risk >20%	<100 mg/dL	≥100 mg/dL	≥100 mg/dL
Very high risk*	<70 mg/dL	≥70 mg/dL	<100 mg/dL, consider drug options
Moderately high risk: more than 2 risk factors, 10-year risk is 10%–20%	<130 mg/dL	≥130 mg/dL	≥130 mg/dL (100–129 mg/dL, consider drug options)
Moderate risk: more than 2 risk factors, 10-year risk <10%	<130 mg/dL	≥130 mg/dL	≥160 mg/dL
Lower risk: 0–1 risk factor	<160 mg/dL	≥160 mg/dL	≥190 mg/dL (160–189 mg/dl, consider drug options)

*Very high risk patients have established ASCVD plus the following: (1) multiple major risk factors, especially diabetes; (2) severe and poorly controlled risk factors, especially continued cigarette smoking; (3) multiple risk factors of the metabolic syndrome, especially high triglycerides ≥200 mg/dL plus non-HDL cholesterol ≥130 mg/dL with HDL cholesterol <40 mg/dL; and (4) acute coronary syndromes.
LDL, low-density lipoprotein; TLC, therapeutic lifestyle changes; CHD, coronary heart disease.

revealed that the rate of MI in diabetic patients without a history of CHD is similar to the rate of recurrent MI in patients who have suffered such an ASCVD event.[14] The ATP-III update adds a classification of "very high risk," which includes patients who warrant intense lipid-modifying treatment. This risk cohort includes patients in the immediate post-MI interval, diabetic patients with CHD, and patients with established ASCVD and multiple or poorly controlled risk factors.

The presence of multiple ASCVD risk factors alone may place an individual in the CHD-risk-equivalent class. To identify these patients, who are at a 20% risk of MI over the next 10 years, the Framingham risk calculator is employed (Table 6-6). In an individual with two or more major risk factors, this risk projection tool can better define candidates for aggressive lipid-modifying treatment. The clinical variables considered by this instrument include age, gender, blood pressure, cigarette smoking, and total cholesterol and HDL levels. Patients are classified into 10-year-risk categories of less than 10%, 10% to 20%, or greater than 20%; this last class represents patients who are CHD risk equivalent (Table 6-5). As individuals with no or only one major risk determinant are rarely candidates for intensive interventions, Framingham scoring is not necessary in these lower risk patients. Thus, ATP-III recommends a two-step process for refining risk assessments in individuals without preexisting ASCVD: Count major risk factors and then employ the Framingham calculator.

RELATED RISK FACTORS

Several "emerging" ASCVD risk factors have been identified that are not formally included in the Framingham or other risk-stratification tools. These factors have not yet been demonstrated to be beneficial targets for therapeutic intervention. They include homocysteine, proinflammatory factors, lipoprotein(a) (Lp[a]), and subclinical atherosclerotic disease. Homocysteine is a byproduct of protein metabolism and is believed to be prothrombotic; high-sensitivity C-reactive protein is a readily available marker of systemic inflammation; Lp(a) is an LDL-like and plasminogen-like atherogenic particle; and noninvasive assessments of carotid artery intimal medial thickness can yield objective measures of vascular dysfunction.[15] There is no consensus regarding the use of these studies as screening tests, and they are not used to categorically set lower LDL goals. However, they may impact clinical judgment and modify dyslipidemia therapy in patients on the cusp of treatment set points.

Many dyslipidemia patients also meet diagnostic criteria for the metabolic syndrome. This concurrence of independent risk factors increases the risk for ASCVD events at any LDL level. The metabolic syndrome is characterized by visceral adiposity, insulin resistance, and an atherogenic lipid profile.[16] Although criteria for the diagnosis are not uniform, the ATP-III report offers a widely utilized definition (Table 6-7). The metabolic syndrome is considered a secondary target for risk-reducing therapy, after a patient's LDL goal is achieved. Because the underlying cause of the metabolic syndrome appears to be obesity and physical inactivity, weight reduction and increased exercise are essential to treatment. After these "life–habit risk factors" have been addressed, drug therapy to reduce elevated triglycerides level or increase HDL levels may be clinically indicated.

NON-HDL CHOLESTEROL

Elevated triglyceride levels are independent risk factors for the development of ASCVD and are associated with incident CHD events. Hypertriglyceridemia may result from lifestyle factors, medical comorbidities, and prescription drug use, as well as from genetic predisposition (Table 6-2). For very high triglyceride levels, equal to or greater than 500 mg/dL, immediate treatment is required to prevent acute pancreatitis. For more modest elevations, 200–499 mg/dL, therapy can be considered and should be directed at ASCVD risk amelioration. Whereas some authorities delineate specific triglyceride goals, the ATP-III report focuses on the atherogenic lipid profile associated with hypertriglyceridemia. Atherogenic remnant lipoproteins, which represent degraded VLDL particles, are elevated in hypertriglyceridemia; thus, elevated VLDL cholesterol can be used as a marker of the risk conferred by elevated triglyceride levels. A measure of VLDL can be calculated from a nonfasting assessment of total cholesterol and HDL. Subtraction of the value of the latter from the former yields the "non-HDL cholesterol" level. This calculated value is an aggregate measure of all circulating atherogenic particles. As VLDL levels less than 30 mg/dL are considered normal, the ATP-III recommends non-HDL cholesterol goals to be no more than 30 mg/dL higher than the corresponding LDL targets (Table 6-5). That is, ATP-III considers non-HDL cholesterol to be another secondary target of lipid-modifying therapy, after the LDL goal is achieved. As needed, dyslipidemia therapy is intensified to achieve the non-HDL cholesterol goal, in patients with triglyceride levels of 200 mg/dL or greater. Treatment recommendations for reaching the non-HDL cholesterol goal may include diet intervention, exercise prescription, and pharmacologic therapy. Combination drug regimens are often necessary to reach non-HDL targets. Whereas a low HDL level is recognized as an independent risk factor for

Table 6-6. Framingham Risk Calculator

Age and Gender

Age (y)	Points for Men	Points for Women
20–34	−9	−7
35–39	−4	−3
40–44	0	0
45–49	3	3
50–54	6	6
55–59	8	8
60–64	10	10
65–69	11	12
70–74	12	14
75–79	13	16

Age and Total Cholesterol for Men

	Points				
Men: Total Cholesterol (mg/dL)	Age 20–39 y	Age 40–49 y	Age 50–59 y	Age 60–69 y	Age 70–79 y
<160	0	0	0	0	0
160–199	4	3	2	1	0
200–239	7	5	3	1	0
240–279	9	6	4	2	1
≥280	11	8	5	3	1

Age and Total Cholesterol for Women

	Points				
Women: Total Cholesterol (mg/dL)	Age 20–39 y	Age 40–49 y	Age 50–59 y	Age 60–69 y	Age 70–79 y
<160	0	0	0	0	0
160–199	4	3	2	1	1
200–239	8	6	4	3	1
240–279	11	8	5	3	2
≥280	13	10	7	4	2

Smoking Status

	Points for Different Age Groups				
Age (y)	20–39	40–49	50–59	60–69	70–79
Nonsmoker	0	0	0	0	0
Male smoker	8	5	3	1	1
Female smoker	9	7	4	2	1

HDL Cholesterol

HDL (mg/dL)	Points for Men or Women
≥60	−1
50–59	0
40–49	1
<40	2

Blood Pressure Control and Gender

	Points			
Systolic Blood Pressure (mm/Hg)	Men Untreated	Men Treated	Women Untreated	Women Treated
<120	0	0	0	0
120–129	0	1	1	3
130–139	1	2	2	4
140–159	1	2	3	5
≥160	2	3	4	6

(continued)

Table 6-6. Framingham Risk Calculator *(continued)*

10-year Risk Score for Men		10-year Risk Score for Women	
Total Points	**10-year Risk in %**	**Total Points**	**10-year Risk in %**
<0	<1	<9	<1
0	1	9	1
1	1	10	1
2	1	11	1
3	1	12	1
4	1	13	2
5	2	14	2
6	2	15	3
7	3	16	4
8	4	17	5
9	5	18	6
10	6	19	8
11	8	20	11
12	10	21	14
13	12	22	17
14	16	23	22
15	20	24	27
16	25	≥25	≥30
≥17	≥30		

HDL, high-density lipoprotein.

the development of ASCVD and as a predictor of CHD events, the evidence is insufficient to specify a goal for targeted therapy.[17] In patients with low HDL, ATP-III still considers LDL to be the primary target of therapy and non-HDL cholesterol to be a secondary priority.

TREATMENT OF DYSLIPIDEMIA

NONPHARMACOLOGIC TREATMENT

Therapeutic lifestyle changes (TLC) should be initiated for all individuals with dyslipidemia. Weight management, diet modification, and increased exercise are first-line interventions for patients who are prescribed drug therapy. Two-thirds of U.S. adults are overweight, and weight control can improve all lipid parameters and the components of the metabolic syndrome. Dys-

Table 6-7. Metabolic Syndrome Clinical Criteria*

Risk Factor	Defining Level
Abdominal obesity	Waist circumference
Men	>102 cm (>40 in.)
Women	>88 cm (>35 in.)
Triglycerides	≥150 mg/dL
HDL cholesterol	
Men	<40 mg/dL
Women	<50 mg/dL
Blood pressure	≥130/≥85 mm Hg
Fasting glucose	≥110 mg/dL

*Diagnosis is made when three or more risk factors are identified.
HDL, high-density lipoprotein.

lipidemia patients should be stratified by body mass index to assess the need for caloric restriction and increased physical activity. Determination of waist circumference provides an easily obtained measure of metabolically detrimental visceral adiposity. Regardless of weight, dyslipidemia patients should limit total fat, saturated and trans fats, and cholesterol in their diets. The ATP-III diet recommends limiting saturated fat in the diet to less than 7% of total calories and decreasing total cholesterol intake to less than 200 mg per day. This TLC diet also encourages the intake of soluble fiber and plant stanols or sterols to lower LDL levels. Stanols and sterols are essential components of plant cell membranes, and when ingested, they reduce the dietary cholesterol absorption by disrupting the formation of intestinal mixed micelles.[18] The so-called Mediterranean diet, which emphasizes consumption of monounsaturated fats, such as olive oil, whole grains, vegetables, and fish can also be recommended to reduce ASCVD risk.[19]

Physical activity can be recommended for all adults, especially dyslipidemia patients who are overweight. At least 30 minutes of moderate aerobic exercise on most days of the week should be encouraged. Prescribed physical activity need not be part of a structured exercise program or accrued all at one time. Activities such as running, cycling, or swimming produce cardiovascular benefit, but walking, gardening, housework, and stair climbing are also beneficial. To yield a maximum advantage, exercise should be intense enough to raise the heart rate. Regular physical activity can raise HDL levels, while decreasing blood pressure and insulin resistance. Exercise also assists smoking cessation, which can have an added beneficial impact on HDL values.

PHARMACOLOGIC TREATMENT

Lipid-modifying drug therapies have demonstrated an ability to slow the progression of atherosclerotic disease, stabilize rupture-prone atheromatous plaques, and improve cardiovascular outcomes. They confer these benefits through their favorable impact on lipid profiles and through drug-specific actions, vasodilatory actions, anti-inflammatory actions, and antithrombotic actions, which are often referred to as their pleiotropic effects.[20] Pharmacologic treatment should be considered an adjunct to diet and lifestyle changes. In stable, low-risk patients, drug interventions may follow a 3-month trial of TLC, but in higher risk patients, they must be considered an initial intervention.

Six drug classes are used to treat dyslipidemia. Lipid-modifying medications differ in their impact on lipid parameters, their relative and absolute contraindications, and their tolerability (Table 6-8). Safety concerns may be paramount when drugs are used in combination strategies. This increased risk of adverse events requires appropriate patient counseling, and close clinical and laboratory monitoring. Pharmacologic treatment must be taken indefinitely to maintain its benefit, thus the prescribed regimens must also be well tolerated to enhance persistence with therapy (Figure 6-1).

STATINS

Statins, or more formally, 3-hydroxy-3-methylglutaryl coenzyme A (HMG-CoA) reductase inhibitors, competitively inhibit the rate-limiting step in hepatic cholesterol synthesis. By decreasing intrahepatic cholesterol, they facilitate LDL clearance from the circulation through an upregulated expression of liver-associated LDL receptors. They also exert a favorable impact on triglyceride and HDL levels. Clinical trials reveal that statins reduce cardiovascular event rates and all-cause mortality in a broad range of demographic and risk populations.[21] Six statins are currently available in the United States; cerivastatin (Baycol®) was withdrawn from the market due to excess rates of morbidity (Table 6-9). Statins not only differ in LDL-lowering efficacy, but also in their metabolic fates, and thus in their potential for drug and disease interactions (Table 6-10).[22] They are generally well tolerated, though they are associated with dose-dependent elevations in liver transaminases. Patients with liver disease should be monitored closely, as medication withdrawal usually leads to resolution. Muscle cramping, or myalgia, is common, but muscle toxicity is rare and is indicated by more severe pain, weakness, and elevations in creatine kinase. Rhabdomyolysis with renal failure or death is more common with higher doses, in combination drug therapies and in certain patient cohorts (Table 6-11).[23] Statins are classified as category X in pregnancy; they should be used cautiously in women of child-bearing potential.

BILE-ACID SEQUESTRANTS

The use of bile-acid sequestrants, sometimes referred to as anion-exchange resins, is complicated by tolerability and compliance issues, as well as their modest LDL-lowering effects. Bile acids emulsify dietary fats to facilitate their absorption in the small intestine. These cholesterol-rich compounds are reabsorbed in the ileum and enterohepatically circulated back to the duodenum. Sequestrants prevent their resorption, by increasing their excretion in the stools, and increase the need for hepatic synthesis of bile acids from cholesterol and thus facilitate the occasional removal of cholesterol from the circulation. Coadministration with a statin can yield additive LDL-lowering benefits, and may obviate the modest triglyceride elevations sometimes seen with sequestrant use. Resins are not systemically absorbed; their adverse-effect profile is limited to gastrointestinal disturbances such as bloating, flatulence, and constipation. Tolerability can be enhanced by gradual dose titration and by increasing fluid and fiber intake. Bile acid sequestrants can bind many orally administered medications, including other-lipid modifying treatments,

Table 6-8. Medication Classes and Effect on Lipid Parameters

Medication Class	LDL	Triglycerides	HDL
Statins	Decrease by 20%–60%	Decrease by 10%–30%	Increase by 5%–15%
Bile-acid sequestrants	Decrease by 15%–30%	No change or increase	Increase by 5%
Niacin	Decrease by 5%–25%	Decrease by 20%–50%	Increase by 15%–35%
Fibrates	Decrease by 5%–20%	Decrease by 20%–50%	Increase by 10%–20%
Cholesterol-absorption inhibitors	Decrease by 15%–20%	Decrease by 5%–15%	Increase by 5%
Fish oil	No change or increase	Decrease by 20%–50%	Increase by 5%–10%

LDL, low-density lipoprotein; HDL, high-density lipoprotein.

Table 6-9. Statins and Combination Agents

Statin	Available Dose (mg)	Generic	LDL Decrease (%)
Atorvastatin (Lipitor®)	10, 20, 40, 80	No	39–60
Fluvastatin (Lescol®)	20, 40 maximum dose 80 mg (40 mg bid)	No	22–36
Fluvastatin extended release (Lescol XL®)	80	No	35
Lovastatin (Mevacor®)	10, 20, 40 maximum dose 80 mg (40 mg BID)	Yes	21–42
Lovastatin extended release (Altocor®)	10, 20, 40, 60	No	24–41
Pravastatin (Pravachol®)	10, 20, 40, 80	Yes	22–37
Rosuvastatin (Crestor®)	5, 10, 20, 40	No	45–63
Simvastatin (Zocor®)	5, 10, 20, 40, 80	Yes	26–47
Simvastatin/Ezetimibe (Vytorin®)	10/10, 10/20, 10/40, 10/80	No	45–60
Niacin extended release/ Lovastatin (Advicor®)	500/20, 1000/20 Dose 1000/20 to maximum dose 2000/40	No	30–42

LDL, low-density lipoprotein.
Data abstracted from Manufacturers' Prescribing Information.

thus decreasing the bioavailability of these drugs and detrimentally impacting their efficacy. Coadministered medications should be taken 1 hour before or 4 to 6 hours after resins are ingested. A more palatable, tablet form of sequestrant, colesevelam (Welchol®), does not impair the absorption of other drugs and is purported to be better tolerated than granular agents. Colesevelam is rated category B in pregnancy.

FIBRATES

Fibric-acid derivatives lower elevated triglyceride levels by increasing LPL activity, and increase HDL levels through peroxisome proliferator-activated receptor α binding. No predictable impact on LDL levels is seen, though LDL particle composition may be rendered less atherogenic. Clinical trial benefit has been variably

Table 6-10. Drug–Drug Interactions with HMG-CoA Reductase Inhibitors

Statin	CYP Metabolism	Major Drug Interactions	Other Potential Interactions
Atorvastatin	3A4: Substrate	Cyclosporine, Azole antifungals, erythromycin, clarithromycin, protease inhibitors, grapefruit juice, nefazodone	
Fluvastatin	2C9: Inhibitor	Warfarin	
Lovastatin	3A4: Substrate	Cyclosporine, Azole antifungals, erythromycin, clarithromycin, protease inhibitors, grapefruit juice, nefazodone	
Pravastatin	None	None significant	
Rosuvastatin	2C9: Substrate	Warfarin	Do not exceed 5 mg/d cyclosporine. Lower dose in Asian patients.
Simvastatin	3A4: Substrate	Cyclosporine, Azole antifungals, erythromycin, clarithromycin, protease inhibitors, grapefruit juice, nefazodone	Do not exceed 10 mg/d when used with gemfibrozil, or cyclosporine. Do not exceed 20 mg/d when used with amiodarone or verapamil.

CYP, cytochrome P450.

Table 6-11. Increase Statin-Associated Myopathy Risk

Factors that Increase Risk for Statin Myopathy

Advanced age (especially >80 y)
Female gender
Small body frame, frailty
Multisystem disease (e.g., chronic kidney disease in diabetes mellitus)
Perioperative period
Alcohol abuse
Concomitant medication use (especially cytochrome interactions)

demonstrated; their benefit on cardiovascular outcomes has not been extended to a decrease in total mortality. Fibrates are well tolerated, though myopathy and rhabdomyolysis can be a concern, especially with concurrent statin use. Fenofibrate (Tricor®) has less of an impact on statin metabolism and is the preferred agent in combination regimens. Fibrates are hepatically metabolized and eliminated in the urine; use in patients with moderate to severe liver and kidney disease should be avoided. There is an increased risk of gallstone formation with fibrate use. Fenofibrate belongs to category C as a pregnancy risk factor.

NIACIN

The mechanism by which nicotinic acid, or more commonly niacin, mediates its beneficial lipid effects is poorly understood. It is believed to inhibit lipolysis, decrease the release of free fatty acids into the circulation, and thus lower VLDL levels. Its use favorably impacts multiple lipid parameters: Niacin decreases LDL, triglycerides, and Lp(a) levels and increases HDL cholesterol. Niacin is an ideal drug for patients with mixed lipid disorders. It is available in a nonprescription, immediate-release formulation as well as a branded, extended-release formulation (Niaspan®). Widespread utilization is hindered by tolerability and dose-titration issues. Niacin usually causes cutaneous flushing, a prostaglandin-mediated event that can be symptomatically ameliorated with prior aspirin administration. Flushing can also be diminished with gradual dose titration over weeks and the use of the extended-release formulation. Niacin use should be closely monitored in patients with diabetes mellitus, as it can impair glucose tolerance.[24] It can also lead to hyperuricemia or precipitate gouty arthritis. Niacin can cause gastrointestinal distress, and should be avoided in patients with a history of peptic ulcer. Elevations in liver enzymes are rare, but more common when it is used in combination with a statin. Given these tolerability and disease and drug interactions, patient counseling is especially important to achieve target niacin doses and to maintain patient adherence with treatment. Pharmacologic doses of niacin are considered a category C pregnancy risk.

CHOLESTEROL-ABSORPTION INHIBITORS

Ezetimibe (Zetia®) is the first in a novel class of lipid-modifying medications, the selective cholesterol absorption inhibitors. Ezetimibe inhibits the intestinal absorption of cholesterol from exogenous sources, cholesterol in food, and endogenous sources, biliary free cholesterol. This inhibition is selective, in that there is no detrimental impact on administered steroids or fat-soluble vitamins. Ezetimibe use leads to a decrease in intestinal cholesterol delivered to the liver and a subsequent increase in the clearance of cholesterol from the circulation. Ezetimibe benefits all lipid parameters, but its impact on LDL levels is modest as a monotherapy. No dietary or anthropometric factors predict its efficacy. Its mechanism of action is complementary to statins, and it is approved by Food and Drug Administration (FDA) for adjunctive therapy.[25] Ezetimibe has also demonstrated additive lipid-modifying effects when used in combination with fenofibrate and colesevelam. Ezetimibe requires no dosage titration, or adjustment with renal disease or mild hepatic insufficiency. It is administered once daily, regardless of meals. Use is well tolerated and no adverse biochemical effect monitoring is mandated for monotherapy. However, elevated liver transaminases occur more frequently when ezetimibe is used in combination drug regimens, though prompt resolution with drug withdrawal is the rule. It is considered a category C agent in regard to pregnancy risk.

FISH OILS

Long-chain, highly unsaturated omega-3 fatty acid supplements can be used to treat hypertriglyceridemia. High doses of the fish oils like docosahexaenoic acid and eicosahexaenoic acid reduce VLDL production, though their impact on triglyceride levels are less pronounced than that of fibrates or niacin. Supplementation may produce less atherogenic LDL particles as well as yield antioxidant or antithrombotic effects (See Fig. 6-1). Clinical trial data are limited, but omega-3 fatty acids have been demonstrated to reduce sudden cardiac death.[26] Many proprietary formulations are available over the counter, though patients should be advised to identify product potency and to dose titrate based upon docosahexaenoic acid/eicosahexaenoic acid content. The FDA recently approved a prescription compound (Lovaza®) that provides a standardized omega-3-acid ethyl ester content. Adverse effects are limited to dyspepsia and

Clinical Pearls

1. The LDL goal for patients with ischemic heart disease and diabetes is <100 mg/dL; an OPTIONAL LDL goal of <70 relates to patients at very high risk such as acute coronary syndrome (ACS)[12]

2. The incidence of rhabdomyolysis is very low with moderate dose (simva 40 or equivalent) statin therapy (0.023%)[21]

3. Patients should receive additional liver function tests prior to titration and 3 months after titration to the 80-mg dose of a statin, and periodically thereafter (e.g., semiannually) for the first year of treatment.

4. Niaspan is an extended-release formulation of niacin that is associated with less flushing and itching than other forms of niacin; patients should take nonenteric coated aspirin (ASA) 325 mg 30 minutes prior to dose

5. The combination of statin and fibrate therapy increases the risk of rhabdomyolysis up to 5% [number needed to harm (NNH) 20]

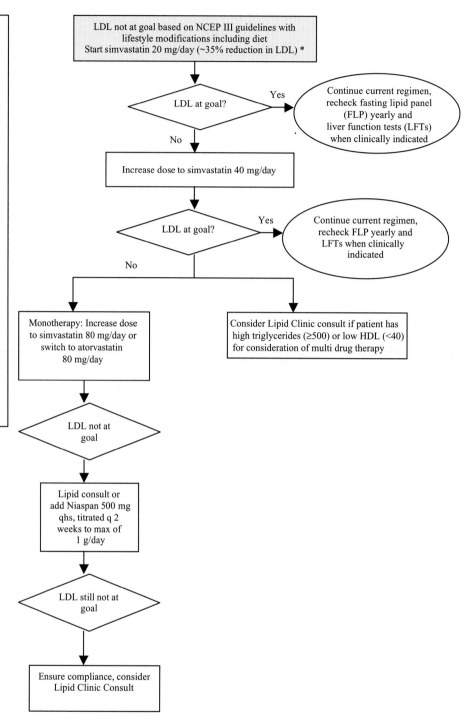

Figure 6-1. LDL reduction algorithm.

*Check baseline liver function tests prior to initiation of treatment and when clinically indicated thereafter. Simvastatin was chosen because it is now available generically.

reports of a fishy taste or fishy burps. Multiple times per day dosing is generally required of all products. No significant drug interactions are noted. Use in patients with sensitivity or allergies to fish is contraindicated. High-dose supplementation is assigned category C in regard to pregnancy risk.

COMBINATION THERAPY

Many patients will require combination lipid-modifying treatments to achieve optimal lipid management. Emerging clinical trial evidence supports lower LDL targets and intensified therapy for triglyceride and HDL abnormalities.[27,28] To meet these more stringent goals, combination therapy is often necessary. Use of a statin with an enteric agent, either a bile-acid sequestrant or ezetimibe, may decrease the rate of adverse effects experienced when doses of statins are titrated upwards. Combination therapy with a statin and an agent beneficially impacting triglycerides or HDL levels, either a fibrate or niacin, is often required in patients with mixed lipid disorders or with the metabolic syndrome. Familial dyslipidemia may warrant triple-drug therapy. Pharmaceutical manufacturers have responded by introducing fixed-dose combination drugs (Table 6-9).[29] However, such combination regimens have not demonstrated CHD outcome benefits in clinical trials. Regardless of FDA labeling, the use of combination therapy requires additional patient education, more vigilant biochemical monitoring, and a greater scrutiny of potential disease and drug interactions. Such close monitoring may be best conducted in a specialized dyslipidemia clinic staffed by trained physicians, advanced-practice nurses, and pharmacists.

FUTURE THERAPY

Novel mechanisms for treating dyslipidemia are under active investigation. It is likely that as our understanding of lipoprotein metabolism and transport evolves, more pathophysiologic targets for pharmacologic therapy will be identified. Intense scrutiny is currently focused on reverse cholesterol transport by HDL. Thus far, drugs that inhibit cholesteryl ester transfer protein and raise HDL levels have been clinically disappointing. Medications that inhibit acyl-coenzyme A:cholesterol acyltransferase and microsomal transfer protein, thus preventing the enterocyte from assembling chylomicrons, and drugs that directly inhibit ileal bile-acid transport, thus preventing their enterohepatic circulation and so depleting hepatic cholesterol stores, are early in their development and no clinical judgments can be made.

EVIDENCE-BASED SUMMARY

- Dyslipidemia is a prerequisite risk factor in the development of ASCVD, and treatment can reduce ASCVD events and mortality.
- ASCVD risk assessment is necessary to determine lipid-modifying-treatment goals, which are primarily stated in terms of LDL.
- The metabolic syndrome and non-HDL cholesterol are considered secondary targets of dyslipidemia therapy.
- Pharmacologic treatment is an adjunct to TLC, and should be individualized based upon global ASCVD risk and medical comorbidities.
- Expanded indications for intensive dyslipidemia interventions, including use of combination drug therapies, require diligent patient education and vigilant symptom and biochemical monitoring.

REFERENCES

1. Lloyd-Jones DM, Larson MG, Beiser A, et al. Lifetime risk of developing coronary heart disease. *Lancet.* 1999; 353:89.
2. Law MR, Wald NJ, Rudnicka AR. Quantifying effect of statins on low-density lipoprotein cholesterol, ischaemic heart disease, and stroke: Systematic review and meta-analysis. *BMJ.* 2003;326:1423.
3. Pearson TA, Laurora I, Chu H, et al. The Lipid Treatment Assessment Project (L-TAP): A multicenter survey to evaluate the percentages of dyslipidemic patients receiving lipid-lowering therapy and achieving low-density lipoprotein cholesterol goals. *Arch Intern Med.* 2000;160:459.
4. Executive summary of the Third Report of the National Cholesterol Education Program (NCEP) expert panel on detection, evaluation, and treatment of high blood cholesterol in adults (Adult Treatment Panel III). *JAMA.* 2001;285:2486.
5. Buse JB, Ginsberg HN, Bakris GL, et al. Primary prevention of cardiovascular disease in people with diabetes mellitus: A scientific statement from the American Heart Association and the American Diabetes Association. *Diabetes Care.* 2007;30:162.
6. Snow V, Aronson MD, Hornbake ER, et al. Lipid control in the management of type 2 diabetes mellitus: A clinical practice guideline from the American College of Physicians. *Ann Intern Med.* 2004;140:644.
7. Grundy SM, Cleeman JI, Bairey-Merz CN, et al. Implications of recent clinical trials for the National Cholesterol Education Program Adult Treatment Panel III Guidelines. *Circulation.* 2004;110:227.
8. Nam BH, Kannel WB, D'Agostino RB. Search for an optimal atherogenic lipid risk profile: From the Framingham Study. *Am J Cardiol.* 2006;97:372.

9. Shepard J, Blauw GJ, Murphy MB, et al. Pravastatin in elderly individuals at risk of vascular disease (PROSPER): A randomized controlled trial. Prospective study of pravastatin in the elderly at risk. *Lancet.* 2002;360:1623.

10. Baigent C, Keech A, Kerney PM, et al. Efficacy and safety of cholesterol-lowering treatment: Prospective meta-analysis of data from 90,056 participants in 14 randomized trials of statins. *Lancet.* 2005;366:1267.

11. Wilt T, Bloomfield H, MacDonald R, et al. Effectiveness of statin therapy in adults with coronary heart disease. *Arch Intern Med.* 2004;164:1427.

12. Smith SC, Jr., Allen J, Blair SN, et al. AHA/ACC Guidelines for secondary prevention for patients with coronary and other atherosclerotic vascular disease: 2006 update. *Circulation.* 2006;113:2363.

13. Wilson PW, D'Agostino RB, Levy D, et al. Prediction of coronary heart disease using risk factor categories. *Circulation.* 1998;97:1837.

14. Haffner SM, Lehto S, Ronnemaa T, et al. Mortality from coronary heart disease in subjects with type 2 diabetes and in nondiabetic subjects with and without prior myocardial infarction. *N Engl J Med.* 1998;339:229.

15. Ridker PM, Cannon CP, Morrow D, et al. C-reactive protein levels and outcomes after statin therapy. *N Engl J Med.* 2005;352:20.

16. Kahn R, Buse J, Ferrannini E, Stern M. The metabolic syndrome: Time for a critical appraisal: Joint statement from the American Diabetes Association and the European Association for the Study of Diabetes. *Diabetes Care.* 2005;28:2289.

17. Dean BB, Borenstein JE, Henning JM, et al. Can change in HDL-cholesterol reduce cardiovascular risk? *Am Heart J.* 2004;147:966.

18. Katan MB, Grundy SM, Jones P, et al. Efficacy and safety of plant stanols and sterols in the management of blood cholesterol levels. *Mayo Clin Proc.* 2003;78:965.

19. Lichtenstein AH, Appel LJ, Brands M, et al. Diet and lifestyle recommendations revision 2006: A scientific statement from the American Heart Association Nutrition Committee. *Circulation.* 2006;114:82.

20. Hayward RA, Hofer TP, Vijan S. Narrative review: Lack of evidence for recommended low-density lipoprotein treatment targets: A solvable problem. *Ann Intern Med.* 2006;145:520.

21. Collins R, Armitage J, Parish S. MRC/BHF Heart Protection Study of cholesterol-lowering with simvastatin in 5963 people with diabetes: A randomized placebo-controlled trial. *Lancet.* 2003;361:2005.

22. Jones PH, Davidson MH, Stein EA, et al. Comparison of the efficacy and safety of rosuvastatin versus atorvastatin, simvastatin, and pravastatin across doses (STELLAR Trial). *Am J Cardiol.* 2003;92:152.

23. Pasternak RC, Smith, Jr., SC, Bairey-Merz CN, et al. ACC/AHA/NHLBI clinical advisory on the use and safety of statins. *Circulation.* 2002;106:1024.

24. Haffner SM. American Diabetes Association: Dyslipidemia management in adults with diabetes. *Diabetes Care.* 200427:S68.

25. Davidson MH, McGarry T, Bettis R, et al. Ezetimibe coadministered with simvastatin in patients with primary hypercholesterolemia. *J Am Coll Cardiol.* 2002;40:2125.

26. Marchioli R, Barzi F, Bomba E, et al. Early protection against sudden death by n-3 polyunsaturated fatty acids after myocardial infarction: Time–course analysis of the results of the Grippo Italiano per lo Studio della Sopravvivenza nell'Infarto Miocardico (GISSI)-Prevenzione trial. *Circulation.* 2002;105:1897.

27. Cannon CP, Braunwald E, McCabe CH, et al. Intensive versus moderate lipid lowering with statins after acute coronary syndromes. *N Engl J Med.* 2004;350:1495.

28. Waters DD, Guyton JR, Herrington DM, et al. Treating to new targets (TNT) study: Does lowering low-density lipoprotein cholesterol levels below currently recommended guidelines yield incremental clinical benefit? *Am J Cardiol.* 2004;93:154.

29. Bays HE, Dujovne RCA, McGovern ME, et al. Advicor versus other cholesterol-modulating agents trial evaluation (ADVOCATE). *Am J Cardiol.* 2003;91:667.

Chapter 7

Peripheral Arterial Disease

Barbara Jean Hoeben

SEARCH STRATEGY

A systematic search of the medical literature was performed in January 2008. The search, limited to human subjects and English language journals, included the National Guideline Clearinghouse, the Cochrane database, PubMed, UpToDate®, and PIER®. The current American College of Cardiology/American Heart Association 2006 Guidelines for the management of patients with peripheral arterial disease can be found at www.acc.org

Peripheral arterial disease (PAD), the most common form of peripheral vascular disease, is a manifestation of progressive narrowing of arteries caused by atherosclerosis.[1] PAD can be used to designate occlusive, stenotic, and aneurysmal diseases of the aorta and its branch arteries.[2] This chapter will focus on lower extremity PAD. PAD is associated with elevated risk of cardiovascular disease (CVD) morbidity and mortality, even in the absence of prior history of acute myocardial infarction (AMI), stroke or other manifestations of CVD.[1,3] Patients with PAD have approximately the same relative risk of death from CVD as do patients with a history of coronary or cerebrovascular disease and PAD should be considered a surrogate marker of subclinical coronary artery disease (CAD) and other vascular territories.[1,4,5] The treatment of PAD focuses on decreasing the functional impairment caused by symptoms of intermittent claudication (IC) through nonpharmacologic and pharmacologic therapy and by minimizing the impact of other cardiovascular risk factors.[6,7]

CLINICAL PRESENTATION

PAD is most commonly a manifestation of systemic atherosclerosis in which the arterial lumen of the lower extremities becomes progressively occluded by atherosclerotic plaque.[8] The major risk factors for the development of atherosclerosis are older age (greater than 70 years), cigarette smoking, diabetes mellitus, hypercholesterolemia, hypertension (HTN), and hyperhomocysteinemia.[2,8,9] Additionally, patients less than 50 years of age are at risk if they have been diagnosed with diabetes and one additional atherosclerotic risk factor, as well as patients more than age 50 who have a history of diabetes or smoking.[2] The arteries most commonly involved, in order of occurrence, are the femoropopliteral-tibial, aortoiliac, carotid and vertebral, splanchnic and renal, and brachiocephalic.[10] Familial hypercholesterolemia (FH) leading to hypercholesterolemia and elevated low-density lipoprotein (LDL) levels is associated with accelerated development of atherosclerosis earlier and with more severe symptoms (e.g., IC) and abnormal blood flow studies compared to controls.[11] Intima-media thickness can be used as a surrogate phenotype for cardiovascular risk in FH and carotid and/or femoral artery atherosclerosis results in increased intima-media thickness and it is correlated to cardiovascular risk in FH patients compared with normolipidemic individuals.[7]

PHYSICAL FINDINGS

The clinical presentation of PAD is variable and includes a range of symptoms from no symptoms at all (typically early in the disease, with 5% to 10% developing symptoms more than 5 years[12,13]) to pain and discomfort. The two most common characteristics of PAD are IC and pain at rest in the lower extremities.[14–16] IC is generally regarded as the primary indicator of PAD and has been described as fatigue, discomfort, cramping, pain, or numbness in the affected extremities (typically the buttock, thigh, or calf) during exercise and is resolved within a few minutes by resting.[14,15,17–19] Rest pain typically occurs later in the disease when the blood supply is not adequate to perfuse the extremity (critical limb ischemia). This most often can be felt at night, while the patient is lying in bed, in the feet (typically the toes or heel).[7,14–16]

DIAGNOSTIC EVALUATION

An important criterion for the accurate diagnosis of PAD is the exclusion of other conditions that possess similar signs and symptoms. A differential diagnosis should rule out other neurological conditions (i.e., peripheral neuropathy), inflammatory conditions (i.e., arthritis), and vascular conditions (i.e., deep venous thrombosis) which may mimic PAD.[7,15,19,20]

MEDICAL HISTORY/PATIENT INTERVIEW

A detailed medical history and interview with the patient is the first step in providing information that may help to determine a differential diagnosis of PAD. Does the patient have a history of walking impairment, poorly healing wounds of the legs or feet, or pain at rest localized to the lower extremities? Does the medical history include a diagnosis of diabetes, obesity, HTN, and/or hypercholesterolemia? Does the social history include current, or past, smoking of tobacco products?[2] Detailed documentation of this information may help to determine the diagnosis of PAD, either in the present with patient complaining of symptoms, or in the future if the patient presents without symptoms.

PHYSICAL EXAMINATION

As with any good medical encounter, a detailed patient history of symptoms and atherosclerosis risk factors can be helpful in the diagnosis of PAD. Unfortunately, as illustrated by the Peripheral Arterial Disease Awareness, Risk, and Treatment: New Resources for Survival program, providers who rely on a history alone will miss approximately 85% to 90% of patients with PAD.[17] Therefore, a complete medical examination of the patient is vital to proper diagnosis.[7]

Requesting that the patient remove socks and shoes may reveal nonspecific signs of decreased blood low to the extremities (i.e., cool skin temperature, shiny skin, decreased pulses, thickened toenails, lack of hair on the calf, feet and/or toes) or, in severe cases, visible sores or ulcers that are slow to heal and may even be black in appearance.[2,7,14–16,21,22]

ANKLE-BRACHIAL INDEX (ABI)

The ankle-brachial index (ABI) is a simple, noninvasive, quantitative test that has been proven to be a highly sensitive and specific (≥90%) tool in the diagnosis of PAD.[13,17,23–25] To measure the ABI, the patient lies in the supine position as the systolic blood pressure is measured at the brachial arteries on both arms and the dorsalis pedis and posterior tibial arteries of the legs with a standard sphygmomanometer and a continuous-wave Doppler device. The pressures obtained at the dorsalis pedis and posterior tibial arteries are averaged and divided by the mean measurement taken at the left and right brachial arteries.[9,21,26,27] An ABI of 1 is considered normal while a measurement less than 0.9 is consistent with PAD. Further, the range of 0.7 to 0.9 correlates with mild PAD, 0.4 to 0.7 indicates moderate disease, and less than 0.4 denotes severe PAD.[7,8,18,26]

The ABI can also be useful after a test of exercise tolerance (i.e., 5–6 min on a treadmill or 30–50 repetitions of heel raises). Patients with PAD will have a significant drop in the ABI after exercise while pain with a normal or unchanged ABI can rule out PAD and suggest to the provider that an alternate diagnosis exists.[8,18,21] In addition to providing diagnostic information, the ABI measurement has been shown to be a strong predictor of future cardiovascular events associated with PAD.[7,28] Alternatively, arteriography is an expensive, invasive test that may be used to diagnose PAD. However, as ABI is a sufficient means of diagnosis, arteriography is not necessary or encouraged.[7,14,19,24] Repeat ABI measurements should be assessed at each patient visit to determine if there has been stabilization, or progression, of the disease process.[7]

OTHER USEFUL DIAGNOSTIC TOOLS

Other noninvasive tools are available for the diagnosis of PAD. Handheld Dopplers are becoming more readily available and may serve to aid in the diagnosis of PAD at the bedside. One study has suggested a calculation that takes into consideration the patient's history of AMI and the number of auscultated and palpated posterior tibial arteries.[29,30] Magnetic resonance angiography can be used to examine the presence and location of significant stenosis, or lack thereof, and is a reasonable option in patients who are being considered for surgical revascularization.[2] Similarly, computed tomographic angiography can be used to determine the presence of significant stenosis and soft tissue diagnostic information that may be associated with PAD (i.e., aneurysms).[2] A provider must determine if the benefits of these additional tests will outweigh their limitations (i.e., magnetic resonance angiography can overestimate the degree of stenosis and computed tomographic angiography requires iodinated contrast[2]) and justify the additional costs.

LABORATORY TESTS

There are no specific laboratory tests for the diagnosis of PAD. However, tests that screen for risk factors of other atherosclerotic conditions can lend useful information (i.e., complete lipid panel demonstrating elevated LDL, elevated total cholesterol and/or low HDL, elevated blood glucose, and hemoglobin A-1C, etc.)[7]

RISK STRATIFICATION

The National Health and Nutrition Examination Survey found that the prevalence of PAD among adults aged 40 years and older in the United States was 4.3% using the definition of an ABI of less than 0.9 in either leg.[3] The prevalence of PAD is highly dependent on age, being infrequent in younger individuals and common in older individuals. In age- and gender-adjusted logistic regression analyses, black race/ethnicity (odds ratio [OR] 2.83), current smoking (OR 4.46), diabetes (OR 2.71), HTN (OR 1.75), hypercholesterolemia (OR 1.68), and impaired renal function (estimated glomerular filtration rate less than 60 mL/min per 1.73 m^2) (OR 2.00) were associated with more prevalent PAD.[3,31] The relative risk of death from CVD in patients with PAD is reported to range from 2.0 to 5.1 in patients with or without CVD and 2.9 to 5.7 in patients with known CVD.[9] CVD accounts for 75% of all deaths in patients with PAD.[8] It is important to recognize that the risk of death is approximately the same in men and women and is elevated even in asymptomatic patients. Patients with critical leg ischemia who have the lowest ABI values have an annual mortality of 25%.[7,32]

MANAGEMENT

NONPHARMACOLOGIC THERAPY

Smoking Cessation

It has been thoroughly documented that cigarette smoking not only increases the risk of developing PAD and other cardiovascular disorders, but that the duration and quantity smoked can negatively impact disease progression (i.e., increase the risk of amputation) and increase mortality.[9,20,28,33–37] As a result, providers must advise patients to quit and should offer nonpharmacologic and pharmacologic means to aid the patient to that goal. Individual or group behavior modification therapy with or without the addition of certain antidepressants (i.e., bupropion) or nicotine replacement therapies (i.e., gum or patches) has been proven effective in numerous studies. Reassessment of smoking status and progress encouragement at each encounter can help to reemphasize to the patient the vital importance of this lifestyle change.[7]

Exercise

Walking exercise programs for patients with PAD have been proven to result in an increase in walking duration and distance, an increase pain-free walking, and a delayed onset of claudication by 179%.[20,22,34,35,38–43] Other benefits of exercise programs include improving diabetes and lipid management, reducing weight, improving blood viscosity and flow, and reducing blood pressure.[6] The type of aerobic activity recommended, as well as the duration and frequency of the activity, should be individually designed on a patient-to-patient basis. The 2006 American College of Cardiology and American Heart Association Guidelines for the Management of PAD recommends supervised exercise training for patients with IC, for a minimum of 30 to 45 minutes, to be performed at least 3 times per week.[2] A recent prospective, observational study has concluded that PAD patients with higher physical activity (as measured with a vertical accelerometer) have reduced mortality and cardiovascular events compared to those with low physical activity, regardless of confounders.[44] Repeat exercise treadmill walking testing should be repeated at regular intervals (i.e., quarterly to biannually) to assess improvement or decline in walking duration and distance, as well as the time to pain onset while performing this activity.[7]

PHARMACOLOGIC ANTIPLATELET THERAPY

See Table 7-1.

ASPIRIN

By far, the most compelling evidence for the use of any pharmacologic agent in PAD can be found with aspirin (ASA). The Antithrombotic Trialists' Collaboration (ATC) conducted a meta-analysis of 195 randomized trials, composed of more than 135 000 patients at high risk for occlusive arterial disease, and concluded that low-dose ASA (75–160 mg) and medium-dose ASA (160–325 mg/d) lead to a significant reduction in serious vascular events (12%) in "high-risk" patients, such as those with PAD.[45] It was also noted in this analysis that the risk of major extracranial bleed was similar between the low-dose and medium-dose regimens.

The recommendations of the Seventh American College of Chest Physicians (ACCP) Conference on Antithrombolitic and Thrombolytic Therapy recommend

Table 7-1. Pharmacotherapy Options for Patients with PAD[1–15]

Agent	Daily Dose (Oral)	MOA	Side Effects	Contraindications	Level of Evidence
Aspirin (ASA)	81–325 mg	Irreversibly inhibits prostaglandin cyclooxygenase in platelets, prevents formation of thromboxane A_2	Gastrointestinal upset and/or bleeding	Active bleeding; Hemophilia; Thrombocytopenia	With coronary or cerebrovascular (Grade 1A), without (Grade 1C+)
Dipyridamole ER	400 mg (+ASA 50 mg)	May act by inhibiting platelet aggregation (complete MOA unknown)	Angina; Dyspnea; Hypotension; Headache; Dizziness	Active bleeding; CAD ("coronary steal syndrome")	Recommendation for use not specified in report
Cilostazol (Pletal®)*	100 mg BID	Phosphodiesterase inhibitor, suppresses platelet aggregation; direct artery vasodialator	Fever; Infection; Tachycardia	All CHF patients (decreased survival)	With IC (Grade 2A)
Clopidogrel (Plavix®)	75 mg	Inhibits binding of ADP analogues to its platelet receptor causing irreversible inhibition of platelets	Chest pain; Purpura Generalized pain; Rash	Active pathological bleeding (i.e., peptic ulcer, intracranial hemorrhage)	Recommend clopidogrel over no antiplatelet therapy (Grade 1C+)
Pentoxifylline (Trental®)	1.2 g	Alters RBC flexibility; decreases platelet adhesion; reduces blood viscosity; decreases fibrinogen concentration	Dyspnea; Nausea; Vomiting; Headache; Dizziness	Recent retinal or cerebral hemorrhage; active bleeding	Not recommended in patients with IC (Grade 1B)
Ticlopidine (Ticlid®)	500 mg	Inhibits binding of ADP analogues to its platelet receptor causing irreversible inhibition of platelets	Leukopenia; Rash Thrombocytopenia; Neutropenia; Agranulocytosis; Aplastic anemia	Active bleeding; Hemophilia; Thrombocytopenia	Clopidogrel recommended over ticlopidine (Grade 1C+)

* Cilostazol should be used in combination with antiplatelet therapy.
 Grades of recommendation for antithrombotic and thrombolytic therapy is part of the Seventh ACCP Conference on Antithrombotic and Thrombolytic Therapy[16]
ASA, aspirin; ER, extended-release; mg, milligrams; g, grams; BID, twice-daily; ADP, adenosine 5'-diphosphate; RBC, red blood cell; CAD, coronary artery disease; CHF, congestive heart failure; IC, intermittent claudication.

lifelong ASA (75–325 mg/d) over clopidogrine, and no antithrombolitic therapy in patients with PAD.[46] Unfortunately, no data are currently available from large, clinical, randomized trials that ASA, or any other antiplatelet therapies, can actually prevent or delay the progression of PAD.[7,46]

ASA ± DIPYRIDIMOLE EXTENDED-RELEASE

The ATC also examined the use of dipyridamole extended-release in combination with ASA in "high risk" patients, such as those with PAD. Their meta-analysis of 25 trials (more than 10 000 patients) concluded that the addition of dipyridamole to aspirin led to an additional reduction in serious vascular events over ASA alone (6%); however, this reduction was unable to reach statistical significance ($p = 0.32$).[45,47] It should also be taken into consideration that most of the reduction in

nonfatal stoke in this analysis came from one trial, and these data are not replicated in the other studies.[45,48,49] The addition of dipyridamole to ASA may cause an increased risk of bleeding and gastrointestinal side effects when compared to placebo and should not be used in with CAD.[7,49]

CLOPIDOGREL (PLAVIX®)

The ATC meta-analysis also reviewed the effectiveness of clopidogrel 75 mg per day in "high-risk" patients, including those with PAD. The Collaboration concluded that although clopidogrel was able to reduce serious vascular events by 10%, this was significantly less than the reduction seen with ASA (12%, $p = 0.03$), as described previously.[45] Included in this meta-analysis was the report from the Clopidogrel versus ASA in Patients at Risk of Ischemic Events trial which had concluded that clopidogrel (75 mg daily) was more effective than ASA (325 mg daily) in preventing vascular events in "high-risk" patients with an overall reduction in ischemic stroke, MI or vascular death from 5.83% to 5.32% ($p = 0.043$). This difference was even more pronounced in the subgroup analysis of PAD patients (clopidogrel therapy led to a significant reduction of 4.86% vs. 3.71% in the ASA group, $p = 0.0028$).[5,23,28] It must be noted that clopidogrel is significantly more expensive than ASA therapy, not only in drug costs, but clopidogrel remains a by-prescription only medication and, thus, requires a physician visit to obtain a prescription for the medication. It is for all these reasons that the current recommendations list clopidogrel as first-line agent, but only in cases where ASA therapy is either not tolerated or contraindicated.[7,45,48]

TICLOPIDINE (TICLID®)

Although ticlopidine has the same mechanism of action (MOA) as clopidogrel and possesses a similar molecular structure, the once promising results seen with ticlopidine therapy have now been overshadowed by the severe hematological side effects unique to this agent. Other agents, namely, clopidogrel, are now used in its stead.[7,9,20,35]

PHARMACOLOGIC THERAPY OF IC

See Table 7-1.

CILOSTAZOL (PLETAL®)

In a head-to-head, randomized, placebo-controlled study in 698 patients with moderate-to-severe claudication, Dawson et al.[50] assigned patients to cilostazol (100 mg twice a day), pentoxifylline (400 mg 3 times a day), or placebo in an effort to improve maximal walking distance. After 24 weeks, the cilostazol group demonstrated a 54% mean increase in distance versus pentoxifylline which demonstrated only a 30% mean increase ($p < 0.001$).[50] Similarly, a meta-analysis of eight randomized, double-blind, placebo-controlled, parallel-design trials supported this conclusion with a reported increase in maximal walking distance and pain-free walking distance over placebo with cilostazol at doses of 50 mg and 100 mg twice-daily ($p < 0.05$ for all).[51] Regrettably, improvement in walking distance has appeared to come with a price (in addition to the high drug cost); cilostazol has a "black box" warning from the U.S. Food and Drug Administration warning providers not to use this medication in patients with PAD and coexisting heart failure.[33] If patients with PAD are not candidates for surgical interventions to improve

severe IC, and after appropriate exercise therapy and therapeutic lifestyle changes have been implemented, the Seventh ACCP Conference on Antithrombotic and Thrombolytic Therapy then suggests the use of this agent.[7,46]

PENTOXIFYLLINE (TRENTAL®)

Unlike cilostazol, pentoxifylline has produced less promising results in clinical trials. An illustration of this is the randomized, placebo-controlled trial by Dawson et al.[50] mentioned above. Not only did cilostazol outperform pentoxifylline in improvement in walking distance, the improvement seen with pentoxifylline was no different from placebo ($p = 0.82$).[50] This nonsignificant improvement in walking distance has been observed in other studies as well.[9,52] Meanwhile, other meta-analyses of pentoxifylline in comparison to placebo for the improvement of maximal walking distance, have shown some minimal improvement over placebo, but the average effects were relatively small.[9,53–56] For these reasons, the Seventh ACCP Conference on Antithrombotic and Thrombolytic Therapy does not recommend the use of this agent.[7,46]

VASCULAR SURGERY CONSULTATION

See Table 7-2.

Various surgical procedures are available for patients with severe, debilitating claudication who have attempted, and failed, other means of nonpharmacologic and pharmacologic therapy. However, surgical intervention is not indicated as a means of *preventing* the progression to limb-threatening ischemia in patients with IC.[2] For patients with severe IC resulting in critical leg ischemia, physicians may need to discuss alternate surgical interventions including aortofemoral bypass, femoralpopliteal bypass, or even amputation.[14,15,34] However, the TransAtlantic Inter-Society Consensus (TASC) document on PAD is very clear on the recommendations for invasive therapy.[22] The decision to attempt percutaneous revascularization is often made

Table 7-2. The TASC Recommendations for Invasive Therapy of IC17

There must be a lack of adequate response to exercise therapy and risk factor modification.
The patient must have severe disability from IC resulting in impairment of daily activities.
There must be a thorough evaluation of the risks versus benefits of an invasive intervention including probability of success, the anticipated future course of the disease if an intervention is not performed, as well as an evaluation of concomitant disease states.

with the guidance of diagnostic angiography. Angiography can help to identify the location and size of lesions and provide valuable information as to the likelihood of success with surgical revascularization.[7,22]

PERCUTANEOUS TRANSLUMINAL ANGIOPLASTY

Percutaneous transluminal angioplasty (PTA) is an example of an invasive treatment for PAD. A randomized controlled clinical trial performed by Whyman et al.[57] determined that, at 2 years postintervention, the PTA outcomes on maximum walking distance and ABI and were not significantly different than in patients that had only received daily low-dose ASA ($p > 0.05$). Nevertheless, patients who had received PTA had significantly fewer occluded arteries ($p = 0.003$), but the true clinical significance of this finding was not able to be realized in the time allotted for the study.[7]

STENT PLACEMENT

Stent placement in PAD patients has also been an area of study and controversy. A meta-analysis examining the use of stent placement versus PTA for the treatment of aortoiliac occlusive disease determined that, although stent placement and PTA yielded similar complication and mortality rates, posttreatment ABI were more improved with stents (0.87 with PTA and 0.76 with stents, $p < 0.03$) and the risk of long-term failure was 39% less with stent placement.[58] However, other studies have not demonstrated improvement in patency rates in peripheral arteries versus PTA alone.[14] The TASC document provides specific recommendations for PTA, with or without stenting, depending on the how diffuse the disease process is, the number and size of the lesions, and the location of the lesions.[7,22]

PHARMACOLOGIC THERAPY OF COMORBID DISEASE STATES

HYPERTENSION

HTN is a major risk factor for PAD and can lead to AMI, stroke, heart failure, and death.[43] Current guidelines recommend the treatment goal for blood pressure in patients with PAD to mirror those in patients with documented CVD, 130/85 mm Hg.[33,43] Although, the Heart Outcomes Prevention Evaluation study (HOPE trial), demonstrated that angiotensin-converting-enzyme (ACE) inhibitors reduced not only blood pressure, but other cardiovascular events (i.e., AMI, stroke and death) in high-risk patients, including those with PAD, no specific class of antihypertensives are recommended over another for the treatment of HTN in patients with PAD. Therefore, selection of drug therapy for HTN should be made on the basis of comorbid disease states, drug costs and availability, drug allergies, or other possible limiting factors.[7]

HYPERLIPIDEMIA

PAD is considered by the Expert Panel on Detection, Evaluation, and Treatment of High Blood Cholesterol in Adults (Adult Treatment Panel III, or ATP III) to be in the category of highest risk, or a coronary heart disease risk equivalent. Therefore, it was recommended by the Expert Panel that levels of LDL be maintained at <100 mg/dL and non-high-density lipoprotein (HDL) levels (total cholesterol–HDL cholesterol) at <130 mg/dL.[59] Clinical trials have been conducted since the time of this recommendation, specifically the Heart Protection Study[60] and the Pravastatin or Atorvastatin Evaluation and Infection—Thrombolysis in Myocardial Infarction[61] trial, that have lead many clinical experts to now recommend an optional LDL goal of <70 mg/dL for additional retardation of atherosclerotic plaque formation in persons considered to be at very high risk, including patients with PAD.[62] Several options are available for the initiation of drug therapy for LDL-lowering in patients with PAD. Statins, bile acid sequestrants, and nicotinic acid are all effective treatment options. However, in most cases, statins are the preferred starting agent in this patient population.[2,7,17,34,59,60]

DIABETES MELLITUS

A recent meta-analysis of more than 95 000 diabetic patients demonstrated an increasing risk of death from cardiovascular events as blood glucose concentrations increased, thus providing additional support for the accepted premise that glycemic control serves as a risk factor for CVD.[63] Because of the high prevalence of PAD among diabetic patients, the American Diabetes Association recommends ABI screening of all diabetics above 50 years of age for PAD.[64] Because of the presence of peripheral neuropathy, patients with diabetes may be less likely to experience or report symptoms of PAD and the first sign may be as drastic as the appearance of a gangrenous foot ulcer. Therefore, although there is currently a lack of randomized-controlled studies illustrating that the degree of glycemic control is predictive of the extent of PAD present, it is recommended that all patients with concomitant diabetes and PAD maintain good glycemic control, as evidenced by a hemoglobin A-1c level of <7%.[7,15,20,22,33,35,64,65]

EVIDENCE-BASED SUMMARY

- PAD is most commonly a manifestation of systemic atherosclerosis in which the arterial lumen of the lower extremities becomes progressively occluded by atherosclerotic plaque
- Risk factors for PAD are age more than 40 years, cigarette smoking, diabetes mellitus, hypercholesterolemia, HTN, and hyperhomocysteinemia
- Clinical presentation of PAD is variable and includes a range of symptoms from no symptoms at all (typically early in the disease) to pain and discomfort
- The two most common characteristics of PAD are pain at rest in the lower extremities and IC, described as fatigue, discomfort, cramping, pain, or numbness in the affected extremities during exercise and is resolved by rest
- ABI is the most useful tool in establishing the diagnosis of PAD: 1 is considered normal, 0.7 to 0.9 correlates with mild PAD, 0.4 to 0.7 indicates moderate disease, and below 0.4 denotes severe PAD
- Every effort must be made, via pharmacologic and nonpharmacologic means, to control comorbid conditions such as diabetes, obesity, HTN, and hyperlipidemia
- Aspirin is the pharmacologic agent that has the most compelling evidence for use in PAD
- Various surgical procedures, such as PTA and stent placement, are available for patients with severe, debilitating claudication who have attempted, and failed, other means of nonpharmacologic and pharmacologic therapy

REFERENCES

1. Hiatt WR. Sounding the PAD alarm. GPs can diagnose peripheral artery disease with a simple ankle-and-arm blood pressure test. *Health News*, April 2004:10(4).
2. Hirsch AT, Haskal ZJ, Hertzer NR, et al. ACC/AHA Guidelines for The Management of Patients with Peripheral Arterial Disease (Lower Extremity, Renal, Mesenteric, and Abdominal Aortic): Executive summary: A Collaborative Report from the American Association for Vascular Surgery/Society for Vascular Surgery, Society for Vascular Medicine and Biology, Society of Interventional Radiology, and the ACC/AHA Task Force on Practice Guidelines (Writing Committee to Develop Guidelines for the Management of Patients with Peripheral Arterial Disease [Lower Extremity, Renal, Mesenteric, and Abdominal Aortic]). *J Am Coll Cardiol*. 2006;1–75. www.ace.org
3. Selvin E, Erlinger TP. Prevalence of and risk factors for peripheral arterial disease in the United States. Results from the National Health and Nutrition Examination Survey, 1999–2000. *Circulation*. 2004;110:738–743.
4. Newman AB, et al. Ankle-arm index as a predictor of cardiovascular disease and mortality in the cardiovascular health study. The Cardiovascular Health Study Group. *Arterioscler Thromb Vasc Biol*. 1999;19(3):538–545.
5. CAPRIE Steering Committee. A randomised, blinded, trial of clopidogrel versus aspirin in patients at risk of ischaemic events (CAPRIE). *Lancet*. 1996;348(9038):1329–1339.
6. Stewart KJ, et al. Exercise training for claudication. *N Engl J Med*. 2002;347(24):1941–1951.
7. DiPiro JT, et al. eds. *Pharmacotherapy: A Pathophysiologic Approach*, 6th ed. New York, NY: McGraw-Hill; 2005: 2801.
8. Mohler ER III. Peripheral arterial disease. Identification and implications. *Arch Intern Med*. 2003;163:2306–2314.
9. Hiatt WR. Medical treatment of peripheral arterial disease and claudication. *N Engl J Med*. 2001;344(21):1608–1621.
10. Jackson M, Clagett G. Antithrombotic therapy in peripheral arterial occlusive disease. *Chest*. 2001;119(Suppl):283S–299S.
11. Hutter C, Austin M, Humphries S. Familial hypercholesterolemia, peripheral arterial disease, and stroke: A HuGE minireview. *Am J Epidemiol*. 2004;160(5):430–435.
12. Hooi JD, et al. The prognosis of non-critical limb ischaemia: A systematic review of population-based evidence. *Br J Gen Pract*. 1999;49(438):49–55.
13. Hankey G, Norman P, Eikelboom JW. Medical tratmant of peripheral arterial disease. *JAMA*. 2006;295(5):547–553.
14. Creager MA. Peripheral Arterial Disease. In: Federman DD, Dale DC (eds). *ACP Medicine*. New York: Web MD Corporation; 2004.
15. Hiatt W, Nehler MR. Peripheral Arterial Disease. In: Cassel CK (ed). *Geriatric Medicine: An Evidence Based Approach*. New York: Spring-Verlag; 2003.
16. Hiatt WR. Preventing atherothrombotic events in peripheral arterial disease: The use of antiplatelet therapy. *J Intern Med*. 2002;251(3):193–206.
17. Hirsch AT, et al. Peripheral arterial disease detection, awareness, and treatment in primary care. *JAMA*. 2001;286(11):1317–1324.
18. Dormandy JA, Rutherford RB. Management of peripheral arterial disease (PAD). TASC Working Group. TransAtlantic Inter-Society Concensus (TASC). *J Vasc Surg*. 2000;31(1 Pt 2):S1–S296.
19. Carman TL, Fernandez BB, Jr. A primary care approach to the patient with claudication. *Am Fam Physician*. 2000;61(4):1027–1032, 1034.
20. Gey DC, Lesho EP, Manngold J. Management of peripheral arterial disease. *Am Fam Physician*. 2004;69(3):525–532.
21. Schmieder FA, Comerota AJ. Intermittent claudication: Magnitude of the problem, patient evaluation, and therapeutic strategies. *Am J Cardiol*. 2001;87(12A):3D–13D.
22. Group TW. Management of peripheral arterial disease (PAD). TransAtlantic Inter-Society Consensus (TASC). Section B: Intermittent claudication. *Eur J Vasc Endovasc Surg*. 2000;19(Suppl A):S47–S114.

23. Aronow W. Management of peripheral arterial disease of the lower extremities in elderly patients. *J Gerontol.* 2004;59A(2):172–177.

24. Criqui MH. Systemic atherosclerosis risk and the mandate for intervention in atherosclerotic peripheral arterial disease. *Am J Cardiol.* 2001;88(7B):43J–47J.

25. Yao ST, Hobbs JT, Irvine WT. Ankle systolic pressure measurements in arterial disease affecting the lower extremities. *Br J Surg.* 1969;56:676–679.

26. McDermott MM, et al. The ankle brachial index is associated with leg function and physical activity: The Walking and Leg Circulation Study. *Ann Intern Med.* 2002;136(12): 873–883.

27. McDermott MM, et al. Lower ankle/brachial index, as calculated by averaging the dorsalis pedis and posterior tibial arterial pressures, and association with leg functioning in peripheral arterial disease. *J Vasc Surg.* 2000;32(6): 1164–1171.

28. Belch JJ, et al. Critical issues in peripheral arterial disease detection and management: A call to action. *Arch Intern Med* 2003;163(8):884–892.

29. Farkouh ME. Improving the clinical examination for a low ankle-brachial index. *Int J Angiol.* 2002;11:41–45.

30. Khan NA, et al. Does the clinical examination predict lower extremity peripheral arterial disease? *JAMA.* 2006;295(5):536–546.

31. O'Hare AM, et al. High prevalence of peripheral arterial disease in persons with renal insufficiency: Results from the National Health and Nutrition Examination Survey 1999–2000. *Circulation.* 2004;109(3):320–323.

32. Dormandy JA, Murray GD. The fate of the claudicant—a prospective study of 1969 claudicants. *Eur J Vasc Surg.* 1991;5(2):131–133.

33. Hiatt WR. Pharmacologic therapy for peripheral arterial disease and claudication. *J Vasc Surg.* 2002;36(6):1283–1291.

34. Burns P, Gough S, Bradbury AW. Management of peripheral arterial disease in primary care. *BMJ.* 2003;326 (7389):584–588.

35. Regensteiner JG, Hiatt WR. Current medical therapies for patients with peripheral arterial disease: A critical review. *Am J Med.* 2002;112(1):49–57.

36. Kannel WB, Shurtleff D. National Heart and Lung Institute, National Institutes of Health. The Framingham Study: Cigarettes and the development of intermittent claudication. *Geriatrics.* 1973;28:61–68.

37. Tierney S, Fennessy F, Hayes DB. ABC of arterial and vascular disease: Secondary prevention of peripheral vascular disease. *BMJ.* 2000;320:1262–1265.

38. Gardner AW, et al. Effects of long-term exercise rehabilitation on claudication distances in patients with peripheral arterial disease: A randomized controlled trial. *J Cardiopulm Rehabil.* 2002;22(3):192–198.

39. Gardner AW, et al. Exercise rehabilitation improves functional outcomes and peripheral circulation in patients with intermittent claudication: A randomized controlled trial. *J Am Geriatr Soc.* 2001;49(6):755–762.

40. Langbein WE, et al. Increasing exercise tolerance of persons limited by claudication pain using polestriding. *J Vasc Surg.* 2002;35(5):887–893.

41. Falcone RA, et al. Peripheral arterial disease rehabilitation: A review. *J Cardiopulm Rehabil.* 2003;23(3):170–175.

42. Tan KH, De Cossart L, Edwards PR. Exercise training and peripheral vascular disease. *Br J Surg.* 2000;87(5):553–562.

43. Chobanian AV, et al. The Seventh Report of the Joint National Committee on Prevention, Detection, Evaluation, and Treatment of High blood pressure: The JNC 7 Report. *JAMA.* 2003;289(19):2560–2571.

44. Garg PK, et al. Physical activity during daily life and mortality in patients with peripheral arterial disease. *Circulation.* 2006;114:242–248.

45. Collaboration AT. Collaborative meta-analysis of randomised trials of antiplatelet therapy for prevention of death, myocardial infarction, and stroke in high risk patients. *BMJ.* 2002;324(7329):71–86.

46. Clagett GP, et al. Antithrombotic therapy in peripheral arterial occlusive disease: The Seventh ACCP Conference on Antithrombotic and Thrombolytic Therapy. *Chest.* 2004;126(Suppl 3):609S–626S.

47. Tran H, Anand SS. Oral antiplatelet therapy in cerebrovascular disease, coronary artery disease, and peripheral arterial disease. *JAMA.* 2004;292(15):1867–1874.

48. Moore TD, Linn WD, O'Rourke RA. Hot Topic: Current evidence for the use of antiplatelet therapy in cerebrovascular ideas, coronary artery disease, and peripheral arterial disease. McGraw-Hill. 2004.

49. Diener HC, et al. European Stroke Prevention Study 2. Dipyridamole and acetylsalicylic acid in the secondary prevention of stroke. *J Neurol Sci.* 1996;143(1–2):1–13.

50. Dawson DL, et al. A comparison of cilostazol and pentoxifylline for treating intermittent claudication. *Am J Med.* 2000;109(7):523–530.

51. Thompson PD, et al. Meta-analysis of results from eight randomized, placebo-controlled trials on the effect of cilostazol on patients with intermittent claudication. *Am J Cardiol.* 2002;90(12):1314–1319.

52. Lindgarde F, et al. Conservative drug treatment in patients with moderately severe chronic occlusive peripheral arterial disease. Scandinavian Study Group. *Circulation.* 1989; 80(6):1549–1556.

53. Girolami B, et al. Treatment of intermittent claudication with physical training, smoking cessation, pentoxifylline, or nafronyl: A meta-analysis.[see comment]. *Arch Intern Med.* 1999;159(4):337–345.

54. Radack K, Wyderski RJ. Conservative management of intermittent claudication. *Ann Intern Med.* 1990;113(2): 135–146.

55. Ernst E. Pentoxifylline for intermittent claudication. A critical review. *Angiology.* 1994;45(5):339–345.

56. Hood SC, Moher D, Barber GG. Management of intermittent claudication with pentoxifylline: Meta-analysis of randomized controlled trials. *CMAJ.* 1996;155(8): 1053–1059.

57. Whyman MR, et al. Is intermittent claudication improved by percutaneous transluminal angioplasty? A randomized controlled trial. *J Vasc Surg.* 1997;26(4):551–557.

58. Bosch J, Hunink M. Meta-analysis of the results of percutaneous transluminal angioplasty and stent placement for aortoiliac occlusive disease [published erratum appears in

Radiology 1997 Nov;205(2):584]. *Radiology.* 1997;204(1): 87–96.

59. Expert Panel on Detection, Evaluation, and Treatment of High Blood Cholesterol in Adults. Executive Summary of the Third Report of the National Cholesterol Education Program (NCEP) Expert Panel on Detection, Evaluation, and Treatment of High Blood Cholesterol in Adults (Adult Treatment Panel III). *JAMA.* 2001;285(19): 2486–2497.

60. MRC/BHF Heart Protection Study of cholesterol lowering with simvastatin in 20536 high-risk individuals: A randomised placebo-controlled trial. *Lancet.* 2002;360(9326): 7–22.

61. Cannon CP, et al. Intensive versus Moderate Lipid Lowering with Statins after Acute Coronary Syndromes. *N Engl J Med.* 2004;350(15):1495–1504.

62. Grundy S, et al. Implications of Recent Clinical Trials for the National Cholesterol Education Program Adult Treatment Panel III Guidelines. *Circulation.* 2004;110(2): 227–239.

63. Coutinho M, et al. The relationship between glucose and incident cardiovascular events. A metaregression analysis of published data from 20 studies of 95,783 individuals followed for 12.4 years. *Diabetes Care.* 1999;22(2):233–240.

64. American Diabetes Association, Peripheral arterial disease in people with diabetes. *Diabetes Care.* 2003;26(12): 3333–3341.

65. Creager MA, et al. Diabetes and vascular disease: Pathophysiology, clinical consequences, and medical therapy: Part I. *Circulation.* 2003;108(12):1527–1532.

FURTHER READING

1. Mills DC, Puri R, Hu CJ, Clopidogrel inhibits the binding of ADP analogues to the receptor mediating inhibition of platelet adenylate cyclase. *Arterioscler Thromb.* 1992;12: 430–436.

2. Plavix package insert. New York, NY: Bristol-Myers. Squibb/Sanofi-Synthelabo Pharmaceuticals Partnership. Rev 11/97, Rec 2/98.

3. Salicylates (systemic) Monographs. Aspirin. In: U.D.E. Group, ed. *USP DI® Drug Information for the Health Care Professional.* Taunton, MA: Micromedex Inc.; 2004.

4. Dipyridamole (Systemic) Monographs. U.D.E. Group, ed. In *USP DI® Drug Information for the Health Care Professional,* Taunton, MA: Micromedex Inc.; 2004.

5. Pentoxifylline (Systemic) Monographs. U.D.E. Group, ed. In *USP DI® Drug Information for the Health Care Professional,* Taunton, MA: Micromedex Inc.; 2004.

6. Cilostazol (Systemic) Monographs. U.D.E. Group, ed. In *USP DI® Drug Information for the Health Care Professional,* Taunton, MA: Micromedex Inc.; 2004.

7. Guyatt G, et al., Applying the Grades of Recommendation for Antithrombotic and Thrombolytic Therapy: The Seventh ACCP Conference on Antithrombotic and Thrombolytic Therapy. *Chest.* 2004;126(Suppl 3):179S–187.

8. TransAtlantic Inter-Society Consensus (TASC) Working Group. Management of peripheral arterial disease (PAD). Section B: Intermittent claudication. *Eur J Vasc Endovasc Surg.* 2000;19(Suppl A):S47–114.

PART 2

Respiratory Disorders

CHAPTERS

Chapter 8

Asthma Management

Michelle S. Harkins and H. William Kelly

SEARCH STRATEGY

A systematic review of the literature was performed and included the Cochrane database, PubMed, UpToDate®, the National Heart, Lung, and Blood Institute and Global Initiative for Asthma Web Sites, and the National Institute of Health's National Asthma Education and Prevention Program (NAEPP) Expert Panel documents. Much of the contents of this chapter are available online at www.nhlbi.nih.gov and www.ginasthma.com.

Asthma is a chronic inflammatory disease of the airways affecting 20 million Americans. Despite continuing research and development of new drugs, asthma is responsible for approximately 500 000 hospitalizations per year and between 5000 and 6000 deaths per year. It is the third leading cause of preventable hospitalizations in the United States. The incidence and prevalence of this disease are rising for a variety of reasons.

This is a complex disease with both genetic and environmental contributors. There are a variety of asthma phenotypes in susceptible individuals, for example, exercise-induced asthma, cough-variant asthma, nocturnal asthma, and a spectrum of mild to severe disease. The underlying problem is inflammation of the airways and airway hyperresponsiveness mediated by substances produced by many different cells (eosinophils, neutrophils, epithelial cells).[1–4] Environmental factors such as viral infections, irritants, aeroallergens, and stress can precipitate exacerbations in the inflamed airway. The principal clinical consequence of this acute and chronic inflammation is the development of asthma exacerbations, characterized by bronchial smooth-muscle contraction, increased mucus secretion and mucosal edema with desquamation of airway epithelium.[1,2] Exacerbations of asthma are an important clinical marker of disease control and progression. Exacerbations are probably the most important outcome from a humanistic and health economics viewpoint. Thirty-seven percent of the total costs for asthma, $2.7 billion, resulted from medical care of severe acute exacerbations.[5] The National Institutes of Health's NAEPP and the Global Initiative for Asthma have provided guidelines and resources for optimal asthma management, the most recent of which were evidence-based.[3,4] Since primary care providers deal with the vast majority of asthma patients, it is vital that they recognize and appropriately manage asthma in both the chronic-maintenance phase as well as the acute-exacerbation phase.

CLINICAL PRESENTATION[2,3,4]

Patients may present with recurrent episodes of wheezing, chest tightness, difficulty breathing, and cough at any age; the majority of patients with asthma are diagnosed during childhood (about 80%). Epidemiological studies of children with asthma in many populations reveal that approximately one-third have symptoms only during childhood, one-third have a period of quiescence during adolescence and then have return of their symptoms later in life, and one-third have unremitting symptoms. Adult-onset asthma is less likely to remit. Although the diagnosis is clinical, it can be challenging; *not all that wheezes is asthma.* Table 8-1 outlines the key indicators for the diagnosis of asthma. A personal or family history of atopy, eczema, or allergic rhinitis, although not a key indicator, is often associated with asthma.

Table 8-2 includes the differential diagnosis for asthma. Of note, sinus disease and reflux should always be considered, as they may mimic asthma; also, reflux is associated with asthma, and can worsen disease control.

Table 8-1. Key Indicators in the Diagnosis of Asthma

One or more attacks of wheezing
A normal chest examination does not rule out asthma
Symptoms occur or worsen at night, awakening the patient
History of any of the following:
    cough, worse particularly at night
    recurrent wheezing
    recurrent difficult breathing
    recurrent chest tightness
Colds "go to the chest" or take more than 10 d to clear up
Symptoms occur or worsen in the presence of
    exercise
    viral infection
    animals with fur
    smoke (tobacco or wood)
    temperature changes
    pollen
    strong emotional expression
    aerosol chemicals
    menses
    drugs (ASA, sulfites, β-blockers)
    house dust mite exposure
Symptoms improved by appropriate anti-asthma treatment
Reversible and variable airflow limitation—as measured by peak
    expiratory flow in any of the following ways:
        Peak expiratory flow increases by more than 15%, 15–20
        min after inhalation of a short-acting β$_2$-agonist, varies
        between measurement upon arising and measurement in
        the afternoon by 20%, if on bronchodilators, 10%, if not
        on bronchodilators, or decreases by more than 15% after
        exercise

ASA, acetylsalicylic acid.

During acute asthma attack, patients may demonstrate wheezing, accessory muscle use, nasal flaring (important in children), tachypnea, and pulsus paradoxus, depending on the severity of exacerbation. Chest examination findings may include hyperinflation, wheezing, and prolonged expiratory phase.

DIAGNOSTIC TESTING[2,3,4]

Spirometry measures of FEV$_1$ (forced expiratory volume in 1 second), FVC (forced vital capacity), and the FEV$_1$/FVC ratio are undertaken pre- and postinhalation of a short-acting β$_2$-agonist to evaluate reversible airflow obstruction, the hallmark of asthma. An obstructive defect is defined when FEV$_1$ becomes lesser than FVC and thus the FEV$_1$/FVC ratio goes below the predicted value (less than 70%). These measures may be normal, may show fixed airway obstruction, or may show reversibility (12% increase in value, postbronchodilator), depending on the time for which they were performed and the severity of the disease. Typically, spirometry is valid in children 6 years of age and older.

Additional studies are occasionally done to confirm or exclude the diagnosis. A chest X-ray may be needed to rule out other disorders. Additional pulmonary function testing, including diffusion capacity for carbon monoxide, full lung volumes, or maximal inspiratory or expiratory pressures may distinguish asthma from emphysema, a restrictive lung disease or neuromuscular weakness.

Table 8-2. Differential Diagnosis for Asthma

Infants and Children		
Upper Airway Obstruction	**Large Airway Obstruction**	**Small Airway Obstruction**
Allergic rhinitis	Foreign body	Viral bronchiolitis
Sinusitis	Vocal cord dysfunction	Bronchopulmonary dysplasia
Other	Vascular rings/webs	Cystic fibrosis
Chronic cough	Tracheomalacia/stenosis	Heart disease
Aspiration/GERD	Enlarged lymph nodes/tumor	
Adults		
Chronic obstructive pulmonary disease	Vocal cord dysfunction	
Cough secondary to drugs (ACE inhibitors)	Pulmonary embolus	
Pulmonary infiltrates with eosinophilia	Congestive heart failure	
Mechanical obstruction due to tumor/mass	Laryngeal dysfunction	
Allergic rhinitis/sinusitis	GERD	
Chronic cough		

GERD, gastroesophageal reflux disease; ACE, angiotensin converting enzyme.

If the spirometry is normal and the diagnosis is in question, bronchoprovocation with methacholine, histamine, or exercise may be useful. This test can exclude the diagnosis of asthma if the patient does not exhibit a 20% drop in the FEV_1 with subsequent increasing doses of the inhaled challenge. Testing should not be performed on subjects with a FEV_1 of less than 65% of the predicted value or be done by untrained personnel. Alternatively, measuring diurnal variations in the peak expiratory flow over 1 to 2 weeks can support the suspected diagnosis of asthma when baseline spirometry is normal.

Currently, both the national (NAEPP) and international (Global Initiative for Asthma) guidelines for the management of asthma recommend spirometry and peak-expiratory-flow monitoring as objective measures of asthma stability. However, the standard measures of lung function such as FEV_1 and peak expiratory flow only assess airway patency and not necessarily airway inflammation. They do not reliably predict asthma exacerbation.

NONPHARMACOLOGIC THERAPY[2,3,4,6]

The key components for asthma management are listed in Table 8-3. The NAEPP emphasizes the partnership of health care providers and patients in understanding and managing the disease. First, providers should help patients to identify and control precipitants of exacerbations. By avoiding triggers, asthma control is improved

Table 8-3. Major Components of Asthma Management

1) **Avoidance of Contributing Factors**
   Skin testing to identify allergens
   Controlling household and workplace allergens and irritants
   Prevention and treatment of viral infections
   Prevention and treatment of gastroesophageal reflux
2) **Patient Education**
   Provide basic asthma education regarding underlying disease, triggers, medications used
   Teach and reinforce inhaler and peak-flow technique
   Develop action plans
   Encourage self-management
3) **Periodic Assessment and Monitoring**
   Monitor signs and symptoms of asthma
   Monitor pulmonary function (spirometry, peak-flow monitoring)
   Monitor quality of life and functional status
   Monitor asthma exacerbations
   Monitor pharmacotherapy (adverse effects, inhaler technique, and frequency of quick-reliever use)
   Monitor patient–provider communication and patient satisfaction
4) **Pharmacotherapy**
   Explain and reinforce role of medications (quick relief, long-term agents)
   Stepwise therapy recommended with provision for step-up and step-down in therapy

and medication use is decreased. Second, providers should educate patients to recognize symptoms and take appropriate steps to control them. This is especially important in patients with severe asthma who may have a blunted perception of airflow obstruction and dyspnea and underestimate the severity of their disease or delay action until symptoms are quite advanced. The NAEPP guidelines also suggest a written asthma-management plan outlining medications for long-term control of asthma and for exacerbations. This dynamic plan should be updated through the course of treatment. An example of an action plan is depicted in Fig. 8-1. Finally, repeated instruction by the provider on the appropriate techniques for medication delivery is necessary to assure that patients take them correctly.

REFERRAL TO A SPECIALIST[2]

Any patients with risk factors for death from asthma (Table 8-4), patients with severe persistent or moderate persistent asthma (steps 3 and higher in Table 8-5), and patients with a poor response to therapy should be referred to a trained allergist or pulmonologist.

Referral is also appropriate if the diagnosis is unclear, if an occupational etiology is suspected, or if immunotherapy is contemplated. If significant environmental triggers are identified and avoidance of the allergen is not possible, immunotherapy should be considered. This should only be done in patients with mild to moderate disease under the direct care of an allergist.

Patients on high doses of inhaled corticosteroids, continuous oral corticosteroids or frequent oral steroid bursts should be referred for subspecialty evaluation.

PHARMACOTHERAPY[3,4]

Inhaled corticosteroids are the mainstay of treatment to reduce inflammation, prevent exacerbations, and gain control of symptoms, even in the mild persistent asthma patient. Despite the advent of newer classes of drugs, inhaled corticosteroids remain the best treatment for inflammation. The NAEPP presented an update of guidelines in 2007 for the stepwise treatment of patients based on the severity and control of disease (Table 8-5). It is important to note that patients may move up or down along a continuum of severity rather than remaining in a clearly defined step. In addition, patients with similar levels of severity may require different levels of therapy for achieving control. Assessing disease control is a major focus in the most recent NAEPP guidelines. The level of control can be classified by the impairment depending on the symptoms, use of rescue medications, and lung function and the risk of exacerbations and potential side effects. The severity classification is determined by the

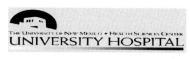

Asthma Action Plan

Name: Date: **Doctor:**

My Best Peak Flow Reading is:

GREEN   Peak Flow Above _____

Breathing is good. You can work and play. This is where you should be every day.
Take these medicines everyday, good days, and bad days. Use spacer with metered-dose inhalers.

Medicine	How Much to Take	When to take it
1.		
2.		
3.		
4.		

Yellow   **Peak Flow Between _____ and _____**

This is **NOT** where you should be. There may be coughing, wheezing, and mild shortness of breath. Sleep and usual activities may be disturbed.

- Keep taking green-zone medicines. Use spacer with metered-dose inhalers.
- **Add quick relief medicine: albuterol 2 to 4 puffs every 4 hours**
- If you improve completely after 2 to 3 treatments, continue your quick-relief medicine 4 times per day for the next 24 hours. Call for further advice.
- **If your peak flow is not back to Green Zone after using quick-relief medication. Add Prednisone ____ mg per day for 4 days.** Call for further advice.
- If you improve completely after 2 to 3 treatments, continue your quick-relief medicine 4 times per day for the next 24 hours. Call for further advice.
- NOTE: Call your doctor if you keep dropping into the yellow zone. The green-zone plan may need to be changed to prevent this.

RED   **Peak Flow Below_____   GET HELP NOW!**

**Your asthma is out of control. Quick-relief medication is not working.
Breathing is hard and fast. Can't walk and talk well.**

Call your doctor now. Call for an ambulance or go to the hospital if
- you are still in the red zone after 15 minutes AND
- you have not reached your doctor.

Repeat quick-relief medications every 20 minutes on your way to the hospital.

PATIENT LABEL

Figure 8-1. Example of a written asthma-management plan that includes the home management of an acute exacerbation.

worst parameter in any given category. Table 8-5 provides an example of recommendations for adults. The reader should refer to the NAEPP guidelines for recommendations for children of 0 to 4 years and 5 to 11 years.[2]

AEROSOL DELIVERY DEVICES[7,8]

Many of the most effective therapies for acute and chronic asthma are delivered by inhalation, improving both safety and efficacy. Delivery devices used include metered-dose inhalers pressurized with chlorofluorocarbons and hydrofluoroalkanes, and single-dose and multiple-dose breath-actuated dry-powder inhalers and nebulizers (jet or air powered and ultrasonic). Different devices within a category have different delivery characteristics so that delivery of one cannot be extrapolated to another. Delivery to the lung is generally 10% to 50% of the labeled dose.

Most chlorofluorocarbon-powered metered-dose inhalers will be discontinued in 2008 due to the adverse effect of chlorofluorocarbons on the ozone layer. Inhalation with a metered-dose inhaler requires hand–lung coordination and a slow, deep inhalation (15–30 L/min or 5 seconds for the entire inhalation).

Table 8-4. Risk Factors for Asthma Mortality

Near fatal asthma: Prior intubation or ICU admission
History of sudden severe exacerbations
≥ 3 emergency department visits for asthma in the last year
> 2 hospitalizations for asthma in the last year
Emergency department visit or hospital admission in the last
  month
Usage of > 2 canisters of β-agonist MDI/mo
Current oral steroid use or recent taper
Illicit drug use
Urban environment and low socioeconomic status
Poor perception of airflow obstruction or its severity
Comorbid illness
Serious psychiatric disease
Sensitivity to *Alternaria*

MDI = metered-dose inhalers.

Spacer devices can be attached to metered-dose inhalers to enhance delivery and decrease oropharyngeal deposition. Of these, the one-way-valved holding-chamber spacer is preferred. Addition of a one-way-valved holding chamber to a metered-dose inhaler allows the patient to actuate the device and then inhale requiring less coordination. As the speed of inhalation helps break up the particles in a dry-powder inhaler, a deep inhalation technique/approximately 60 L/min) is generally required.

Nebulizers usually only require tidal breathing from the patients but occasional deep breaths will enhance delivery. Since they are a suspension, inhaled corticosteroids can only be given by jet nebulizers; ultrasonic nebulizers cannot deliver suspensions.

Both the nebulizers and one-way-valved holding chambers can have soft face masks attached to facilitate the delivery of aerosols to infants, elderly, or patients in severe distress. Use of face masks reduces delivery by one-half as drug is filtered out by nasal inhalation.

Short-Acting Inhaled β_2-Agonists[3,4,9,10]

The rapid onset and potent smooth-muscle-relaxation properties make these drugs ideal for reversing or preventing acute bronchospasm in asthma. They are functional antagonists; they reverse bronchospasm induced by any mechanism. They do not possess clinically significant

Table 8-5. Stepwise Approach to Managing Asthma Long Term for Adults and Children of More Than 11 Years of Age[2]

Type of Asthma/Control	Days With Symptoms or as Needed Short-acting β_2 Agonist Use	Nights with Symptoms	FEV$_1$ or PEF FEV$_1$/FVC	Long-Term Control—Daily Medications*
Step 6 Severe persistent	Continual Limit activity	Frequent often nightly	<60% reduced >5%	ICS (high dose) + LABA + oral corticosteroids, generally not to exceed 60 mg/d and consider omalizumab for patients with allergies
Step 5 Moderate persistent; uncontrolled on Step 4	>2/wk on Step 4 therapy	>2/month on Step 4 therapy	<80% predicted/ personal best on Step 4 therapy	High dose ICS + LABA and consider omalizumab for patients with allergies
Step 4 Moderate persistent; uncontrolled on Step 3	>2/wk on Step 3 therapy	>2/month on Step 3 therapy	<80% predicted/ personal best on Step 3 therapy	Medium dose ICS + LABA preferred or Medium dose ICS + either LTM or theophylline
Step 3 Moderate persistent	Daily Affect activity	$\geq$1/week but not nightly	>60%-<80% reduced 5%	Low dose ICS + LABA or medium dose ICS preferred or low dose ICS + either LTM or sustained-release theophylline
Step 2 Mild persistent	3–6/wk with minor limitation	3–4/mo	$\geq$80% Normal	Inhaled steroid (low dose) or cromolyn, LTM, nedocromil, or sustained-release theophylline
Step 1 Mild	$\leq$2/wk	$\leq$2/mo	$\geq$80% Normal	No daily medications as needed short-acting β_2 agonists

*All patients: 2–4 puffs of short-acting inhaled β_2-agonists for rescue medication, consider use of a spacer with MDIs for patients unable to coordinate actuation and inhalation, allergen avoidance.
PEF, peak expiratory flow; FEV$_1$, forced expiratory volume in 1 second; ICS, inhaled corticosteroid; LABA, long-acting inhaled β_2-agonist; LTM, leukotriene modifier.
Adapted from: National Institutes of Health: National Heart, Lung, and Blood Institute. National Asthma Education and Prevention Program. Expert Panel Report 3: Guidelines for the diagnosis and management of asthma. 2007.

anti-inflammatory activity. The selective β_2-agonists produce less cardiac stimulation than nonselective agents and are the preferred therapy for acute bronchospasm and the prevention of exercise-induced bronchospasm. For severe acute-asthma exacerbations, selective β_2-agonists are given in higher doses and more frequently. β_2-Agonists administered systemically or by wet nebulization are not superior to the metered-dose inhaler plus one-way-valved holding-chamber spacer device in severe acute exacerbations. All of the short-acting inhaled β_2-agonists appear to be equally effective and tolerable when administered in equivalent doses. Regularly scheduled use of β_2-agonists does not provide benefit beyond use as needed for symptoms, and regular administration leads to a shorter duration of action of 2 to 4 hours.

The frequency of need of short-acting inhaled β_2-agonists provides a measure of symptom control. Use that exceeds 2 times in a week for symptoms (not including prevention for exercise-induced bronchospasm) indicates a need for initiation or increase in long-term controller therapy. Use of two or more metered-dose-inhaler canisters per month indicates a high risk for severe life-threatening asthma exacerbations. At usual recommended outpatient doses, β_2-agonists are well tolerated, but in high doses, they may cause tachycardia, decreased potassium levels, and increased glucose and lactic acid levels.

Long-Acting Inhaled β_2-Agonists[3,4,11]

When taken regularly, both salmeterol and formoterol are effective for at least 12 hours for bronchodilation and 4 hours for prevention of exercise-induced bronchospasm. As an adjunct to inhaled corticosteroids, long-acting inhaled β_2-agonists (LABAs) significantly reduce the rate of severe asthma exacerbations and are associated with lower doses of inhaled corticosteroids. The combination of LABAs and inhaled corticosteroids is the most effective combination and is the preferred therapy for moderate-to-severe persistent asthma. However, LABAs do not possess any clinically significant anti-inflammatory activity. They should only be used in conjunction with inhaled corticosteroids. There is some evidence that the use of monotherapy may result in deterioration of asthma and increased risk of severe life-threatening exacerbations and death. Currently, it is not recommended to use LABAs in the management of acute symptoms.

Anticholinergics[3,4,12,13]

Neither ipratropium bromide, administered 3 times daily, nor tiotropium, administered once daily, are indicated for the outpatient treatment of asthma. They are selective antagonists of muscarinic receptors and thus reverse only the bronchospasm that is mediated through cholinergic input. However, ipratropium bromide administered in frequent doses either by metered-dose inhalers or nebulizers to patients presenting to the emergency department provides additive bronchodilation to short-acting inhaled β_2-agonists and reduces hospital admissions. Therefore, it is recommended for patients not responding completely to the first few doses of short-acting inhaled β_2-agonists or those presenting with peak flows less than 35% of the patient's baseline normal values. These highly bronchoselective agents have few side effects, producing only mouth dryness or accommodation problems (if accidentally administered in the eye).

Inhaled Corticosteroids[3,4,14,15]

The inhaled corticosteroids are the preferred therapy for patients with any level of persistent asthma. They are the most effective long-term control drugs for the treatment of asthma due to their broad range of anti-inflammatory activity. They improve all outcome measures in asthma and are the only long-term control agents demonstrated to reduce the risk of death from asthma.

In low-to-medium doses, as recommended by the NAEPP guidelines, they are safe (Table 8-6). High doses increase the risk of significant systemic side effects such as adrenal suppression, decreased bone mineral density, growth suppression, and dermal thinning and bruising. Long-term high doses may produce an increased risk of cataracts, osteoporosis, and growth failure. In prepubertal children, use of low-to-medium doses is associated with a noncumulative growth retardation of about 1 cm, but the final predicted adult height does not appear to be affected. When administered in equipotent doses in the low-to-medium dose range, side effect profiles are similar; however, at high doses, differences in systemic activity may exist. Inhaled corticosteroids are available as metered-dose inhalers and dry-powder inhalers. Nebulizer suspension is approved for infants. It is recommended that patients use a one-way-valved holding-chamber spacer with metered-dose inhalers and also that patients rinse, gargle, and spit following dry-powder inhalers and nebulizer use to prevent thrush and hoarseness. Infants who require a face mask should have their face washed following the treatment.

The addition of LABAs, leukotriene modifiers, or theophylline can reduce the dose of inhaled corticosteroid required to control symptoms. The addition of LABAs is often more effective than doubling the dose of the inhaled corticosteroid, but this is not true for leukotriene modifiers or theophylline. However, none of these medicines should replace inhaled corticosteroids.

Systemic Corticosteroids[3,4,16,17]

Three- to ten-day courses of oral corticosteroids are the most effective anti-inflammatory therapy for severe asthma exacerbations not responsive to usual doses of short-acting inhaled β_2-agonists. They are more effective

Table 8-6. Comparable Daily Doses in Micrograms for Children 5–11 Years of Age and and Adults and Children >11 Years of Age[2]

Medication	Low Dose Child/Adult	Medium Dose Child/Adult	High Dose Child/Adult
Beclomethasone dipropionate			
HFA-MDI (40 and 80 µg/actuation)	80–160/80–240	>160–320/>240–480	>320/>480
Budesonide			
DPI (90 and 180 µg/inhalation)	180–360/200–600	>360–720/>540–1080	>720/>1080
Nebules (200 and 500 µg/ampule)	500/Unknown	500–1000/Unknown	>1000/Unknown
Flunisolide			
CFC-MDI (250 µg/actuation)	500–750/500–1000	>750–1250/>1000–2000	>1250/>2000
Fluticasone propionate			
HFA-MDI (44, 110, and 220 µg/actuation)	88–176/88–264	>176–440/>264–660	>440/>660
DPIs (50, 100, and 250 µg/inhalation)	100–200/100–300	>200–400/>300–600	>400/>600
Mometasone furoate			
DPI 200 µg/inhalation	Unknown/200	Unknown/400	Unknown/>400
Triamcinolone acetonide			
CFC-MDI (75 µg/actuation)	300–600/300–750	>600–900/>750–1,500	>900/>1,00

CFC, chlorofluorocarbons; MDI, metered-dose inhalers; HFA, hyrofluoroalkanes; DPI, dry powedered inhaler.
Adapted from: National Institutes of Health: National Heart, Lung, and Blood Institute. National Asthma Education and Prevention Program. Expert Panel Report 3: Guidelines for the diagnosis and management of asthma. 2007.

than high-dose inhaled corticosteroids and they have been shown to reduce admission to the hospital and prevent relapse. The usual dose of prednisone is 40 to 60 mg daily or 1 to 2 mg/kg in young children, in divided doses. This is continued until the patient reaches 80% of personal best peak flow or symptoms dissipate. A tapering dose is not required if the patient is begun on inhaled corticosteroids. Patients who require more that four courses of systemic prednisone per year may experience long-term corticosteroid induced toxicities such as adrenal suppression, osteoporosis, and growth suppression. Need for frequent courses of oral steroids is an indication for referral to a specialist.

Leukotriene Modifiers[3,4,11,18]

Stimulation of the leukotriene D4 receptor produces bronchospasm, mucus secretion, microvascular permeability, and airway edema. Zileuton inhibits the synthesis of leukotrienes from arachadonic acid. Montelukast and zafirlukast competitively inhibit the leukotriene D4 receptor. The leukotriene receptor antagonists are more commonly used as they require once- or twice-daily oral dosing and do not require liver-function monitoring, as does zileuton. All these drugs produce moderate bronchodilation and mild anti-inflammatory activity. They attenuate but do not block exercise-induced bronchospasm. They are significantly less effective than inhaled corticosteroids at all levels of asthma severity. When given in combination with inhaled corticosteroids they do allow reduction in the inhaled-corticosteroid dose, but to a lesser extent than LABAs. They are safe with remarkably few side effects.

Chromones[3,4]

Cromolyn sodium and nedocromil are prophylactic inhaled drugs that primarily function as mast cell stabilizers preventing the activation of mast cells after allergen exposure. They are significantly less-effective anti-inflammatory agents than the inhaled corticosteroids but are equally effective to the leukotriene modifiers and theophylline for maintenance therapy. They can effectively inhibit exercise-induced bronchospasm when administered 5 to 10 minutes prior to exercise. They have an excellent safety profile. Since the chromones require multiple daily dosing (3–4 times daily), they have been largely replaced by the leukotriene receptor antagonists as an alternative to the inhaled corticosteroids in mild persistent asthma.

Theophyllines[3,4,19]

Theophylline, a nonselective phosphodiesterase inhibitor, is a moderately potent bronchodilator with mild anti-inflammatory activity. In addition, it is a competitive antagonist of adenosine and stimulates endogenous catecholamine release leading to dose-related central nervous system and cardiovascular toxicities. It is important to maintain serum concentration between 5 and 15 µg/mL for safe use.

This narrow therapeutic range as well as multiple drug interactions has limited the use of theophylline. The leukotriene receptor antagonists have largely replaced the use of oral sustained-release theophylline due to similar efficacy and greater safety profile. In addition, theophylline lowers the esophageal sphincter tone and may promote gastric reflux, a factor known to potentiate asthma symptoms. Its ethylenediamine complex, aminophylline, has been used in severe acute-asthma exacerbations but has been largely replaced by more intensive use of high-dose inhaled β_2-agonists and ipratropium bromide.

Omalizumab[20]

This drug is a humanized monoclonal antibody to the Fc portion of IgE. It binds to and reduces the circulation of free IgE and prevents interaction with the high-affinity FcεRI receptors on mast cells and basophils. This eventually reduces the number of FcεRI receptors on mast cells. Omalizumab is injected subcutaneously every 2 to 4 weeks, depending on the patient's weight and IgE level. In severe allergic asthma patients, use of omalizumab allows the reduction of inhaled corticosteroids and discontinuation of oral corticosteroids in 30% to 40% of

oral-corticosteroid-dependent patients. Omalizumab has not been compared to other treatments for reduction of inhaled corticosteroids in moderate-to-severe persistent allergic patients but is the only therapy that has been shown to provide added benefit to those patients on high-dose inhaled corticosteroids and LABAs.[2] Principal side effects are irritation at the injection sites.

ACUTE EXACERBATION MANAGEMENT[3,4,16,17,21,22]

Despite appropriate therapy, some patients still experience exacerbations. Prompt treatment with intensive inhaled β_2-agonists and timely initiation of corticosteroids improves symptoms and may lead to decreased hospital admission. Correction of hypoxemia with oxygen and frequent monitoring of therapeutic response are paramount. Figure 8-2 outlines the

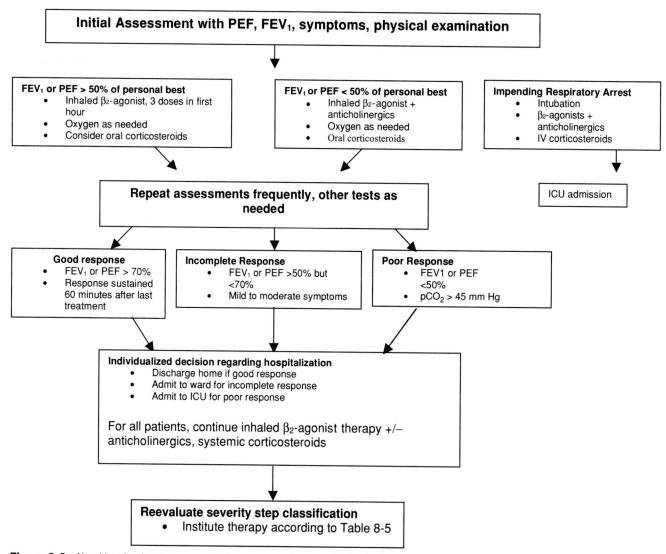

Figure 8-2. Algorithm for the management of a severe acute exacerbation in the emergency department and hospital from the National Asthma Education and Prevention Program Guidelines.[2]

stepwise treatment for an asthma exacerbation in the hospital. The recommended doses of drugs for exacerbations in both children and adults are found in Table 8-7. Although intravenous magnesium sulfate has been used during exacerbation, there is no evidence that it has any beneficial effect. Likewise, sedatives, aminophylline, and antihistamines do not have a role in the therapy of acute exacerbation. Antibiotics should be reserved for those patients with evidence of bacterial infection.

Table 8-7. Dosages of Drugs for Asthma Exacerbations in Emergency Medical Care or Hospital

Medication	Adult Dose	Child* Dose	Comments
Inhaled β$_2$-agonists			
Albuterol Nebulizer solutions (5.0 mg/mL, 2.5 mg/3mL, 1.25 mg/3mL, 0.63 mg/3mL)	2.5–5 mg every 20 min for 3 doses, then 2.5–10 mg every 1–4 h as needed, or 10–15 mg/h continuously	0.15 mg/kg (minimum dose = 2.5 mg) every 20 min for 3 doses, then 0.15–0.3 mg/kg up to 10 mg every 1–4 h as needed, or 0.5 mg/kg/h by continuous nebulization	Only selective β$_2$-agonists are recommended. For optimal delivery, dilute aerosols to 3 mL at a gas flow of 6–8 L/min. Use a face mask for children of age <6 y.
MDI (90 mcg/puff)	4–8 puffs every 20 min up to 4 h, then every 1–4 h as needed	4–8 puffs every 20 min for 3 doses, then every 1–4 h as needed. Use holding-chamber-type spacer	It is as effective as intermittent nebulization therapy if patient is able to coordinate inhalation maneuver.
Levalbuterol Nebulizer solution (0.63 mg/3mL, 1.25 mg/3mL)	1.25–2.5 mg every 20 min for 3 doses, then 1.25–5 mg every 1–4 h as needed, or 5–7.5 mg/h continuously	0.075 mg/kg (minimum dose = 1.25 mg) every 20 min for 3 doses, then 0.075–0.15 mg/kg up to 5 mg every 1–4 h as needed, or 0.25 mg/kg/h by continuous nebulization	It is the single active R isomer of albuterol and has not been adequately studied in acute severe asthma. Thus, doses are based upon one-half of the racemic albuterol doses.
Systemic (injected) β$_2$-agonists			
Epinephrine 1:1000 (1 mg/mL)	0.3–0.5 mg every 20 min for 3 doses subcutaneously	0.01 mg/kg up to 0.3–0.5 mg every 20 min for 3 doses subcutaneously	No proven advantage over aerosol therapy.
Terbutaline (1 mg/mL)	0.25 mg every 20 min for 3 doses subcutaneously	0.01 mg/kg every 20 min for 3 doses then every 2–6 h as needed subcutaneously	No proven advantage over aerosol therapy.
Anticholinergics			
Ipratropium bromide Nebulizer solution (0.25 mg/mL)	0.5 mg every 30 min for 3 doses then every 2–4 h as needed	0.25 mg every 30 min for 3 doses then every 2–4 h as needed	May mix in the same nebulizer with albuterol.
MDI (18 mcg/puff)	4–8 puffs as needed	4–8 puffs as needed	It should not be used as first-line therapy; should be added to β$_2$-agonist therapy.
Ipratropium with albuterol Nebulizer solution (0.5 mg Ipratropium + 2.5 mg albuterol/3 mL)	3 mL every 30 min for 3 doses then every 2–4 h as needed	1.5 mL every 30 min for 3 doses then every 2–4 h as needed	Dose delivered in MDI is low and has not been adequately studied in asthma exacerbations.
MDI (each puff contains 18 mcg ipratropium and 90 mcg albuterol)	4–8 puffs as needed	4–8 puffs as needed	Contains EDTA to prevent discoloration. This additive does not induce bronchospasm.
Systemic corticosteroids†			
Methylprednisolone Prednisolone Prednisone	120–180 mg/d in 3–4 divided doses for 48 h, then 60–80 mg/d until PEF reaches 70% of predicted or personal best	1 mg/kg every 6 h for 48 h then 1–2 mg/kg/d (maximum = 60 mg/d) in 2 divided doses until PEF 70% of predicted or personal best	For outpatient "burst" use 40–60 mg in single or 2 divided doses for adults (children: 1–2 mg/kg/d, maximum = 60 mg/d) for 3–10 d.

*Children of age ≤ 12 years.
†No advantage has been found for higher-dose corticosteroids in severe asthma exacerbations. There is no advantage for intravenous over oral therapy unless gastrointestinal transit time or absorption is impaired. The usual regimen is continued, multiple daily doses, until the patient achieves an FEV1 or PEF of 50% of predicted or personal best and then the dose is decreased to twice daily. This usually occurs within 48 hours. Therapy following a hospitalization or emergency-department visit may last 3–10 days. If patients are then started on inhaled corticosteroids, studies indicate there is no need to taper the systemic corticosteroid dose. If systemic corticosteroids are given once daily, one study indicates that it may be more clinically effective to give the dose at 3 PM, with no increase in adrenal suppression.
MDI, metered-dose inhaler; EDTA, ethylenediamine tetraacetic acid; PEF, peak expiratory flow.
Adapted from: National Institutes of Health: National Heart, Lung, and Blood Institute. National Asthma Education and Prevention Program. Expert Panel Report 3: Guidelines for the diagnosis and management of asthma. 2007

FUTURE DIRECTIONS

To date, immune modulation therapies have been somewhat disappointing. Nevertheless, many immunologic targets exist and there is hope that new agents will counteract the immune and neuroimmune systems responsible for propagating the chronic inflammation in asthma. Additionally, the new field of pharmacogenomics holds promise for finding the genetic basis for a patient's response to various drug therapies.

EVIDENCE-BASED SUMMARY

- Asthma is a complex disease with strong genetic and environmental components affecting disease presentation.
- Asthma is a chronic inflammatory disease of the airways with acute episodic exacerbations.
- There is an overlap with allergic rhinitis and other atopic diseases.
- Airflow obstruction is reversible initially but over time may lead to fixed obstruction secondary to airway remodeling.
- Inhaled corticosteroids are the most effective anti-inflammatory therapy.
- The addition of LABAs is the most effective adjunctive therapy improving control of asthma and allowing lower doses of inhaled corticosteroids.

REFERENCES

1. Bousquet J, Jeffery PK, Busse WW, Johnson M, Vignola AM. Asthma. From bronchoconstriction to airways inflammation and remodeling. *Am J Respir Crit Care Med.* 2000;161(5):1720.
2. NIH. *National Asthma Education and Prevention Program Expert Panel Report 3: Guidelines for the Diagnosis and Management of Asthma.* NIH publication 07–4051. Bethesda, MD: National Heart, Lung and Blood Institute; 2007. Available at http://www.nhlbi.nih.gov/guidelines/asthma. Accessed August 29, 2007.
3. National Institutes of Health: National Heart, Lung, and Blood Institute. National Asthma Education and Prevention Program. Expert Panel Report: Guidelines for the diagnosis and management of asthma update on selected topics 2002. *J Allergy Clin Immunol.* 2002;110:S142–S219.
4. Global Initiative for Asthma (GINA). *Global Strategy for Asthma Management and Prevention.* NHLBI/WHO Workshop Report. 2002. Bethesda, MD: NIH Publication No 02–3659; 2002.
5. Weiss KB, Sullivan SD. The health economics of asthma and rhinitis I. Assessing the economic impact. *J Allergy Clin Immunol.* 2001;107:3–8.
6. Gibson PG, Powell H, Coughlan J, et al. Self-management education and regular practitioner review for adults with asthma. *Cochrane Database Syst Rev.* 2002;3:CD001117.
7. Dolovich MA, MacIntyre NR, Dhand R, et al. Consensus conference on aerosols and delivery devices. *Respir Care.* 2000;45:588–776.
8. Cates CC, Bara A, Crilly JA, Rowe BH. Holding chambers versus nebulisers for beta-agonist treatment of acute asthma. *Cochrane Database Syst Rev.* 2003;3:CD000052.
9. Ram FS, Brocklebank DM, White J, Wright JP, Jones PW. Pressurised metered dose inhalers versus all other hand-held inhaler devices to deliver beta-2 agonist bronchodilators for non-acute asthma. *Cochrane Database Syst Rev.* 2002;1:CD002158.
10. Travers AH, Rowe BH, Barker S, Jones A, Camargo CA, Jr. The effectiveness of IV beta-agonists in treating patients with acute asthma in the emergency department: A meta-analysis. *Chest.* 2002:122(4):1200–1207.
11. Ram FSF, Cates CJ, Ducharme FM. Long-acting beta2-agonists versus anti-leukotrienes as add-on therapy to inhaled corticosteroids for chronic asthma. *Cochrane Database Syst Rev.* 2005;1:CD003137.
12. Westby M, Benson M, Gibson P. Anticholinergics for chronic asthma in adults. *Cochrane Database Syst Rev.* 2004;3:CD003269.
13. Rodrigo GJ, Rodrigo C. The role of anticholinergics in acute asthma treatment: An evidence-based evaluation. *Chest.* 2002;121:1977–1987.
14. Adams N, Bestall JM, Lasserson TJ, et al. Inhaled fluticasone versus inhaled beclomethasone or inhaled budesonide for chronic asthma. *Cochrane Database Syst Rev.* 2004;2:CD002310.
15. Kelly HW, Nelson HS. Potential adverse effects of the inhaled corticosteroids. *J Allergy Clin Immunol.* 2003;112:469–478.
16. McFadden ER, Jr. Acute severe asthma. *Am J Respir Crit Care Med.* 2003;168(7):740–759.
17. Rowe BH, Edmonds ML, Spooner CH, Diner B, Camargo CA, Jr. Corticosteroid therapy for acute asthma. *Respir Med.* 2004;98(4):275–284.
18. Ducharme FM, Di Salvio F. Anti-leukotriene agents compared to inhaled corticosteroids in the management of recurrent and/or chronic asthma in adults and children. *Cochrane Databae Syst Rev.* 2004;1:CD002314.
19. Parameswaran K, Belda J, Rowe BH. Addition of intravenous aminophylline to beta2-agonists in adults with acute asthma. *Cochrane Database Syst Rev.* 2000;4:CD002742.
20. Walker S, Monteil M, Phelan K, et al. Anti-IgE for chronic asthma in adults and children. *Cochrane Database Syst Rev.* 2004;2:CD003559.
21. Graham V, Lasserson T, Rowe, BH. Antibiotics for acute asthma. *Cochrane Database Syst Rev.* 2001;3:CD002741.
22. Manser R, Reid D, Abramson M. Corticosteroids for acute severe asthma in hospitalised patients. *Cochrane Database Syst Rev.* 2001;1:CD001740.

Chapter 9

Management of Chronic Obstructive Pulmonary Disease

Patrick F. Walsh and Michael L. Ayers

SEARCH STRATEGY

A comprehensive search of the medical literature was performed from January 1985 to December 2006. The search, limited to human subjects and English language journals, included UpToDate, Ovid, MEDLINE®, PubMed, and the Cochrane Database of Systematic Reviews.

INTRODUCTION

Chronic obstructive pulmonary disease (COPD) is a chronic disease of the airways characterized by significant morbidity and mortality. It represents a substantial, global economic and societal burden. COPD is the fourth leading cause of death in the United States and Europe and is projected to be the third leading cause of death for both men and women by 2020.[1] In contrast to other leading chronic diseases including cardiac disease, cerebrovascular disease, and cancer, COPD is the only major disease with an increasing mortality. In the United States, 122 283 patients died from COPD in 2003. It is estimated that 1.4 million Americans had COPD in 2004. The prevalence data is misleading because most patients with COPD do not seek medical attention until later in the disease course when their symptoms have become apparent. Unfortunately, by the time their symptoms arise, the disease is typically advanced. Women and whites have a higher incidence of the disease.[2] Since 2002, more women have died from COPD than men. In 2003, more than 63 000 women died of COPD compared to 59 000 men.

The economic burden of COPD is high. In the United States, there were about 726 000 hospitalizations for COPD patients and 1.5 million emergency-department visits in adults in 2000. In 2004, the disease cost the United States a sum of $37.2 billion, of which $20.9 billion were direct expenditures and $16.3 billion were indirect costs.[3] Unfortunately, due to increasing cigarette smoking in adolescents, women, and those from developing countries as well as increases in population and life expectancy, further increases in the prevalence, morbidity, mortality, and economic burden of COPD are expected in the years to come.

DEFINITION

Traditionally, the term COPD has referred to a number of different obstructive airway diseases including emphysema, chronic bronchitis, bronchiectasis, and cystic fibrosis. Today, the term COPD refers primarily to emphysema and chronic bronchitis or a combination of the two. Asthma is a separate entity with a distinct pathogenesis and pathology different from that of COPD. The pharmacotherapy of asthma has been discussed in Chapter 8.

Updated definitions of COPD have been provided by a number of medical societies and organizations. Of note, the terms emphysema and chronic bronchitis are no longer included in these definitions. The Global Initiative for Obstructive Lung Disease (GOLD) guidelines, a report prepared by a joint expert panel from the National Heart, Lung, and Blood Institute and the World Health Organization, defined COPD as "a disease state characterized by airflow limitation that is not fully reversible. The airflow limitation is usually both progressive and associated with an abnormal inflammatory response of the lungs to noxious particles or gases."[4] Another expert panel from a joint commission of the American Thoracic Society and the European Respiratory Society, stresses that COPD is a preventable and treatable disease and includes the new concept that it not only affects the lungs but also produces systemic consequences.[5] The systemic effects of COPD include systemic inflammation, skeletal muscle dysfunction, weight loss, cardiovascular disease, dementia, depression, and cancer.[6]

RISK FACTORS

Cigarette smoking is the most important etiologic factor in the development of COPD. It is believed that 15% to 20% of smokers develop COPD.[7] Other risk factors include air pollution or environmental and occupational exposures. Perinatal events and childhood illness predispose patients to the potential development of COPD later in life. In addition, COPD has been linked to socioeconomic status and diet. Asthma is also believed to be a risk factor. Asthma patients can lose lung function as they age at a rate similar to cigarette smokers.[8] Genetic factors also play a role in the development of COPD. Although rare, α-1 antitrypsin deficiency is the only known genetic risk factor for COPD; it accounts for less than 5% of COPD patients.[9]

CLINICAL PRESENTATION

COPD is characterized by a progressive, insidious course over many years; most patients present usually between the age of 50 and 70. The diagnosis is based on clinical presentation, radiographic findings, and pulmonary-function testing. Typical symptoms include chronic cough, sputum production, wheezing, and exertional dyspnea. Although not very sensitive for the diagnosis, chest radiography may demonstrate hyperinflated lungs, bullous disease, an increased retrosternal airspace, or flattened diaphragms. In advanced COPD, chest radiography may reveal enlarged pulmonary arteries and cardiomegaly indicative of the development of cor pulmonale or pulmonary hypertension. Spirometry confirms the diagnosis of COPD. The GOLD guidelines define airflow obstruction as a reduced forced expiratory volume/forced vital capacity (FEV_1/FVC) ratio less than 0.70 in combination with a post-bronchodilator FEV_1 that is less than 0.80 of the predicted normal value.[4] In addition, the GOLD guidelines have classified the severity of COPD in four cate-

gories or stages based on symptoms and spirometry. The classification of the severity of disease is helpful in discussions of the quality of life and prognosis. All stages are characterized by an FEV_1/FVC ratio of ≤ 0.70. Stage 1 or "mild disease" is characterized by the presence or absence of chronic symptoms (cough, sputum production) with an FEV_1 of ≥ 0.80 of the predicted normal value. Stage 2 or "moderate disease" is characterized by the presence or absence of chronic symptoms with an FEV_1 of ≥ 0.50 and ≤ 0.80 of the predicted normal value. Stage 3 or "severe disease" is defined as the presence or absence of chronic symptoms along with an FEV_1 of ≥ 0.30 and ≤ 0.80 of the predicted normal value. Finally, stage 4 or "very severe disease" is characterized by an FEV_1 of < 0.30 or an FEV_1 of < 0.50 in combination with chronic respiratory failure.[4] Another severity classification scoring system, which employs the *B*ody mass index, airway *O*bstruction (FEV_1), *D*yspnea assessment, and *E*xercise capacity (BODE index). Celli and colleagues devised the score to incorporate all these parameters into a multivariate component. The BODE index was shown to be a better predictor than FEV_1 alone for the risk of hospitalization and death in COPD patients.[10]

NONPHARMACOLOGIC THERAPY

Although pharmacologic therapy is the mainstay of therapy for patients with COPD, there are a number of nonpharmacologic options. Smoking cessation and supplemental oxygen therapy are the only interventions with a proven impact on survival in patients with COPD.[11,12] Other nonpharmacologic therapies include vaccinations, pulmonary rehabilitation, and surgical therapies.

SMOKING CESSATION

Although a difficult task for many smokers, smoking cessation is imperative. Smoking cessation has been shown to reduce the rate of decline in FEV_1, COPD exacerbations, and mortality.[11] Smoking-cessation strategies should include counseling patients and implementation of nicotine-replacement agents (nicotine gum, transdermal patch, nicotine inhaler, lozenges, and antidepressants such as bupropion) when counseling is ineffective. Bupropion, a non-nicotine agent, in combination with the nicotine patch has been shown to increase smoking cessation.[13] Varenicline, the newest smoking-cessation agent, is a nicotine-receptor antagonist. Head-to-head studies with other smoking-cessation agents are underway.

OXYGEN

The Nocturnal Oxygen Therapy Trial, a large multicenter randomized trial, demonstrated that selected COPD patients with severe hypoxemia ($PaO_2 < 55$ mmHg) have an improved mortality when they use daily supplemental oxygen therapy for 15 hours or more per day.[12] Long-term oxygen therapy has also been shown to enhance hemodynamics, exercise capacity, lung mechanics, and cognitive performance. It reduces the polycythemia and pulmonary hypertension that can be caused by chronic hypoxemia.[14]

VACCINATIONS

The pneumococcal and influenza vaccines are two injectable vaccines universally recommended in the elderly and high-risk patients. One goal of COPD management is to prevent acute exacerbations. Acute exacerbations can be precipitated by common viral and bacterial infections. Although the use of the pneumococcal vaccine has not been clearly shown to be useful specifically in COPD patients, it is suggested.[4,15] The influenza vaccine, on the other hand, has been shown in a number of studies to result in a 50% reduction in serious illness and death in patients with COPD.[16,17]

PULMONARY REHABILITATION

Pulmonary rehabilitation programs involve patient education, pharmacologic interventions, nutrition counseling, and development of an exercise program suited to the individual patient with COPD. These programs have been shown to improve patient's quality of life and exercise capacity, reduce dyspnea and fatigue, and decrease the number of hospitalizations and length of hospital stay.[18] Pulmonary rehabilitation has not been shown to impact disease progression or mortality.

SURGICAL THERAPY

There are a number of potential surgical options for selected patients with advanced COPD. The options include bullectomy, lung volume reduction surgery (LVRS), and transplantation. Many patients with COPD are elderly and have significant comorbidities making them poor surgical candidates. The National Emphysema Treatment Trial studied the role of LVRS versus medical management (pharmacologic interventions and pulmonary rehabilitation). Overall, the study did not show that LVRS resulted in an improved mortality However, it was demonstrated that in a select group of patients with predominantly upper lobe disease and a significantly reduced exercise capacity LVRS

resulted in improved exercise capacity, quality of life, and survival after surgery. LVRS was shown to increase mortality in a subgroup of patients who had an FEV_1 of ≤ 0.20 of the predicted normal value and either a homogeneous disease or a carbon-monoxide diffusing capacity of $\leq 20\%$ of the predicted normal value.[19] Any form of surgery for patients with COPD should be reserved as a last resort after all medical management has been exhausted.

PHARMACOTHERAPY

BRONCHODILATORS

Short-Acting β_2-Agonist

Short-acting agonists increase cyclic adenosine monophosphate (cAMP) and increase bronchodilation. However, the effects are short lived and necessitate frequent dosing, resulting in decreased compliance. Albuterol is the most commonly used short-acting β_2-agonist and is available as a metered-dose inhaler and a solution for nebulization. Short-acting β_2-agonists have not been shown to improve the quality of life or decrease exacerbations. They are useful for acute exacerbations or on an as-needed basis in patients with intermittent symptoms and mild COPD (defined as $FEV_1/FVC < 0.7$ with $FEV_1\%$ predicted being $>80\%$).[20]

Long-Acting β_2-Agonists

Formoterol and salmeterol are β_2 selective, long-acting β_2-agonists that are more effective in COPD than similar agents with a shorter half-life. The increased duration of action is due to a prolonged dissociation time from the receptor, as both agents are lipophilic. Stimulation of the β_2 receptor activates adenyl cyclase, converting ATP to cAMP resulting in bronchodilation. The pathophysiology of COPD differs from asthma. By definition, the FEV_1 in COPD does not improve more than 12% in response to the administration of a bronchodilator; however, the long-acting β_2-agonists are still effective in the treatment of COPD. There are several proposed mechanisms for this, including the effect on neutrophil burst, airway leak, increased mucociliary clearance, and, probably the most important, a decrease in total lung volume. Studies have demonstrated reduced dynamic hyperinflation and an increase in exercise tolerance in patients with COPD treated with β_2-agonists.[21–23]

Adverse affects include tachycardia, increased QTc interval, and decreased serum potassium. Serious adverse events are rare. Long-acting β_2-agonists have been shown to improve the quality of life, exercise endurance, total lung volumes, FEV_1, dyspnea, and the number of acute exacerbations. The pharmacologic properties increasing the duration of action of these agents can also delay their onset of action; therefore, these agents should not be used for the treatment of an acute exacerbation of COPD. No study to date has demonstrated a significant difference in the efficacy between these agents when utilized as chronic therapy for COPD. Formoterol and salmeterol are administered every 12 hours and each is available as a single agent in a dry-powder formulation along with a unique delivery device. These agents are also available in combination with an inhaled corticosteroid to increase compliance with a multidrug regimen.[24,25]

ANTICHOLINERGIC AGENTS

Short-Acting Anticholinergic Therapy

Anticholinergic agents including belladonna and stramonium have been utilized since antiquity, and anticholinergics remain a mainstay of treatment for COPD today. An increase in parasympathetic tone results in activation of muscarinic receptors and so causes bronchoconstriction. Acetylcholine binds to all five types of muscarinic receptors; however, binding to the M3 receptor is responsible for the majority of bronchoconstriction. Older generation, tertiary anticholinergic drugs antagonized many acetylcholine receptors and penetrated the central nervous system (CNS) resulting in many untoward effects. Ipratropium is a quaternary compound specifically developed to decrease the CNS effects and to interact more selectively with the muscarinic receptors. The drug antagonizes all of the muscarinic receptors, but blocking of the M3 receptor accounts for the bronchodilator effect. Combination of ipratropium with the short-acting β_2-agonist albuterol results in greater bronchodilation than either agent alone. The benefits of this combination are well established and most experts recommend the combination for acute exacerbations and treatment of mild disease. Ipratropium is available as a single agent or in combination with albuterol as a metered-dose inhaler (Combivent) or solution for nebulization (Duoneb).[20,21]

Long-Acting Anticholinergic Therapy

Tiotropium is a structural analogue of ipratropium. It has an affinity for all muscarinic receptors, but dissociates more slowly from the M3 receptor. Binding studies confirm that tiotropium dissociates from M2 more rapidly than M3, and these dissociation kinetics allow for the once-daily dosing of tiotropium. The administration of tiotropium as a single agent in COPD results in a significant increase in FEV_1 and inspiratory capacity both at rest and during exercise, resulting in less-dynamic hyperinflation. (Inspiratory capacity, as opposed to FEV_1, correlates more consistently with patient-centered outcomes such as dyspnea.) The beneficial effects on dyspnea, number of exacerbations, hyperinflation, and increase in exercise tolerance appear long lived in studies over 12 months.

A recent meta-analysis demonstrated the superiority of anticholinergic compounds over long-acting β_2-agonists in the treatment of COPD. The study contained a few flaws limiting the strength of the conclusions. It highlights the need for an original study comparing tiotropium to long-acting β_2-agonists. Tiotropium given once a day is more effective than ipratropium given four times a day, and combination with a long-acting β_2-agonist provides additional improvement than either agent alone.[26–28]

THEOPHYLLINE

Caffeine, a xanthine derivative found in kola nuts, tea, and coffee beans, has been used for centuries as a CNS stimulant, diuretic, and bronchodilator. Theophylline, a methylated xanthine structurally similar to caffeine, has been utilized since the 1940s to treat COPD. In recent years, its use has declined because of adverse events and questionable therapeutic benefits.

Theophylline acts by inhibition of the enzyme phosphodiesterase, thereby blocking the conversion of cAMP to ATP. This results in an increase of intracellular level of cAMP, causing bronchodilation. In the past, a serum level of 10 to 20 mcg/mL was believed to be the optimum range to achieve maximal bronchodilatory effect. These serum levels are also associated with serious side effects including seizures and fatal arrhythmias leading. As safer agents became available, there was a decline in use of theophylline.

Over recent years there has been an upsurge in the use of theophylline at lower doses, aiming for serum levels of 5 to 10 mcg/mL. Unique mechanisms of action favorable to the treatment of COPD have been noted at these lower levels. Some of the proposed mechanisms include increased apoptosis, increased catecholamine release, inhibition of intracellular calcium release, inhibition of tumor necrosis factors, adenosine receptor antagonism, and a synergistic effect with steroids on inflammatory gene expression.

The metabolism and clearance of the drug is affected by multiple physiologic conditions and interactions with numerous other agents. Low doses should be prescribed and a plasma concentration of 5 to 10 mcg/mL should not be exceeded, as this concentration is sufficient for expression of the immunomodulatory and anti-inflammatory effects of theophylline.[29–33]

CORTICOSTEROIDS

Oral Corticosteroids

The long-term use of oral corticosteroids has no role in the treatment of COPD, but short courses provide moderate benefit by *decreasing* the time to the next exacerbation, hospital readmission from the emergency department, and overall length of hospital stay. The optimum dose is uncertain but recent studies show no significant benefit beyond 40 mg of prednisone per day (or equivalent) or duration of treatment beyond 14 days.[20]

Inhaled Corticosteroids

Controversy has long existed regarding the benefit of inhaled corticosteroids in patients with COPD and their role is still being defined. Large studies of inhaled corticosteroids combined with long-acting bronchodilators in patients with $FEV_1 < 50\%$ of the predicted normal value showed fewer exacerbations and a decrease in the rate of deterioration in health status. Inhaled corticosteroids do not affect the rate of change in FEV_1 and no trial to date has shown an improvement in mortality. Long-acting β_2-agonists may reverse corticosteroid resistance. Inhaled corticosteroids mediate the benefit by increasing the expression of β_2 receptors, not through anti-inflammatory effects. Inhaled corticosteroids have no significant anti-inflammatory effect when used alone in COPD. A randomized, double-blinded study demonstrated a significant decrease in the occurrence of COPD exacerbations with salmeterol and fluticasone compared to salmeterol alone. The study patients had severe COPD and a history of two or more exacerbations in the prior year, which is consistent with the current GOLD recommendations for the utilization of inhaled corticosteroids (Table 9-1).[35,36]

When considering inhaled corticosteroids, side effects including candidiasis, infection, and osteoporosis should be considered and appropriate patient education be provided.

ANTIBIOTICS

Evidence suggests that many exacerbations are precipitated by viral or bacterial infections of the respiratory tract, and COPD patients have a faster recovery with antimicrobial therapy. The studies utilized older agents including doxycycline, amoxicillin, and trimethoprim–sulfamethoxazole and all the agents showed benefit in patients with purulent sputum. Antibiotics are suggested in patients with worsening cough and dyspnea along with increased volume or purulence of sputum,

Table 9-1. Summary Based on Global Initiative for Chronic Obstructive Lung Disease (GOLD) Guidelines

All patients	One or more attacks of wheezing Smoking cessation Annual influenza vaccination Pneumococcal vaccination
Mild (with or without symptoms) $FEV_1/FVC < 0.70$ $FEV_1 > 0.80$ of predicted value	Use of short-acting bronchodilator as needed β_2-agonist, anticholinergic agent (alone or combined)
Persistent symptoms	Regular use of bronchodilators
Moderate IIA $FEV_1/FVC < 0.70$ $FEV_1 = 0.50$–0.80 of predicted value	Regular use of one or more bronchodilators Consider initial use of tiotropium Add long-acting β_2-agonist if symptoms persist
IIB $FEV_1/FVC < 0.70$ $FEV_1 = 0.30$–0.50 of predicted value	Use of inhaled corticosteroids if there are significant symptoms and/or frequent exacerbations May consider steroids for IIA for frequent symptoms and exacerbations Pulmonary rehabilitation
Severe $FEV_1/FVC < 0.70$ $FEV_1 < 0.30$ of predicted value	Rehabilitation, consider surgical options, long-term oxygen therapy, may consider addition of theophylline

Adapted from: GOLD Workshop. Global Strategy for the Diagnosis, Management, and Prevention of Chronic Obstructive Pulmonary Disease. *Am J Respir Crit Care Med.* 2001;163:1256–1276.

and local resistance patterns should be considered when selecting an antibiotic.[37]

The above pharmacologic agents do not impact mortality. The agents are focused on decreasing exacerbations, hospitalizations, dyspnea, and hyperinflation, increasing exercise tolerance, and improving quality of life. The long-acting bronchodilators are expensive, which is problematic for many COPD patients. It is important to provide close patient follow-up to determine which long-acting bronchodilator is best suited for each patient. Anticholinergic agents are becoming the first-line long-acting bronchodilators for use in COPD; however, some patients may benefit more from a β_2-agonist or a combination of both long-acting agents.

Unfortunately, clinical features and physiologic measurements do not accurately identify those few COPD patients who will benefit from aggressive life support. Therefore, it is important that the physician, patient, and family maintain an ongoing dialogue regarding goals of care. Limitations on life support should be clearly documented and shared by all of the health care professionals providing care for the patient.

CONCLUSION

COPD was once associated with a nihilistic approach. Today, the disease is considered preventable and treatable. There have been considerable advances in the epidemiology, pathophysiology, and therapy of COPD in recent years. Despite these advances, the disease continues to have a significant morbidity and societal burden. In addition, it has an increasing mortality. However, there remains room for optimism. Newer medications are under development, like the phosphodiesterase-4 inhibitors, another class of anti-inflammatory agents, as well as other combination pharmacologic agents. Advances continue in smoking prevention and cessation (varenicline and combination therapies). Surgical and bronchoscopic treatment options for lung volume reduction continue to be developed. Clearly, there are many existing pharmacologic and nonpharmacologic therapies in our armamentarium for the management of COPD, and there are newer therapies on the horizon.

REFERENCES

1. Murray CJL, Lopez AD, eds. *The Global Burden of Disease: A Comprehensive Assessment of Mortality and Disability from Diseases, Injuries, and Risk Factors, in 1990 and projected to 2020.* Cambridge, MA: Harvard University Press; 1996.
2. Mannino DM, Homma DM, Akinbami LJ, Ford ES, Redd SC. Chronic obstructive pulmonary disease surveillance—United States, 1971–2000. *MMWR Surveill Summ.* 2002;51: 1–16.
3. National Heart, Lung, and Blood Institute. *Morbidity and Mortality: 2004 Chartbook on Cardiovascular, Lung, and Blood Diseases.* Available at www.nhlbi.nih.gov/resources/docs/ 04_chtbk.pdf. Accessed November 21–26, 2006.
4. Global Initiative for Chronic Obstructive Lung Disease. *Global Strategy for the Diagnosis, Management, and Prevention of Chronic Obstructive Pulmonary Disease.* Bethesda, MD: National Institutes of Health, National Heart, Lung, and Blood Institute; 2005 (updated). Available at www.gold-copd.com. Accessed November 21–26, 2006.
5. American Thoracic Society. *Standards for the Diagnosis and Treatment of Patients with Chronic Obstructive Pulmonary Disease*; 2004. Available at www-test.thoracic.org/copd/pdf/ copddoc.pdf. Accessed November 21–26, 2006.
6. Agusti AGN, Noguera A, Sauleda J, et al. Systemic effects of chronic obstructive pulmonary disease. *Eur Respir J.* 2003;21:347–360.
7. Fletcher C, Peto R. The natural history of chronic airflow obstruction. *Br Med J.* 1977;1:1645–1648.
8. Lange P, Parner J, Vestbo J, et al. A 15-year follow up study of ventilatory function in adults with asthma. *N Engl J Med.* 1998;339:1194–1200.
9. American Thoracic Society/European Respiratory Society. American Thoracic Society/European Respiratory Soci-

ety Statement: Standards for the diagnosis and management of individuals with α-1 antitrypsin deficiency. *Am J Respir Crit Care Med.* 2003;168:818–900.
10. Celli BR, Cote CG, Martin JM. The body-mass index, airflow obstruction, dyspnea, and exercise capacity index in chronic obstructive pulmonary disease. *N Engl J Med.* 2004;350:1005–1012.
11. Anthonisen NR, Skeans MA, Wise RA, et al. The effects of smoking cessation intervention on 14.5 year mortality: A randomized clinical trial. *Ann Intern Med.* 2005;142:233–239.
12. Nocturnal Oxygen Therapy Trial Group. Continuous or nocturnal oxygen therapy in hypoxemic chronic obstructive lung disease: A clinical trial. *Ann Intern Med.* 1980;93: 391–398.
13. Jorenby DE, Leischow SJ, Nides MA, et al. A controlled trial of sustained-release buproprion, a nicotine patch, or both for smoking cessation. *N Engl J Med.* 1999;340:685–691.
14. Tarpy SP, Celli BR. Long-term oxygen therapy. *N Engl J Med.* 1995;333:10–14.
15. Celli BR, MacNee W. Standards for the diagnosis and treatment of patients with COPD: A summary of the ATS/ERS position paper. *Eur Respir J.* 2004;23:932–946.
16. Wongsurakiat P, Maranetra KN, Wasi C, et al. Acute respiratory illness in patients with COPD and the effectiveness of influenza vaccination: A randomized controlled study. *Chest.* 2004;125:2011–2020.
17. Nichol KL, Margolis KL, Wuorenma J, et al. The efficacy and cost effectiveness of vaccination against influenza among elderly persons living in the community. *N Engl J Med.* 1994;331:778–784.
18. Ries AL, Kaplan RM, Limberg TM, Prewitt LM, et al. Effects of pulmonary rehabilitation on physiologic and psychosocial outcomes in patients with chronic obstructive pulmonary disease. *Ann Intern Med.* 1995;122:823–832.
19. National Emphysema Treatment Trial Research Group. A randomized trial comparing lung volume reduction surgery with medical therapy for severe emphysema. *N Engl J Med.* 2003;348:2059–2073.
20. Barnes PJ, Stockley RA. COPD: Current therapeutic interventions and future approaches. *Eur Respir J.* 2005;25: 1084–1103.
21. Tashkin DP, Cooper CB. The role of long-acting bronchodilators in the management of stable COPD. *Chest.* 2004;125:249–259.
22. Appleton S, Poole P, Smith B, et al. Long-acting β_2-agonists for chronic obstructive pulmonary disease patients with poorly reversible airflow limitation. *Cochrane Database Syst Rev.* 2002;3:CD001104.
23. Reid DW, Ward C, Wang N, et al. Possible anti-inflammatory effect of salmeterol against interleukin-8 and neutrophil activation in asthma *in vivo. Eur Resp J.* 2002;21. 994–999.
24. Anderson GP. Long acting inhaled β-adrenoceptor agonists. The comparative pharmacology of formoterol and salmeterol. *New Drugs in Allergy and Asthma.* 1993;2:34–38.
25. vanNoord JA, Smeets JJ, Raaijmakers JAM, et al. Salmeterol versus formoterol in patients with moderately severe asthma: Onset and duration of action. *Eur Respir J.* 1996;9:878–885.

26. Celli B, ZuWallack R, Wang S, et al. Improvement in resting inspiratory capacity and hyperinflation with tiotropium in COPD patients with increased static lung volumes. *Chest.* 2003;124:1743–1748.

27. Brusasco V, Hodder R, Miravitlles M, et al. Health outcomes following treatment for 6 months with once daily tiotropium compared with twice daily salmeterol in patients with COPD. *Thorax.* 2003;58:399–404.

28. Chapman KR, Arvidsson P, Chuchalin AG, et al. The addition of salmeterol 50 µg bid to anticholinergic treatment in patients with COPD: A randomized, placebo controlled trial. *Can Resp J.* 2002;9:178–185.

29. Culpitt SV, De Matos C, Russell RE, et al. Effect of theophylline on induced sputum inflammatory indices and neutrophil chemotaxis in chronic obstructive pulmonary disease. *Am J Respir Crit Care Med.* 2002;165:1371–1376.

30. Mascali JJ, Cvietusa P, Negri J, et al. Anti-inflammatory effects of theophylline: Modulation of cytokine production. *Ann Allergy Asthma Immunol.* 1996;77:34–38.

31. Rabe KF, Magnussen H, Dent G. Theophylline and selective PDE inhibitors as bronchodilators and smooth muscle relaxants. *Eur Respir J.* 1995;8:637–642.

32. Hansel TT, Tennant RC, Tan AJ, et al. Theophylline: Mechanism of action and use in asthma and chronic obstructive pulmonary disease. *Drugs Today (Barc).* 2004;40:1:647–653.

33. Barnes PJ. Theophylline: New perspectives for an old drug. *Am J Respir Crit Care Med.* 2003;167:813–818.

34. Calverley PM, Boonsawat W, Cseke Z, et al. Maintenance therapy with budesonide and formoterol in chronic obstructive pulmonary disease. *Eur Respir J.* 2003;22:912–919.

35. Mak JCW, Nishikawa M, Shirasaki H, et al. Protective effects of a glucocorticoid on down-regulation of pulmonary β_2-adrenergic receptors *in vivo. J Clin Invest.* 1995;96:99–106.

36. Calverley PM, Boonsawat W, Cseke Z, et al. Maintenance therapy with budesonide and formoterol in chronic obstructive pulmonary disease. *Eur Respir J.* 2003;22:912–919.

37. Anthonisen NR, Manfreda J, Warren CP, et al. Antibiotic therapy in exacerbations of chronic obstructive pulmonary disease. *Ann Intern Med.* 1987;106:196–204.

PART 3

Gastrointestinal Disorders

CHAPTERS

Chapter 10

Gastroesophageal Reflux Disease

Dianne B. Williams and Robert R. Schade

SEARCH STRATEGY

A systematic medline search of the medical literature was performed using Ovid in July 2007. The search was limited to human subjects, English language and the time frame of 1998 to 2007. Subject headings included gastroesophageal reflux disease, guidelines, clinical trials, and review articles.

INTRODUCTION

Gastroesophageal reflux disease (GERD) is a common disorder seen in the primary care setting. It is described as symptoms or mucosal damage that occurs when the gastric contents are abnormally refluxed into the esophagus.[1] A defective lower esophageal sphincter pressure plays an important role in the development of GERD. Other contributing factors include defects of the normal mucosal "defense mechanisms" such as anatomic factors, esophageal clearance, mucosal resistance, and gastric emptying. In addition, "aggressive factors," such as gastric acid, pepsin, bile acids, and pancreatic enzymes may play a role in the development of GERD.

The prevalence and incidence of GERD are hard to predict because of many patients not going to their health care provider for evaluation, symptoms not always correlating with disease severity, and the lack of a universal method for diagnosing the disease.[2] Most patients can be characterized as having (1) nonerosive reflux disease, (2) erosive esophagitis, or (3) Barrett's esophagus.[3] Nonerosive reflux disease, also known as endoscopy-negative GERD or "symptomatic" GERD, occurs in patients experiencing GERD symptoms with no evidence of mucosal damage per endoscopy.

Patients with nonerosive reflux disease may experience symptoms as severe as those with erosive esophagitis and should be treated similarly. Others may present with erosions of the esophagus as a result of repeated exposure of refluxed material for prolonged periods of time (erosive esophagitis). Still others may present with complications of GERD, such as Barrett's esophagus. This occurs when the normal squamous epithelial lining is replaced with specialized columnar-type epithelium during the reparative process. GERD affecting organ systems outside the esophagus is referred to as atypical, or extra-esophageal GERD.

The diagnosis of GERD is generally made based upon symptoms reported to the health care provider by the patient. If these symptoms are relieved by empiric acid-suppressing therapy, a clinical diagnosis of GERD can be made. However, those patients not responding to therapy, or those presenting with atypical or complicated symptoms require further diagnostic evaluation. The primary care provider should recognize the differences in presentation and be prepared to treat appropriately. Patients presenting with complicated or atypical symptoms should be referred to a specialist.

CLINICAL PRESENTATION

GERD symptoms are described as typical, atypical, or complicated[4] (Table 10-1).

Heartburn and regurgitation are common, highly specific symptoms of GERD.[1] These symptoms may be aggravated when the patient is in a recumbent position, bending over, or eating a meal high in fat. Symptom severity does not always correlate with the degree of esophagitis, but it does correlate with the duration of reflux episodes.

Table 10-1. Clinical Presentation Of GERD[4]

Typical symptoms
    Heartburn, regurgitation
    Water brash (hypersalivation)
    Belching
Atypical symptoms
    Nonallergic asthma, chronic cough
    Hoarseness
    Pharyngitis
    Chest pain
    Erosion of tooth enamel
Complicated symptoms
    Continual pain
    Dysphagia, odynophagia
    Bleeding
    Weight loss
    Choking

Atypical GERD symptoms should be distinguished from other diseases, especially when chest pain or pulmonary symptoms are present. Patients presenting with asthma (especially nocturnal) or chronic cough not responding to standard therapy may have extraesophageal GERD.[4]

The presence of complicated symptoms, such as difficulty swallowing (dysphagia), painful swallowing (odynophagia), and weight loss should be further investigated to differentiate from other diseases as the cause and referral to a specialist is appropriate.

PHYSICAL FINDINGS

The physical examination may be normal or provide nonspecific findings, such as hoarseness or erosion of tooth enamel, caused by the reflux of acid on the vocal cords and teeth, respectively. Patients with atypical symptoms may also present with wheezing or cough. Heartburn or regurgitation may be aggravated when the patient is in a recumbent or squatting position.

DIAGNOSTIC EVALUATION

Tests that are useful in diagnosing GERD include clinical history, endoscopy (using either endoscope or Pillcam® ESO capsule), 24-hour ambulatory pH monitoring, proton pump inhibitor as a diagnostic tool, and manometry.

The most useful tool in the diagnosis of gastroesophageal reflux is the clinical history, including both presenting symptoms and associated risk factors. Invasive diagnostic tests are unnecessary in patients presenting with uncomplicated, typical symptoms. These patients usually benefit from an initial trial of lifestyle modifications and acid-suppressing therapy. A clinical diagnosis of GERD can be assumed in patients responding to therapy.[5]

Patients who initially present to the primary care provider with complicated symptoms, such as dysphagia, should be referred for endoscopy. Endoscopy is recommended any time visualization or biopsy of the esophageal mucosa is needed. The presence of erosive esophagitis or Barrett's esophagus can only be determined via endoscopy.[5] Endoscopy should also be performed in the following patients: (1) those not responding to empiric (prescription) anti-suppressing therapy, (2) those with chronic, long-standing symptoms who are at risk for Barrett's esophagus, and (3) those requiring continuous, chronic therapy to relieve symptoms. Patients are characterized as having nonerosive reflux disease if no erosions or Barrett's esophagus are seen on endoscopy and other disease processes have been eliminated as the cause of GERD symptoms. The availability of the new Pillcam® ESO provides a noninvasive method of performing endoscopy via a camera-containing capsule. The capsule is swallowed by the patient and images of the esophagus are transmitted into an external data collector. The procedure takes approximately 15 minutes and can be performed in the physician's office. Eventually, the patient defecates the capsule naturally.

Patients with atypical symptoms, nonerosive disease, or inadequate response to treatment may benefit from 24-hour ambulatory pH monitoring because it is the most reliable method to correlate symptoms with reflux episodes. In addition, it also documents the percentage of time the intraesophageal pH is less than four and determines the frequency and severity of reflux.[5] The empiric use proton pump inhibitors as a diagnostic agent is more convenient and cost effective than ambulatory pH monitoring. However, the lack of a standard dosing regimen and trial duration are limitations to the use of proton pump inhibitors as a diagnostic tool.

More recently a probe has been developed (impedance dual probe) that can detect any gastric refluxate (both acid and nonacid) by measurement of electrical impedance. In addition, this probe has numerous sensors that permit determination of the extent of a reflux event in terms of distance from the lower esophageal sphincter, as well as the duration of the reflux event. The precise diagnostic role for the use of this new impedance technique has yet to be determined.

Patients with GERD who are candidates for antireflux surgery generally receive esophageal manometry to evaluate motility and lower esophageal sphincter pressure.[5] It is also useful in determining the ideal surgical procedure for the patient.

RISK STRATIFICATION

Many factors should be considered when stratifying a patient's risk for developing GERD. The prevalence of

GERD increases in adults older than 40 years of age. Elderly patients are especially at risk because they have decreased host defense mechanisms, such as saliva production. Bicarbonate-containing saliva can buffer any gastric refluxate on the surface of the esophagus and helps maintain a neutral intraesophageal pH. Infants are also at risk as result of developmental immaturity of the lower esophageal sphincter, impaired luminal clearance of gastric acid, or if they have neurological impairment.

Gender plays a role in GERD. Females are more likely to develop nonerosive reflux disease and may experience GERD during pregnancy. Barrett's esophagus is more common in males.

Other factors that may put a patient at risk for developing or worsening GERD include certain foods and medications (Table 10-2). The use of nonsteroidal anti-inflammatory drugs or aspirin has been implicated as a risk factor that may contribute to the development or worsening of esophageal strictures.[6] In addition, lifestyle factors such as smoking and obesity may worsen GERD symptoms.

The patients at the highest risk for developing sequelae from GERD are those who present with atypical symptoms or complicated symptoms. Patients presenting with atypical symptoms may require higher doses and longer treatment courses of acid-suppressing therapies as compared with patients with typical symptoms. Long-term, recurrent reflux symptoms that are not adequately treated increase the patient's risk for developing strictures, Barrett's esophagus and adenocarcinoma.[7] The presence of Barrett's esophagus may also increase the patient's risk of developing adenocarcinoma. In addition, stricture formation can occur in as many as 30% of patients with Barrett's esophagus.

MANAGEMENT

The goals of treatment are to (1) alleviate or eliminate the patient's symptoms, (2) decrease the frequency or recurrence and duration of gastroesophageal reflux, (3) promote healing of the injured mucosa, and (4) prevent the development of complications. Therapy is directed at (1) decreasing the acidity of the refluxate, (2) decreasing the gastric volume available to be refluxed, (3) improving gastric emptying, (4) increasing lower esophageal sphincter pressure, (5) enhancing esophageal acid clearance, and (6) protecting the esophageal mucosa.

The treatment of GERD is categorized into one of the following: (1) lifestyle changes and patient-directed therapy (with over-the-counter H_2-receptor antagonists or proton pump inhibitors), (2) pharmacologic treatment with acid suppressing agents (H_2-receptor antagonists or proton pump inhibitors), (3) anti-reflux surgery, or (4) endoscopic therapies (Table 10-3). Every effort should be made to control symptoms and to prevent relapses early in the course of the patient's disease in order to prevent the complications seen with long-standing symptomatic GERD.[8]

Maintenance therapy may be required in certain patients. Proton pump inhibitors are preferred as maintenance therapy in those with more severe symptoms (with or without esophageal erosions) or in those with complications.

NONPHARMACOLOGIC THERAPY

Lifestyle and Dietary Changes

Lifestyle modifications and dietary changes that may be helpful in managing GERD should be discussed with the patient[5,9,10] (Table 10-4). The importance of maintaining these lifestyle changes throughout the course of GERD therapy should be stressed on a routine basis. Patients not responding to lifestyle changes and patient-directed therapy after 2 weeks should be treated with an acid-suppressing agent.

Anti-Reflux Surgery

Surgical intervention may be appropriate for certain patients with well-documented GERD.[5] The goal of

Table 10-2. Foods and Medications that May Worsen GERD Symptoms[15]

Decrease Lower Esophageal Sphincter Pressure	
Foods	Medications
Chocolate	Anticholinergics
Chili pepper	Barbituates
Coffee, cola, tea,	Benzodiazepines (diazepam)
Fatty meal	Caffeine
Onions, garlic	Dihydropyridine calcium
Peppermint, spearmint	channel blockers
	Dopamine
	Estrogen
	Ethanol
	Isoproterenol
	Narcotics (meperidine, morphine)
	Nicotine (smoking)
	Nitrates
	Phentolamine
	Progesterone
	Theophylline
Direct Irritants to the Esophageal Mucosa	
Foods	Medications
Spicy foods	Alendronate
Orange juice	Aspirin
Tomato juice	Nonsteroidal
Coffee	anti-inflammatory drugs
	Iron
	Potassium chloride
	Tetracycline

Table 10-3. Therapeutic Approach to GERD

Presentation	Treatment Recommendation	Comments
Intermittent, mild heartburn	Lifestyle modifications plus patient-directed therapies Antacids Over-the-counter H_2- receptor antagonists Over-the-counter proton pump inhibitors	Change to standard dose acid-suppressing therapy after 2 weeks if symptoms not relieved.
Symptomatic GERD	Lifestyle modifications plus Standard dose acid-suppressing therapy with an H_2-receptor antagonist × 6–12 weeks or proton pump inhibitor (once daily) × 4–6 weeks	Proton pump inhibitor preferred for moderate–severe symptoms. Patients who relapse may require long-term maintenance therapy.
Erosive Esophagitis or Treatment Failures or Complicated Symptoms	Lifestyle modifications plus Proton pump inhibitor (twice daily) × 4–16 weeks	Long-term maintenance therapy generally required. Anti-reflux surgery or endoscopic therapies are viable options.

antireflux surgery is to reestablish the antireflux barrier, to position the lower esophageal sphincter within the abdomen where it is under positive (intra-abdominal) pressure, and to close any associated hiatal defect.[11] It should be considered in patients (1) who fail to respond to pharmacologic treatment, (2) who opt for surgery despite successful treatment because of lifestyle considerations including age, time, or expense of medications, (3) who have complications of GERD, or (4) who have atypical symptoms and reflux documented on 24-hour

ambulatory pH monitoring.[11] The procedure chosen depends on the surgeon's expertise and preference, as well as on anatomic considerations.[11] Common complications of antireflux surgery include gas bloat syndrome (inability to belch or vomit) and dysphagia.[12]

Endoscopic Therapies

Endoscopic therapies, such as (1) application of radio frequency to the lower esophageal sphincter area, (2) endoscopic suturing, and (3) endoscopic injection of a biopolymer at the gastroesophageal junction are new procedures that look promising but require more experience and study to determine their place in the management of GERD.

PHARMACOLOGIC THERAPY

Antacids and Antacid-Alginic Acid Products

Antacids and antacid–alginic acid combinations relieve mild, infrequent GERD symptoms. The combination of an antacid with alginic acid (Gaviscon®), forms a protective barrier on the esophagus and decreases reflux episodes. However, patients who continue to have symptoms should be treated with prescription acid-suppressing therapy.

Antacids interact with a variety of drugs by altering gastric pH, increasing urinary pH, adsorbing medications to their surfaces, providing a physical barrier to absorption, or forming insoluble complexes with other medications. Clinically significant drug interactions include tetracycline, ferrous sulfate, isoniazid, quinidine, sulfonylureas, and quinolone antibiotics. Antacids require frequent administration to provide adequate acid neutralization throughout the day.

Table 10-4. Nonpharmacologic Treatment of GERD with Lifestyle Modifications

Elevate the head of the bed (increases esophageal clearance). Use 6–8-inch blocks under the head of the bed. Sleep on foam wedge.

Avoid foods that may decrease lower esophageal sphincter pressure or have a direct irritant effect on the esophageal mucosa.

Take drugs that have a direct irritant effect on the esophageal mucosa with plenty of liquid.

Include protein-rich meals into diet (augments lower esophageal sphincter pressure).

Eat small meals and avoid eating within 3 hours of sleeping. (decreases gastric volume).

Lose weight (reduces symptoms).

Stop smoking (decreases spontaneous esophageal sphincter relaxation).

Avoid alcohol (increases amplitude of the lower esophageal sphincter, peristaltic waves, and frequency of contraction)

Avoid tight-fitting clothes.

Adapted from: Kitchin LI, Castell DO. Rationale and efficacy of conservative therapy for gastroesophageal efflux disease. *Arch Intern Med*. 1991;151; 448–454; Richter JE, Castell DO. Drugs, foods and other substances in the cause and treatment of reflux esophagitis. *Med Clin North Am*. 1981;65: 1223–1234.

Acid Suppression with H$_2$-Receptor Antagonists (Cimetidine, Famotidine, Nizatidine, and Ranitidine)

H$_2$-receptor antagonists block the histamine-2 receptors in gastric parietal cells thereby decreasing acid secretion. Symptomatic improvement is seen in approximately 60% of patients after 12 weeks of therapy.[5] However, endoscopic healing rates tend to be lower (50%).[5]

The efficacy of H$_2$-receptor antagonists is similar among the various agents. Factors that influence which agent is chosen include differences in pharmacokinetics, safety profile, and cost. The H$_2$-receptor antagonists are well tolerated. The most common adverse effects include headache, somnolence, fatigue, and dizziness. Cimetidine may inhibit the metabolism of theophylline, warfarin, phenytoin, nifedipine, or propranolol. Select a different H$_2$-receptor antagonist if the patient is on cimetidine and any of these medications.

Acid Suppression with Proton Pump Inhibitors (Esomeprazole, Lansoprazole, Omeprazole Pantoprazole, and Rabeprazole)

Proton pump inhibitors block gastric acid secretion by inhibiting gastric H$^+$ (K$^+$-adenosine triphosphatase in gastric parietal cells.[13] This acid suppressing activity helps maintain the gastric pH above four. There is a correlation between the percentage of time the gastric pH remains above four during the 24-hour period and healing erosive esophagitis. In addition, pepsin, an aggressive factor contributing to GERD, is not active at a pH greater than four. Proton pump inhibitors improve symptoms and heal the esophagus better than H$_2$-receptor antagonists.[14] They are also more cost effective in patients with severe disease. Approximately 83% of patients receiving a proton pump inhibitor obtain symptomatic relief. Healing rates per endoscopy at 8 weeks are 78%.[5] The proton pump inhibitors are generally well tolerated. The most common adverse effects include headache, dizziness, nausea and somnolence. The long-term safety, once a concern, is no longer an issue. The role of *Helicobacter pylori* in GERD remains under investigation.[12]

Esomeprazole, pantoprazole, and rabeprazole, appear less likely to cause significant drug interactions. Drug interactions with omeprazole may be more likely in patients who are considered "slow metabolizers," however, it is hard to predict who may have a problem. In general, all of these agents are safe and effective and the choice of a particular agent will most likely be based on cost.

The proton pump inhibitors degrade in acidic environments. Lansoprazole, esomeprazole, and omeprazole contain enteric-coated (pH-sensitive) granules in a capsule form. The contents of these capsules can be mixed in applesauce or placed in orange juice if needed. Esomeprazole can be mixed with water. Lansoprazole is available in a powder for oral suspension and a delayed-release orally disintegrating tablet. Lansoprazole is the only U.S. Food and Drug Administration-approved proton pump inhibitor for treating GERD in pediatric patients, although there is also clinical data supporting the use of omeprazole in the pediatric population. Patients taking pantoprazole or rabeprazole should be instructed not to crush, chew, or split the delayed-release tablets. Esomeprazole, lansoprazole and pantoprazole are available in an intravenous formulation. However, the intravenous form is not more efficacious than oral proton pump inhibitors and is significantly more expensive.

Ideally, patients should take their proton pump inhibitor in the morning, 30 to 60 minutes before breakfast to improve efficacy, because these agents inhibit only actively secreting proton pumps.[1] If two doses per day are needed, the second dose should be given prior to the evening meal and not at bedtime.[1]

Prokinetic Agents

Prokinetic agents, such as metoclopramide, cisapride, and bethanechol have been studied in GERD but are limited by their adverse effect profile. Cisapride is not routinely available because of life-threatening arrhythmias. Bethanechol is not well tolerated and not routinely prescribed in GERD. Metoclopramide, a dopamine antagonist, has shown limited benefit in GERD but also has a negative adverse effect profile. More study is needed with newer agents, such as tegaserod, to determine their potential place in the management of GERD. Currently, no clinical trials are available.

Mucosal Protectants

Sucralfate is a nonabsorbable aluminum salt of sucrose octasulfate which forms a protective barrier on the gastric mucosa. It is not routinely recommended in the management of GERD.

COMBINATION THERAPY

There is limited data to support combination therapy with an acid-suppressing agent and a prokinetic agent. This approach should not be routinely recommended unless a patient has esophagitis with a known motor dysfunction occurring concurrently. A proton pump inhibitor should be recommended in patients not responding to monotherapy with either an H$_2$-receptor antagonist or prokinetic agent. Proton pump inhibitors not only improve compliance with once-daily dosing but they may also be more cost-effective.

MAINTENANCE THERAPY

The goal of maintenance therapy is to improve quality of life by controlling the patient's symptoms and preventing complications. Patients generally require standard doses of acid suppressing therapy to remain symptom-free and to prevent relapses.

EVIDENCE-BASED SUMMARY

Diagnosis
- Diagnosis is assumed in patients presenting with typical symptoms (e.g., heartburn, regurgitation) who respond to appropriate acid suppressing therapy.
- Patients with atypical or complicated symptoms and those who fail initial course of therapy are diagnosed after other possible disease processes have been eliminated and diagnostic testing (e.g., endoscopy, ambulatory reflux monitoring) confirm mucosal damage or acid reflux episodes.

Initial Evaluation
- Determine the type of symptoms the patient is experiencing (typical, atypical, complicated).
- Perform endoscopy in any patient presenting with complicated symptoms.
- Assess duration of patient's symptoms. Long-term acid reflux that is not adequately treated may increase risk for adenocarcinoma.
- Identify lifestyle preferences that may contribute to symptoms.
- Evaluate what patient has done to manage symptoms to date.

Management
- Lifestyle modifications
- Pharmacotherapy (Treatment and possible maintenance therapy)
  - Acid-suppressing therapy (H2 receptor antagonists, proton pump inhibitors)
  - Antacids
- Endoscopic Therapy
- Surgery

Follow-Up
- Monitor for compliance and safety issues (adverse drug reactions, drug interactions)
- Stress lifestyle modifications
- Monitor for efficacy to determine if long-term maintenance therapy appropriate

CONCLUSION

The short-term goal of therapy is to improve the patient's quality of life by relieving symptoms. Educate patients about lifestyle modifications that should be adhered to throughout the course of therapy. Medications or foods that aggravate GERD should be avoided. The primary care provider should take an active role in educating the patient about potential adverse effects and drug interactions that may occur with drug therapy. The frequency and severity of symptoms should be monitored and patients should be counseled on symptoms that suggest the presence of complications requiring immediate medical attention, such as dysphagia or odynophagia. Patients should also be monitored for the presence of atypical symptoms such as cough, nonallergic asthma, or chest pain. These symptoms require further evaluation.

The second goal is to heal the injured mucosa. Again, lifestyle modifications and the importance of complying with the therapeutic regimen chosen to heal the mucosa should be stressed. Patients should be educated about the risk of relapse and the need for long-term maintenance therapy to prevent recurrence or complications.

The final, more long-term goal of therapy is to decrease the risk of complications (esophagitis, strictures, and Barrett's esophagus). A small subset of patients may continue to fail treatment, despite therapy with high doses of H_2-receptor antagonists or proton pump inhibitor. Maintenance therapy with acid suppressing medication may be indicated in these patients.

In conclusion, GERD is a common disease that classically presents as heartburn. The pathophysiology of reflux is involves both aggressive factors and defense mechanisms. Therapeutic options are designed to minimize the aggressive factors and/or augment defense mechanisms.

REFERENCES

1. Devault KR, Castell DO. Updated guidelines for the diagnosis and treatment of gastroesophageal reflux disease. *Am J Gastroenterol.* 2005;100:190–200.
2. Spechler SJ. Epidemiology and natural history of gastroesophageal reflux disease. *Digestion.* 1992;51(Suppl 1): 24–29.
3. Wong WM, Wong BCY. Definition and diagnosis of gastroesophageal reflux disease. *J Gastroenterol Hepatol.* 2004; 19:S26–S32.
4. Krueger KJ. Changing clinical perspectives toward gastroesophageal reflux. *South Med J.* 1996;89:548–550.
5. Devault KR, Castell DO, Practice Parameters Committee of the American College of Gastroenterology. Updated guidelines for the diagnosis and treatment of gastroesophageal reflux disease. *Am J Gastroenterol.* 1999;94:1434–1442.

6. Orenstein SR. Gastroesophageal reflux disease. *Semin Gastrointest Dis.*1994;5:2–14.

7. Lagergren J, Bergstrom R, Lindgren A, Nyren O. Symptomatic gastroesophageal reflux as a risk factor for esophageal adenocarcinoma. *N Engl J Med.* 1999;340:825–831.

8. Welage LS, Berardi RR. Evaluation of omeprazole, lansoprazole, pantoprazole, and rabeprazole in the treatment of acid-related disorders. *J Am Pharm Assoc.* 2000;40:52–62.

9. Kitchin LI, Castell DO. Rationale and efficacy of conservative therapy for gastroesophageal reflux disease. *Arch Intern Med.* 1991;151:448–454.

10. Richter JE, Castell DO. Drugs, foods and other substances in the cause and treatment of reflux esophagitis. *Med Clin North Am.* 1981;65:1223–1234.

11. Anonymous. Guideline for the surgical treatment of gastroesophageal reflux disease (GERD). *Surg Endosc.* 1998;12: 186–188.

12. Kahrilas PJ. Gastroesophageal reflux disease. *JAMA.* 1996;276:983–988.

13. Horn J. The proton-pump inhibitors: Similarities and differences. *Clin Ther.* 2000;22:266–280.

14. Chiba N, De Cara CJ, Wilkinson JM, Hunt RH. Speed of healing and symptom relief in grade II to IV gastroesophageal reflux disease: A meta-analysis. *Gastroenterology.* 1997;112:1798–1810.

15. Weinberg DS, Kadish, SL. The diagnosis and management of gastroesophageal reflux disease. *Med Clin North Am.* 1996;80(2):411–429.

Chapter 11

Peptic Ulcer Disease

Alexandria A. Dunleavy and Dalia Mack

SEARCH STRATEGY

A systematic search of the medical literature was conducted in January 2008. Databases used in this search were PubMed, UpToDate®, National Guideline Clearinghouse, and SUMSearch. The search was limited to humans and journals published in the English language. Information included in this chapter is current as of January 2008.

BACKGROUND

Peptic ulcer disease (PUD) is characterized by excoriation of the mucosal layer of the stomach (gastric ulcer) or duodenum (duodenal ulcer). Ulcers should be differentiated from erosions in that ulcers extend deep into the muscular mucosae, whereas erosions tend to be superficial and less deep. Patients with peptic ulcers typically present with dyspepsia. However, several gastrointestinal (GI) disorders other than peptic ulcers can cause dyspepsia. Thus, the diagnosis of gastroesophageal reflux disease (GERD, Chapter 10), function dyspepsia (indigestion), and acid-hypersecretory states such as Zollinger–Ellison syndrome need to be considered in patients presenting with upper GI symptoms. Our understanding of the role of *Helicobacter pylori* in the development of peptic ulcers has increased significantly and has had a tremendous impact on the treatment of PUD. Unfortunately, advances in the treatment of peptic ulcers have not altered the rate of complications associated with PUD.[1]

EPIDEMIOLOGY

Approximately 25 million Americans have had PUD during their lifetime.[2] PUD causes an estimated 1 million hospitalizations and 6500 deaths per year.[2] The incidence of complications secondary to peptic ulcer increases with age, possibly due to increased risk for bleeding associated with nonsteroidal anti-inflammatory drug (NSAID) use. The burden of PUD on our healthcare system—although frequently overlooked—is quite substantial. Excluding medication costs, estimated expenditures are $5.65 billion annually.[3]

ETIOLOGY AND PATHOPHYSIOLOGY

Traditionally, the major risk factors for peptic ulcer were thought to be acid hypersecretion, diet, and stress. However, it is now known that causative factors such as infection with *H. pylori* and NSAID use are the primary mechanisms of ulceration.

HELICOBACTER-PYLORI-INDUCED PEPTIC ULCER

H. pylori may induce ulcer formation by several mechanisms.[4] First, the pathogen produces urease, which catalyzes urea to ammonia. Ammonia, which is necessary for the organism to survive the acidic environment of the stomach, is very caustic to the GI mucosa and can lead to epithelial damage. *H. pylori* also secretes various mucolytic enzymes that degrade the protective mucosal layer, exposing the epithelium and increasing the risk for acid-related damage. Finally, the cytokines and other inflammatory factors that are released in response to infection may play a role in ulcer formation.

NSAID-INDUCED PEPTIC ULCER

NSAIDs exert both topical and systemic effects that contribute to the development of PUD.[4] Topically, NSAIDs diffuse across the mucosal layer and into epithelial cells where damage to the cells may occur. Systemically, NSAIDs inhibit the production of prostaglandins that protect epithelial cells in the GI tract from acid-related damage.

CLINICAL EVALUATION

Classic symptoms of PUD include epigastric pain or discomfort, often described as a gnawing or burning sensation. The pain may be relieved or aggravated by eating food. In gastric ulcers, eating may exacerbate the pain whereas with duodenal ulcers the pain seems to worsen on an empty stomach (2–3 hours after meals). Nocturnal symptoms are also common. Patients may experience temporary relief from antacids.

DIAGNOSTIC TESTING

The diagnosis of PUD is based largely on clinical presentation and history. Endoscopy or upper GI radiography can confirm the diagnosis, although these studies are not always necessary if uncomplicated disease is sus-

Table 11-1. Alarm Symptoms in the Evaluation of Dyspepsia[5,6]

Weight loss
Dysphagia
Recurrent vomiting
Gastrointestinal bleeding
Family history of cancer

pected. Differential diagnoses such as GERD, functional dyspepsia, and acid-hypersecretory states such as Zollinger–Ellison syndrome need to be excluded.

Most patients with suspected PUD should be tested for *H. pylori* and treated if results are positive. Individuals who are 55 years of age or older, those with complications, or those who present with alarm symptoms for gastric cancer such as weight loss or dysphagia should be referred for endoscopy.[5] Evaluation for *H. pylori* is unnecessary in patients with documented nonulcer dyspepsia. Table 11-1 and Fig. 11-1 present an approach to determine which patients should be referred for endoscopy.

Several diagnostic tests are available to detect *H. pylori*. These tests can be generally classified as invasive (e.g.,

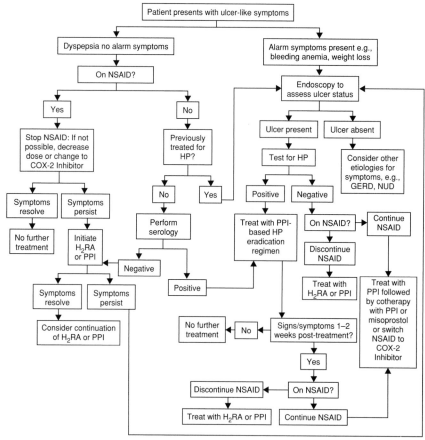

Figure 11-1. Patients to be referred for endoscopy. (Adapted from Berardi RR, Welage LS. Peptic ulcer disease. In: DiPiro JT, Talbert RL, Yee GC, et al, eds. *Pharmacotherapy: A Pathophysiologic Approach.* 6th ed. New York, NY: McGraw-Hill; 2005:629.)

endoscopy) or noninvasive. The choice of diagnostic test depends on the cost, clinical situation, convenience, and use of acid-suppressive therapy.

During endoscopy, biopsy samples are obtained and assessed by histology, urease activity, or culture.[7] Histological examination is the preferred method of assessment because it is highly sensitive (90%) and specific (nearly 100%) for *H. pylori*.[7] False-negative results may occur with urease testing if the patient is on acid-suppressive therapy. Cultures are generally used to determine the sensitivity of the organism to antibiotics rather than to make the diagnosis of infection because of the time duration required to obtain results (approximately 2 weeks).

Noninvasive testing includes serum antibody testing, urease breath testing, and stool antigen testing. Serologic testing for antibodies to *H. pylori* is commonly used as the initial screening tool to indicate infection. Enzyme-linked immunosorbent assay (ELISA) is used to detect IgG antibodies to *H. pylori* in the serum. The sensitivity and specificity of laboratory antibody testing are approximately 90%.[6]

Office-based serologic testing for *H. pylori* is also available. Office-based serologic testing is more convenient, but less accurate than laboratory testing.[6] Since antibodies persist after infection, ELISA serum testing would not be appropriate to confirm eradication of *H. pylori* after treatment. ELISA testing cannot distinguish between active infection and previously eradicated infection.

Urea breath testing can be used to detect active infection with *H. pylori*. For the urea breath test, the patient must drink a radiolabeled carbon isotope. *H. pylori*, if present, will liberate tagged carbon dioxide through the hydrolysis of urea. The radiolabeled carbon is then detected in the breath of the infected patient. The specificity and sensitivity of the urea breath test for active infection with *H. pylori* is greater than 90%.[6] The major limitation of the urea breath test is that patients need to discontinue treatment with antibiotics 4 weeks prior to the test and proton-pump inhibitor (PPI) 1 week prior to the test as these drugs may result in false-negative results.[6,7] Urea breath testing can be used to confirm eradication of *H. pylori* after treatment.

Similar to the urea breath test, the stool antigen test for *H. pylori* can be used to confirm eradication of infection. Antibodies in the stool persist for a limited time (days to a few months); however, false-positive results are possible 4 weeks after treatment.[7] The stool antigen test is office-based, less costly, and as accurate as the urea breath test.

Other tests such as polymerase chain reaction, salivary assays, and urinary assays are available to detect *H. pylori*; these tests are not routinely used in clinical practice.

COMPLICATIONS

Peptic ulcers may lead to serious complications including bleeding, penetration, perforation, and gastric outlet obstruction. Complications can occur with either gastric or duodenal ulcer, and do not seem to be influenced by ulcer etiology. Despite improvements in medical therapy, the incidence of potentially life-threatening ulcer complications has not declined.[1]

BLEEDING

The most common complication of PUD is hemorrhage.[4] Signs and symptoms of hemorrhage include black tarry stools, vomiting of "coffee ground" material, weakness, syncope, and orthostasis. Hematochezia (red blood per rectum), usually related to lower GI bleeding, can occur with massive upper GI bleeding. If upper GI bleeding is suspected, nasogastric lavage should be used to confirm the diagnosis. Those with GI bleeding may require fluid and blood resuscitation, medical treatment with acid-suppressive therapy, or endoscopic intervention. Endoscopic intervention typically involves coagulation of the bleeding site by electrocautery, heater probe, laser, or epinephrine.[4] Embolization of vessels that supply the bleeding site may stop the bleeding. If endoscopic intervention is performed, patients should be treated with acid-suppressive therapy to decrease the risk for rebleeding (see "Treatment").

PENETRATION

Peptic ulcers may penetrate through the stomach or duodenum without leakage of luminal contents into the free peritoneal cavity. Penetration of ulcers into the pancreas, liver, or biliary tract can occur. The pain associated with penetration may be referred to sites other than the abdomen (such as the back) and is typically described as an intense, persistent pain. Radiographic evidence is generally necessary to confirm the diagnosis of penetration. No high-quality studies are available to provide guidance in the management of these patients.

PERFORATION

Perforation of gastric or duodenal ulcer is a serious medical condition requiring immediate attention. Perforation has been described in three phases.[8] During the initial phase of ulcer perforation (within 2 hours of onset), patients may experience symptoms of sudden, intense epigastric pain that quickly spreads throughout the abdomen. Patients often do not want to move because even taking a deep breath is painful. These symptoms reflect the release of acidic fluid into the peritoneal cavity. After this initial phase, a second phase (2–12 hours after onset) occurs in which the pain may partially subside and the patient may appear as if his condition is improving. On physical examination, the abdomen is tender to palpation, the abdominal muscles are rigid, and bowel sounds are decreased or absent. During the third and last phase of perforation (>12 hours after onset), abdominal distention and third-spacing is evident. Peritonitis and septic shock may ensue if there is a delay in diagnosis and medical treatment.

GASTRIC OUTLET OBSTRUCTION

Inflammation, scarring, or spasm associated with peptic ulcer can lead to gastric outlet obstruction.[4] It is the least common complication of PUD. Symptoms suggestive of gastric outlet obstruction include abdominal bloating or fullness, anorexia, and nausea or vomiting, particularly a long time after meals (6 hours or longer after eating). Typically, X-rays are used to confirm obstruction. Treatment involves gastric decompression and acid suppression.

GASTRIC CANCER

H. pylori has been identified as a carcinogen for gastric cancer.[9] Based on estimates from the International Agency on Research for Cancer, *H. pylori* is responsible for 36% to 47% of all gastric cancers. The precise mechanism by which *H. pylori* causes gastric cancer is unknown, and it is not yet clear whether eradication of *H. pylori* reduces the risk for cancer. At this point, routine screening for *H. pylori* as a tool to prevent gastric cancer is not recommended.[6]

TREATMENT

The treatment options for PUD are numerous and the practitioner's choice often depends upon factors such as ulcer etiology and the presence or absence of complications. Treatment for an initial ulcer may also differ compared to treatment for recurrent PUD. The primary goals of therapy include pain relief, ulcer healing, prevention of ulcer recurrence, and reduction of complications. Therapy in *H. pylori*-positive patients with active or previously documented ulcers is aimed at eradicating *H. pylori* and healing the ulcer. The objective of therapy in patients with NSAID-induced PUD is to heal the ulcer and remove the offending agent. These patients may also benefit from switching to a cycloxygenase-2 (COX-2) inhibitor or receiving prophylactic cotherapy for ulcer prevention.[10] Guidelines for the

evaluation and management of patients who present with dyspeptic or ulcer-like symptoms are presented in Fig. 11-1.

NONPHARMACOLOGIC THERAPY

Patients with PUD should eliminate or decrease their exposure to contributing agents such as cigarette smoking and nonselective NSAIDs. Psychosocial and psychological issues should be addressed due to the association between active psychosocial issues and recurrence or persistence of ulcer symptoms.[11] No firm dietary recommendations exist, but patients should generally avoid foods and beverages (e.g., spicy foods, caffeine, and alcohol) that precipitate dyspepsia. The availability of effective options for *H. pylori* eradication and acid suppression has drastically decreased the incidence of elective surgery for PUD.[12] A small subgroup of patients, however, may require surgery in response to dangerous complications such as bleeding, perforation, or obstruction (see "Complications").

PHARMACOLOGIC THERAPY

All ulcer patients infected with *H. pylori* should receive combination therapy with antibiotics and acid-suppressive agents to eradicate the organism due to the high risk of recurrence and ulcer-related complications with conventional ulcer treatments such as an H_2 receptor antagonist (H2RA), PPI, or sucralfate. The most extensively studied antibiotics for eradication of *H. pylori* include amoxicillin, clarithromycin, metronidazole, and tetracycline.[13] Metronidazole should be avoided in patients who chronically consume alcohol and alternatives to amoxicillin should be selected in penicillin-allergic patients.

Regimens that combine two antibiotics and one antisecretory drug (triple therapy) or a bismuth salt, two antibiotics, and an antisecretory drug (quadruple therapy) achieve acceptable eradication rates and decrease the risk of microbial resistance.[11,13] Treatment options for the eradication of *H. pylori* infection are presented in Table 11-2.

PPI-Based Three-Drug Regimens

The most commonly recommended regimen for first-line treatment is triple therapy with a PPI, amoxicillin, and clarithromycin.[11] A prepackaged daily dose kit is currently available for the combination of lansoprazole, amoxicillin, and clarithromycin, Prevpac (TAP Pharmaceuticals). Dual therapy with a PPI and either amoxicillin or clarithromycin has yielded marginal and variable eradication rates in the United States and is not recommended.[11,13] Yet, 2-week dual therapies with a

Table 11-2. Treatment Options for the Eradication of *H. pylori* Infection

Drug 1	Drug 2	Drug 3	Drug 4
PPI-based three-drug regimens* Omeprazole, 20 mg twice daily, or lansoprazole, 30 mg twice daily, or pantoprazole, 40 mg twice daily, or esomeprazole, 40 mg daily, or rabeprazole, 20 mg daily	Clarithromycin, 500 mg twice daily	Amoxicillin, 1 g twice daily, or metronidazole, 500 mg twice daily	
Bismuth-based four-drug regimens† Omeprazole, 40 mg twice daily, or lansoprazole, 30 mg twice daily, or pantoprazole, 40 mg twice daily, or esomeprazole, 40 mg daily, or rabeprazol, 20 mg daily, or standard ulcer-healing dosages of an H_2-receptor antagonist taken for 4–6 wks (see Table 33-9)	Bismuth subsalicy late 525 mg 4 times daily	Metronidazole, 250–500 mg 4 times daily	Tetracycline, 500 mg 4 times daily, or amoxicillin, 500 mg 4 times daily, or clarithromycin, 250–500 mg 4 times daily

*Although treatment is minimally effective if used for 7 days, 10–14 days of treatment is recommended. The antisecretory drug may be continued beyond antimicrobial treatment in the presence of an active ulcer.
†In the setting of an active ulcer, acid suppression is added to hasten pain relief.
Adapted from: Berardi RR, Welage LS. Peptic ulcer disease. In: DiPiro JT, Talbert RL, Yee GC, et al, eds. *Pharmacotherapy: A Pathophysiologic Approach*, 6th ed. New York, NY: McGraw-Hill; 2005:629.

PPI and clarithromycin or amoxicillin are FDA approved in the United States and the latter regimen could be considered in the rare patient who is intolerant to clarithromycin and metronidazole.[11]

The appropriate treatment duration for initial eradication attempts is yet to be determined. Some clinicians favor a 7-day initial regimen, while others prefer a 10- or 14-day-treatment course. While patient compliance may be increased with an abbreviated duration of therapy, eradication rates are lower and the risk of microbial resistance is enhanced.[11,14]

Bismuth-Based Four-Drug Regimens

Eradication rates for a 14-day regimen containing bismuth, metronidazole, tetracycline, and an H_2RA are similar to those of PPI-based regimens.[13] Although effective and relatively inexpensive, quadruple therapy is associated with frequent adverse effects and patient noncompliance.[10] First-line quadruple therapy with a PPI instead of an H_2RA achieves similar eradication rates as those of PPI-based triple therapy and allows for a shorter duration of treatment (7 days).[15] All medications except the PPI should be taken with food and at bedtime. A combination capsule, Pylera, (Axcan ScandiPharma) containing bismuth subcitrate, metronidazole, and tetracycline has been approved for use in the United States.

TREATMENT FAILURES

Initial attempts at eradicating *H. pylori* fail in as many as 20% of infected patients.[11] The incidence of unsuccessful eradication is increased by factors such as poor patient compliance, resistant organisms, low intragastric pH, and high bacterial load.[16,17] Initial treatment failure is often associated with a more difficult repeat attempt and extremely variable eradication rates.[13] Second-line empiric therapy should include antibiotics that were not previously utilized, a drug that has a topical effect such as bismuth, and an extended duration of treatment (10–14 days).[11,18] Therefore, after an unsuccessful initial treatment with a PPI–amoxicillin–clarithromycin regimen, second-line therapy should be initiated with bismuth subsalicylate, metronidazole, tetracycline, and a PPI for 10 to 14 days. Twice daily dosing of PPI is appropriate with second-line bismuth-based therapy.[13,18] Successful eradication has also been achieved with a 10-day course of pantoprazole (40 mg), amoxicillin (1 g), and levofloxacin (250 mg), all given twice daily.[11] Failure of both first- and second-line regimens in primary care may necessitate referral to a specialist.

ANTISECRETORY THERAPY AFTER *H. PYLORI* ERADICATION OR MAINTENANCE THERAPY

Asymptomatic patients, with small (<1 cm), uncomplicated duodenal or gastric ulcers, often do not require further therapy directed at ulcer healing after appropriate *H. pylori* treatment. Current data suggest that eradication of *H. pylori* can lead to ulcer healing without concurrent acid-suppression therapy.[19] There are no firm guidelines regarding continuation of antisecretory therapy after *H. pylori* eradication in patients with a history of complicated PUD. However, two consensus panels recommend maintenance of antisecretory therapy in patients who have suffered GI bleeding in the past until *H. pylori* eradication and complete ulcer healing are confirmed.[20,21] Suppressive therapy may also be continued in patients with a history of giant ulcers (>2 cm) or densely fibrosed ulcer beds. These patients should undergo follow-up endoscopy within 4 to 12 weeks following completion of *H. pylori* treatment to evaluate posttreatment status.[19]

If symptoms persist, despite successful eradication of *H. pylori*, patients may have persisting ulceration or, more commonly, another cause of dyspepsia such as GERD or nonulcer dyspepsia.[20]

Maintenance therapy should always be considered to prevent recurrence in high-risk patients, including those with a history of complications, giant or severely fibrosed ulcers, or frequent recurrences. Maintenance therapy with antisecretory agents is effective in reducing recurrence of duodenal ulcers and ulcer complications. Typical recurrence rates are 20% to 25% with H_2RAs over a period of 1 year compared to 60% to 90% with placebo.[19]

Effective maintenance doses for available H_2RAs are presented in Table 11-3.

Similar efficacy has been noted amongst the four H_2Ras; however, ranitidine may be a more favorable choice over cimetidine due to its superior antisecretory properties and decreased potential for drug–drug interactions.[22]

PPIs are also effective agents for maintenance therapy at appropriate doses. The response to low-dose omeprazole (5–20 mg) is variable.[19] One study noted a recurrence rate of 23% with omeprazole, 20 mg, given three times per week over 6 months, compared to 67% with placebo.[23] Although PPIs are reasonable options for maintenance therapy, there are limited data regarding the most appropriate maintenance doses of these agents. Therefore, it may be appropriate to reserve these agents for patients who do not respond to H_2RA therapy or those with large, severely fibrosed, or refractory ulcers.[19]

Most data on ulcer recurrence rates are related to duodenal ulcers; however, patterns appear to be similar with gastric ulcers. There are no clinical studies to provide insight into the optimal duration for maintenance therapy. The highest rates of recurrence are typically found during the first 3 to 6 months of maintenance therapy. Studies suggest that maintenance therapy may be effective for up to 5 years.[19] Decisions related to duration of maintenance therapy should depend on ulcer severity and whether or not the causal factor can be successfully eliminated.

NSAID-INDUCED ULCERS

Treatment for *H. pylori* is recommended for patients taking NSAIDs who have ulcers and are infected with this organism.[24] Patients with ulcers who test negative for *H. pylori* should still receive appropriate antiulcer

Table 11-3. Oral Drug Regimens Used to Heal Peptic Ulcers or Maintain Ulcer Healing

Drug	Duodenal or Gastric Ulcer Healing	Maintenance of Duodenal or Gastric Ulcer Healing
Proton-pump inhibitors (mg/dose)		
Omeprazole	20–40/daily	20–40/daily
Lansoprazole	15–30/daily	15–30/daily
Rabeprazole	20/daily	20/daily
Pantoprazole	40/daily	40/daily
Esomeprazole	20–40/daily	20–40/daily
H_2-receptor antagonists (mg/dose)		
Cimetidine	300/4 times daily	400–800/at bedtime
	400/twice daily	
	800/at bedtime	
Famotidine	20/twice daily	20–40/at bedtime
	40/at bedtime	
Nizatidine	150/twice daily	150–300/at bedtime
	300/at bedtime	
Ranitidine	150/twice daily	150–300/at bedtime
	300/at bedtime	
Promote mucosal defense (g/dose)		
Sucralfate	1/4 times daily	1–2/twice daily
	2/twice daily	1/4 times daily

Adapted from: Berardi RR, Welage LS. Peptic ulcer disease. In: DiPiro JT, Talbert RL, Yee GC, et al, eds. *Pharmacotherapy: A Pathophysiologic Approach,* 6th ed. New York, NY: McGraw-Hill; 2005:629.

therapy (i.e., antisecretory agent). The first step in treatment of patients with NSAID-induced ulcers is the discontinuation of all nonselective NSAIDs (when possible).[24] The healing rates of NSAID-induced ulcers compare favorably to those of non-NSAID-induced ulcers, provided that the NSAID is discontinued.[24] If the NSAID must be continued in spite of ulceration, consideration should be given to lowering the NSAID dose, switching to acetaminophen, a nonacetylated salicylate, a partially selective COX-2 inhibitor, or a selective COX-2 inhibitor.[25] PPIs are the treatment of choice for NSAID-induced ulcers not only after NSAID discontinuation but also in cases where it is not possible to discontinue the NSAID.[26] PPI treatment is associated with ulcer healing and prevention of relapse in patients requiring long-term NSAID therapy.[27] Therefore, patients with gastroduodenal ulcers or those who must continue NSAID therapy should be treated with a PPI, such as omeprazole or lansoprazole, for 4 to 8 weeks followed by maintenance therapy for as long as the NSAID is used.[11] H2RAs are less effective when NSAID therapy is continued.[24] Sucralfate is effective in the treatment of both NSAID-induced duodenal ulcers and those unrelated to NSAIDs, and the agent appears to be as effective as H2RAs in the healing of non-NSAID-related gastric ulcers. However, sucralfate has no proven benefit in the treatment or prevention of gastric ulcers attributed to NSAIDs.[27] NSAID-related ulcers may be treated effectively with any approved therapy for PUD (see Table 11-3). Studies demonstrate that acceptable healing rates can be obtained with all agents (H2RAs and PPIs) from both 4- and 8-week-treatment durations.[24]

PREVENTION

PRIMARY PREVENTION

Numerous strategies have been implemented to decrease the incidence of NSAID-induced ulcers and gastropathy. Strategies aimed at minimizing the topical irritant effects of NSAIDs such as enteric coating, delayed-release formulation, or prodrugs do not prevent ulcers or serious complications such as perforation and bleeding.[10] Medical cotherapy with misoprostol, a synthetic prostaglandin E1 analog, or a PPI has become increasingly popular and has been proven to decrease the risk of GI ulcerations and complications in high-risk patients.[24,27] Ulcer risk is increased with the concomitant use of NSAIDs and low-dose aspirin, and the GI-protective effects of COX-2 inhibitors are diminished by the addition of low-dose aspirin.[28] Additional factors that have been identified with an increased risk for NSAID-related GI complications are presented in Table 11-4.

Table 11-4. Factors That Have Been Identified with an Increased Risk for NSAID-Related Gastrointestinal Complications[24]

Prior history of gastrointestinal event (ulcer, hemorrhage)
Age > 60 y
High dosage of NSAID
Concurrent use of corticosteroids
Concurrent use of anticoagulants

SECONDARY PREVENTION

The issue of whether or not to choose a PPI and a nonselective NSAID over a selective COX-2 inhibitor with a PPI for secondary prevention in patients who require NSAIDs is the subject of controversy amongst clinicians. The potential for increased cardiovascular risk and higher financial burden associated with the latter regimen are of concern. Patients' cardiovascular risk factors and the cost-effectiveness of these regimens must be considered, but the use of a selective COX-2 inhibitor alone in patients at high risk for re-ulceration is not recommended.[29]

SUMMARY

Peptic ulcer is a GI disease associated with *H. pylori* infection and NSAID use. Serious complications of PUD include bleeding, penetration, perforation, and gastric outlet obstruction. Treatment of peptic ulcer in patients infected with *H. pylori* typically involves combination therapy with two antibiotics and a PPI. In contrast, management of NSAID-induced ulcer focuses on removing the offending agent and treatment with either a PPI or H2RA.

EVIDENCE-BASED SUMMARY

- PUD is characterized by excoriation of the mucosal layer of the stomach or duodenum.
- Infection with *H. pylori* and use of NSAIDs are major causes of PUD.
- Complications of PUD include bleeding, penetration, perforation, and gastric outlet obstruction.
- Treatment of peptic ulcers associated with *H. pylori* involves combination therapy with antibiotics and antisecretory agents.
- Treatment of NSAID-induced peptic ulcers includes discontinuation of the offending agent and treatment with an antisecretory agent.

REFERENCES

1. Kurata JH, Corboy ED. Current time trends in peptic ulcer. An epidemiological profile. *J Clin Gastroenterol.* 1988;10:259–268.

2. Sonnenberg A. Peptic ulcer. In: Everhart JE, ed. *Digestive Diseases in the United States: Epidemiology and Impact.* NIH publication no. 94–1447. Washington, DC: US Department of Health and Human Services, Public Health Service, National Institutes of Health; 1994:359–408.

3. Sonnenberg A, Everhart JE. Health impact of peptic ulcer in the United States. *Am J Gastroenterol.* 1997;92:614–620.

4. Cohen S. Gastritis and Peptic Ulcer Disease. In: Beers MH, Berkow R, eds. *The Merck Manual of Diagnosis and Therapy,* 17th ed. Available at http://www.merck.com/mrkshared/mmanual/home.jsp. Accessed January 29, 2008.

5. American Gastroenterological Association. AGA medical position statement: Evaluation of dyspepsia. *Gastroenterology.* 2005;129:1753–1755.

6. Peterson WL, Frendrick A, Cave DR, et al. *Helicobacter pylori*-related disease: Guidelines for testing and treatment. *Arch Intern Med.* 2000;9:1285–1291.

7. Frendrick A, Forsch RT, Harrison RV, et al. *Peptic Ulcer Disease: Guidelines for Clinical Care.* University of Michigan Health System. Available at http://cme.med.umich.edu/pdf/guideline/PUD05.pdf. Accessed August 8, 2005.

8. Soll, AH. *Complications of Peptic Ulcer Disease.* Available at www.uptodate.com. Accessed August 8, 2006.

9. International Agency for Research on Cancer. Schistosomes, liver flukes and *Helicobacter pylori.* IARC. 1994;61:177. Available at http://www.iarc.fr. Accessed August 8, 2005.

10. Berardi RR, Welage LS. Peptic ulcer disease. In: DiPiro JT, Talbert RL, Yee GC, et al, eds. *Pharmacotherapy: A Pathophysiologic Approach,* 6th ed. New York, NY: McGraw-Hill; 2005:640.

11. Peura DA. *Treatment Regimens for Helicobacter pylori.* www.uptodate.com. Accessed January 14, 2008.

12. Semour NE, Andersen DK. Surgery for peptic ulcer disease and postgastrectomy syndromes. In: Yamada T, Aplers DH, Kaplowitz N, et al, eds. *Textbook of Gastroenterology.* 4th ed. Philadelphia, PA: Lippincott Williams & Wilkins; 2003:1441–1454.

13. Suerbaum S, Michetti P. *Helicobacter pylori* infection. *N Engl J Med.* 2002;347:1175–1186.

14. Calvet X, Garcia N, Lopez T, et al. A meta-analysis of short versus long therapy with a proton pump inhibitor, clarithromycin and either metronidazole or amoxicillin for treating *Helicobacter pylori* infection. *Aliment Pharmacol Ther.* 2000;14:603–609.

15. Gene E, Calvet X, Azagra R, et al. Triple vs quadruple therapy for treating *Helicobacter pylori* infection: A meta-analysis. *Aliment Pharmacol Ther.* 2003;17:1137–1143.

16. Meyer JM, Silliman NP, Wang W, et al. Risk factors for *Helicobacter pylori* resistance in the United States; the Surveillance of *H. pylori* Antimicrobial Resistance Partnership (SHARP) Study, 1993–1999. *Ann Intern Med.* 2003;136:3–20.

17. Vakil N. *Helicobacter pylori*: Factors affecting eradication and recurrence. *Am J Gastroenterol.* 2005;100:2392–2394.

18. Megraud F, Lamouliatte H. Review article: The treatment of refractory *Helicobacter pylori* infection. *Aliment Pharmacol Ther.* 2003;17:1333–1343.

19. Soll AH. Overview of the natural history and treatment of peptic ulcer disease. Available at www.uptodate.com. Accessed January 14, 2008.

20. Professional Advisory Panel (CRAG) and Scottish Intercollegiate Guidelines Network (SIGN). *Helicobacter pylori*-Eradication Therapy in Dyspeptic Disease. A Clinical Guideline. August 1996.

21. Buckley M, Culhane A, Drumm B, et al. Guidelines for the management of *Helicobacter pylori*-related upper gastrointestinal diseases. Irish *Helicobacter Pylori* Study Group. *Ir J Med Sci.* 1996;165(5):1.

22. Dammann HG, Walter TA. Efficacy of continuous therapy for peptic ulcer in controlled clinical trials. *Ailment Pharmacol Ther.* 1993;7(2):17.

23. Lauritsen K, Andersen BN, Laursen LS, et al. Omeprazole 20 mg 3 days a week and 10 mg daily in prevention of duodenal ulcer relapse. Double-blind comparative trial. *Gastroenterology.* 1991;100:663.

24. Lanza FL, et al. A guideline for the treatment and prevention of NSAID-induced ulcers. *Am J Gastroenterol.* 1998;93:2037–2046.

25. Gupta S, McQuaid K. Management of nonsteroidal, anti-inflammatory, drug-associated dyspepsia. *Gastroenterology.* 2005;129:1711–1719.

26. Laine L. Approaches to nonsteroidal anti-inflammatory drug use in the high-risk patient. *Gastroenterology.* 2001;120:594–606.

27. Wolfe MM, Lichtenstein DR. Gastrointestinal toxicity of nonsteroidal anti-inflammatory drugs. *N Engl J Med.* 1999;340:1888–1899.

28. Silverstein FE, Faich G, Goldstein JL, et al. Gastrointestinal toxicity with celecoxib vs nonsteroidal anti-inflammatory drugs for osteoarthritis and rheumatoid arthritis: The CLASS study: A randomized controlled trial. Celecoxib Long-term Arthritis Safety Study. *JAMA.* 2000;284:1247–1255.

29. Feldman, M. NSAIDs (including aspirin): Treatment and secondary prevention of gastroduodenal toxicity. Available at www.uptodate.com. Accessed January 14, 2008.

Chapter 12

Inflammatory Bowel Disease

Alexandria A. Dunleavy

SEARCH STRATEGY

A systematic search of the medical literature was performed on January 9, 2008. The databases used to conduct the search were PubMed, UpToDate®, SUMSearch, PIER, and the National Guideline Clearinghouse. The search was limited to human subjects and journals in the English language. The references of articles obtained through the search were reviewed for additional relevant materials. Medical position statements regarding inflammatory bowel disease are available at www.gastro.org.

Inflammatory bowel disease (IBD) is a gastrointestinal (GI) disorder that includes both ulcerative colitis (UC) and Crohn's disease (CD). UC is characterized by diffused inflammation that is limited to the mucosa of the colon and rectum. CD describes a chronic inflammatory process that is manifested by focal, discontinuous, transmural lesions that may occur anywhere in GI tract from the mouth to the anus.

Patients with IBD are often embarrassed by the symptoms of the disease. The impact of the disease on social functioning and psychological health can be tremendous. Although some patients will experience an exacerbation that requires hospitalization, many will be treated in the community. Primary care providers will likely encounter patients with IBD, and should be prepared to meet the medical, psychological, and social needs of these patients.

EPIDEMIOLOGY

IBD affects approximately 1 million individuals in the United States.[1] The incidences of UC and CD in the United States are approximately 11 per 100 000 and 7 per 100 000 persons, respectively.[2] The incidence of UC has remained stable over several years, whereas the incidence of CD appears to be increasing over the last few decades. UC and CD have a bimodal distribution, with peak incidence occurring in the mid-teens to early thirties and then a second peak in individuals who are 50 years or older. UC is more common among some ethnic groups than others, for instance, Ashkenazi Jews are at higher risk for developing UC whereas blacks and Asians are less likely to develop it. Additionally, IBD is more common in urban areas and is more prevalent in higher socioeconomic classes.[2]

Cigarette smoking has differential effects on UC and CD. For smokers, the risk for developing UC is 40% that of nonsmokers. In contrast, the risk for CD in smokers is twice that of nonsmokers. Interestingly, oral contraceptive use increases the relative risk for CD by 1.9 times.[2]

CLINICAL PRESENTATION

Like many other chronic illnesses, the clinical courses of UC and CD are characterized by disease relapse and remission. Health care providers should educate patients about the chronic nature of IBD. Symptoms are variable and often related to the extent of the disease.

ULCERATIVE COLITIS

UC is classified as mild, moderate, or severe based on presenting symptoms (Table 12-1).[3] The disease is further categorized based on the location of involvement in the colon and/or rectum (Fig. 12-1). The most common sites of involvement are the rectum and sigmoid region of the colon. The following terminology is considered important:

Table 12-1. Classification of Ulcerative Colitis[3]

Disease Severity	Clinical Presentation
Mild	<4 stools/d (+/− blood), no systemic involvement, normal ESR
Moderate	>4–6 stools/d with minimal systemic involvement
Severe	>6 bloody stools/d with systemic involvement (fever, tachycardia, anemia) or elevated ESR
Fulminant	>10 stools/d, continuous bleeding, abdominal tenderness, and distension, requirement of blood transfusion

ESR, erythrocyte sedimentation rate.

- Proctitis describes the disease that is limited to the rectum.
- Proctosigmoiditis describes the disease in the rectum and sigmoid colon.
- Left-sided colitis describes the disease up to the splenic flexure (i.e., junction of the transverse and descending colon)
- Pancolitis describes the disease that extends throughout the colon.

This terminology is important as the extent of disease involvement guides the treatment therapy. Distal disease, which is limited to the areas below the splenic flexure, can generally be managed with topical therapy whereas more extensive disease often requires oral medications.

Mild Disease

Typically those with mild disease, suffer from UC proctitis or proctosigmoiditis. Initially, patients may present with rectal bleeding (often associated with the passage of mucous) and mild diarrhea (up to four

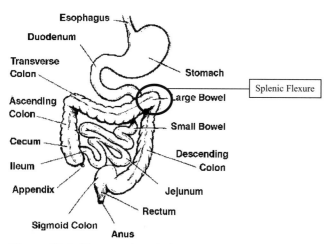

Figure 12-1. The gastrointestinal tract.
(Adapted from Mount Sinai Hospital, Ontario, Canada available at: http://www.mtsinai.on.ca/familialgicancer/Diseases/FAP/where.htm)

bloody stools daily). Tenesmus (urgency with the feeling of incomplete evacuation) and intermittent constipation are common. Severe abdominal pain, fever, and other systemic symptoms are rare.

Moderate Disease

Those with more extensive disease (beyond the splenic flexure) generally experience frequent, loose, bloody stools (four to six bloody stools daily). Some systemic manifestations of moderate UC include anemia (not requiring a blood transfusion), low-grade fever, and abdominal pain.

Severe Disease

Clinical features of severe or fulminant UC include bloody diarrhea (more than six bloody stools daily with the need for blood transfusion), abdominal pain, and distension. Systemic symptoms include fever, tachycardia, weight loss, and anemia. With severe disease, inflammation can penetrate the muscular layer of the colon, leading to impaired motility. Decreased GI motility results in colonic dilation that may progress to toxic megacolon. Plain abdominal films should be obtained in order to exclude toxic megacolon.

CROHN's DISEASE

Similar to UC, the clinical manifestations of CD are variable and related to the site of the disease. CD typically presents in one of the following two patterns: a fibrostenotic-obstructive pattern that results from chronic transmural inflammation or a penetrating-fistulous pattern resulting from sinus tracts that lead to microperforations and fistulae.[2] The most common areas of involvement are the ileum and the cecum where the colon meets the small intestine. This is often referred to as the ileocecal region of the GI tract.

Ileocolitis

Patients with ileocolitis often present with right lower quadrant pain and diarrhea. These symptoms may be accompanied by fever, leucocytosis, and weight loss (10–20% of body weight). On physical examination, the practitioner may palpate an inflammatory mass in the right lower quadrant which consists of inflamed bowel, adherent and indurated mesentery, and enlarged abdominal lymph nodes.[2] This mass can extend and cause obstruction of the bowel and/or bladder. Initially, bowel obstruction is intermittent; however, over time, chronic inflammation slowly progresses to fibrostenotic narrowing.[2]

Inflammation causes thinning of the bowel wall which may lead to microperforation and fistula formation. Fistulas may form on the retroperitoneum, urinary bladder, vagina, skin, or on the adjacent bowel wall. Symptoms correlate to the location of the fistula. For example, enterovaginal fistulae can present as the passage of stool through vagina.

Jejunoileitis

When CD extends into the jejunum, malabsorption of nutrients and steatorrhea can occur. This eventually leads to nutritional deficiencies of certain vitamins and minerals such as niacin, cyanocobalamin, calcium, and vitamin D. Diarrhea is common. Possible causes of diarrhea include (1) bacterial overgrowth in the presence of obstruction or fistulization, (2) malabsorption of bile acids as a result of disease in the ileum, and (3) inflammation with decreased absorption of water and increased secretion of electrolytes.[2]

Colitis and Perianal Disease

Typically, symptoms of CD colitis include fever, diarrhea, abdominal pain, and possibly hematochezia (blood in the stool). Rectal bleeding is not as common in CD colitis as it is in UC. Similar to those with ileocolitis, obstruction and fistulization can occur. Those with perianal CD may present with incontinence, hemorrhoidal tags, anorectal fistulas, and/or anal stricture.

Gastroduodenal Disease

When CD affects the stomach or the duodenum, patients may experience symptoms typical of gastritis, such as epigastric pain, nausea, and vomiting. The gastritis is most often negative for *Helicobacter pylori*. Gastric outlet obstruction can occur with advanced gastroduodenal disease. Similar to UC, CD is classified as mild-to-moderate, moderate-to-severe, or severe to fulminant, based on presenting symptoms (Table 12-2).[4]

Table 12-2. Classification of Crohn's Disease[4]

Disease Severity	Clinical Presentation
Mild/Moderate	Tolerance of oral feeding, no fever, dehydration, abdominal tenderness, <10% weight loss
Moderate/Severe	Failed treatment for mild/moderate disease or fevers, abdominal tenderness, nausea/vomiting, anemia, significant weight loss
Severe/Fulminant	Failed outpatient steroid or high fever, persistent vomiting, evidence of obstruction, rebound tenderness, cachexia, abscess

DIAGNOSIS

The diagnosis of IBD is based on a combination of clinical, endoscopic, and radiological findings. Differential diagnostic features of UC and CD are presented in Table 12-3.

HISTORY AND PHYSICAL EXAMINATION

A comprehensive history should include information about symptoms, family history, current medications, recent travel, and smoking status.[5] In addition, patients should be asked to provide details about stool frequency and consistency, bleeding, abdominal pain, fever, weight loss, or other systemic manifestations of IBD (e.g., arthralgias, ocular symptoms such as photophobia, blurred vision, and dermatologic complications). The examination should include measurement of blood pressure, pulse, temperature, and weight. The abdomen should be palpated and a rectal examination performed if indicated (e.g., in case of

Table 12-3. Differential Clinical Features of Ulcerative Colitis and Crohn's Disease[2]

Clinical	UC	CD
Blood in the stool	Yes	Occasionally
Passage of mucus	Yes	Occasionally
Systemic symptoms	Occasionally	Frequently
Location	Confined to rectum, colon	Anywhere in GI tract
Abdominal mass	Rarely	Yes
Fistulas	No	Yes
Obstruction	Rarely	Yes
Malnutrition/malabsorption	Yes	Yes
Toxic megacolon	Yes	Occasionally
Endoscopic		
Aphthous ulcers	No	Yes
Cobblestone appearance	No	Yes
Rectal sparing	No	Frequently
Disease involvement	Continuous	Discontinuous
Granuloma	No	Occasionally

UC, ulcerative colitis; CD, Crohn's disease; GI, gastrointestinal.

rectal bleeding). Laboratory data, including complete blood count (CBC), serum electrolytes, iron studies, vitamin B_{12} and folate levels erythrocyte sedimentation rate (ESR), C-reactive protein, and liver-function tests should also be obtained. The stool should be tested to rule out infectious causes of diarrhea such as *Clostridium difficile*, *Campylobacter*, ova, and parasites.

COLONOSCOPY WITH ILEOSCOPY

Colonoscopy with intubation of the terminal ileum is the procedure of choice in the initial evaluation of IBD because it enables visualization and biopsy of the rectum, colon, and terminal ileum. This procedure should be performed during the initial evaluation of patients with suspected IBD unless contraindicated because of severe colitis or possible toxic megacolon.[6] Nonsteroidal anti-inflammatory drugs and sodium–phosphate-based bowel preparation should be avoided prior to initial colonoscopy as these agents can cause mucosal changes that mimic IBD. Colonoscopy should be performed prior to the initiation of treatment as therapy may obscure characteristic features such as rectal involvement and segmental involvement that can help distinguish CD from UC and vice versa.

Endoscopy along with other diagnostic tools can differentiate CD from UC in 85% or more patients.[6] Endoscopic features typical of CD include aphthous ulcers adjacent to normal-appearing mucosa ("skip lesions") and areas of linear ulceration that often give the mucosa a cobblestone appearance (the ulcers represent the "cracks" while normal or inflamed tissue represent "stones"). Discontinuous lesions are an important distinguishing feature of CD; this disease pattern is in direct contrast to the continuous ulceration that is characteristic of UC. Additional features that allow clinicians to differentiate CD from UC include rectal sparing (seen in CD) and anal or perianal involvement (seen in CD). In contrast to the deep ulceration that can occur with CD, ulcers associated with UC generally affect only the mucosal layer of the GI tract. Typical endoscopic findings for UC include (1) loss of mucosal vascularity, (2) friablity and granularity, (3) continuous disease involvement, and possibly (4) pseudopolyps.

Ileoscopy is used to establish the extent of the disease. Strictures of the terminal ileum and discrete ulcers are suggestive of CD ileitis. In general, endoscopy appearance correlates poorly with clinical remission, and repeated endoscopy is not used to monitor for inflammation. However, repeat endoscopy can be used as an objective measure to assess response to therapy.

FLEXIBLE SIGMOIDOSCOPY

For patients with severe colitis and suspected UC, sigmoidoscopy may provide sufficient diagnostic information with considerably less risk than colonoscopy. Additionally, sigmoidoscopy can detect other causes of colitis such as infection with cytomegalovirus or *C. difficile* in patients with established disease.[6]

ESOPHAGOGASTRODUODENOSCOPY

CD can affect any part of the GI tract, including the esophagus, stomach, or duodenum. Therefore, esophagogastroduodenoscopy can be useful in the evaluation of IBD. However, most patients with upper GI involvement will also have disease elsewhere in the GI tract. Thus, esophagogastroduodenoscopy is not routinely recommended in individuals with IBD.[6]

CAPSULE ENDOSCOPY

The role of capsule endoscopy in CD is not well established. Capsule endoscopy may detect superficial lesions in the small bowel that are not apparent on endoscopy or radiography. However, there are several limitations to this procedure. First, capsule endoscopy does not allow for tissue sampling or therapeutic intervention. Furthermore, there is the risk that the capsule will be retained in individuals with strictures and obstruction. Therefore, the individuals with evidence of stricture or obstruction should not undergo capsule endoscopy.[6]

RADIOGRAPHY

Radiological evaluation includes diagnostic procedures such as barium enema or upper GI series. These studies can be used to visualize strictures, aphthous lesions, or small perforations with fistulous tracts. During an acute attack, a plain abdominal film should be obtained to assess for toxic dilatation of the colon. Barium studies should not be performed in individuals with suspected obstruction as this may lead to vomiting and aspiration of the contrast dye. Additionally, barium enemas should be avoided in individuals with moderate-to-severe colitis because of the risk for inducing toxic megacolon. Often radiography is used in conjunction with endoscopy (rather than as the primary diagnostic tool) in the evaluation of IBD.

Other diagnostic tests, including computed tomography or magnetic resonance imaging, are not as useful as endoscopy or barium enema but can be used to detect fistulas, abscesses, and sinus tracts in CD.

BIOPSY

Biopsy is an important component of the diagnostic evaluation of IBD. Mucosal biopsy can differentiate IBD from other causes of colitis and help distinguish CD from UC. Features suggestive of IBD include architectural distortion, increased number of transmucosal lamina propria cells, and severe mucin depletion.[6] Granulomas may be detected on biopsy with CD, although this is not particularly specific for CD as granulomas may occur with other diseases such as tuberculosis or sarcoidosis. Primary care providers should share relevant clinical findings with the consulting pathologist in order to obtain the most information from biopsy.

COMPLICATIONS

The complications of IBD can be local or systemic. Local complications of UC include hemorrhage, toxic megacolon, and intestinal perforation. CD can lead to obstruction, acute bowel perforation, fistulas, stricture, and abscess. Some systemic complications associated with both UC and CD include (1) ocular manifestations such as uveitis and episcleritis, (2) dermatologic conditions such as erythema nodosum and pyoderma gangrenosum, (3) hepatobiliary complications such as sclerosing cholangitis and cholelithiasis, and (4) rheumatic diseases such as arthritis and anklylosing spondylitis.

CANCER RISK

Patients with IBD are at higher risk for developing colorectal cancer than the general population. The risk for colorectal cancer is associated with both the duration and extent of the disease. The cancer risk after 10 years of extensive disease is 0.5% to 1% per year; however; patients with proctitis or proctosigmoiditis are not at increased risk for cancer.[3] Although the value of surveillance in reducing morality associated with colorectal cancer has not been established, several major associations recommend routine screening for individuals with IBD.[3,4,6,7] The American Society for Gastrointestinal Endoscopy recommends colonoscopy with multiple biopsies every 1 to 2 years beginning 8 to 10 years after diagnosis for those with UC and extensive Crohn's colitis.[6]

MANAGEMENT

Goals for treatment of IBD include (1) inducing and maintaining disease remission, (2) maintaining and/or improving the quality of life, and (3) controlling systemic manifestations. The treatment approach depends on the extent and severity of the disease. For distal disease (involving the rectum and sigmoid colon), topical therapy or a combination of oral and topical therapy may be appropriate. For extensive disease (beyond the splenic flexure), treatment with aminosalicylates or azathioprine is often necessary to maintain remission. The following sections discuss nonpharmacologic and pharmacologic treatment approaches to UC and CD.

NUTRITION

Although it has been suggested that dietary factors contribute to the development of IBD, there is little evidence to link diet with disease pathogenesis or etiology. Patients may report that certain foods such as nuts, seeds, fruits, or vegetables aggravate the condition; in this case, diet therapies should be tailored to the specific needs of the individual. CD predisposes individuals to malnutrition. Therefore, nutritional status, height, and weight should be monitored on a regular basis in an outpatient status. Nutritional support should be considered for children and adolescents with active small bowel disease, as it can modify the course of the disease.[5] In addition, nutritional support is an appropriate adjunctive therapy for any malnourished patient or anyone who is unable to meet nutritional requirements for 5 to 7 days because of severe disease.

NICOTINE

Smoking is protective against UC, but worsens the clinical course of CD. The mechanism of differential effects of smoking on UC and CD is unclear. Transdermal nicotine is superior to placebo for inducing remission of UC, but does not have any significant advantage when compared to standard treatment, and adverse effects significantly limit the clinical use of nicotine for this purpose.[8] Patients with CD, who smoke should receive counseling on smoking cessation as cessation may translate into fewer disease relapses.

SURGERY

Primary care providers should consider consulting with a gastroenterologist and colorectal surgeon for patients who fail to respond to intensive medical therapy for UC since surgery is sometimes curative.[5] In contrast, surgery is only undertaken for symptom relief of CD, since disease usually recurs after surgery. Surgical options should also be discussed for patients with dysplasia or carcinoma and those with recurrent acute or chronic episodes of UC.

PHARMACOTHERAPY

Pharmacologic agents such as aminosalicylates, corticosteroids, and immunomodulators such as azathioprine are often used to induce and maintain remission. Fortunately, these drugs are available in several formulations, making topical therapy an option for some patients.

Aminosalicylates

Aminosalicylates such as sulfasalazine or mesalamine (5-aminosalicylic acid, 5-ASA) are effective in treating mild-to-moderate UC or CD colitis. Several formulations of 5-ASA are available, including sulfasalazine (Azulfidine), oral mesalamine (Asacol, Pentasa and Lialda), mesalamine suppositories and enemas (Rowasa), olasalazine (Dipentum) and balsalazide (Colazal). These agents appear to have comparable efficacy.[3]

Although effective, side effects limit the use of sulfasalazine. In fact, up to 30% of patients treated with higher doses of sulfasalazine (6–8 g/d) experience serious or intolerable side effects such as allergic reaction, headache, nausea, and vomiting.[2] These side effects are most often related to the sulfa component of the drug. Nonetheless, many practitioners choose to initiate treatment with sulfasalazine given the cost-effectiveness of this medication in comparison to other oral aminosalicylates. If treatment with sulfasalazine is intolerable, then another formulation of 5-ASA is prescribed.

Oral aminosalicylates can be used alone or in combination with topical treatments. Mesalamine suppositories or 5-ASA enemas are a mainstay treatment for ulcerative proctitis and proctosigmoiditis. Often, these topical treatments alone are effective in left-sided colitis as well. Patients should be counseled that it may take 3 to 6 weeks to achieve the maximal benefits of oral aminosalicylates. Doses are gradually increased and then tapered to a minimally effective maintenance dose once remission is achieved. Dosing and other informations on various formulations of aminosalicylate products are presented in Table 12-4.

Corticosteroids

Corticosteroids have potent anti-inflammatory and immunomodulatory effects in UC and CD. Similar to mesalamine, corticosteroids are available in various dosage forms in an effort to optimize response while minimizing systemic toxicity. Steroid suppositories, enemas or foams are alternatives to mesalamine suppositories and 5-ASA enemas in the treatment of ulcerative proctitis, proctosigmoiditis, and left-sided colitis. However, the aminosalicylate products (suppositories and enemas) are preferred to maintain remission. Budesonide is a corticosteroid with poor bioavailability that undergoes extensive first-pass metabolism which limits systemic toxicity. Budesonide is available in a controlled, ileal-release formulation that is useful in the treatment of mild-to-moderate ileal and right-sided colonic CD.[1]

Corticosteroids can be given rectally, orally, or intravenously. Oral prednisone, 40 to 60 mg/d or 1 mg/kg per day, effectively induces remission in patients with moderate-to-severe UC or CD. It is often necessary to continue oral steroids for 7 days to one month in order to induce remission, and then gradually taper the steroid dose. For fulminant disease treatment, intravenous methylprednisolone 48 to 60 mg/d or hydrocortisone 300 to 400 mg/d, is often necessary to induce remission. Treatment with intravenous steroids beyond 7 to 10 days has no proven benefit and increases the risks for adverse events. Corticosteroids are reserved for those with active disease who have failed conventional treatment with agents such as aminosalicylates. Generally, treatment with corticosteroids is an indication of increased disease severity, often requiring intensification of maintenance therapy.

Maintenance Therapy

Corticosteroids have no role in the long-term maintenance treatment of UC or CD. However, short-term (3 months) treatment with budesonide does effectively maintain remission of mild-to-moderate ileocecal CD.[1] These effects are not maintained in the long term (more than 1 year).

Chronic treatment with corticosteroids is associated with serious adverse effects such as osteoporosis, glaucoma, cataracts, cushingoid symptoms, GI injury, and delayed wound healing; for this reason, treatment with corticosteroids should be limited to the shortest duration

Table 12-4. Formulations of Aminosalicylates for Inflammatory Bowel Disease

Generic Name	Brand Name	Formulation	Daily Dose (g)	Site of Action
Sulfasalazine	Azulfidine	Tablet	4–6	Colon
Mesalamine	Rowasa, Pentasa	Enema	1–4	Rectum, sigmoid colon
	Asacol	Delayed-release tablet	2.4–4.8	Ileum, colon
	Lialda			
	Pentasa	Microencapsulated capsule	2–4	Small bowel, colon
Osalazine	Dipenum	Dimer of 5-ASA, capsule	1.5–3	Colon
Balsalazide	Colazal	Capsule	6.75	Colon

5-ASA, 5-aminosalicylic acid.

possible. If corticosteroids are used, a decisive treatment plan should be established, including a strategy to wean the patient off steroids and to treat steroid-refractoriness and dependence.

Corticosteroid Dependence and Refractoriness

Corticosteroid dependence refers to the inability to reduce the dose of steroid without the patient experiencing a disease flare. Corticosteroid refractoriness refers to those who fail to respond to treatment with steroids. Those who are steroid-dependent or refractory, should be considered for treatment with infliximab with or without an immunomodulator. Adalimumab can be considered for those who do not respond to immunomodulors or infliximab.

Antibiotics

Antibiotics may be necessary in some patients with IBD, particularly after surgery or in the treatment of abscess. For fistulous perianal CD, metronidazole, 10 to 20 mg/kg per day in three divided doses, is the treatment of choice. Metronidazole is often continued for 3 months. The major concern for long-term treatment with metronidazole is the development of peripheral neuropathy that may or may not be reversible. Other side effects associated with metronidazole include disulfiram-like reaction, metallic taste, and nausea. An alternative to metronidazole for fistulous CD is ciprofloxacin, 500 mg twice daily.

With the exception of toxic megacolon, antibiotics have no role in the treatment of UC. However, metronidazole, ciprofloxacin, or tetracyclines are effective in the treatment of pouchitis that can occur after surgery for UC.[2]

Thiopurines

Azathioprine (AZA) and mercaptopurine (6-MP) are immunomodulatory agents that are thought to act through the metabolites 6-thioguanine nucleotides.[1] Although the precise mechanism of the thiopurines is not clear, the metabolites of AZA and 6-MP inhibit DNA and RNA synthesis and also induce T-cell apoptosis by modulating cell signaling. AZA is a prodrug of 6-MP and is converted to 6-MP after oral absorption.

The primary role of the thiopurines is to treat patients with UC or CD who are corticosteroid dependent. Thiopurines should be considered for patients with IBD who experience a severe exacerbation requiring corticosteroids. These agents are often used to wean patients with UC or CD off corticosteroids and are effective regardless of the disease distribution. Unless contraindicated, corticosteroid-dependent patients should be treated with AZA, 2.0 to 3.0 mg/kg per day, or with 6-MP, 1.0 to 1.50 mg/kg per day. Some practitioners start patients on these doses immediately as the full therapeutic benefits may not be realized until 3 months after starting treatment, while others prefer to start at lower doses and titrate up. Those corticosteroid-dependent or refractory patients, who cannot tolerate a thiopurine or who have a contraindication to treatment, should be considered for treatment with infliximab.

Maintenance Therapy

Thiopurines are effective maintenance therapy for CD. Treatment with AZA or 6-MP should also be considered for those individuals with refractory ulcerative colitis that has not responded to medical treatment. Thiopurines may prevent recurrences of CD after surgery and should be considered for those who are at risk for postoperative recurrence of CD.[1]

Thiopurines are generally well tolerated. However, patients may experience GI side effects and hypersensitivity reactions that lead to discontinuation of the drug. Pancreatitis occurs in 3% to 4% of patients.[2] Additionally, leukopenia and myelosuppression may occur with treatment. Bone-marrow suppression is often delayed and related to the dose of AZA or 6-MP. For this reason, treatment with AZA or 6-MP requires weekly monitoring of the CBC during dose titration and every 3 months thereafter. Additionally, periodic liver-function tests should be performed in individuals treated with AZA or 6-MP.

The Food and Drug Administration recommends genotype testing for thiopurine methyltransferase (TPMT) enzyme prior to the initiation of AZA or 6-MP. This is the enzyme responsible for metabolism of AZA and 6-MP. Approximately 1 in 300 individuals lack TPMT, and an additional 11% of the population consists of heterozygotes with intermediate activity.[2] Lack or deficiency of TPMT leads to drug accumulation and increases the risk for serious adverse events, including bone-marrow suppression.

Methotrexate

The dihydrofolate-reductase inhibitor, methotrexate, has anti-inflammatory and immunomodulating effects in CD. Methotrexate, when administered in doses of approximately 25 mg intramuscularly each week for up to 16 weeks, effectively induces remission in corticosteroid-dependent CD.[1] Thereafter, methotrexate, 15 mg intramuscularly each week, can be used to effectively maintain remission of CD. Methotrexate can also be used in patients who are intolerant to AZA or 6-MP. Although methotrexate is beneficial for the treatment of CD, evidence to support the use of methotrexate in UC is not well established.

Adverse events associated with methotrexate include leukopenia, nausea and vomiting, hypersensitivity pneumonitis, and hepatic fibrosis. Patients, who are started on methotrexate, require monitoring of CBC, creatinine, and liver-function tests. Liver biopsy may be required to evaluate persistently elevated liver-function tests. Chest X-ray and pulmonary-function tests should also be performed prior to starting therapy. Patients should be counseled that methotrexate can cause GI side effects (nausea, vomiting, diarrhea) and instructed to report these symptoms as they may be reduced by taking folic acid, 5 mg, within a few days of methotrexate.

Cyclosporine

Cyclosporine inhibits calcineurin and prevents T-cell activation. The intravenous form of the drug is used as salvage therapy for patients with severe UC that is refractory to medical treatment with oral or intravenous corticosteroids and for those with fistulizing CD. For those with severe UC, concurrent treatment with corticosteroids and intravenous cyclosporine is recommended to induce remission. Treatment with cyclosporine is often used as a temporary bridge to thiopurine therapy. Once remission is induced with intravenous cyclosporine, treatment with oral cyclosporine is often required for a few months. During this time, corticosteroids should be tapered and therapy with a thiopurine should commence. Although cyclosporine is useful in the management of IBD, this agent is associated with several adverse effects such as infection (caused by immunosuppression), hypertension, nausea, dyspepsia, and renal dysfunction. Treatment with cyclosporine requires monitoring of blood pressure, pulse, renal function, serum electrolytes, and cyclosporine levels.

Infliximab

Infliximab is a chimeric monoclonal antibody against tumor necrosis factor that possesses beneficial effects in active and in fistulizing CD. Additionally, recent studies have established the benefits of infliximab in UC.[9] The Active Ulcerative Colitis Trials 1 and 2 found that 64% to 69% of patients with moderate-to-severe UC responded to treatment with infliximab compared to about a 30% response rate with placebo. Patients were treated with three doses of infliximab at either 5 mg/kg or 10 mg/kg at weeks 0, 2, and 6, followed by maintenance infusions every 8 weeks. Clinical guidelines indicate that patients with IBD who do not respond to conventional treatment with aminosalicylates, antibiotics, corticosteroids, or immunomodulators are ideal candidates for infliximab.[1,4] Those who do respond to treatment should receive maintenance therapy with infliximab every 8 weeks.

Infliximab increases the risk of tuberculosis and other infections; therefore, all patients should have tuberculin skin testing and a chest X-ray prior to start-ing therapy. Individuals should be counseled to promptly report signs or symptoms of infections, such as sore throat or fever. Infusion-related reactions may occur with infliximab. These generally respond to decreasing the infusion rate or premedicating with acetaminophen and/or antihistamines.

Adalimumab

Like infliximab, adalimumab is an antibody directed against tumor necrosis factor. Adalimumab effectively induces and maintains remission in those individuals with moderate-to-severe CD. Generally, adalimumab is reserved for patients whose disease is refractory to other treatments (i.e., AZA, methotrexate) or fails to respond to treatment with infliximab. An initial induction dose of adalimumab 160 mg (4 injections) is administered subcutaneously, followed by 80 mg (2 injections) 2 weeks later and then a maintenance dose of 40mg every other week. Adalimumab carries the same risks and warnings for infection as infliximab.

EVIDENCE-BASED SUMMARY

- CD is characterized by discontinuous, transmural lesions that may involve any area in the GI tract from the mouth to the anus.
- UC is characterized by diffused, continuous inflammation of the mucosa that is confined to the rectum and colon.
- Complications of IBD may be local or systemic, including anemia, rectal fissure, fistula, perforation, and toxic megacolon.
- Treatment of IBD depends on the extent and severity of the disease.
- Aminosalicylates effectively treat and maintain remission of UC.
- Thiopurines are effective maintenance treatment for CD.
- Long-term treatment with corticosteroids is not recommended to maintain remission of IBD.

REFERENCES

1. Lichtenstein GR, Abreu MT, Cohen R, et al. American Gastroenterological Association Institute. Technical review on corticosteroids, immunomodulators and infliximab in inflammatory bowel disease. *Gastroenterology.* 2006;130: 940–987.
2. Inflammatory Bowel Disease. In: Harrison's Internal Medicine. McGraw-Hill Access Medicine. 2006. McGraw-Hill. Available at: www.accessmedicine.com.

3. Kornbluth A, Sachar DB. Ulcerative colitis practice guidelines in adults (update): American College of Gastroenterology, Practice Parameters Committee. *Am J Gastroenterol.* 2004;1371–1385.

4. Hanauer SB, Sandborn W. Management of Crohn's disease in adults. *Am J Gastroenterol.* 2001;635–643.

5. Carter MJ, Lobo AJ, Travis SP, et al. Guidelines for the management of inflammatory bowel disease in adults. *Gut.* 2004;53:v1–v16.

6. Leighton JA, Shen B, Baron TH, et al. Standards of Practice Committee, American Society for Gastrointestinal Endoscopy. ASGE guideline: Endoscopy in the diagnosis and treatment of inflammatory bowel disease. *Gastrointest Endosc.* 2006;63:558–565.

7. Eaden JA, Mayberry JF. Guidelines for screening and surveillance of asymptomatic colorectal cancer in patients with inflammatory bowel disease. *Gut.* 2002;51(S5):v10–v12.

8. McGrath J, McDonald JW, Macdonald JK. Transdermal nicotine for induction of remission in ulcerative colitis. *Cochrane Database Syst Rev.* 2004;4:CD004722.

9. Rutgeerts P, Sandborn WJ, Feagan BG, et al. Infliximab for induction and maintenance therapy for ulcerative colitis. *N Engl J Med.* 2005;2462–2476.

Chapter 13

Nausea and Vomiting

Rebecca E. Greene and Trevor McKibbin

SEARCH STRATEGY

A systematic search of medical literature was performed in January 2008. The search was limited to human subjects and journals in English language. Keywords included nausea, vomiting, emesis, antiemetic, chemotherapy, pregnancy, motion sickness, postoperative nausea and vomiting. Databases searched included Ovid, PubMed, National Guideline Clearinghouse, and the Cochrane database.

Nausea and vomiting are generalized symptoms that accompany a wide array of disorders and therapies (Tables 13-1 and 13-2). Although severe or prolonged vomiting may signal a complex clinical problem, more commonly, it is a self-limiting, unwanted side effect of medications, medical conditions, or procedures. Nausea and vomiting may be associated with gastrointestinal (GI) diseases, infections, neurologic or metabolic processes, cardiovascular disorders, pregnancy, chemotherapy, and surgical procedures.[1,2] Nausea and vomiting pose a significant expense to society as it has been estimated that pregnancy-induced nausea and vomiting account for 8.5 million days of work lost per year and postoperative nausea and vomiting (PONV) increase hospital costs by over $400 per patient.[1]

PATHOPHYSIOLOGY

Nausea, vomiting, and retching are three distinct phases involved in the process of emesis. Nausea is the subjective awareness of the urge to vomit and may be associated with flushing, tachycardia, diaphoresis, and salivation. Vomiting involves contraction of the abdominal muscles, descent of the diaphragm, and opening of the gastric cardia leading to expulsion of gastric contents through the mouth. Retching may precede or alternate with vomiting and involves spasmodic contractions of the thoracic and abdominal muscles as well as the diaphragm without expulsion of stomach contents.[1,2]

The vomiting center (VC), located in the reticular formation of the medulla, is the final common pathway mediating vomiting from most causes.[2,3] It is a diffuse, interconnecting neural network that, upon stimulation, coordinates the respiratory, GI, and abdominal musculature involved in emesis. The VC may be stimulated by several means including receiving afferent impulses from the cerebral cortex and higher brainstem, the vestibular system, the chemoreceptor trigger zone (CTZ), and via visceral afferents from the pharynx and GI tract.[2] The stimulation is mediated most commonly by dopamine, 5-hydroxytryptamine 3 (5HT3), opiate, histamine, muscarinic, and neurokinin-1 (NK-1) receptors (Table 13-3).[2,3]

The GI tract stimulates the VC through the nucleus tractus solitarius in which the vagal nerve afferents terminate. The CTZ is located in the area postrema in the floor of the fourth ventricle, effectively outside the blood–brain barrier where it is vulnerable to circulating emetogenic substances in the blood or cerebrospinal fluid.[2] The vestibular cause of vomiting is thought to be from stimulation of the eighth cranial nerve and involves muscarinic and histamine receptors.[1] The ability of higher brain centers to stimulate vomiting is the least-understood pathway. Vomiting from emotional stimuli or learned responses such as anticipatory nausea and vomiting associated with chemotherapy are thought to be mediated through the cortex but receptors and neurotransmitters involved are yet to be determined.

Table 13-1. Medications Causing Nausea and Vomiting

Class	Examples
Chemotherapy	Cisplatin, dacarbazine, cyclophosphamide, doxorubicin, carboplatin
Opioids	Morphine, oxycodone, codeine
Antibiotics	Erythromycin, sulfonamides, tetracycline
Anti-inflammatory	Aspirin, ibuprofen, ketorolac, naproxen
Hormonal therapies	Oral contraceptives, estrogen
Cardiovascular	Digoxin, beta-blockers, calcium-channel blockers
Miscellaneous	Nicotine, theophylline, colchicine, iron preparations, amifostine, L-dopa

Table 13-2. Other Etiologies of Nausea and Vomiting

Gastrointestinal Causes	Central Nervous System Causes
Obstruction	Migraine
Constipation	Increased intracranial
Gastroparesis	pressure
Irritable bowel	Malignancy, hemorrhage,
syndrome	meningitis, hydrocephalus,
Pancreatitis	trauma, pseudotumor
Pancreatic	cerebri
adenocarcinoma	Seizure disorder
Peptic ulcer disease	Emotional distress
Cholecystitis	Labyrinth disorders
Hepatitis	Motion sickness, tumor,
Gastroenteritis	Meniere's
Chronic intestinal	disease
pseudo-obstruction	Psychological
	Anorexia, bulimia,
	depression,
	pain, anxiety
	Endocrine and Metabolic
Cardiovascular Causes	**Causes**
Acute myocardial infarction	Pregnancy
Congestive heart failure	Diabetic ketoacidosis
Shock	Hyperthyroid
	Hyperparathyroid
	Hypoparathyroid
	Uremia
	Hypercalcemia
Operative Procedures	**Miscellaneous**
Gynecologic	Radiation therapy
Inner ear	Tube feeding
Tonsillectomy	
Laproscopic	

ASSESSMENT

The large number of diverse pathologic and physiologic causes of nausea and vomiting can make the evaluation of the underlying etiology difficult. Therefore, appropriate assessment is critical in providing recommendation for treatment.[1] Often patients with acute vomiting may require no treatment, particularly when vomiting is related to a viral infection, food poisoning, or excessive intake of food or alcohol. Vomiting associated with blood in the vomitus, fever, severe headache, trauma, or abdominal pain or distention should be referred for further workup and is beyond the scope of this chapter. Therefore, knowledge of onset and duration, precipitating and alleviating factors, medication history including over-the-counter or herbal supplements, food and liquid ingestion, sick contacts, or other medical conditions is crucial. The management of patients with nausea and vomiting includes identification of the underlying cause, treatment of any adverse sequelae that may result, and suppression of symptoms if the primary cause is self-limiting or cannot be eliminated. In cases where nausea and vomiting are anticipated outcomes, as in surgical procedures or chemotherapy, the focus should be on prevention on the basis of the most likely neurotransmitters and receptors involved.

TREATMENT

Although there is a large volume of literature on the treatment and prevention of nausea and vomiting, there is a surprising lack of controlled trials of pharmacologic therapies for the most common causes of nausea and vomiting. Most clinical trials have focused on specific clinical scenarios with a high risk for nausea and vomiting such as surgery, chemotherapy, and radiotherapy. Risk factors for PONV, chemotherapy-induced

Table 13-3. Receptor Location and Therapies

Afferent Origination	Receptors Involved	Target Therapies
Gastrointestinal	5HT3, DA	5HT3 antagonists, DA antagonists
Nucleus tractus solitarius	5HT3, DA, H2, NK-1, M	5HT3 antagonists, DA antagonists, antihistamines, NK-1 antagonists, anticholinergic
Chemoreceptor trigger zone	DA, 5HT3	DA antagonists, 5HT3 antagonists
Vestibular	H2, M	Antihistamines, anticholinergic
Cortex	Unknown	Benzodiazepines

5HT3, 5-hydroxytryptamine 3; DA, dopamine; H2, histamine; NK-1, neurokinin-1; M, muscarinic.

Table 13-4. Risk Factors for Nausea and Vomiting

Pregnancy	Chemotherapy/Radiation	Postoperative
History of motion sickness	Emetogenicity of chemotherapy	Female
History of migraines	Female	Nonsmoker
Nausea/vomiting with previous pregnancy	Young age	History of motion sickness
Mother or sister with nausea/vomiting of pregnancy	Chronic alcohol (decreases risk)	History of PONV
	History of motion sickness	Use of volatile anesthetics, nitrous oxide, or opioids
	Nausea/vomiting with previous chemotherapy	Duration of surgery
	Whole-body radiation	Type of surgery (laparoscopy, ear–nose–throat, neurosurgery, breast, laparotomy, plastic surgery, strabismus)
	Upper abdomen radiation	

PONV, postoperative nausea and vomiting.

nausea and vomiting (CINV), and radiation-induced emesis often help in identifying patients who are most likely to suffer from nausea and vomiting and who, therefore, would benefit from antiemetic prophylaxis (Table 13-4).[3–5]

Given the different neurohormonal mechanisms for the nonspecific symptoms of nausea and vomiting, it may not be appropriate to extrapolate results from a trial of these specific indications to a different clinical scenario.[1] In these situations, knowledge of the underlying pathophysiology, as outlined above, as well as the pharmacology of medications is used to aid in prescribing appropriate treatment. In those areas where much research is available, the principal drug classes used to treat and prevent nausea and vomiting include anticholinergics, antihistamines, phenothiazines, benzamides, 5HT3 antagonists, cannabinoids, benzodiazapines, corticosteroids, and butyrophenones (Table 13-5). Alternative therapies including acupressure/acupuncture, ginger, and pyridoxine (vitamin B6) have more limited support in the literature.

ANTICHOLINERGIC/ANTIHISTAMINES

Medications with anticholinergic and antihistamine activity are most commonly used to prevent nausea and vomiting associated with motion sickness and vertigo. These medications act upon muscarinic and histamine receptors in the VC and areas related to the vestibular system but have little effect on other causes of nausea and vomiting. Scopolamine, diphenhydramine, dimenhydrinate, meclizine, and hydroxyzine are the primary medications used in these classes. Scopolamine appears to be the most effective agent. A recent Cochrane review identified five studies comparing scopolamine to placebo for prevention of nausea and vomiting from motion sickness.[6] Transdermal scopo-

lamine was superior to placebo in preventing nausea with a pooled odds ratio of 0.25. In other studies that were reviewed, scopolamine was superior to meclizine in one study and equivalent to dimenhydrinate in another.[6] Although scopolamine is effective for the prevention of nausea and vomiting when compared to placebo, the studies were small and contained methodological quality issues. Common adverse effects associated with anticholinergic and antihistamine medications include dry mouth, drowsiness, dilated pupils, urinary retention, and blurred vision.[7] Their relatively low cost and lack of serious side effects make them good choices for nausea and vomiting associated with motion sickness.

BENZAMIDES

Metoclopramide, a substituted benzamide, exerts its action on both dopamine and serotonin receptors, depending on the dose. At low doses (0.15–0.5 mg/kg), metoclopramide is a powerful dopamine antagonist. At higher doses, it has 5HT3 antagonistic action.[8] In addition, metoclopramide enhances gastric peristalsis and emptying of the upper GI tract, thereby minimizing stasis, which may precede and exacerbate nausea and vomiting. Metoclopramide may be particularly useful in the treatment of nausea due to gastroparesis. It has also been extensively evaluated for CINV as well as PONV. At higher doses, metoclopramide may cause extrapyramidal symptoms (EPS), which should be prevented or treated with diphenhydramine or benzotropine. Other side effects include drowsiness, fatigue, diarrhea, and restlessness.[1]

When used in the setting of CINV, multiple dosages and dosing intervals have been evaluated. Due to the different combinations of therapy and the different

Table 13-5. Antiemetic Dosing

Medications	PONV	CINV	Motion Sickness	Receptor(s)	ADE
5HT3 antagonists				5HT3	Headache, dizziness
Dolasetron	IV: 12.5 mg	IV/PO: 100 mg	—		
Granisetron	IV: 1 mg	IV: 1 mg; PO: 2 mg	—		
Ondansetron	IV: 4 mg	IV: 8 mg; PO: 8–32 mg	—		
Palonosetron		IV: 0.25			
Anticholinergic	1.5 mg transdermal	—	1.5 mg transdermal	Muscarinic	Sedation, blurred vision,
Scopolamine	patch, apply 4 h prior to procedure		patch		dry mouth, urinary retention
Antihistamines					
Diphenhydramine	—	—	PO: 25–50 mg	Histamine	Sedation, blurred vision,
Dimenhydrinate	—	—	PO: 10 mg		dry mouth, urinary
Hydroxyzine	—	—	PO: 25–100 mg		retention
Meclizine	—	—	PO:25–50 mg		
Aprepitant	—	PO: 125 mg on day 1 then 80 mg PO on days 2–3	—	Neurokinin-1	Sedation, hiccups, constipation
Benazodiazepines	—		—		
Lorazepam	—	PO: 0.5–2 mg tid		Unknown	Sedation
Alprazolam	—	PO: 0.5–2 mg tid			
Dronabinol	—	PO: 5–10 mg Q 6 h	—	Unknown	Sedation, hallucinations, paranoia
Droperidol	0.625–1.25 mg	1.25–2.5 mg q 4–6 h	—	Dopamine	Sedation, dizziness, QT
Haloperidol		PO/IV: 1–3 mg q 4–6 h			interval prolongation
Corticosteroids			—	Unknown	Hyperglycemia, insomnia,
Dexamethasone	PO/IV: 4 mg	PO/IV: 12–20 mg			leukocytosis, adrenal suppression
Phenothiazines			—	Dopamine,	Sedation, hypotension,
Prochlorperazine	PO/IV: 5–10 mg	PO/IV/PR: 10 mg		histamine	
Promethazine	PO/IV: 12.5–25 mg	PO/IV/PR: 12.5–25 mg			
Metoclopramide	PO/IV: 10–20 mg	PO/IV: 20 mg Q 4–6 h up to 1–3 mg/kg Q 3 h	—	Dopamine, 5HT3	Diarrhea, sedation

PONV, postoperative nausea and vomiting; CINV, chemotherapy-induced nausea and vomiting; ADE, adverse drug events; 5HT3, serotonin receptor; IV, intravenous; PO, oral; PR, per rectum; tid, three times a day; q, every.

outcomes measured, it is difficult to determine which of these regimens is the most appropriate. In the setting of acute CINV, metoclopramide can be used in doses of 1 to 3 mg/kg every 3 hours for three doses starting 1/2 hour prior to the administration of chemotherapy. To prevent delayed CINV, doses of 0.5 mg/kg can be given every 6 hours until the risk of CINV has passed. At these doses, side effects attributable to the multiple mechanisms of action become more apparent.[3] Diarrhea due to the cholinergic effects has been reported at an incidence of 25% to 30%, as well as EPS in approximately 5% of patients.

Metoclopramide is approved by the Food and Drug Administration for the prevention of PONV at a dose of 10 to 20 mg just prior to the completion of the procedure. Results from clinical trials have been inconclusive regarding the most effective regimen, and despite being on the market for over 40 years, a scientific dose-finding study is yet to be performed. Consensus guidelines, published in 2003 for PONV, list metoclopramide

as having "lack of evidence" and the majority of members agreed that it should not be recommended.[4]

PHENOTHIAZINES

Phenothiazines, including promethazine, prochlorperazine, chlorpromazine, and perphenazine, treat nausea and vomiting via antidopamenergic mechanism, most likely in the CTZ. These agents are inexpensive and come in a variety of dosage forms including intravenous, oral, and rectal. Prochlorperazine and promethazine are the agents most widely used for nausea and vomiting.[1] They are commonly used to prevent nausea and vomiting in low to moderate emetogenic chemotherapy and also to prevent breakthrough nausea and vomiting in chemotherapy.[3] They have also demonstrated efficacy in PONV when given at the end of surgery.[4] Common adverse events to these medications include sedation and orthostatic hypotension, and less commonly EPS; there are also rare reports of hypersensitivity, neuroleptic malignant syndrome, and blood dyscrasias.[1]

SEROTONIN ANTAGONISTS

The selective serotonin-receptor antagonists include ondansetron, granisetron, dolasetron, and palonosetron. These agents act by selectively inhibiting serotonin, an important neurotransmitter in acute CINV at the 5HT3 receptor in the small bowel, vagus nerve, and CTZ. Each agent has relative differences in potency, half-life, metabolism, and availability of an oral-dosage form (Table 13-5).

The 5HT3 antagonists have been extensively studied in CINV and PONV. These agents with the exception of palonosetron have not been shown to be effective beyond the first 16 to 24 hours of CINV. This highlights the different neurotransmitters responsible for acute CINV as compared to delayed CINV. Due to their efficacy in acute CINV, their use is warranted for prevention of CINV due to both highly and moderately emetogenic chemotherapy. Dosing and guidelines for use have been extensively studied and published elsewhere.[3]

Ondansetron, dolasetron, and granisetron are commonly used in the prevention and treatment of PONV. As a group, they are effective agents in preventing PONV; however, their routine use is not cost effective. The use of these agents should be based on individual risk factors of the patient, the type of procedure, and the type of anesthesia. According to recent guidelines, patients at high risk for PONV should receive combination prophylaxis, which may include a 5HT3 antagonist with droperidol, dexamethasone, or promethazine. For those with moderate risk, monotherapy with a 5HT3 antagonist may be considered.[4] No routine prophylaxis is used for patients with a low risk of PONV. Patients who did not receive a 5HT3 antagonist for PONV prophylaxis and then experience PONV may then receive treatment with a 5HT3 antagonist. In patients who received a 5HT3 antagonist for prevention of PONV, initiation of a 5HT3 antagonist for treatment within 6 hours provides no additional benefit and alternative agents should be considered.[4]

Due to the limited indications in which randomized controlled trials have been performed and the added expense of these agents compared to the phenothiazines and metoclopramide, their use may not be justified outside of PONV and CINV. With the exception of palonosetron, the majority of comparative trials has found these agents to be interchangeable; they are often chosen on the basis of cost. Side effects include headache, dizziness, and less commonly, QTc interval prolongation.[1]

BUTYROPHENONES

Haloperidol and droperidol are antidopaminergic medications that have shown to be useful in managing nausea and vomiting. They are commonly utilized in both CINV and PONV. A meta-analysis published in 2004 evaluated the use of haloperidol for nausea and vomiting related to operative procedures, chemotherapy, and GI diseases. Haloperidol was effective in preventing and treating PONV at doses ranging from 0.5 mg to 5 mg given either intravenously or intramuscularly. There was also evidence to suggest that haloperidol is effective at treating nausea and vomiting related to GI diseases. Its use in chemotherapy and radiation-induced nausea and vomiting, however, was less clear due to lack of placebo-controlled trials and inconsistent endpoint reporting.[9] The Consensus guidelines for PONV state that less than 1 mg of droperidol is equivalent to ondansetron in preventing PONV.[4] However, due to a recent Food and Drug Administration "black box" warning for death or life-threatening events associated with QT prolongation, its use has decreased. Other adverse effects of these medications include EPS, sedation, and drowsiness.

BENZODIAZEPINES

Benzodiazepines have been used traditionally for the treatment of anticipatory CINV and as an adjuvant agent treating CINV refractory to other agents. Alprazolam and lorazepam are the most commonly used agents. Recently, alprazolam showed efficacy in the prevention of CINV when added to a 5HT3 inhibitor. Sedation as well as amnesia is common in patients treated with benzodiazepines.[3] Dependence is usually not a concern given the short duration of treatment.

CORTICOSTEROIDS

Corticosteroids have been shown to be more active than placebo in the prevention of CINV and PONV, though the exact mechanism of action is not fully understood. The most widely studied of the corticosteroids in these settings is dexamethasone, which readily crosses the blood–brain barrier. The addition of corticosteroids to 5HT3 antagonists are more effective in the prevention of CINV than either agent alone, and this combination has formed the backbone of treatment for moderately and highly emetogenic chemotherapy.[3] In the prevention of PONV, a one-time dose of 5 to 10 mg of dexamethasone can be given prior to induction and is utilized in combination with a 5HT3 antagonist in patients at high risk for PONV.[4] Side effects associated with short-term use of corticosteroids include hyperglycemia, leukocytosis, insomnia, and mood disorders.

SUBSTANCE P/NK-1 ANTAGONIST

A recent development in the prevention of CINV is aprepitant, a synthetic NK-1 receptor antagonist. In a three-drug regimen, that included ondansetron and dexamethasone, aprepitant provided a statistically significant prevention of acute and delayed nausea caused by the use cisplatin. Aprepitant is normally well tolerated with the most frequent adverse events being asthenia and fatigue which occurred in a numerically higher percentage of patients treated with aprepitant compared to placebo but did not reach statistical significance.[10] Drug interactions are of concern because aprepitant is a substrate, moderate inducer, and moderate inhibitor of cytochrome P450 enzyme 3A4 (CYP3A4). Aprepitant also induces CYP2C9. Chemotherapy agents known to be metabolized by CYP3A4 include docetaxel, paclitaxel, etoposide, irinotecan, ifosfamide, imatinib, vinorelbine, vinblastine, and vincristine. In studies evaluating aprepitant, the prechemotherapy dose of dexamethasone was adjusted from 20 mg to 12 mg. However, the chemotherapy doses were not adjusted for potential drug interactions. Caution is urged, because of the small number of patients overall.[10]

CANNABINOIDS

Dronabinol is a synthetic oral form of tetrahydrocannabinol and has been found to be more active than placebo in the treatment of nausea and vomiting. The specific mechanism of action remains unknown. Cannabinoids are generally reserved for CINV, which is unresponsive to other agents, and have no role in PONV.[1,4] Side effects include sedation or drowsiness, euphoria, dysphoria, depression, dizziness, hallucinations, paranoia, and hypotension.

OLANZAPINE

Olanzapine is an antipsychotic drug that has action at numerous neurotransmitters receptors including dopamine D1, D2, D3, and D4, and serotonin at 5HT2a, 5HT2c, 5HT3, and 5HT6. The effects on D2 and 5HT3 receptors, which are involved in nausea and emesis pathways, make it likely to have a significant antiemetic effect. A recent phase II trial by Navari and colleagues demonstrated a regimen of olanzapine used to prevent nausea and vomiting associated with moderately and highly emetogenic chemotherapy.[11] Their regimen of 5 mg daily for 2 days prior to chemotherapy and 10 mg daily for 2 to 4 days, in addition to standard corticosteroids and granisetron, showed a high complete response rate, but the study was limited by the lack of a control arm and small population size. Larger controlled studies are still needed to confirm its use in CINV.[11]

PREGNANCY

It is estimated that 70% to 85% of women may experience nausea and vomiting during pregnancy with 0.5% to 2% progressing to hyperemesis gravidarum.[5] The pathogenesis is not well understood but likely due to hormonal changes. Although mild to moderate nausea and vomiting are generally self-limiting with little effect on pregnancy outcomes, many women experience significant psychosocial morbidity including depression and report poor support by family. Hyperemesis gravidarum has been associated with low birth weight and other complications including Wernicke's encephalopathy, splenic avulsion, and esophageal rupture.[5] The American College of Obstetricians and Gynecologists published guidelines for the treatment of PINV. Pyridoxine, 30 to 100 mg daily, is recommended first line with the addition of doxylamine, 12.5 mg 3 to 4 times per day, if symptoms persist. Other possible therapies include promethazine, dimenhydrinate, metoclopramide, and ondansetron. Methylprednisolone is reserved as a last-resort therapy due to an association with oral clefts when used in the first trimester.[5] Other alternative therapies include ginger, which has been found to be more effective than placebo in preventing early nausea and vomiting of pregnancy, and acupressure or electrical stimulation at the P6 point.[5]

EVIDENCE-BASED SUMMARY

- Nausea and vomiting are generalized symptoms that accompany a wide array of disorders and therapies.
- Nausea and vomiting involve complicated interactions between neurotransmitters and receptors. The most common receptors involved include dopamine, 5HT3, NK-1, histamine, and opiate.
- When nausea and vomiting are expected outcomes of medications or procedures, prevention is the goal of therapy.
- Guidelines for CINV and PONV suggest prevention on the basis of risk factors.

REFERENCES

1. AGA. Technical review on nausea and vomiting. *Gastroenterology.* 2001;120:263.
2. DiPiro CV, Taylor AT. Nausea and vomiting. In: DiPiro JT, Talbert RL, Yee GC, Matzke GR, Wells BG, Posey LM, eds. *Pharmacotherapy: A Pathophysiologic Approach.* 6th ed. New York, NY: McGraw-Hill; 2005:665.
3. National Comprehensive Cancer Network. *Clinical Practice Guidelines in Oncology.* Antiemesis version1. 2005. Available at www.nccn.org. Accessed October 2005.
4. Gan TJ, Meyer T, Apfel CC, et al. Consensus guidelines for managing post operative nausea and vomiting. *Anesth Analg.* 2003;97:62–71.
5. ACOG Practice Bulletin. Clinical management guidelines for obstetrician-gynecologists, nausea and vomiting of pregnancy. *Obstet Gynecol.* 2004;52:803.
6. Spinks AB, Wasiak J, Villanueva EV, Bernath V. Scopolamine for preventing and treating motion sickness. *Cochrane Database Syst Rev.* 2004;3:1–17.
7. Flake ZA, Scalley RD, Bailey AG. Practical selection of antiemetics. *Am Fam Physician.* 2004;69:1169.
8. Saller R, Hellenbrecht D, Hellstern A, Hess H. Improved benefit/risk ratio of higher-dose metoclopramide therapy during cisplatin induced emesis. *Eur J Clin Pharmacol.* 1985;29:311–312.
9. Büttner M, Walder B, von Elm E, et al. Is low-dose haloperidol a useful antiemetic? A meta-analysis of published and unpublished randomized trials. *Anesthesiology.* 2004;101:1454.
10. Dandno TM, Perry CM. Aprepitant: A review of its use in the prevention of chemotherapy-induced nausea and vomiting. *Drugs.* 2004;64:777–794.
11. Navari RM, Einhorn LH, Passik SD. A phase II trial of olanzapine for the prevention of chemotherapy-induced nausea and vomiting: A Hoosier Oncology Group Study. *Support Care Cancer.* 2005;13:529–534.

Chapter 14

Constipation and Diarrhea

Nicole L. McMaster-Baxter and Sharon A. Jung Tschirhart

SEARCH STRATEGY

A systematic search of the medical literature was performed on September 1, 2005. The search, limited to human subjects and journals in English language, included the National Guidelines Clearinghouse, the Cochrane database, PubMed, and UpToDate®.

CONSTIPATION

Constipation is a highly prevalent condition, especially in the older adult population. It is estimated that the prevalence of chronic constipation in North America varies between 2% and 27%.[1] Constipation is generally more common in women, older adults, nonwhites, and patients of lower socioeconomic status.[1]

SYMPTOMS

Constipation can be assessed by using several variables such as stool frequency, stool size or consistency, and other related symptoms. It is important to keep in mind that all patients have individual bowel habits. Therefore, the frequency of bowel movements may not be the most reliable method to assess constipation.[1] The Rome II criteria is a standardized tool that diagnoses functional constipation as two or more of the criteria listed in Table 14-1 for at least 12 weeks during the preceding year with symptoms occurring at least 25% of the time.[2]

The knowledge of the criteria given in Table 14-1 can be used as a guide in the clinic setting. However, it is important to remember that symptoms can vary depending upon the individual bowel habits of the patients. Patients having daily bowel movements may complain of occasional constipation.[3] Symptoms of con-

stipation may arise secondary to other conditions such as primary diseases of the colon, metabolic disturbances, and neurologic disorders as listed in Table 14-2.[3–5]

ETIOLOGY[3]

Constipation arises from two disorders of colorectal motility. The first disorder, slow-transit constipation, or "colonic inertia," refers to slower-than-normal movement of fecal contents from the proximal to the distal colon and rectum. There are two proposed mechanisms that lead to slow colonic transit: (1) decreased peristaltic contractions and (2) uncoordinated motor activity in the distal colon. Pelvic floor dysfunction is another major disorder of colorectal motility. This condition leads to an inability to evacuate contents from the rectum adequately. Combination syndromes can also occur, in which a patient exhibits both slow transit and disorders of evacuation.

EVALUATION

When a patient complains of symptoms of constipation, a thorough history should be taken including the following: past medical history, associated symptoms, usual bowel patterns, current therapies used, frequency of current bowel movements and consistency of stools, dietary habits, and current medications including both prescription and over-the-counter drugs. There are several risk factors that can predispose a patient to developing constipation (Table 14-3).

Symptoms of bloating, pain, and/or malaise between infrequent bowel movements may be suggestive of irritable bowel syndrome.[3] Pelvic floor dysfunction should be suspected if a patient reports prolonged straining before elimination or the need for direct digital evacuation; this condition may not respond well to standard laxative

Table 14-1. Rome II Criteria for Functional Constipation

- Straining at defecation
- Lumpy or hard stools at defecation
- Sensation of incomplete evacuation
- Sensation of anorectal obstruction or blockage at defecation
- Manual maneuvers to facilitate defecation (e.g., digital evacuation)
- Less than three defecations per week

Adapted from: Thompson WG, Longstreth D, Drossman KW, et al. Functional bowel disorders and functional abdominal pain. *Gut.* 1999;45(II):II43–II47.

therapies.[3] A physical examination of the abdomen and rectum should be performed to rule out any abdominal mass, fecal impaction, hemorrhoids, and so on. Screening tests such as fecal occult blood tests, complete blood count, thyroid-stimulating hormone, serum glucose, serum creatinine, and serum calcium can also be performed, especially if the patient presents with symptoms of chronic constipation (persisting for more than 3 months) that do not have an identifiable cause.[1,3,6]

When a patient presents with complaints of constipation, alarm symptoms listed in Table 14-4 warrant further testing including, but not limited to, the following: flexible sigmoidoscopy, colonoscopy, or barium enema.[1] Routine use of colon cancer screening tools is recommended for all patients 50 years and older with colorectal risk factors.[1] According to expert opinion, no further initial workup may be needed in healthy adults presenting with acute constipation due to an identifiable cause who meet the following criteria: under the age of 50 years with no risk factors for colorectal cancer, a negative fecal occult blood and normal initial laboratory tests, negative abdominal and rectal examinations, and adequate response to initial therapy.[1,6]

Untreated constipation can lead to serious consequences such as fecal incontinence, bowel obstruction, irritability, hypertension, hemorrhoids, and tachycardia.

MANAGEMENT

Nonpharmacologic Therapies

Patient education programs should focus on reducing constipation and promoting bowel health.[7] Education

Table 14-2. Organic Diseases Associated with Constipation[3–5]

- Autonomic neuropathy
- Hypothyroidism
- Hypercalcemia
- Spinal cord injury
- Parkinsonism
- Bowel obstruction
- Paralytic ileus
- Cancer
- Diabetes mellitus
- Depression

Table 14-3. Risk Factors for Constipation[3,6]

- Low-fiber diet
- Low fluid intake
- Reduced mobility
- Contributing medications
  - Analgesics
  - Anticholinergics
  - Calcium-containing antacids
  - Calcium-channel blockers
  - Iron supplements
  - Clonidine
  - Diuretics

should include lifestyle recommendations such as the following: adequate fluid intake (1500–2000 mL/d), avoidance of caffeinated and alcoholic beverages, increased physical activity, increased dietary fiber (25–30 g/d), and regular toileting throughout the day.[7] Patients should be encouraged to keep a log of bowel activity including frequency, character, and amount of bowel movements, in order to recognize the need for pharmacologic therapy.[7]

Pelvic floor retraining involves biofeedback and relaxation training to assist patient in relaxing the pelvic floor muscles during straining.[3] This type of nonpharmacologic therapy is generally more effective for treating patients with slow-transit constipation or impaired evacuation when other treatments have failed.[4]

Surgical treatment of slow-transit constipation is a last-line option that involves total colectomy with ileorectal anastomosis. This procedure is designed to treat the symptoms of constipation and achieve regular defecation.[3] However, other symptoms such as abdominal pain and bloating may not be alleviated.[3]

Pharmacologic Therapies

Pharmacologic therapies involve the use of laxatives. Table 14-5 lists dosage recommendations for a variety of laxative preparations.

Bulk Laxatives.[1,6] Psyllium (e.g., Metamucil®, Konsyl®), methylcellulose (e.g., Citrucel®), and polycarbophil (e.g., FiberCon®) increase colonic residue and stimulate peristalsis. These agents should not be given to

Table 14-4. Alarm Symptoms

- Hematochezia
- Weight loss ≥10 lb
- Family history of colon cancer or inflammatory bowel disease
- Anemia
- Positive fecal occult blood tests
- Acute onset of constipation in older patients

Adapted from: American College of Gastroenterology Chronic Constipation Task Force. An evidence-based approach to the management of chronic constipation in North America. *Am J Gastroenterol.* 2005;100(S1).

Table 14-5. Dosage Recommendations

Agents that Cause Softening of Feces in 1–3 d
  Bulk-forming agents
    Methylcellulose: 4–6 g/d
    Polycarbophil: 4–6 g/d
    Psyllium: varies with formulation
  Emollients
    Docusate sodium: 50–360 mg/d
    Docusate calcium: 50–360 mg/d
    Docusate potassium: 100–300 mg/d
  Lactulose: 15–30 mL orally
  Sorbitol: 30–50 g/d orally
  Mineral oil: 15–30 mL orally
  Chloride Channel Activators
    Lubiprostone: 24 mcg orally twice daily with food
Agents that Result in Softened Stool in 6–12 h
  Bisacodyl (oral): 5–15 mg orally
  Phenolphthalein: 30–270 mg orally
  Cascara sagrada: varies with formulation
  Senna: varies with formulation
  Magnesium sulfate: <10 g orally
Agents that Cause Watery Evacuation in 1–6 h
  Magnesium citrate: 18 g/300 mL solution
  Magnesium hydroxide: 2.4–4.8 g orally
  Magnesium sulfate: 10–30 g orally
  Sodium phosphates: varies with formulation
  Bisacodyl: 10 mg rectally
  Polyethylene glycol preparations: 4 L

Adapted from: DiPiro JT, Talbert RL, Yee GC, et al. *Pharmacotherapy: A Patho-physiologic Approach.* New York, NY: McGraw-Hill; 2005.

patients with inadequate fluid intake, as they have to be taken with plenty of water to avoid intestinal obstruction.

Osmotic Laxatives.[1,5,6] Lactulose, glycerin, and sorbitol can be administered rectally or orally. These agents increase osmotic activity in the lumen, which draws fluid into the colon to produce soft, formed stools. The expected onset of action after oral ingestion is 12 to 72 hours, whereas the onset of action after rectal administration is 30 minutes. Lactulose (e.g., Kristalose®) is usually more expensive than other agents, but has been shown to be effective at increasing stool frequency and stool consistency in patients with chronic constipation. Polyethylene glycol (e.g., Miralax®) has also been shown to be effective at increasing stool frequency and stool consistency in patients with chronic constipation. However, high doses of polyethylene glycol may lead to diarrhea, nausea, and cramping.

Saline Osmotic Laxatives.[1,5,6] Magnesium hydroxide, magnesium citrate, and sodium phosphate are primarily used for acute management of constipation and followed with bulk or osmotic laxatives for maintenance therapy. These agents may cause fluid and electrolyte depletion and hence should be used with caution in patients with renal and cardiac diseases.

Stimulant Laxatives.[1,5,6] Senna (e.g., Senokot®, Ex-lax®) and bisacodyl (e.g., Dulcolax®, Correctol®) are approved by the Food and Drug Administration for the treatment of occasional constipation, and are the most commonly used ingredients in stimulant laxatives in the United States. These agents appear to act by altering the transport of electrolytes within the intestinal mucosa, causing water retention, and stimulating peristalsis. The use of these agents would be an appropriate choice to patients taking chronic opioids. However, continuous daily use can lead to diarrhea, hyponatremia, hypokalemia, and dehydration.

Surfactant Laxatives.[1,5] Castor oil, docusate sodium (e.g., Colace®), and docusate calcium (e.g., Surfak®) are anionic surfactants that act as stool-softening agents by altering intestinal permeability, which stimulates peristalsis. Although docusates have minimal laxative effects, they are useful for patients with painful defecation due to hemorrhoids. Castor oil has strong purgative actions, which induce bowel movements within 1 to 3 hours. Castor oil should not be recommended for routine treatment of constipation.

Suppositories and Enemas.[1,5] Water, saline, sodium phosphate, lactulose, and mineral oil have all been used as enemas. Water enemas should be used with caution in older patients due to increased risk of acute water intoxication. Glycerin and bisacodyl suppositories are often used in the hospital setting to stimulate bowel activity.

Chloride Channel Activators.[8,9] Lubiprostone (Amitiza®) is a new agent that acts locally on the apical membrane of gastrointestinal tract to increase intestinal fluid secretion. It is approved by the Food and Drug Administration for the treatment of chronic, idiopathic constipation. In placebo-controlled trials, lubiprostone demonstrated an increase in spontaneous bowel movements throughout duration of therapy. However, long-term safety remains to be established. This agent should be reserved for patients with severe constipation despite use of other agents. Be aware that doses may need to be reduced if patients develop nausea. A baseline negative pregnancy test must be obtained prior to use in women of childbearing age.

DIARRHEA

Diarrheal diseases are one of the top five causes of death worldwide.[10] An estimated 211 to 375 million episodes of acute diarrhea occur annually in the United States, accounting for more than 900,000 hospitalizations and 6000 deaths per year.[11]

DEFINITION/ETIOLOGY

Several definitions of diarrhea exist, including references to increased frequency of stools (more than three per day), increased liquidity of stools, and stool weight greater than 200 g/d.[12] An increased frequency of defecation (three or more times per day or at least 200 g of stool per day) lasting for less than 14 days is one accepted definition of acute diarrhea. Abdominal cramping, nausea and vomiting, malnutrition, or clinically significant systemic symptoms may also be present.[11] The major causes of acute gastrointestinal illness in otherwise healthy individuals in developed countries are viruses, bacteria, and less often, protozoa.[13] Most cases are probably viral in nature with many patients choosing not to seek medical attention.[10] Cases of severe diarrhea (greater than or equal to four fluid stools per day for more than 3 days) are usually caused by bacteria.[10] The most common pathogens implicated in causing acute diarrhea in 2002 were salmonella, campylobacter, shigella, *Escherichia coli* O157:H7, and cryptosporidium. *Clostridium difficile* is the most common pathogen implicated in nosocomial diarrhea.[11] Chronic diarrhea is defined as the production of loose stools with or without increased stool frequency for more than 4 weeks and occurs at a prevalence of approximately 3% to 5% in the United States.[14]

EVALUATION

Limited evidence is available to guide the evaluation and treatment of diarrhea.[12] The initial clinical evaluation of acute diarrhea should evaluate the severity of the illness and the requirement for rehydration, and also identify the likely causes of diarrhea on the basis of a thorough history and clinical findings.[11] Most cases of acute diarrhea are usually self-limited, regardless of whether the cause is due to an infection, viruses, or noninfectious. Because most cases of diarrhea are self-limited and nearly 50% of cases persist for less than 1 day, microbiologic investigation is usually unnecessary for patients who present within 24 hours after the onset of diarrhea. However, if patients present with dehydration, are febrile, have blood or pus in their stool, or have other indications for medical evaluation (see Table 14-6), further workup is indicated.[10,11]

Obtaining an accurate medical history is an important key in the evaluation of diarrhea (Table 14-7).[14] Fecal testing for Shiga toxin is recommended, as well as cultures for *E. coli* O157:H7, in individuals with a sudden onset of bloody diarrhea (especially if afebrile) or the hemolytic-uremic syndrome.[11] Travelers' diarrhea occurs in an individual, normally residing in an industrialized region, who travels to a devel-

Table 14-6. Indications for Medical Evaluation

Profuse watery diarrhea with signs of hypovolemia	Passage of > 6 unformed stools per 24 h or a duration of illness of >48 h
Passage of many small volume stools containing blood and mucus	Severe abdominal pain
Bloody diarrhea	Recent use of antibiotics or hospitalized patients
Temperature ≥38.5°C	Diarrhea in older adults (≥70 y of age) or the immunocompromised

Adapted from: Wanke CA. *Approach to the Patient with Acute Diarrhea.* UpToDate online 13.2 Available at www.uptodate.com.Accessed April 2005.

oping tropical or semitropical country. The passage of at least three unformed stools in a 24-hour period with accompanying symptoms of nausea, vomiting, abdominal pain or cramps, fecal urgency, tenesmus,

Table 14-7. Obtaining Accurate Medical History

Onset of Diarrhea Congenital, abrupt, or gradual	Presence of Weight Loss Substantial weight loss more likely caused by nutrient malabsorption, ischemia, or neoplasm
Pattern of Diarrhea Continuous or intermittent loose stools	Assess for Aggravating Factors Diet, stress
Duration of Symptoms	Mitigating Factors Alteration of diet, use of prescription or over-the-counter drugs
Epidemiological Factors Travel before onset, potential exposure to food or water, illness in family	Review Previous Evaluations of Diarrhea Objective records, radiograms, biopsy specimens
Stool Characteristics Watery, bloody, or fatty	Investigate for Iatrogenic Causes Obtain detailed medication history, surgical history, and radiation history
Presence or Absence of Fecal Incontinence	Evaluate for Factitious Diarrhea Caused by surreptitious laxative ingestion
Presence or Absence of Abdominal Pain Pain often present in irritable bowel syndrome, inflammatory bowel disease, mesenteric ischemia	Review of Systems Hyperthyroidism, diabetes mellitus, collagen-vascular diseases and other inflammatory conditions, tumor syndromes, acquired immunodeficiency syndrome, and other immune problems

Adapted from: Musher DM, Musher BL. Contagious Acute gastrointestinal infections. *NEJM.* 2004;351:2417–2427.

or the passage of bloody or mucoid stools is included in the definition of travelers' diarrhea. The illness usually occurs during the first 7 to 10 days after returning home and consists of the passage of between three and ten unformed stools daily for 3 to 5 days. About 10% to 20% of cases are accompanied by abdominal pain and cramps, fever, vomiting, and the passage of bloody stools (dysentery). Diarrhea lasts longer than 1 week in 10% of patients and longer than 1 month in 2% of patients.[15] Treatment generally includes rehydration and antibiotics. Travelers may be given a prescription for an antibiotic prior to travel, in the event of diarrheal episodes. Antibiotics are generally reserved for moderate to severe cases (more than four unformed stools daily, fever, blood, pus, or mucus in the stool).[16] Fluoroquinolones (generally ciprofloxacin 500 mg twice a day for 1 or 2 days) and azithromycin 1000 mg as a single dose, have been shown to be effective in the treatment of travelers' diarrhea.[16] Patients should be advised to seek medical attention if they develop high fever, abdominal pain, bloody diarrhea, or vomiting.

Antibiotics (Table 14-8) have been implicated in causing diarrhea ranging from colitis (potentially progressive and serious) to "nuisance diarrhea" (frequent loose and watery stools with no other complications). Antibiotic-associated colitis can produce fever, abdominal cramping, leukocytosis, hypoalbuminemia, fecal leukocytes, and colonic thickening on computed tomography.[17] Other medications have been implicated in causing diarrhea as shown in Table 14-9.

C. difficile infection is only responsible for 10% to 20% of cases of antibiotic-associated diarrhea, but accounts for the majority of cases of antibiotic-associated colitis.[17] For patients hospitalized for more than 72 hours or those with recent exposure to antibiotics, toxigenic *C. difficile*, the most common recognized cause of nosocomial diarrhea, should be suspected.[11] Clindamycin, cephalosporins, and penicillins are the most commonly implicated antibiotics causing *C. difficile* diarrhea.[17] Individuals with bloody diarrhea (especially if

Table 14-9. Drugs Causing Diarrhea

Laxatives
Antacids containing magnesium
Antineoplastics
Auranofin (gold salt)
Antibiotics
- Clindamycin
- Tetracyclines
- Sulfonamides
- Broad-spectrum antibiotics
Antihypertensives
- Reserpine
- Guanethidine
- Methyldopa
- Guanabenz
- Gaunadrel
Cholinergics
- Bethanechol
- Neostigmine
Cardiac agents
- Quinidine
- Digitalis
- Digoxin
Nonsteroidal anti-inflammatory drugs
Prostaglandins
Colchicine

Adapted from: DiPiro JT, Talbert RL, Yee GC, et al. *Pharmacotherapy: A Pathophysiologic Approach.* New York, NY: McGraw-Hill; 2005.

afebrile) and a history of eating seed sprouts or rare hamburger meat should be evaluated for Shiga toxin-producing *E. coli* infection. Fecal testing is recommended for cases where diarrhea is persistent or recurring or if the history (for instance, of fever or tenesmus) is equivocal. Inflammatory bowel disease should be suspected if fecal evidence of inflammation is present (see Chapter 12).[11]

MANAGEMENT

Since most cases of diarrhea usually last for 1 to 3 days and are self-limited, supportive fluid therapy is usually indicated as initial therapy. Oral rehydration solutions with a glucose-based electrolyte solution as recommended by the World Health Organization are preferred. Most adults with acute diarrhea in developed countries are advised to drink fluids and take in salt from soups and salted crackers.[11] Although there are nearly 400 over-the-counter preparations in the United States promoted for their antidiarrheal properties, few have proven their effectiveness in randomized, controlled trials (Table 14-10).

Loperamide, bismuth subsalicylate, and kaolin have proven evidence of efficacy and safety as antidiarrheals. Loperamide inhibits intestinal peristalsis and is considered a first-line antimotility drug for adults. Antimotility agents should not be utilized in individuals presenting

Table 14-8. Antibiotic-Associated Diarrhea

Rates of Occurrence (%)	Antibiotics
15–20	Cefixime
10–25	Amoxicillin-clavulanate
5–10	Ampicillin
2–5	Cephalosporins, fluoroquinolones, azithromycin, clarithromycin, erythromycin, tetracyclines

Adapted from: Bartlett JG. Antibiotic-associated diarrhea. *NEJM.* 2002;346: 334–339.

Table 14-10. Antidiarrheal Preparations

Agent	Dosage Form	Adult Dose
Antimotility		
Diphenoxylate	2.5 mg/tablet	5 mg 3 to 4 times daily; do not exceed 20 mg/d
	2.5 mg/5 mL	
Loperamide	2 mg/capsule	Initially 4 mg, then 2 mg after each loose stool;
	1 mg/5 mL	do not exceed 16 mg/d
Paregoric	2 mg/5 mL (morphine)	5–10 mL, 1–4 times daily
Opium tincture	5 mg/mL (morphine)	0.6 mL, 4 times daily
Difenoxin	1 mg/tablet	2 tablets, then 1 tablet after each loose stool;
		up to 8 tablets/d
Adsorbents		
Kaolin–pectin mixture	5.7 g kaolin + 130.2 mg pectin/ 30 mL	30–120 mL after each loose stool
Polycarbophil	500 mg/tablet	Chew 2 tablets 4 times daily with 8 oz of fluid or after each loose stool; do not exceed 12 tablets/d
Attapulgite	750 mg/15 mL	1200–1500 mg after each loose stool or every 2 h; do not exceed 9000 mg/d
	300 mg/7.5 mL	
	750 mg/tablet	
	600 mg/tablet	
	300 mg/tablet	
Antisecretory		
Bismuth sulfate	1050 mg/30 mL	2 tablets or 30 mL every 30 min to 1 h as needed; do not exceed 8 doses/d
	262 mg/15 mL	
	524 mg/15 mL	
	262 mg/tablet	
Enzymes (lactase)	1250 neutral lactase units/4 drops	3–4 drops taken with milk or dairy product
	3300 FCC lactase units per tablet	1 or 2 tablets as above
Bacterial replacement		2 tablets or 1 granule packet (*Lactobacillus acidophilus*, *L. bulgaricus*), 3–4 times daily; given with milk, juice, or water
Octreotide	0.05 mg/mL	Initial: 50 mcg subcutaneously, 1–2 times daily; titrate dose based on indication up to 600 mcg/d in 2–4 divided doses
	0.1 mg/mL	
	0.5 mg/mL	

FCC, Food Chemical Codex.
Adapted from: DiPiro JT, Talbert RL, Yee GC, et al. *Pharmacotherapy: A Pathophysiologic Approach.* New York, NY: McGraw-Hill; 2005.

with bloody diarrhea or suspected inflammatory diarrhea. Bismuth subsalicylate has proven inferior to loperamide in clinical trials, but is noted to alleviate symptoms of nausea, abdominal pain, and diarrhea in individuals suffering from traveler's diarrhea. Kaolin–pectin, an adsorbent, has limited evidence to support its use. The use of antimicrobial therapy needs to be based upon the cause and duration of diarrhea, risk of adverse reactions, benefit versus cost, and risk of eradicating normal flora.[11]

Empirical therapy for chronic diarrhea is used as a temporizing or initial treatment before diagnostic testing, after diagnostic testing has failed to confirm a diagnosis, or when a diagnosis has been made but no specific treatment is available or specific treatment fails to affect a cure.[12] Individuals with chronic diarrhea

should maintain a lactose-free diet for several days to rule out lactase deficiency.[18] Medications may be responsible for almost 4% of cases of chronic diarrhea, especially magnesium-containing products, theophylline, antibiotics, antihypertensives, nonsteroidal anti-inflammatory drugs, antineoplastic agents, antiarrhythmics, and food additives such as fructose and sorbitol.[19] Adequate hydration is a mainstay of treatment. An empiric trial of antimicrobial therapy may be utilized in environments with a high prevalence of bacterial or protozoal infection. Use of bile-acid-binding resins, such as cholestyramine, can aid in the diagnosis of bile-acid-induced diarrhea. Diphenoxylate and loperamide may be used in certain cases of less severe diarrhea. Opiates are nonspecific antidiarrheal agents used in the treatment of severe chronic diarrhea and octreotide, a somatostatin analog, should be reserved as a second-line agent in the management of chronic idiopathic diarrhea. Psyllium or other stool modifiers typically do not decrease stool weight, but may modify stool consistency.[12]

EVIDENCE-BASED SUMMARY

- Constipation is a common condition that can lead to serious consequences if left untreated.
- It is important to recognize symptoms that differentiate constipation from other disease states that would warrant diagnostic testing.
- Effective treatment and prevention of constipation are important including lifestyle modifications, patient education, and proper use of pharmacologic therapies.
- Proper assessment and monitoring of constipation symptoms will lead to patient satisfaction regarding their health care and improved quality of life.
- Diarrhea is associated with significant morbidity and mortality worldwide and in the United States.
- An increased frequency of defecation (3 or more times per day or at least 200 g of stool per day) lasting for less than 14 days is one accepted definition of acute diarrhea, whereas chronic diarrhea is defined as the production of loose stools with or without increased stool frequency for more than 4 weeks.
- The key to evaluating the cause of diarrhea is obtaining a thorough medical history and clinical evaluation.
- Limited evidence is available to guide the evaluation and management of diarrhea, but one of the most important concepts in the management of diarrhea is maintaining adequate hydration.

REFERENCES

1. American College of Gastroenterology Chronic Constipation Task Force. An evidence-based approach to the management of chronic constipation in North America. *Am J Gastroenterol.* 2005;100(S1–4).

2. Thompson WG, Longstreth D, Drossman KW, et al. Functional bowel disorders and functional abdominal pain. *Gut.* 1999;45(II):II43–II47.

3. Locke GR, Pemberton JH, Phillips SF. American Gastroenterological Association Medical Position Statement: Guidelines on constipation. *Gastroenterology.* 2000; 119(6):1761–6 .

4. Kamm MA. Constipation and its management. *Br Med J.* 2003;327:459.

5. DiPiro JT, Talbert RL, Yee GC, et al. *Pharmacotherapy: A Pathophysiologic Approach.* New York, NY: McGraw-Hill; 2005.

6. Folden SL, Backer JH, Maynard F, et al. *Practice Guidelines for the Management of Constipation in Adults.* Glenview, IL: Association of Rehabilitation Nurses; 2002.

7. Registered Nurses Association of Ontario (RNAO). *Prevention of Constipation in the Older Adult Population.* Toronto, Ontario, Canada: Registered Nurses Association of Ontario (RNAO); 2002:38.

8. Amitiza® Package Insert. Available at www.amitiza.com. Accessed January 16, 2008.

9. Wald, A. Treatment of Chronic Constipation in Adults. UpToDate online. 2007. Available at www.uptodate.com

10. Wanke CA. *Approach to the Patient with Acute Diarrhea.* UpToDate online 13.2 Available at www.uptodate.com. Accessed April 2005.

11. Thielman NM, Guerrant RL. Acute infectious diarrhea. *NEJM.* 2004;350:38–47.

12. American Gastroenterological Association Clinical Practice and Practice Economics Committee. AGA technical review on the evaluation and management of chronic diarrhea. *Gastroenterology.* 1999;116:1464–1486.

13. Musher DM, Musher BL. Contagious acute gastrointestinal infections. *NEJM.* 2004;351:2417–2427.

14. American Gastroenterological Association. AGA Medical Position Statement: Guidelines for the evaluation and management of chronic diarrhea. *Gastroenterology.* 1999; 116:1461–1463.

15. DuPont HL, Ericsson CD. Prevention and treatment of traveler's diarrhea. *NEJM.* 1993;328:1821–1827.

16. Wanke CA. *Travelers' Diarrhea.* UpToDate online 14.1. Available at www.uptodate.com. Accessed April 2006.

17. Bartlett JG. Antibiotic-associated diarrhea. *NEJM.* 2002; 346:334–339.

18. Donowitz M, Kokke FT, Saidi R. Current Concepts: Evaluation of patients with chronic diarrhea. *NEJM.* 1995;332: 725–729.

19. Thomas PD, Forbes A, Green J, et al. Guidelines for the investigation of chronic diarrhoea, 2nd edition. *Gut.* 2003;52:1–15.

PART 4

Neurologic Disorders

CHAPTERS

Chapter 15

Epilepsy

Susan J. Rogers

SEARCH STRATEGY

A systematic search of the literature was performed on June 30, 2005. The search, limited to human subjects and journals in the English language, included PubMed (including Practice Guidelines), MD Consults, UpTo-Date®, and EBM Reviews (2000–2005): Cochrane database, DARE, and ACP Journal Club.

INTRODUCTION

Epilepsy is a common chronic neurological disorder with an age-adjusted incidence of approximately 44 per 100 000 person-years, a prevalence of 6 to 8 per 1000, and a cumulative incidence, through age 74, of 3.1%.[1,2] There is a bimodal distribution of the first seizure, with one peak occurring in newborn and young children and the second in patients older than 65 years.[3]

It is important to recognize and optimally treat epileptic patients since epilepsy can significantly impact their quality of life; it can affect their chances of employment, social relationships, and feelings of self-worth. Epilepsy may be responsible for significant morbidity including psychological distress, anxiety and depression, and mortality.

Unfortunately up to 30% of the population develops drug-resistant epilepsy, especially people with partial onset seizures. The failure to respond to three or more antiepileptic drugs (AEDs) denotes drug-resistant or intractable epilepsy.

To optimally manage a patient with epilepsy, the physician must first determine the type of epilepsy. This is based on the clinical history (both from the patient and observers), radiographic information, and electroencephalogram (EEG) results. The International League Against Epilepsy (ILAE) developed a seizure-classification scheme, which is used today (Table 15-1)[4]. This scheme categorizes seizures as partial, generalized, or unclassified. Partial seizures are further subdivided into simple partial seizures (typified by no impairment of consciousness), complex partial seizures (impairment of consciousness present), and partial seizures developing into secondarily generalized seizures. Generalized seizures are subdivided into nonconvulsive (absence of convulsions) and convulsive seizures.

Additionally, the ILAE devised a second method of categorizing epilepsy by syndromes, taking into account the age of onset of the seizures, family history of epilepsy, seizure type(s), and associated neurological symptoms and signs. After grouping epilepsy into generalized and focal syndromes, the ILAE classifies epilepsies as idiopathic, cryptogenic (those with unknown but suspected cause) or secondary, and symptomatic epilepsies. A modified working version of the ILAE 1989 classification is provided in Table 15-2.[5]

CLINICAL PRESENTATION

EVENTS MIMICKING SEIZURE

In evaluation for possible epilepsy it is important to consider nonepileptic paroxysmal events such as transient ischemic attacks, pseudoseizures, movement disorders, migraine, syncope, cardiac arrhythmias, fugue states, transient global amnesia, panic attacks, night terrors, narcolepsy, and hyperventilation. Frontal lobe seizures can be especially difficult to differentiate from pseudoseizures as a result of their unusual presentation.

Table 15-1. International Classification of Epileptic Seizures

I. Partial (Focal Seizures)
   A. Simple partial seizures (consciousness not impaired)
      1. With motor signs (including Jacksonian, versive, and postural)
      2. With sensory symptoms (including visual, somatosensory, auditory, olfactory, gustatory, and vertiginous)
      3. With psychic symptoms (including dysphasic, dysmnesic, hallucinatory, and affective changes)
      4. With autonomic symptoms (including epigastric sensation, pallor, flushing, papillary change)
   B. Complex partial seizures (consciousness is impaired)
      1. Simple partial onset followed by impaired consciousness
      2. With impairment of consciousness at onset
      3. With automatisms
   C. Partial seizures evolving to secondarily generalized seizures
II. Generalized Seizures of Nonfocal Origin (convulsive or nonconvulsive)
   A. Absence seizures
      1. With impaired consciousness only
      2. With one or more of the following: atonic components, tonic components, automatisms, autonomic components
   B. Myoclonic jerks (single or multiple)
   C. Tonic–clonic seizures (may include clonic–tonic–clonic seizures)
   D. Tonic seizures
   E. Atonic seizures
III. Unclassified Epileptic Seizures

Adapted from: Pedley TA. Classification of seizures and epilepsy. In: Resor SR, Jr., Kutt H, eds. *The Medical Treatment of Epilepsy.* New York, NY: Marcel Dekker; 1992:11.

Table 15-2. Operational Classification of Epileptic Syndromes

I. Idiopathic Epilepsy Syndromes
   A. Benign neonatal convulsions
      1. Familial
      2. Nonfamilial
   B. Benign childhood epilepsy
      1. With central-midtemporal spikes
      2. With occipital spikes
   C. Childhood/juvenile absence epilepsy
   D. JME (including generalized tonic–clonic seizures on awakening)
   E. Idiopathic epilepsy, otherwise unspecified
II. Symptomatic Epilepsy Syndromes
   A. West syndrome (infantile spasms)
   B. Lennox–Gastaut syndrome
   C. Early myoclonic encephalopathy
   D. Epilepsia partialis continua
      1. Rasmussen's syndrome (encephalitic form)
      2. Restricted form
   E. Acquired epileptic aphasia (Landau–Kleffner syndrome)
   F. Temporal lobe epilepsy
   G. Extratemporal focal epilepsy, not specified
   H. Other symptomatic epilepsy, focal or generalized, not specified
III. Other Epilepsy Syndromes of Uncertain or Mixed Classification
   A. Neonatal seizures
   B. Febrile seizures
   C. Reflex epilepsy
   D. Other unspecified

Adapted from: Pedley TA. Classification of seizures and epilepsy. In: Resor SR, Jr., Kutt H, eds. *The Medical Treatment of Epilepsy.* New York, NY: Marcel Dekker; 1992:11.

NONNEUROLOGIC CAUSES OF A SEIZURE

Epileptic seizures can occur as a result of a nonneurologic etiology such as sleep deprivation, hypoglycemia, hyponatremia, metabolic encephalopathy, alcohol or drug withdrawal, drug abuse, or drug toxicity. These seizures should not be treated with an AED. A recent publication is available that provides clinical policy on critical issues facing the emergency department health care provider in assessing a person who has experienced a new onset seizure (see Table 15-3).[6]

TYPES OF SEIZURES

Partial Seizures

Partial seizures can be either simple or complex. Simple partial seizures are characterized by no loss of consciousness, so the patient is aware of his symptoms. The presentation varies depending on the location of the epileptic focus. For example, an epileptic focus in the sensory cortex leads to a sensory distur-bance, while a focus in the motor cortex causes movement of an extremity or the face contralateral to the focus. A focus in the occipital lobe causes visual hallucinations or simply flashing lights. A simple partial seizure may precede a complex partial seizure or a secondarily generalized seizure and is commonly referred to as the aura.

Complex partial seizures result in an alteration of consciousness, but only involve a specific part of the brain. There may be repetitive, semi-purposeful movements called automatisms such as lip smacking, chewing, repeating words or phrases, or staring, or the patient may be nonresponsive but awake. Impairment of consciousness usually lasts for less than 3 minutes. The postictal state may last for minutes or a few hours during which time the patient is lethargic, sleepy, confused, or dazed. The patient does not realize having had a seizure. Either type of seizure may secondarily generalize and the patient will experience a loss of consciousness along with tonic–clonic, tonic, or clonic movements. When a partial seizure secondarily generalizes, the postictal state is usually longer in duration, and the postictal symptoms may be more severe.

Table 15-3. Patient Management Recommendations in Adult Patients Presenting to the Emergency Department with a Seizure

Clinical Issue Level of Evidence*	Specific Recommendation
Laboratory Tests[†,‡]	
B	Serum glucose
	Serum sodium
	Pregnancy test in woman of childbearing age
	Lumbar puncture (after CT scan) in immunocompromised patient
CT[†]	
B	First-time seizure patient. (May be deferred to outpatient when reliable follow-up is available)
Admission to Hospital[†]	
C	Abnormal neurological examination
Antiepileptic Drugs[†]	
C	Abnormal neurological examination, comorbidities, structural brain lesion
Dosing of Phenytoin or Fosphenytoin (in Patients with Subtherapeutic Drug Level)	
C	IV or oral loading dose, restart oral maintenance dose (phenytoin), IV/IM loading dose (fosphenytoin)
Patient in Status Epileptics (Already Given Phenytoin and Benzodiazepine)	
C	*Give* one of these agents intravenously: high-dose phenytoin (24–30 mg/kg), phenobarbital, valproic acid, infusion of midazolam pentobarbital or propofol
EEG	
C	Patient who may be in nonconvulsive status epilepticus or in subtle convulsive status epilepticus, or patient who has received long-acting paralytic, or patient in drug-induced coma

*Level of evidence: A, high degree of clinical certainty; B, moderate clinical certainty; C, based on preliminary, inconclusive, or conflicting evidence, or based on consensus of members in the Clinical Policies Committee.
[†]New onset seizure patient who has returned to baseline.
[‡]Patient with no comorbidities.
CT, computed tomography; IV, intravenous; IM, intramuscular; EEG, electroencephalography.

Frontal lobe seizures are often simple partial or complex partial with secondary generalization. The presentation reflects the anatomical area of onset. Patients can present with unusual behavioral or motor manifestations that may be mistaken for a psychiatric disorder or pseudoseizure. The postictal state may last for several seconds instead of minutes or hours. Status epilepticus is associated more commonly with frontal lobe seizures than with seizures arising from other areas of the cortex.[7]

Todd's Paralysis. Postictal paresis, also known as Todd's paralysis, is a transient paralysis that can occur after a partial seizure. The classical presentation is weakness of a hand, arm, or leg after focal motor seizure activity involving one limb or side of the body. Although study data on postictal paresis are sparse, the following characteristics were noted in one retrospective observational study:

- Postictal paresis always occurred unilateral and contralateral to the seizure focus.
- The most common ictal lateralizing sign was unilateral clonic activity but ictal dystonic posturing was also seen.
- About 20% of patients displayed slight or no ictal motor activity.[8]

Generalized Seizures

Generalized seizures involve both parts of the brain; hence, they cause loss of consciousness. Generalized seizures may be tonic with stiffening of the limbs, clonic with convulsions of the body, or most commonly both tonic and clonic. A patient experiencing a tonic–clonic seizure may frequently let out a cry right before the seizure and there may be tongue or mouth biting, or urinary incontinence during the seizure.

Atonic seizures are another type of generalized seizure, characterized by a sudden loss of muscle tone and falls. This frequently results in head or face trauma if protective gear is not worn. Another type of generalized seizure is the myoclonic seizure—sudden, brief contractions of a single muscle or a group of muscles, affecting any group of muscles. Absence seizures are a generalized-type seizure most common in young children, consisting of a brief staring spell often accompanied by lip smacking or eye blinking. These usually present in clusters and last for 5 to 10 seconds. A patient may have several hundred seizures in a day. The EEG shows a 3-Hz spike-and-wave pattern. Absence seizures are often inherited.

EPILEPSY SYNDROMES

The more common epilepsies in the general population are benign rolandic epilepsy, juvenile myoclonic epilepsy (JME), febrile convulsions, infantile spasms, and Lennox–Gastaut syndrome. Of these, the primary care physician is most likely to come into contact with JME. JME is often misdiagnosed resulting in inappropriate treatment. It presents in adolescence with the patient experiencing mild myoclonic jerks of the arms and shoulders that generally occur first thing in the morning when arising from sleep. As the patient gets older, he may develop tonic–clonic or clonic–tonic–clonic seizures. In about 30% of the patients, brief lapses of awareness (absence seizures) may develop early. This epilepsy syndrome is characterized on the EEG tracing by a 3.5-Hz generalized spike-and-wave pattern. JME has a strong genetic component and rarely goes away with treatment. Fortunately, this syndrome usually responds to low doses of select AEDs (valproic acid, ethosuximide, topiramate, lamotrigine). Some AEDs (carbamazepine, phenytoin) may worsen control of JME.

SEIZURES IN OLDER ADULTS

New onset seizures in patients older than 60 years are commonly partial seizures, either simple or complex with possible secondary generalization. Older patients may display atypical clinical findings such as dizziness and confusion. Auras and automatisms are less commonly seen in older patients with a complex partial seizure.[9] Postictal symptoms such as confusion, sleepiness, and lethargy that last several days to weeks instead of hours are seen. The most common etiology for partial epilepsy in older adults is a cerebrovascular event, accounting for 40% to 50% of new onset symptomatic epilepsy.[9,10] If a structural lesion is suspected, it may be prudent to begin AED treatment after the first seizure.

PHYSICAL FINDINGS

There are no diagnostic physical findings in epilepsy. Localizing abnormalities in patients with seizures may indicate a structural lesion as the cause of seizure.

DIAGNOSTIC EVALUATION

USEFUL TESTS

Two tests are used to support the diagnosis of epilepsy. Magnetic resonance imaging (MRI) is useful in identifying structural lesions such as cortical dysplasias, infarcts, or tumors responsible for focal epileptic activity. When an MRI is contraindicated or unobtainable, computed tomography may be useful. However, computed tomography is not as sensitive as an MRI except in the identification of a hemorrhage.

An EEG is obtained to detect and localize interictal activity. In 50% of patients with epilepsy, a routine EEG will reveal no epileptiform activity. To increase the yield, activation procedures such as hyperventilation, photic stimulation, sleep, and sleep deprivation are used. Obtaining an EEG during sleep is particularly useful when a partial seizure disorder is suspected. AEDs minimally affect interictal epileptiform activity and so EEG is not used to follow drug efficacy. An exception to this rule is the use of EEG to quantify spike–wave episodes in evaluating treatment of absence epilepsy.[11]

Continuous EEG video monitoring for days, or until the patient has a typical spell, is particularly useful when clinical examination, eyewitness accounts, and clinical history fail to elucidate the diagnosis of epilepsy. EEG video monitoring can be invaluable for differentiating seizures from pseudoseizures, especially in a patient with an established history of epilepsy.

It is important to note that most experts will not make the diagnosis of epilepsy on the basis of a single seizure episode.

RISK STRATIFICATION

Risk factors make it more likely that a patient may develop epilepsy; some of the risk factors associated with epilepsy are discussed in Table 15-4.[12]

MANAGEMENT

WHEN TO START TREATMENT

One of the major dilemmas in the treatment of epilepsy is the timing of therapy. AEDs have significant side effects affecting quality of life. The initiation of treatment can also have far-ranging effects on self-esteem, social acceptance, employment, and financial future. Numerous studies have shown that treatment with an AED after the first seizure, either partial or generalized, reduces the chance of another seizure occurring during treatment. However, many of these studies were of short duration. Two studies of treatment for 1 to 2 years showed that immediate, but not long-term treatment, reduced the occurrence of seizures.[13,14]

There are a number of factors to be considered before making the decision to start an AED after the first unprovoked seizure (Table 15-5).[15]

Table 15-4. Risk Factors for Recurrent Epileptic Seizures

Increased Risk
- Known symptomatic cause
- Partial seizures
- Family history of epilepsy
- Abnormal electroencephalogram (particularly generalized spike-and-slow wave)
- Abnormal findings on neurologic examination
- Abnormal imaging findings

Decreased Risk
- Idiopathic cause
- Generalized seizure
- No family history of epilepsy
- Normal electroencephalogram
- Normal findings on neurologic examination

Adapted from: Sirven JI. Antiepileptic drug therapy for adults; when to initiate and how to choose. *Mayo Clin Proc.* 2002;77:1367–1375.

Table 15-5. Suggested Treatment Plan in Patients with First Unprovoked Seizure

Factors to Consider for Starting Treatment*
- Abnormal EEG (especially those with epileptiform abnormalities)
- Age 15–60 y
- Known cause (presence of a tumor or occurrence of a stroke)
- Primary/secondary generalized tonic–clonic seizure
- High-risk occupation (driver, pilot, etc.)
- No disease interfering with drug metabolism

Factors to Consider for not Starting Treatment†
- Normal EEG
- Age <15 y or >60 y
- Unknown cause
- Partial seizure
- Seizure during sleep or upon awakening
- Presence of blood, liver, kidney disease
- Alcohol or drug-related seizures
- Pregnancy
- Aura/prodromal symptoms

*Presence of multiple factors increases likelihood of another seizures.
†Treatment should be deferred in the presence of any of the above conditions.
EEG, electroencephalography.
Adapted from: Beghi E, Berg AT, Hauser WA. Treatment of single seizures. In: Engel J, Jr., Pedley TA, eds. *Epilepsy: A Comprehensive Textbook.* Vol. 2. Philadelphia, PA: Lippincott–Raven Publishers; 1997:1287–1294.

FACTORS THAT MAY EXACERBATE EPILEPSY

The physician should make every effort to identify and alleviate factors exacerbating the frequency and duration of seizures in the individual patient. Intense exercise, illness, fever, hyperventilation, lack of sleep, increased emotional stress, hormonal changes, alcohol, drugs, fluid or electrolyte imbalance, and flashing lights all may increase seizures.

DRUG TREATMENT

Guidelines

Currently in the United States, there are 15 major AEDs. Carbamazepine, ethosuximide, phenobarbital, phenytoin, primidone, and valproic acid were developed before 1990 and are considered the "older agents." With the exception of ethosuximide and valproic acid, these drugs are hepatic enzyme inducers. Ethosuximide is used only in the treatment of absence seizures. Since 1990, eight new drugs have been introduced into the US market, namely, gabapentin, lamotrigine, levetiracetam, oxcarbazepine, tiagabine, topiramate, zonisamide, and felbamate. Pregabalin has also been approved for treatment of epilepsy. Since the completion of this chapter pregabalin has been introduced into the US market for the treatment of partial seizures. Two recent evidence-based guidelines, one from the United Kingdom[16,17] and one from the United States,[18,19] evaluated the safety

and efficacy of most of the newer agents. The UK guideline did not include felbamate due to its liver and bone marrow toxicity, while the US guideline excluded the drug as its usage had already been published in a previous US guideline (Table 15-6).[20]

The US guideline addressed treatment of new onset epilepsy and refractory epilepsy (defined by the failure of a patient to respond to three or more drugs) in adults and children. For new onset epilepsy, the US guideline determined that gabapentin, lamotrigine, topiramate, and oxcarbazepine are effective as monotherapy agents in newly diagnosed adolescents and adults, with either partial or mixed seizure disorders. In addition, patients

Table 15-6. AAN and AES Practice Advisory Recommendations for Felbamate*

Risk-to-Benefit Ratio Supports Use In the Following Cases:
- Lennox–Gastaut patients >4 y, unresponsive to primary AEDs
- Intractable partial seizure patients for >18 y who failed standard AEDs at therapeutic levels (use felbamate as monotherapy since lesser risk-to-benefit ratio)
- Patients on felbamate for >18 mo

Risk-to-Benefit Ratio Does not Support Use In the Following Cases:
- New onset epilepsy in adults or children
- Patients who have experienced significant prior hematologic adverse events
- Patients in whom follow-up and compliance will not allow careful monitoring
- Patients unable to discuss risks/benefits (e.g., those with mental retardation, developmental disability) and for whom no parent or legal guardian is available to provide consent

Risk-to-Benefit Ratio is Unclear, but under Certain Circumstances Depending on Nature and Severity of Patient's Seizure Disorder, Use May be Appropriate as In the Following Cases:
- Children with intractable partial epilepsy
- Other generalized epilepsies unresponsive to primary agents
- Patients who experience unacceptable sedative or cognitive side effects with traditional AEDs
- Lennox–Gastaut syndrome under the age of 4 y, unresponsive to other AEDs

Risk Management:
- Constantly assess risk-to-benefit ratio as therapy continues
- Educate patient to early signs of potentially serious hepatic and hematopoietic side effects (easy bruising, prolonged excessive bleeding, change in skin color, fatigue, fever, change in stool color, change in the color of the whites of the eye)
- Although not proven efficacious, FDA and manufacturer of drug recommend following laboratory monitoring: liver function tests at baseline and every 1–2 wk for first year; CBC may identify hematologic changes before symptoms occur; after first year, risk of aplastic anemia drops and need for laboratory monitoring is less clear
- Advise patient regarding the above laboratory recommendations

*AAN, American Academy of Neurology; AES, American Epilepsy Society. AED, antiepileptic drug; FDA, U.S. Food and Drug Administration; CBC, complete blood count.

can be treated with the older agents such as carbamazepine, phenytoin, valproic acid, or phenobarbital. Choice of agent should be dictated by the characteristics of the individual patient. The guideline also stated that the new AEDs have not been definitively shown to be effective.

The US guideline determined that all the new AEDs are appropriate for adjunctive treatment of partial seizures in adults with refractory epilepsy. Oxcarbazepine, topiramate, or lamotrigine can be used as monotherapy in adults with refractory partial epilepsy. In children, gabapentin is effective as adjunctive treatment of mixed seizure disorders, while gabapentin, lamotrigine, oxcarbazepine, and topiramate are effective as adjunctive treatment for refractory partial seizures. Limited evidence suggests that topiramate and lamotrigine are effective for adjunctive treatment of idiopathic generalized epilepsy in adults and children, as well as treatment of the Lennox–Gastaut syndrome.

The UK guideline recommended the initial use of the older AEDs (preferably carbamazepine or valproic acid) as monotherapy in the treatment of newly diagnosed partial epilepsy in adults or children except when the following situations exist:

- a contraindication to the drug,
- an interaction of the older AED with another drug being taken by the patient,
- the older AED is known to be poorly tolerated by the patient, and
- the patient is female and of childbearing potential.

Repeated monotherapy with older AEDs was recommended in adults and children with partial epilepsy prior to adjunctive treatment. As with the US guideline, the UK guideline recommended the newer AEDs in the adjunctive treatment of refractory partial epilepsy. The UK guideline recommends using cost of the agent as the deciding factor when agents have equal efficacy.

For refractory generalized epilepsy, the UK guideline recommended using the older AEDs first, but did point out that limited data indicate that lamotrigine and topiramate are effective in adults and children older than 2 years.

The UK guideline also recommended vigabatrin as first-line therapy for the management of infantile spasms (West syndrome).

A summary of the US and UK guidelines is provided in Table 15-7.[21] Since the publication of the US guidelines, topiramate has been approved by the U.S. Food and Drug Administration as initial monotherapy for patients older

Table 15-7. Summary of US and UK Guideline Recommendations for Use of New AEDs*

| | Newly Diagnosed Epilepsy | | | | Refractory Epilepsy | | | | | | | |
| | Partial, Mixed | | Absence | | Partial | | Partial Monotherapy | | Idiopathic Generalized | | Symptomatic Generalized | |
Drug	US	UK	US	UK	US	UK	US	UK	US	UK	US	UK
Felbamate†	No	NA	No	NA	Yes‡	NA	Yes	NA	No	NA	Yes§	NA
Gabapentin	Yes¶	No	No	No	Yes	Yes**	No	No	No	No	No	No
Lamotrigine	Yes¶	Yes††	Yes¶	Yes††	Yes	Yes‡‡	Yes	Yes	No	Yes‡‡	No	Yes‡‡
Levetiracetam	No	No	No	No	Yes	Yes§§	No	No	No	No	Yes	Yes‡‡
Oxcarbazepine	Yes	Yes**	No	No	Yes	Yes**	Yes	Yes**	No	No	No	No
Tiagabine	No	No	No	No	Yes	Yes††	No	No	No	No	No	No
Topiramate	Yes¶	Yes**	No	No	Yes	Yes‡‡	Yes¶	Yes**	Yes¶¶	Yes¶¶	Yes	Yes‡‡
Vigabatrin***	NA	No	NA	No	NA	Yes	NA	No	NA	No	NA	Yes†††
Zonisamide	No	NA	No	NA	Yes‡‡‡	NA	No	NA	No	NA	No	NA

*None of the new drugs is recommended as first choice in newly diagnosed epilepsy by the UK guidelines.
†For patients unresponsive to standard drugs in whom the risk-to-benefit ratio supports the use of AED.
‡Only patients >18 years of age.
§Only patients >4 years of age with Lennox–Gastaut syndrome.
¶Indication not approved by U.S. Food and Drug Administration.
**Only patients ≥6 years of age.
††Only patients ≥12 years of age.
‡‡Only patients >2 years of age.
§§Only patients ≥16 years of age.
¶¶Only for generalized tonic–clonic seizures.
***In the UK, the indications are limited to adjunctive use after failure of all other appropriate drug combinations.
†††Only for West syndrome.
‡‡‡Only for adults.
NA, not available.
Adapted from: Beghi E. Efficacy and tolerability of the new antiepileptic drugs: Comparison of two recent guidelines. *Lancet Neurol.* 2004;3:618–621.

Table 15-8. Effects of Comorbid Conditions or Their Treatments on AED

Effects	Antiepileptic Drug
Metabolic disorder may increase risk of hepatoxicity	VPA
Increased risk of hyponatremia	CBZ, OXC
Measurable increase in free-drug fraction with hypoalbuminemia	PHT, VPA
Metabolism affected by renal disease	PB, GBP, LEV, TPM
Metabolism affected by liver disease	CBZ, PHT, VPA, LTG, ZNS, OXC, TGB

VPA, valproic acid; CBZ, carbamazepine; OXC, oxcarbazepine; PHT, phenytoin; PB, phenobarbital; GBP, gabapentin; LEV, levetiracetam; TPM, topiramate; LTG, lamotrigine; ZNS, zonisamide; TGB, tiagabine.

than 9 years of age with partial or generalized tonic–clonic seizures, and levetiracetam has been approved as adjunctive therapy for partial seizures in children older than 3 years of age. Since the completion of this chapter levetiracetam has also been approved as adjunctive treatment for myoclonic seizures in patients with JME.

The US guideline also delineates the more important side effects, drug interactions, and pharmacokinetics of the newer agents. It provides additional clinical information on the effect of comorbid conditions or their treatment on the adverse effect or pharmacokinetics of older and newer AEDs (Table 15-8).

OTHER MANAGEMENT ISSUES

Monotherapy Versus Polytherapy

It is currently believed that monotherapy is the best approach to the treatment of epilepsy. Most experts agree that a low starting dose and slow upward titration lessens the chance of side effects. Levetiracetam is an exception to this rule, with good tolerance even with rapid dose escalation.

There is no evidence in support of the common practice of pushing the dose of the AED to the maximum, or until side effects prevent a further increase, before trying another agent. In addition, there is no evidence to support the selection of a second agent having a different mechanism of action although this is a common practice. The primary and secondary mechanisms of action for the AEDs are provided in Table 15-9.[22] Most of these agents have additional mechanisms of action that have not been listed.

METABOLIC AED ISSUES

Effect on Bone Mineral Density

Hepatic-enzyme-inducing agents, specifically phenytoin, phenobarbital, oxcarbazepine, and carbamazepine,

Table 15-9. Mechanism of Action of Antiepileptic Agents

Primary Mechanism of Action*	Secondary Mechanism of Action
Blockade of voltage-dependent sodium channels	
Carbamazepine	
Phenytoin	
Felbamate	
Lamotrigine	
Oxcarbazepine	
Topiramate	
Zonisamide	
Blockade of calcium channels	
Ethosuximide (T type)	Carbamazepine (L type)
Gabapentin (N, P/Q type)	Valproic Acid (T type)
Lamotrigine (N, P/Q, R, T type)	Felbamate (L type)
Pregabalin (N, P/Q type)	Levetiracetam (N type)
Zonisamide (N, P, T type)	Oxcarbazepine (N, P type)
	Topiramate (L type)
Increase in brain or synaptic GABA levels	
Tiagabine	Phenobarbital
	Valproic acid
	Felbamate
	Lamotrigine
	Topiramate
Selective potentiation of GABA-A-mediated responses	
Benzodiazepines	Phenobarbital
	Felbamate
	Levetiracetam
	Topiramate
Direct facilitation of chloride-ion influx	
Phenobarbital	
Modulation of SV2A synaptic vesicle protein	
Levetiracetam	

*Antiepileptic drugs with sodium-channel blockade as their sole primary mechanism of action may aggravate absence and myoclonic seizures.
T, L, N, P, Q, R, GABA, GABA-A, synaptic vessel protein 2A.
Adapted from: Perucca E. An introduction to antiepileptic drugs. *Epilepsia.* 2005;46(s4):31–37.

have been associated with a reduction in bone mineral density. Enzyme induction increases the clearance of vitamin D, which can lead to secondary hypoparathyroidism and a resultant decrease in bone mineral density. However, reduced bone mineral density has also been noted in patients on enzyme inducers that are not deficient in vitamin D. In addition, valproic acid, a nonenzyme inducer, has been noted to decrease bone mineral density in some patients. This is believed to be related to the drug's effect on osteoblasts.[23] Currently, it is not known whether most of the newer agents have an effect on bone mineral density. Bone-specific alkaline phosphatase is often elevated and calcium and 25-hydroxy vitamin D are often decreased in patients on enzyme inducers causing decreased bone mineral density.

Metabolic Acidosis and Renal Stones

Zonisamide, topiramate, and acetazolamide are carbonic-anhydrase-inhibiting AEDs that can cause metabolic acidosis and renal tubular acidosis. Risk factors are renal disease, severe respiratory disorders, status epilepticus, diarrhea, surgery, ketogenic diet, and certain drugs. Zonisamide, topiramate, and acetazolamide can predispose epileptic patients to calcium or urate renal stone formation, because of their weak carbonic-anhydrase-inhibiting effect. Increased fluid intake is generally recommended to try and avoid stone formation.

SPECIAL AED ISSUES IN WOMEN

Oral Contraceptives

Several of the older AEDs decrease levels of oral contraceptives via P450 hepatic enzyme induction of estradiol and progesterone (phenytoin, primidone, phenobarbital, and carbamazepine). At higher doses, both topiramate and oxcarbazepine can lower contraceptive levels. AEDs that do not affect contraceptive levels are gabapentin, lamotrigine, tiagabine, levetiracetam, and valproic acid. Recently, it has been determined that contraceptives can decrease the plasma level of lamotrigine by 40% to 50%.

Polycystic Ovary Syndrome

Reproductive endocrine disorders occur quite frequently in women with epilepsy and include sexual dysfunction, menstrual irregularities, and possibly an increased risk of polycystic ovary syndrome. Although not proven, an apparent increased incidence of polycystic ovary syndrome has been suggested in women with epilepsy who are taking valproic acid, especially in polytherapy AED regimens. The mechanism is thought to be inhibition of sex-steroid metabolism leading to an increased testosterone level arresting follicular maturation.[24]

Pregnancy

Guidelines for the treatment of women of childbearing age recommend at least 0.4 mg of oral folic acid, continued through pregnancy, to decrease the chance of neural tube and other defects in utero.[25] In addition, the guidelines recommend monotherapy and prepregnancy counseling on specific issues.

The possibility of congenital defects in infants of women on AEDs is a major cause of nonadherence. The original observational study showing an increased risk of malformed fetuses in women on enzyme inducers included many patients on multiple agents. Malformations were twice as common in these infants, and included hypertelorism, microcephaly, low-set ears, transverse palmar creases, short neck, trigonocephaly, and other minor skeletal abnormalities. More recent monotherapy data suggest a significant risk of fetal malformation for valproic acid and carbamazepine (Table 15-10).[26] In addition, caution should be used in treating pregnant patients with phenobarbital or phenytoin. For other agents, sufficient data are not available to make recommendations for use in pregnant patients. Preliminary data suggest that valproic acid and others may affect cognition in infants. However, more data are needed before definite conclusions can be drawn.

DISCONTINUING AED THERAPY IN THE EPILEPTIC PATIENT

After 2 to 5 years without a seizure, discontinuation of drug therapy should be considered, except in patients with JME. This epileptic syndrome has a very a high reoccurence rate regardless of the time elapsed since the last seizure. Factors associated with seizure recurrence are summarized in Table 15-11.

A 6-month taper is suggested for most agents, including barbiturates.[27] Recurrent seizures are most common during the first year. Stroke or structural brain lesions in older adults are associated with high recurrence rate and should prompt consideration of continued therapy.

MANAGEMENT OPTIONS IN DRUG-RESISTANT PATIENTS

Temporal Lobe and Other Brain Surgeries

Surgery is an option for some patients with drug-resistant partial epilepsy, especially mesial temporal lobe epilepsy, a form of drug refractory temporal lobe epilepsy associated with hippocampal sclerosis. Surgery has also been utilized for intractable neocortical epilepsy especially with discrete, easily resectable lesions. In fact, frontal cortical resection is the most common extratemporal cortical resection for intractable epilepsy. The American Academy of Neurology in association with the American Epilepsy Society and the American Association of Neurological Surgeons recommended anteromesial temporal lobe resection over AED treatment for disabling complex partial seizures in appropriately selected patients.[28] Surgical risk was comparable to drug treatment, and approximately two-thirds of patients had only simple partial seizures or no seizures after surgery. About 10% to 15% of the patients did not benefit from surgery. The panel recommended further study of the benefit of surgery in neocortical seizures and noted that there was insufficient data to provide recommendations regarding the safety, efficacy, and timing of multilobar resections, hemispherectomies, corpus callosotomies, lesionectomies, and multiple subpial transections.

Table 15-10. AED-Monotherapy-Associated Malformation Data

AED	Registry/Study	Malformation (Major)	Exposed Numbers
PB	North American	4/6 heart defects; 1/6 cleft lip and palate; 6.5% vs. 1.62% (controls)	77 infants
PHT	Several sources	Increase in fetal AED syndrome malformations especially nails and joints	
VPA	North American	Cardiac abnormalities and neural tube defects; 8.8% vs. 2.8% (comparison to other monotherapies using internal controls—relative risk 5.43; 95% CI, 3.9–9.55)	123 infants
	European Prospective Study group	Neural tube defects (pooled data); relative risk, 4.9 (95% CI, 1.6%–15); absolute risk, 3.8% (>1 g VPA/d)	
CBZ	Canadian and US Case-Control Study	Neural tube defects (odds ratio, 6.9; [95% CI, 1.9–25.7])	1200 infants
	European Collaborative Study	Neural tube defects; relative risk, 4.9 (95% CI, 1.3–18.0)	
	Prospective studies; (pooled data)	Cardiac abnormalities, neural tube defects urinary tract problems; 6.7% vs. 2.34% (controls number 3756); odds ratio, 3.02 (95% CI, 2.56–4.56)	1255 children
GBP	Prospective and retrospective (pooled data)	No malformations seen (monotherapy) 4.5% (monotherapy + polytherapy)	11 infants 44 infants
LTG	Lamotrigine Pregnancy registry	10 malformations (first trimester exposure); 2.8% vs. 3% (control)	360 infants
OXC	Argentine study	No malformations	35 pregnancies
ZNS		No malformations except those on polytherapy	26 pregnancies

PB, phenobarbital; PHT, phenytoin; VPA, valproic acid; CBZ, carbamazepine; AED, antiepileptic drug; CI, confidence interval; GBP, gabapentin; LTG, lamotrigine; OXC, oxcarbazepine; ZNS, zonisamide.
Adapted from: Kaplan PW. Reproductive health effects and teratogenicity of antiepileptic drugs. *Neurology.* 2004;63(4);S13–S23.

Vagal Nerve Stimulation

Vagal nerve stimulation is also used for patients with refractory seizures, although the mechanism is not known. It has been postulated that intermittent stimulation of the vagus may decrease cortical epileptiform activity indirectly by influencing the reticular activating system.

Table 15-11. Unfavorable Prognostic Factors for Antiepileptic Drug Withdrawal

Age at onset is >10–12 y
Symptomatic vs. idiopathic etiology
Mental retardation
Abnormal neurologic examination
Family history of epilepsy
Poor response to initial treatment
More than one drug being used at time of withdrawal
Epileptiform EEG changes
Slowing on EEG
Emergence of EEG abnormalities during drug withdrawal
JME (and some other syndromes)
Structural brain lesion or scar tissue

EEG, electroencephalography.
Adapted from: Britton JW. Antiepileptic drug withdrawal: Literature review. *Mayo Clin Proc.* 2002;77:1378–1388.

Vagal nerve stimulation causes changes in blood flow in the cerebellum, thalamus, and cortex and may activate inhibitory structures in the brain.[29] In July 1997, the U.S. Food and Drug Administration approved vagal nerve stimulation as an adjunctive treatment of refractory partial epilepsy in adults and adolescents older than 12 years. Currently, it is also used off-label in the treatment of generalized epilepsy. Data from uncontrolled studies suggest that vagal nerve stimulation is useful in treatment of idiopathic and symptomatic generalized epilepsies in addition to partial epilepsies.[30] In partial epilepsy, approximately a 50% decrease in seizure frequency was noted in 40% of the patients. However, there are no long-term randomized controlled outcome data available. A Cochrane Database of Systematic Review (up to March 2003) found vagal nerve stimulation treatment for partial seizures to be an effective and well-tolerated treatment. With low stimulation, significant adverse events included hoarseness, cough, pain, and paresthesias. With high stimulation, they were hoarseness and dyspnea. Dropouts from the trials were rare. Vocal cord paralysis and infection occurs in about 1% of the patients. Studies have not identified the best candidates for vagal nerve stimulation.

EVIDENCE-BASED SUMMARY

- Differentiate seizures from events that mimic seizures.
- Determine if seizures are a result of non-neurological causes.
- EEG and MRI are useful in the diagnosis and management of epilepsy.
- Determine if partial versus generalized seizure disorder is present.
- Identify and try to eliminate any factors that may impede the control of seizures.
- Individualize drug treatment according to age, concomitant medical problems, financial resources, compliance, and type of epilepsy.
- Surgery may be an option in drug-resistant epilepsy, especially in temporal lobe epilepsy.
- Vagal nerve stimulation is a treatment option in patients suboptimally controlled with drug therapy.

REFERENCES

1. Hauser WA, Annegers JF, Kurland LT. Incidence of epilepsy and unprovoked seizures in Rochester, Minnesota: 1935–1984. *Epilepsia.* 1993;34:453–468.
2. Hauser WA, Annegers JF, Kurland LT. Prevalence of epilepsy in Rochester, Minnesota: 1940–1980. *Epilepsia.* 1991;32:429–445.
3. Gidal BE, Garnett WR. Epilepsy. In: Dipiro JT, Talbert RL, Yee GC, et al, eds. *Pharmacotherapy: A Pathophysiologic Approach.* 6th ed. New York, NY: McGraw-Hill; 2005: 1023–1048.
4. Commission on Classification and Terminology of the International League Against Epilepsy. Proposal for revised clinical and electroencephalographic classification of epileptic seizures. *Epilepsia.* 1981;22:489–501.
5. Pedley TA. Classification of seizures and epilepsy. In: Resor SR, Jr., Kutt H, eds. *The Medical Treatment of Epilepsy.* New York, NY: Marcel Dekker; 1992:11.
6. American College of Emergency Physicians. Clinical policy: Critical issues in the evaluation and management of adult patients presenting to the emergency department with seizures. *Ann Emerg Med.* 2004;43:605–625.
7. Haut S. Frontal lobe epilepsy. eMedicine [databse on the Internet]. Omaha (NE): WebMD (US).C1996-2006 [updated 2007 Jan 9; cited August 1 2005]. Available at: http://www.imedicine.com/printopic.asp?bookid=7&topic=141
8. Gallmetzer P, Leutmezer F, Serles W, et al. Postictal paresis in focal epilepsies—Incidence, duration, and causes: A video-EEG monitoring study. *Neurology.* 2004;62:2160–2164.
9. Ramsay RE, Rowan AJ, Pryor FM. Special considerations in treating the elderly patient with epilepsy. *Neurology.* 2004;62(2):S24–S29.
10. Asconape JJ, Penry JK. Poststroke seizures in the elderly. *Clin Geriatr Med.* 1991;7:483–492.
11. Flink R, Pedersen B, Guekht AB, et al. Guidelines for the use of EEG methodology in the diagnosis of epilepsy. *Acta Neurol Scand.* 2002;106:1–7.
12. Sirven JI. Antiepileptic drug therapy for adults; when to initiate and how to choose. *Mayo Clin Proc.* 2002;77:1367–1375.
13. Marson A, Jacoby A, Johnson A, et al. Immediate versus deferred antiepileptic drug treatment for early epilepsy and single seizures: A randomized controlled trial. *Lancet.* 2005;365:2007–2013.
14. Musicco M, Beghi E, Solari A, et al. Treatment of the first seizure does not improve the prognosis of epilepsy. *Neurology.* 1997;49:991–998.
15. Beghi E, Berg AT, Hauser WA. Treatment of single seizures. In: Engel J, Jr., Pedley TA, eds. *Epilepsy: A Comprehensive Textbook.* Vol. 2. Philadelphia, PA: Lippincott–Raven Publishers; 1997:1287–1294.
16. National Institute for Health and Clinical Excellence. Epilepsy (adults)-newer drugs. Updated March 1, 2004. Available at: http://www.nice.org.uk/guidance/index.jsp?action=byID&o=11528. Accessed August 1, 2005.
17. National Institute for Health and Clinical Excellence. Epilepsy (children)-newer drugs. Updated Apr 1, 2004 Available at: http://www.nice.org.uk/guidance/index.jsp?action=byID&o=11532. Accessed August 1, 2005.
18. French JA, Kanner AM, Bautista J, et al. Efficacy and tolerability of the new antiepileptic drugs I: Treatment of new onset epilepsy. *Neurology.* 2004;62:1252–1260.
19. French JA, Kanner AM, Bautista J, et al. Efficacy and tolerability of the new antiepileptic drugs II: Treatment of refractory epilepsy. *Neurology.* 2004;62:1261–1273.
20. French J, Smith M, Faught E, Brown L. Practice advisory: The use of felbamate in the treatment of patients with intractable epilepsy: Report of the quality standards subcommittee of the American Academy of Neurology and the American Epilepsy Society. *Neurology.* 1999;52:1540–1545.
21. Beghi E. Efficacy and tolerability of the new antiepileptic drugs: Comparison of two recent guidelines. *Lancet Neurol.* 2004;3:618–621.
22. Perucca E. An introduction to antiepileptic drugs. *Epilepsia.* 2005;46(s4):31–37.
23. Sheth RD. Metabolic concerns associated with antiepileptic medications. *Neurology.* 2004;63(4):S24–S29.
24. Betts T, Dutton N, Yarrow H. Epilepsy and the ovary (cutting out the hysteria). *Seizure.* 2001;10:220–228.
25. Quality Standard Subcommittee of the American Academy of Neurology. Practice parameter: Management issues for women with epilepsy (summary statement). Report. *Neurology.* 1998;51:944–948.
26. Kaplan PW. Reproductive health effects and teratogenicity of antiepileptic drugs. *Neurology.* 2004;63(4);S13–S23.
27. Britton JW. Antiepileptic drug withdrawal: Literature review. *Mayo Clin Proc.* 2002;77:1378–1388.
28. Engel J, Jr., Wiebe S, French J, et al. Practice parameter: Temporal lobe and localized neocortical resections for epilepsy. *Neurology.* 2003;60:538–547.
29. Rielo D. Vagus nerve stimulation. Updated February 2007. Available at: http://www.imedicine.com/DisplayTopic.asp?bookid=7& topic=559. Accessed August 1, 2005.
30. Ng M, Devinsky O. Vagus nerve stimulation for refractory idiopathic generalized epilepsy. *Seizure.* 2004;13:176–178.

Chapter 16

Stroke and Transient Ischemic Attacks

Susan C. Fagan and Shyamal Mehta

SEARCH STRATEGY

A systematic Medline search of the medical literature was performed in January 2008 using Ovid. Subject headings included Cerebrovascular Accident/Prevention and Control, Drug Therapy, Surgery, Therapy.

INTRODUCTION

Stroke is a common diagnosis in primary care and it is the third leading cause of death in Americans. Primary care clinicians provide stroke care to three main groups of patients: (1) patients at high risk of stroke requiring primary prevention, (2) patients with a history of stroke requiring secondary prevention, or (3) patients with signs and symptoms consistent with acute stroke, requiring urgent care. The purpose of this chapter is to review the risk factors, the clinical presentation and diagnosis of stroke and the recommended approach to acute treatment and prevention.

Stroke can be either ischemic or hemorrhagic. Ischemic stroke is the most common, representing 87% of the more than 700,000 strokes reported in the United States.[1] The classification of stroke is illustrated in Fig. 16-1. Understanding the etiopathogenesis of the stroke is paramount in determining the correct treatment, intervention and/or prevention strategies.

The presentation and etiologies of ischemic stroke vary based on the vessels affected. Atherosclerosis of large, medium, and small arteries can result in ischemic stroke. Aortic, carotid, and vertebral artery plaque can be a source of emboli to the brain leading to stroke.

Atherosclerosis can cause stenosis and impede further blood flow. Lipohyalinosis usually affects the small penetrating arteries and accounts for lacunar (small, deep) infarcts. Cardiac diseases such as atrial fibrillation (which predisposes to embolic phenomenon), acute myocardial infarction, cardiomypopathy, and valvular disease are a few of the many conditions that can predispose to a stroke. Hypotension can cause borderzone infarcts in different vascular territories. Other causes such as hypercoagulable states, vasculitis, and dissections also should be sought. In spite of an exhaustive work up, at times the etiology or cause of the stroke remains elusive. These cryptogenic strokes account for 30% of ischemic strokes.

Hemorrhagic strokes are most commonly caused by uncontrolled hypertension and usually affect penetrating arteries in the putamen, thalamus, pons, and cerebellum. Amyloid angiopathy in the elderly is another cause of hemorrhagic stroke and is often responsible for hemorrhages in the parietal or occipital lobes. Hemorrhage in a young patient without the history of hypertension should raise suspicion of other causes such as drug abuse (e.g., cocaine, amphetamines, methylphenidate, etc.), arteriovenous malformations, and brain tumors. Medications such as thrombolytic therapy (e.g., tissue plasminogen activator [tPA]), or anticoagulants (e.g., warfarin) are also associated with the development of hemorrhagic stroke. Hemorrhagic transformation of an ischemic stroke is seen most often in embolic strokes, large infarcts, middle cerebral artery stem occlusion, and also in the setting of uncontrolled hypertension and early use of anticoagulants.

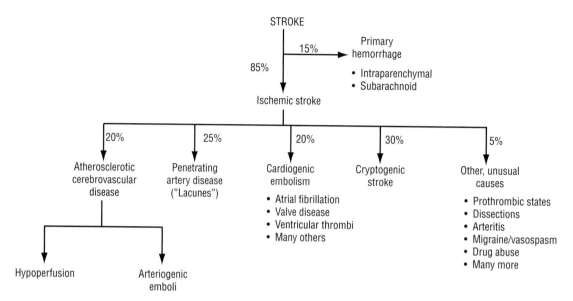

Figure 16-1. Classification of stroke. The types of stroke are illustrated, showing their location and prevalence.

Mortality (30 days) with hemorrhagic stroke is up to 38%, compared to 12% with ischemic stroke. Stroke is the leading cause of adult disability in the United States and is a common cause of nursing home admission. Great strides have been made in decreasing the consequences and recurrence of stroke in the past several decades through careful reduction of risk factors, acute intervention, and secondary prevention.

RISK FACTORS[2–5]

The most important risk factor for both ischemic and hemorrhagic stroke is hypertension. Other important risk factors for ischemic stroke, with their relative risks, are given in Table 16-1.

PRIMARY PREVENTION[5]

Strategies proven to reduce the risk of a first ischemic stroke are illustrated in Table 16-2. Other recommendations including increasing physical activity to 30 minutes most days of the week, a diet of at least 4 to 5 servings of fresh fruits and vegetables daily, restriction of alcohol to 1 to 2 drinks daily, and cessation of substance abuse are also thought to reduce stroke risk.

CLINICAL PRESENTATION OF STROKE AND TRANSIENT ISCHEMIC ATTACK[6–8]

A stroke is defined as an abrupt onset focal neurologic deficit of presumed vascular origin. Some of the most

Table 16-1. Risk Factors for Ischemic Stroke

Risk Factor	Relative Risk
Chronic atrial fibrillation	2.6–4.5
Hypertension	1.4–4
Diabetes mellitus	1.8–6
Smoking (current)	1.8
Carotid stenosis	2.0
Hyperlipidemia	1.8–2.6
Obesity	1.75–2.37
Alcohol abuse	1.6–1.8
Hyperhomocysteinemia	1.3–2.3

Adapted from: Goldstein LB, Adams R, Alberts MJ, et al. *Primary prevention of ischemic stroke. A guideline from the American Heart Association/American Stroke Association Stroke Council. Cosponsored by the Atherosclerotic Peripheral Vascular Disease Interdisciplinary Working Group; Cardiovascular Nursing Council; Clinical Cardiology Council; Nutrition, Physical Activity, and Metabolism Council; and the Quality of Care and Outcomes Research Interdisciplinary Working Group. Stroke.* 2006; 37:1583–1633.

Table 16-2. Strategies for the Primary Prevention of Stroke

Strategy	Population	Risk Reduction (%)
BP lowering	Hypertensives	38
Smoking cessation		50 within first year
Carotid endarterectomy	Asymptomatic carotid stenosis	50
Transfusion	High risk sickle cell disease	91
HMG CoA reductase inhibitors	Hyperlipidemia	20–30
Warfarin	Atrial fibrillation	68

Adapted from: Goldstein LB, Adams R, Alberts MJ, et al. *Primary prevention of ischemic stroke. A guideline from the American Heart Association/American Stroke Association Stroke Council. Cosponsored by the Atherosclerotic Peripheral Vascular Disease Interdisciplinary Working Group; Cardiovascular Nursing Council; Clinical Cardiology Council; Nutrition, Physical Activity, and Metabolism Council; and the Quality of Care and Outcomes Research Interdisciplinary Working Group. Stroke.* 2006; 37:1583–1633.

Table 16-3. Common Presenting Symptoms of Acute Stroke

Symptom	Patients Reporting (%)
Weakness	18.6–23.6
Sensory	17.5–18.8
Imbalance	15.2–19.9
Change in level of conciousness	12–17.4
Dysarthria	16.2–15.6
Aphasia	10.5–11.1
Gait	7.6–10.7
Dizziness/vertigo	8.1–9.6
Pain	8.4–12.0

Adapted from: Labiche LA, Chan W, Saldin KR, Morgenstern LB. Sex and acute stroke presentation. *Ann Emerg Med.* 2002;40:5:453–460.

Table 16-4. Diagnostic Studies for Stroke

Urgent	Nonurgent
Brain CT (MRI in some qualified centers)	Carotid duplex dopplers
Electrocardiogram	Echocardiogram
Blood glucose	
Serum electrolytes	
Renal function tests	
Complete blood count, including platelets	
Prothrombin time/INR	
Activated partial thromboplastin time	

Adapted from: Adams HP, delZoppo G, Alberts MJ, et al. Guidelines for the early management of patients with ischemic stroke: A guideline from the American Heart Association/American Stroke Association Stroke Council, Clinical Cardiology Council, Cardiovascular Radiology and Intervention Council, and the Atherosclerotic Peripheral Vascular Disease and Quality of Care Outcomes in Research Interdisciplinary Working Groups. *Stroke.* 2007;38:1655–1711;34:1056–1083.

common presenting symptoms of stroke are given in Table 16-3. Rapid recognition of these symptoms will improve the appropriate treatment of these patients. Even if the symptoms resolve within the first 24 hours (usually the first 10 minutes), the patient is considered to have experienced a transient ischemic attack (TIA), and requires immediate medical attention. The risk of developing a stroke after a hemispheric TIA is as high as 20% in the first month and highest in the first 48 hours. A neurovascular work-up and prescription of secondary prevention should occur as soon as possible (within one day).

DIAGNOSTIC EVALUATION[6,7]

Although certain symptoms and signs are more common in hemorrhagic than ischemic stroke (for example, headache and loss of consciousness), in the acute stage the two can only be differentiated through imaging. A (noncontrast) CT scan sensitively detects acute hemorrhage and should be performed as soon as possible. Emergency imaging studies to guide intervention are indicated if the duration of symptoms is only a few hours. In acute ischemic strokes, intravenous tPA can be considered at qualified centers when symptoms are present 3 hours or less. Hence, a thorough, yet expedited work-up, is essential. The recommended immediate diagnostic studies in a patient with suspected acute ischemic stroke are given in Table 16-4.

After the diagnosis of acute stroke is made, further diagnostic tests are performed to determine the etiology of the stroke and design appropriate secondary prevention strategies. These include assessments of the intracranial and extracranial arteries and the heart.

ACUTE TREATMENT[2,6,7,9]

Ischemia

Intravenous tPA has been shown to reduce the disability caused by ischemic stroke when administered within 3 hours of the onset of symptoms in eligible patients. To minimize the risk of symptomatic intracranial hemorrhage, it is very important to follow a strict protocol for administration of tPA. Specialized centers with highly-trained rapid response teams are required to safely and effectively use tPA for stroke. In clinical trials, tPA was associated with a 30% increase in the likelihood of an excellent outcome at 90 days, despite a 6.4% incidence of symptomatic intracerebral hemorrhage. Several smaller trials have demonstrated the safety and efficacy of reperfusion therapy beyond 3 hours after onset, but they require imaging- or angiography-guided patient selection. The inclusion and exclusion criteria for tPA use in acute ischemic stroke are given in Table 16-5. At some centers with trained neurointerventionalists, intraarterial tPA is used within 6 hours of symptom onset in the case of angiographically demonstrated MCA occlusion or acute basilar artery thrombosis with no signs of infarction on baseline CT scan.

Hemorrhage

To date, no intervention has been shown to reduce the ultimate disability caused by primary intracerebral hemorrhage. Although acute surgical intervention has been shown to reduce rebleed and mortality in subarachnoid hemorrhage, no benefit of early surgery in primary intracerebral hemorrhages has been shown.

Table 16-5. Inclusion and Exclusion Therapy for tPA in Acute Stroke[6]

Inclusion
   Diagnosis of ischemic stroke with measurable neurologic deficit
   Neurologic signs not rapidly improving
   Neurologic signs not minor and isolated
   Symptoms not suggestive of subarachnoid hemorrhage
   Onset of symptoms <3 h before beginning treatment
Exclusion
   Head trauma or stroke within past 3 months
   Myocardial infarction within past 3 months
   Gastrointestinal or urinary tract hemorrhage within 21 d
   Major surgery within 14 d
   Arterial puncture at noncompressible site within 7 d
   Previous intracranial hemorrhage
   BP > 185 mm Hg systolic or >110 mm Hg diastolic
   Active bleeding or acute trauma on examination
   Oral anticoagulant and INR ≥1,5
   Heparin in previous 48 h and aPTT elevated
   Platelet count <100,000
   Blood Glucose < 50 mg/dL
   Seizure with postictal neurological impairments
   CT shows > 1/3 cerebral hemisphere infracted

Adapted from: Adams HP, delZoppo G, Alberts MJ, et al. Guidelines for the early management of patients with ischemic stroke: A guideline from the American Heart Association/American Stroke Association Stroke Council, Clinical Cardiology Council, Cardiovascular Radiology and Intervention Council, and the Atherosclerotic Peripheral Vascular Disease and Quality of Care Outcomes in Research Interdisciplinary Working Groups. *Stroke.* 2007;38:1655–1711;34:1056–1083.

SECONDARY PREVENTION[3,4,10–17]

Patients who have had a stroke or TIA remain at high risk of recurrence (up to 45% at 5 years) and should receive aggressive secondary stroke prevention measures.

Blood Pressure Control

All patients who have had a stroke (ischemic or hemorrhagic) should have their blood pressure (BP) monitored and reduced to 120/80.[3,4] A thiazide diuretic and an angiotensin converting enzyme (ACE) inhibitor should be used, unless there are contraindications.[14] Patients unable to tolerate an ACE inhibitor should receive an angiotensin receptor blocker (ARB).[18]

Antithrombotic Therapy

All patients with a history of ischemic stroke or TIA should receive anticoagulation or antiplatelet therapy. All patients who have had an ischemic stroke or TIA (noncardioembolic) should receive either low-dose aspirin (50–325 mg daily), clopidogrel (75 mg daily) or the combination of aspirin and extended release dipyridamole (25/200 mg twice daily).[2–4] Patients allergic to aspirin should receive clopidogrel. Use of the combination of clopidogrel and aspirin for secondary stroke prevention is associated with an increase in serious bleeding without increased efficacy over clopidogrel alone.[19]

Anticoagulation with warfarin (International Normalized Ratio [INR] 2.5) should be used in patients with paroxysmal or persistent atrial fibrillation or other compelling source of cardiac embolism.[2–4,12] Anticoagulation should not be initiated until brain imaging has ruled out a hemorrhagic lesion and not until 5 to 14 days have passed if the patient has had a major stroke. Close monitoring of the INR (at least once monthly) and follow-up are necessary to assure the safe and effective use of warfarin for stroke prevention.

HMG CoA Reductase Inhibitors

Treatment with a hydroxymethylglutaryl-coenzyme A (HMG CoA) reductase inhibitor should be considered in all patients with prior ischemic stroke or TIA, regardless of their baseline cholesterol values.[15,16]

Surgery

In patients with ipsilateral carotid artery stenosis ≥60%, carotid endarterectomy to remove the offending plaque, combined with aspirin, should be performed in all eligible patients.[3,4]

Other Interventions

All patients should receive counseling and assistance with smoking cessation, increasing physical activity, adopting a low-salt, low-fat diet rich in fruits and vegetables and avoiding alcohol. Table 16-6 summarizes the important secondary prevention strategies to be recommended.

Table 16-6. Secondary Prevention Strategies

Intervention	Type of Stroke	Comments
BP lowering	Hemorrhagic/ ischemic	ACE inh + thiazide
Anticoagulation	Ischemic (atrial fibrillation)	Warfarin (INR = 2.5)
Antiplatelet	Ischemic (most)	Aspirin Clopidogrel ASA/ERDP
Statin	Ischemic (all)	
Carotid endarterectomy	Ischemic (ipsilateral)	70–99% stenosis

EVIDENCE-BASED SUMMARY

- Ischemic and hemorrhagic stroke can only be differentiated by urgent imaging (computed tomography).
- The most common and important modifiable risk factors for stroke include hypertension, atrial fibrillation, diabetes, and hyperlipidemia.
- Common symptoms of stroke include *sudden onset* weakness, sensory change, imbalance, and speech changes.
- Early recognition and treatment of stroke and TIA is essential to administer effective reperfusion therapy in eligible patients and for the institution of secondary prevention strategies.
- BP lowering is one of the most effective strategies in decreasing both ischemic and hemorrhagic stroke incidence.
- Antiplatelet therapy (aspirin, clopidogrel, or aspirin/extended release dipyridamole) should be prescribed for all patients with a previous noncardioembolic ischemic stroke or TIA.
- Warfarin therapy (INR = 2.5) should only be used in ischemic stroke patients with a history of paroxysmal or persistent atrial fibrillation.
- BP lowering with an ACE inhibitor and a diuretic should be instituted in all stroke patients for secondary prevention.
- HMG CoA reductase inhibitor should be given to all ischemic stroke patients for secondary stroke prevention, regardless of cholesterol values.
- Carotid endarterectomy should be considered in all ischemic stroke patients with significant carotid stenosis.

REFERENCES

1. American Heart Association. *Heart Disease and Stroke Statistics–2008 Update.* Dallas, TX: American Heart Association; 2008.
2. Albers GW, Amerenco P, Easton JD, Sacco RL, Teal P. Antithrombotic and thrombolytic therapy for ischemic stroke. *Chest.* 2004;126:483S–512S.
3. Straus SE, Majumdar SR, McAlister FA. New evidence for stroke prevention. Scientific review. *JAMA.* 2002;288:1388–1395.
4. Sacco RL, Adams R, Albers, G et al. Guidelines for prevention of stroke in patients with ischemic stroke or transient ischemic attack. *Circulation.* 2006;113:409–449.
5. Goldstein LB, Adams R, Alberts MJ, et al. Primary prevention of ischemic stroke. A Guideline from the American Heart Association/American Stroke Association Stroke Council. Cosponsored by the Atherosclerotic Peripheral Vascular Disease Interdisciplinary Working Group; Cardiovascular Nursing Council; Clinical Cardiology Council; Nutrition, Physical Activity, and Metabolism Council; and the Quality of Care and Outcomes Research Interdisciplinary Working Group. *Stroke.* 2006;37:1583–1633.
6. Broderick JP, Adams HP, Barsan W, et al. Guidelines for the management of spontaneous intracerebral hemorrhage in adults: 2007 Update. A guideline from the American Heart Association/American Stroke Association Stroke Council, High Blood Pressure Research Council, and the Quality of Care and Outcomes in Research Interdisciplinary Working Group. *Stroke.* 2007;38:2001–2023; 30:905–915.
7. Adams HP, delZoppo G, Alberts MJ, et al. Guidelines for the early management of patients with ischemic stroke: A guideline from the American Heart Association/American Stroke Association Stroke Council, Clinical Cardiology Council, Cardiovascular Radiology and Intervention Council, and the Atherosclerotic Peripheral Vascular Disease and Quality of Care Outcomes in Research Interdisciplinary Working Groups. *Stroke.* 2007;38:1655–1711; 34:1056–1083.
8. The Intercollegiate Working Party for Stroke, Royal College of Physicians. National Clinical Guidelines for Stroke (Primary Care Concise Guidelines for Stroke), 2nd ed. London, UK: Royal College of Physicians; 2004.
9. The National Institute of Neurological Disorders and Stroke rt-PA stroke study group. Tissue plasminogen activator for acute ischemic stroke. *N Engl J Med.* 1995;333:1581–1587.
10. Cina CA, Clase CM, Haynes RB. Carotid endarterectomy for symptomatic carotid stenosis. Oxford, England: Cochrane Library; CD001081.
11. Antithrombotic Trialists' Collaboration. Collaborative meta-analysis of randomized trials of antiplatelet therapy for prevention of death, myocardial infarction, and stroke in high risk patients. *BMJ.* 2002;324:71–86.
12. Hart RG, Benevente O, McBride R, Pearce LA. Antithrombotic therapy to prevent stroke in patients with atrial fibrillation: A meta-analysis. *Ann Intern Med.* 1999;131:492–501.
13. Mohr JP, Thompson JLP, Lazar RM, et al. A comparison of warfarin and aspirin for the prevention of recurrent ischemic stroke. *N Engl J Med.* 2001;345:1444–1451.
14. PROGRESS Collaborative Group. Randomized trial of perindopril-based blood-pressure-lowering regimen among 6105 individuals with previous stroke or transient ischaemic attack. *Lancet.* 2001;358:1033–1041.
15. Heart Protection Study Collaborative Group. MRC/BHF Heart Protection Study of cholesterol lowering with simvastatin in 20,536 high-risk individuals: A randomized placebo-control trial. *Lancet.* 2002;360:7–22.
16. The Stroke Prevention by Aggressive Reduction in Cholesterol Levels (SPARCL) Investigators. High-dose atorvastatin

after stroke or transient ischemic attack. *N Engl J Med.* 2006;355:549–559.

17. Labiche LA, Chan W, Saldin KR, Morgenstern LB. Sex and acute stroke presentation. *Ann Emerg Med.* 2002;40:5: 453–460.

18. Dahlof B, Devereaux RB, Kjeldsen SE, et al. Cardiovascular morbidity and mortality in the Losartan Intervention for Endpoint reduction in hypertension study (LIFE): A randomized trial against atenolol. *Lancet.* 2002;359:995–1003.

19. Diener HC, Bogousslavsky J, Brass LM, et al. Aspirin and clopidogrel compared with clopidogrel alone after recent ischaemic stroke or transient ischaemic attack in high-risk patients (MATCH): Randomized, double-blind, placebo-controlled trial. *Lancet.* 2004;364:331–337.

Chapter 17

Parkinson Disease

Peter A. LeWitt and Richard C. Berchou

SEARCH STRATEGY

A systematic search of the medical literature was performed in January, 2008. The search, limited to human subjects and English language journals, included the National Guideline Clearinghouse, the Cochrane database, PubMed, UpToDate®, and PIER.

INTRODUCTION

One of the most common neurological disorders of the aging population, Parkinson disease (PD) is the best understood with respect to the specific neurochemical and pathological changes in the brain. The characteristic motor impairments are mostly the consequence of the selective loss of several hundred thousand neurons in the substantia nigra,[1] but the cause of this loss is unknown. PD has a number of treatment options ranging from medications to surgical treatments.[2]

CLINICAL PRESENTATION

The clinical presentation can be distinctive but is not always diagnostic, even when the full Parkinsonian syndrome is present. Parkinsonian syndrome consists of PD or others disorders with similar motor impairments. It is characterized by one or more of the following: tremors of a limb or face at rest, cogwheel-type rigidity, slowed movements with diminished dexterity, facial masking, forward flexed posture, and imbalance.[3]

Idiopathic PD is the most common etiology when signs and symptoms develop slowly.[4] Often, PD starts on one side just with a resting tremor. Other presentations quite distinctive for PD include handwriting that trails off (micrographia), decreased arm swing, and a shuffling gait. It is not necessary for all symptoms to be present to make a diagnosis of PD. Conversely, a diagnosis of PD cannot be made on the basis of symptoms alone. Additional information from medical history and medication response may be necessary. PD should not cause increased muscle stretch reflexes (hyperreflexia), Babinski signs, eye movement disturbance, impairment of cerebellar system function, or cognitive decline as early features. Neuroimaging studies such as head CT or MRI scans are normal in idiopathic PD, and can be used to assess for other syndromes with Parkinsonian symptoms, including strokes, normal pressure (communicating) hydrocephalus, or a structural lesion such as a subdural hematoma.

PD can present a diagnostic challenge because the deficits evolve gradually and can caricature other illnesses often associated with advanced age.[5] The forward flexed posture can resemble changes in the spine in osteoporosis. Decreased arm swing can mimic frozen shoulder. The decreased clarity of voice and diminished facial animation can resemble depression. Tremors in the hand and elsewhere can resemble side effects of medications or essential tremor. PD subjects often complain of generalized weakness and easy fatigue although formal testing generally reveals slowed movements with decreased dexterity rather than loss of muscle power.

There is no pathognomonic testing for PD outside of research settings, in which radiotracer neuroimaging can explore the dopaminergic lesion in vivo.[6] However, responsiveness to medications like levodopa can help greatly in making the diagnosis. Such medication trials are especially important for differentiating PD from Parkinson-plus disorders (Table 17-1). In the initial stages, these disorders, including progressive

Table 17-1. Differential Diagnosis of Parkinsonism

Idiopathic Parkinson's Disease (Parkinsonism with Lewy bodies)
Genetically-determined Parkinsonism (α-synuclein mutations,
  parkin gene, others)
Secondary Parkinsonism
  Drug-Induced
    Antipsychotics (phenothiazines, butyrophenones,
      risperidone, others)
    Antiemetics (metoclopramide, prochlorperazine)
    Other drugs (reserpine, alpha-methyldopa)
  Toxin-induced
    Carbon monoxide
    Hydrogen sulfide
    Manganese
    Methanol
    MPTP (1-methyl-4-phenyl-1-2-5-6-tetrahydropyridine)
    Petrochemicals
  Parkinsonism following viral encephalitis
    Lesions (neoplasm, stroke, or A-V malformations interrupting
      nigrostriatal pathways)
  Traumatic lesions interrupting substantia nigra projections
  Normal pressure (communicating) hydrocephalus
Parkinsonism associated with other types of neuronal
  degeneration
  Wilson disease (hepatolenticular degeneration)
  Progressive supranuclear palsy
  Pallidonigral degeneration
  Corticobasal degeneration
  Alzheimer disease
  Frontotemporal dementia
  Huntington disease (rarely)
  Dentatorubropallidoluysian atrophy
  Pantothenate kinase-associated neurodegenerated
  Spinocerebellar atrophy type-1
  Multiple system atrophy
    Striatonigral degeneration
    Shy-Drager syndrome
    Olivopontocerebellar atrophy

supranuclear palsy, multiple system atrophy and corticobasal degeneration, mimic PD. Other conditions sometimes displaying Parkinsonian features include Alzheimer's disease, diffuse Lewy body disease, Huntington disease, frontotemporal dementia with Parkinsonism, primary pallidal atrophy, Wilson's disease, Parkinsonism acquired from the regular use of dopamine-blocking medications, and rarely metabolic, infectious, or toxic disorders. In recent years, several families with a genetic basis for Parkinsonism have been identified. Mutations in genes for constituent protein, alpha-synuclein, and 5 additional genes have been identified among the 11 genetic patterns of neurodegeneration closely resembling PD.[7] Most of these syndromes lack the full clinical or pathological picture of idiopathic PD.

Most PD appears to be of sporadic origin, as shown by the lack of concordance of disease in identical twin pairs. In younger patients, there is a greater chance for a genetic basis. PD typically develops in the sixth decade

of life, although up to 5% of patients have onset before the age of 50. Resting tremor and predominantly unilateral involvement carry a better prognosis. Disability is rare in the first 3 years and typically is characterized by imbalance (especially falling backwards), "freezing" of gait, and medication side effects including levodopa-induced involuntary movements (dyskinesia) and confusional states including hallucinations. PD patients, especially those with late onset, are at increased risk for dementia.[8] Depression also is more common in PD patients than the general population. Despite all the negative outcomes facing PD patients, the disorder is not inevitably disabling. Therapies offer most patients lasting benefit and a quality of life approaching the norm.

TREATMENT OPTIONS

The satisfactory control of disability and discomforts of PD is generally achievable with medications (Tables 17-2 and 17-3). Medications include levodopa, the dopaminergic agonists, the anticholinergics, and amantadine. What regimen is best for the newly diagnosed patient?[5,9] This question presupposes all patients have similar needs and resources (such as the finances to afford costly medications as well as willingness to take more than one drug several times daily).[10] For the most common presentation, resting tremor, anticholinergic medications like benztropine and trihexyphenidyl provide excellent relief. Side effects are often minimal, including dry mouth, constipation, urinary retention and forgetfulness. The dry mouth can be therapeutic in patients prone to drooling. Amantadine is also a good starting medicine when primary symptom is tremor. Although it is less potent than levodopa, it benefits rigidity and slowed movement and helps in controlling levodopa-induced dyskinesia.

Disability or discomfort is usually experienced in the first or second year and often calls for dopaminergic treatment. Levodopa is the most effective but dyskinesia occurs in up to half the patients in 5 years.[9] Monotherapy with a dopamine agonist sometimes yields results close to those of levodopa but with less risk for dyskinesia or motor fluctuations. Fortunately, the combination of levodopa with a dopaminergic agonist appears to be better than levodopa alone and is probably the best option for patients facing many years of living with PD.[11,12]

The most prominent neurochemical change in PD is a major loss of dopamine, a catecholamine neurotransmitter synthesized in the substantia nigra and projected to regions of the basal ganglia (striatum). Dopamine may be reduced to as little as 40% of normal in nigrostriatal projections before the first clinical

Table 17-2. Drugs for Treatment of Parkinsonism

Drug Name	Dose Forms (mg)	Typical Daily Intake (mg)
Carbidopa/levodopa	10/100, 25/100, 25/250	300–1000 (levodopa)
Carbidopa/levodopa (sustained or controlled release product)	25/100, 50/200	300–1000 (levodopa)
Carbidopa/levodopa/entacapone	212.5/50/300, 25/100/200, 37.5/150/200	300–1000 (levodopa)
Entacapone	200	600–1600
Tolcapone	100	300
Amantadine	100, 50 (per mL)	100–300
Trihexyphenidyl	2, 5	3–15
Benztropine	0.5, 1, 2	1.5–6
Selegiline	5	5–10
Rasagiline	0.5, 1	0.5–1
Pergolide	0.5, 0.25, 1	1.5–6
Bromocriptine	2.5, 5	20–80
Pramipexole	0.125, 0.25, 0.5, 1, 1.5	0.75–6
Ropinirole	0.25, 0.5, 1, 2, 3, 4, 5	6–24
Apomorphine	Variable s.c. injected dose	1–8 per dose prn

features of Parkinsonism are evident.[1] Treatments restoring dopaminergic neurotransmission have been developed, and levodopa is the most effective. Levodopa was hailed as a cure when first released, as it is an amino acid precursor of dopamine. The dramatic reversal of all features of Parkinsonism can be a major reassurance to patients and clinicians. In the best of circumstances, levodopa is a highly effective therapy lasting beyond 10 years.[9] Levodopa therapy radically changed progressive disability to a very manageable condition for most patients.

Chronic levodopa therapy has many side effects. To minimize peripheral side effects such as nausea and hypotension, levodopa is generally combined with carbidopa. Carbidopa inhibits peripheral decarboxylation, thereby preventing the conversion of levodopa to dopamine systemically. At least 75 mg/d of carbidopa is needed and typically 25 mg is given for every 100 mg of levodopa.[2] Central side effects are not diminished by carbidopa, and include vivid dreams and hallucinations.

Additional options for control of side effects of levodopa abound. Symptomatic postural hypotension can be treated by increased salt and water intake, or with fludrocortisone, midodrine, indomethacin or dihydroergotamine. Hallucinations and vivid dreaming can be managed by reducing total or nighttime dose. Chronic levodopa therapy was suspected in the past of potentially accelerating the progression of PD through a potential toxic mechanism but more recent studies have shown this is not the case.[13,14]

Table 17-3. Side Effects of Drugs Used for Parkinsonism

Class of Drugs	Examples	Common	Less Common
Levodopa	Carbidopa/levodopa (immediate- and sustained release)	Nausea, vomiting, lightheadedness, hypotension, sedation	Rash, vivid dreams, hallucination
Dopaminergic agonists	Pergolide, bromocriptine, pramipexole, ropinirole, apomorphine	Nausea, vomiting, lightheadedness, hypotension, sedation, pedal edema, site injection nodules (with apomorphine)	Rash, vivid dreams, hallucination, compulsive behaviors, fibrotic disorders (ergot-structure compounds)
Monoamine oxidase inhibitors	Selegiline, rasagiline	Increased dyskinesia hypertensive	"Cheese" (tyramine) hypertensive effect
Catechol-O-methyltransferase inhibitors	Entacapone, tolcapone	Increased dyskinesia	Diarrhea, hepatic toxicity (tolcapone)
Anti-cholinergic drugs	Trihexyphenidyl, benztropine	Dry mouth, dry eyes, constipation, urinary retention, sedation	Forgetfulness, confusion
Amantadine	Amantadine	Dry mouth, sedation	Pedal edema, hallucination

PD patients should avoid most of the neuroleptic medications because they can exacerbate the Parkinsonian state. However, quetiapine does not, and can be quite effective at control of otherwise disabling and distressing hallucinations, thus permitting continued use of dopaminergic drugs.[15] Quetiapine-unresponsive patients can next try clozapine, the only other neuroleptic medication that does not exacerbate Parkinsonism. Clozapine requires frequent monitoring of the white blood cell count to guard against the occurrence of severe but extremely rare agranulocytosis. If the drug does not control the hallucinations well in the first few weeks, the risk and frequent monitoring are probably not justified. Patients with excessive sedation from PD medications often need to cut back on dosage. Other options include caffeine tablets or the use of modafinil during the day, as well as medications to improve nighttime sleep.

Multiple daily doses of carbidopa-levodopa at 3 to 5 hours intervals generally provide inexpensive and well-tolerated symptom control. Initially, levodopa normalizes clinical features of the disorder in many patients. After several years, however, a significant number develop fluctuations in benefit.[16] Typically the therapeutic effect wanes from the expected 4 hours after approximately 3 years of therapy. This clinical response pattern appears to closely follow the peripheral blood concentrations of levodopa.[17] Levodopa, a large neutral amino acid is absorbed in the small intestine by amino acid facilitated transport mechanisms. Meals, especially large protein intake, can compete for uptake resulting in "off" states during which medication seems not to be working. Strategies to improve the situation include closer spacing of doses, use of sustained-release carbidopa-levodopa, or concomitant use of a catechol-O-methyltransferase inhibitor (COMT-I) such as entacapone or tolcapone.[12] These drugs slow the breakdown of levodopa peripherally by extending its pharmacokinetic profile. The COMT-I most commonly used today is entacapone, used at doses of 200 mg together with each dose of levodopa. Tolcapone, another COMT-I, is more potent but less commonly used because of the extremely rare risk of hepatic toxicity.

When patients become sensitive to medications and experience drowsiness or dyskinesia, it can be useful to extend the dosage interval or even skip a dose. Lengthening the dosing interval but providing extra doses as needed is another useful option. The absorption of levodopa by the GI tract is not always uniform and certain doses can fail to produce benefit. In this situation, a patient can take an extra dose, as needed, an hour or so after the failure of an earlier dose to provide an anti-Parkinson effect. Patient should be aware that meals could compete with levodopa and other medications

from leaving the stomach to their absorption sites. As a result, taking medications 30 minutes before or 60 minutes after a meal may achieve the best pattern of response for medications. The dopaminergic drugs often come from the pharmacy with a label recommending that these medications be taken with meals. While this may be good advice for their startup, eventually patients should adjust mealtimes and dosing intervals accordingly. Because neither sustained release levodopa preparations, monoamine oxidase inhibitors, or COMT inhibition results in much extension of levodopa effect, keeping up with the timing of medication is probably the best way to deal with dose-by-dose response patterns. For this situation, signaling devices offering regular reminders for dosing can perform a valuable role.

Unfortunately, some patients develop Parkinsonian symptoms unresponsive to levodopa. Among these are the typical balance disorder of PD (falling backwards, or retropulsion), a new resting tremor, start hesitation, or freezing in specific situations such as reaching a doorway or leaving a group.[18]

After 2 years or more, patients on levodopa can develop involuntary movements termed dyskinesia.[19] These adverse reactions generally develop during the dose cycle of each dose of levodopa as a peak-effect phenomenon. Dyskinesias appear to be dose related, suggestive of supersensitivity to the drug. Dyskinesias seem to be a unique consequence of levodopa therapy, as they have not been described from the chronic use of anticholinergic drugs or amantadine. The involuntary movements can be slow, writhing limb or trunk movements, facial grimacing, or flailing. They are usually mild and well tolerated, but sometimes are as disabling as the underlying Parkinsonian disorder. Once they develop, they are irreversible and may limit the dose. Thus, clinicians should use the lowest effective dose of levodopa, usually between 300 and 800 mg daily.

Another effective strategy to limit the side effects of levodopa is the use of dopaminergic agonists alone or in combination with levodopa.[11] Dopaminergic agonists available in the United States include bromocriptine, pergolide, pramipexole, and ropinirole. Although less potent, long-term outcomes of dopaminergic agonists can be superior to levodopa.[11] In combination with levodopa, the risk of dyskinesia and motor fluctuation such as start hesitation and freezing is lower and symptom control may improve. Dopaminergic agonists are not subject to enzymatic degradation in the brain and their half-life is longer than levodopa. Overnight use can reduce early morning symptoms, especially cramping of feet and toes.

The dopaminergic agonists are similar in effect; one is not consistently superior. Patients who do not respond well to one may benefit from a trial of another. They differ somewhat in benefit and side effects. All may cause more side effects than levodopa, including drowsiness, nausea, lightheadedness, pedal edema, vivid dreams, and hallucinations. Bromocriptine and pergolide (with ergot or ergoline chemical structures) bear the risk of rare idiosyncratic reactions such as pleural and cardiac valve fibrosis. For patients with prolonged delays in onset of action of medication (or when immobile when waking at night), a subcutaneously injectable dopaminergic agonist, apomorphine, can effect a rapid "rescue" from the "off" state. This medication requires training of the patient for safe and effective use and determining optimal dose. Nevertheless, apomorphine can be extremely beneficial as a supplement to oral medications, even if used only infrequently.

The optimal and maximum tolerated doses of the oral dopaminergic agonists vary greatly among patients. The typical range for bromocriptine is 20 to 80 mg per day; for pergolide and pramipexole it is 1.5 to 6 mg per day and for ropinirole it is from 6 to 24 mg per day, in divided doses. These medicines should be titrated up gradually over several weeks optimal dose selected based on clinical improvement. It is not clear whether low doses provide protection from the dyskinesias of levodopa. Dopaminergic agonists are costly and this limits their usefulness. Sometimes a combination of medications and careful attention to their dosing interval results in the best outcomes.

Drugs that block central acetylcholine neurotransmission were the first available for treatment of Parkinsonism. Benztropine and trihexyphenidyl are the main drugs of this class, and are primarily effective against resting tremor and rigidity, with little benefit for slowed movements. Anticholinergic drugs are a cost-effective treatment for tremor, especially as an adjunct to dopaminergic therapy, but side effects such as constipation, dry mouth and confusion may limit use.[2]

Amantadine can also be quite effective for relief of resting tremor. At doses of 100 to 300 mg daily, it may also suppress the dyskinesias of levodopa therapy.

RESEARCH INTO NEW MEDICATION THERAPIES

There are many promising new therapies for PD. New preparations of levodopa and dopaminergic agonists with longer duration of action are under evaluation. Drugs acting on the adenosine receptor have shown potential for augmenting responses achieved with conventional medications.[20] Methods of preventing the onset or slowing the progression of PD are being sought and tested in a number of clinical trials.[21,22] Among compounds being tested currently are rasagiline (which

is, like selegiline, a selective inhibitor of monoamine oxidase type B), creatine, coenzyme Q-10, and experimental drugs with neurotrophin-like properties. Long-term studies have suggested that pramipexole and ropinirole might also have neuroprotective properties in addition to their symptomatic actions.[23] An alternate explanation is that the dopaminergic agonists are not neuroprotective, but rather that levodopa accelerates the disease. This explanation is challenged by a later study of various doses of levodopa, showing no worsening of the disease.[24,25]

NEUROSURGICAL TREATMENT

Beyond medications, there are several surgical options for relief of Parkinsonian disabilities. Early procedures included brain lesioning at the globus pallidus and/or the thalamus. Interrupting brain pathways at these sites improved control of Parkinsonian symptoms in some patients. The strategy most commonly used today is deep brain stimulation (DBS).[24] This procedure, based on the earlier brain lesioning, involves localized application of high frequency electric current. Performed bilaterally for most patients, DBS involves placing an electrode in the subthalamic nucleus of the basal ganglia. The fine wire electrodes are connected subcutaneously to battery-operated devices implanted in the upper chest, which are programmed to optimize results. By blocking output through the subthalamic nucleus DBS may result in remarkable improvements of motor control, and abolish tremor and dyskinesia. Results are superior to the earlier lesioning procedures, and DBS has supplanted their use. It has a high success rate, and may provide symptom control superior to all medications. However, most patients who undergo DBS receive further benefit from continued medicine, and DBS rarely provides improvement in imbalance and speech disorders.

Intracranial implantation of DBS electrodes poses only a small risk for serious complications such as bleeding or infection. For patients with disabling PD and limited medication responsiveness, DBS of the subthalamic nucleus has provided new hope for recovery from disability.[19]

In the future, intervention with cell-based treatments may also become possible. Clinical trials are exploring the implantation of dopamine-generating minute plastic beads into the striatum to normalize dopaminergic neurotransmission. It is hoped that this will relieve symptoms with fewer side effects than the current therapeutic options of dopaminergic drugs.

OTHER AIDS TO PD CARE

One of the most important therapies to preserve safe mobility is the use of rolling walking frames or walkers.

When specially equipped with wheels and a handbrake, these devices reduce falls significantly. For PD patients, leaning forward while walk with a rolling walking frame reduces the consequences of the impaired balance reflexes or episodic stumbling. The handbrakes prevent runaway forward propulsion. These walkers can offer greatly improved safety to mobility and a greatly increased opportunity for exercise and independence. Canes (conventional or the 4-prong variety) can also be helpful in the quest to avoid falls but are less reliable. PD patients also benefit from motorized lift chairs, elevated toilet seats with side-handles, and a railing in their bed to assist in positioning. Catalogues from medical supply stores and consultations from visiting nurse associations can introduce patients to the full range of aids available for the physical disabilities. Many of these are approved for Medicare reimbursement.

Sometimes the momentary impairments of gait such as freezing can be overcome by various "tricks."[18] These include counting out loud or stepping over an imaginary log in front of the feet. Also helpful is a laser light beam projecting a target in front of the patient's feet, for the next step

Physical and occupational therapy can also be effective. Specific goals include gait and balance training, skills for overcoming impaired dexterity, and strategies to assist in daily activities such as dressing, washing, arising from a chair, turning in bed, and freezing of gait. Speech therapy may be helpful for hypophonia, dysarthria and swallowing disorders. The Lee Silverman Voice Training[26] is specifically designed for patients with speech problems from PD.

PD patients greatly benefit from information about their disease. In addition to advice, they gain knowledge of promising research, and realistic hope and encouragement. Some of the most informative sources are the websites of the national PD lay organizations such as the National Parkinson Foundation (www.parkinson.org), the American Parkinson Disease Foundation (www.apdaparkinson.org), the Parkinson Disease Foundation (www.pdf.org), the Michael J. Fox Foundation for Parkinson's Research (michaeljfox.org), WEMOVE (www.wemove.org), and smaller local organizations. They provide newsletters with up-to-date articles on common problems of PD, highlights of new products and research, and a forum for activism to enhance research support, increase awareness of PD, or improve services. Participation in local support groups provides valuable contacts and personalized help in coping with the disabilities of this chronic illness. In some locations, volunteer support groups meet frequently and are coordinated by professional organizations. Support groups also provide patients with information as to community resources and physicians with special expertise and interest in PD.

EVIDENCE-BASED SUMMARY

- Diagnosis of PD can be difficult and a response to levodopa can be helpful.
- PD progresses slowly and many patients retain good function for many years.
- Dopaminergic agonists are the mainstay of therapy.
- Neurosurgical treatment such as deep brain stimulation has a high success rate.

REFERENCES

1. Jellinger KA. Cell death mechanism in Parkinson's disease. *J Neural Transm.* 2000;107:1–27.
2. Nelson MV, Berchou RB, LeWitt PA. Parkinson's Disease. In: DiPiro JT, Talbert RL, Yee GC, Matzke GR, Wells BG, Posey LM (eds), *Pharmacotherapy: A Pathophysiologic Approach.* 5th ed. Stamford, CT: Appleton & Lange; 2005:1089–1102.
3. Lang AE, Lozano AM. Parkinson's disease (first and second parts). *N Engl J Med.* 1998;339:1044–1053 and 1130–1143.
4. Suchowersky O, Reich S, Perlmutter J, et al. Practice Parameter: Diagnosis and prognosis of new onset Parkinson disease (an evidence-based review). Report of the Quality Standards Subcommittee of the American Academy of Neurology. *Neurology.* 2006;66:968–975.
5. LeWitt PA. The challenge of managing mild Parkinson's disease. *Pharmacotherapy.* 2000;20(pt 2):2S–7S.
6. Jennings DL, Seibyl JP, Oakes D, et al. [^{123}I]β-CIT and SPECT imaging versus clinical evaluation in Parkinsonian syndrome: Unmasking an early diagnosis. *Arch Neurol.* 2004;61:1224–1229.
7. Farrer MJ. Genetics of Parkinson disease: Paradigm shifts and future prospects. *Nat Rev Genet.* 2006;7:306–318.
8. Miyasaki JM, Shannon K, Voon V, et al. Practice Parameter: Evaluation and treatment of depression, psychosis, and dementia in Parkinson disease (an evidence-based review). Report of the Quality Standards Subcommittee of the American Academy of Neurology. *Neurology.* 2006;66:996–1002.
9. Nutt JG, Wooten GF. Clinical practice. Diagnosis and initial management of Parkinson's disease. *N Engl J Med.* 2005;353:1021–1017.
10. Noyes K, Dick AW, Holloway RG, Parkinson Study Group. Pramipexole and levodopa in early Parkinson's disease: Dynamic changes in cost effectiveness. *Pharmacoeconomics.* 2005;23:1257–1270.
11. LeWitt PA. Pharmacology of dopaminergic agonists for Parkinson's disease. In: LeWitt PA, Oertel WH (eds). *Parkinson's Disease: The Treatment Options.* London, UK: Martin Dunitz Publishers; 1999:159–186.
12. LeWitt PA. Extending the action of levodopa's effects. In: LeWitt PA, Oertel WH (eds). *Parkinson's Disease: The Treatment Options.* London, UK: Martin Dunitz Publishers; 1999:141–158.

13. Olanow CW, Agid Y, Mizuno Y, et al. Levodopa in the treatment of Parkinson's disease: Current controversies. *Mov Disord.* 2004;19:997–1005.

14. Fahn S, Parkinson Study Group. Does levodopa slow or hasten the rate of progression of Parkinson's disease? *J Neurol.* 2005;252(Suppl 4):IV37–IV42.

15. Ondo WG, Tintner R, Voung KD, et al. Double-blind, placebo-controlled, unforced titration parallel trial of quetiapine for dopaminergic-induced hallucinations in Parkinson's disease. *Mov Disord.* 2005;20:958–963.

16. Ahlskog JE, Muenter MD. Frequency of levodopa-related dyskinesias and motor fluctuations as estimated from the cumulative literature. *Mov Disord.* 2001;16:448–458.

17. Nutt JG. Long-term L-DOPA therapy: Challenges to our understanding and for the care of people with Parkinson's disease. *Exp Neurol.* 2003;184:9–13.

18. Stern GM, Lander CM, Lees AJ. Akinetic freezing and trick movements in Parkinson's disease. *J Neural Transm.* 1980; 16(Suppl):137–141.

19. Pahwa R, Factor SA, Lyons KE, et al. Practice Parameter: Treatment of Parkinson disease with motor fluctuations and dyskinesia (an evidence-based review). Report of the Quality Standards Subcommittee of the American Academy of Neurology. *Neurology.* 2006;66:983–995.

20. Bara-Jimenez W, Sherzai A, Dimitrova T, et al. Adenosine A(2A) receptor antagonist treatment of Parkinson's disease. *Neurology.* 2003;61:293–296.

21. Suchowersky O, Gronseth G, Perlmutter J, et al. Practice Parameter: Neuroprotective strategies and alternative therapies for Parkinson disease (an evidence-based review). Report of the Quality Standards Subcommittee of the American Academy of Neurology. *Neurology.* 2006;66: 976–982.

22. LeWitt PA. Clinical trials of neuroprotection for Parkinson's disease. *Neurology.* 2004;63(Suppl 2):S23–S31.

23. Marek K, Jennings D, Seibyl J. Do dopamine agonists or levodopa modify Parkinson's disease progression? *Eur J Neurol.* 2002;9(Suppl 3):15–22.

24. Rodriguez-Oroz MC, Obeso JA, Lang AE, et al. Bilateral deep brain stimulation in Parkinson's disease: A multicentre study with 4 years follow-up. *Brain.* 2005;128:240–2249.

25. Hely MA, Morris JG, Reid WG, Trafficante R. Sydney Multicenter Study of Parkinson's disease: Non-L-dopa-responsive problems dominate at 15 years. *Mov Disord.* 2005; 20:190–199.

26. Trail M, Fox C, Ramig LO, Sapir S, et al. Speech treatment for Parkinson's disease. *NeuroRehabilitation.* 2005;20: 205–221.

Chapter 18

Persistent Pain

Julianna Burzynski and Scott Strassels

SEARCH STRATEGY

A systematic search of the medical literature was performed in April and May of 2006. The search, limited to human subjects, and English language journals included the Cochrane database, PubMed, and the National Guideline Clearinghouse.

Pain is a common reason for individuals to seek medical care. In 2003, three of the 20 most frequently mentioned reasons for outpatient department visits in the United States were related to stomach, head, or back pain.[1] Similarly, in a 1998 study, 21.5% of persons in a multinational sample across Asia, Africa, Europe, and the Americas reported pain most of the time during the previous 6 months.[2] In a study of more than 46 000 European and Israeli persons, the prevalence of chronic pain ranged from 12% to 30%, with a weighted average of 19%.[3] In the United States, pain is often suboptimally treated in persons of all ages and a wide variety of conditions.[4–12] Important clinical, human, and economic consequences of this shortcoming include altered immune-system functioning, diminished ability to function, increased risk of chronic pain, needless suffering, and higher healthcare costs.[13–22] In the United States, 2002 costs of lost productive time caused by pain have been estimated at $61.2 billion.[23] A sample of individuals with neuropathic pain disorders incurred charges of more than $17 000 during calendar year 2000 compared to approximately $5 715 in a matched control group without neuropathic pain.[24] An analysis of symptomatic diabetic peripheral neuropathy and its associated complications found that 2001 costs were approximately $237 million.[25]

DEFINITIONS

Terms used to define and describe pain are emotionally charged and often used incorrectly or unclearly. As a result, it is important to begin discussions of pain by building a foundation of commonly agreed upon terms and concepts. A simplified taxonomy of pain follows; the reader is referred to the International Association for the Study of Pain for a more complete list.[26] Pain is a subjective, unpleasant, sensory, and emotional experience associated with actual or potential tissue damage, or described in terms of such damage. More simply put, "pain is what the person says it is, existing whenever he says it does."[27] The core of these definitions is that pain is subjective, has multiple dimensions, without a clear relationship between the intensity of the sensation and tissue damage.[28] Clinicians also need to be aware that individuals may have pain even if communication is difficult or impossible. Because pain is a subjective experience, it is critically important that patients' reports of pain be taken seriously.[26]

Pain is commonly described in terms of duration (e.g., acute or chronic) and pathophysiology (e.g., nociceptive or neuropathic). These constructs can be helpful, suggesting treatments that are likely to be effective, but they can also be misleading. For example, acute pain is often described as being of recent onset and limited duration, with a tendency to decrease over time, while chronic pain is often described as lasting for some undetermined, subjective period of time beyond that expected to be needed to heal.[29] Yet, acute pain from an injury may last much longer than expected, and the biochemical and cellular changes that accompany chronic pain begin shortly after an injury.[30] Nociceptive pain is the result of noxious stimuli that may

Table 18-1. Selected Pain Terminology[26]

Term	IASP Definition
Allodynia	Pain caused by a stimulus that does not normally cause pain
Dysesthesia	Unpleasant abnormal sensation, spontaneous or evoked
Hyperalgesia	Increased response to a stimulus that is normally nonpainful
Hyperesthesia	Increased sensitivity to stimulation, excluding special senses
Hypoalgesia	Diminished pain in response to a normally painful stimulus
Paresthesia	An abnormal sensation, whether spontaneous or evoked

IASP, International Association for the Study of Pain.

damage normal tissue (i.e., pressure, temperature, and chemical stimuli), and can be further delineated into somatic or visceral subtypes.[26,27] Somatic pain originates in the skin, bones, muscle, and connective tissue, and is usually specifically located, while visceral pain originates in internal body structures and organs, and is more generally located. Patients typically describe somatic pain as dull, aching, throbbing, or sharp. In contrast, neuropathic pain results from nervous-system dysfunction or lesions on nerves and is often described as burning, tingling, stinging, or shooting. Table 18-1 includes some common terminology to describe pain.

Pain is a normal, natural reaction to noxious stimuli. In its acute form, pain is a protective mechanism that indicates the risk or presence of an injury. When pain becomes persistent, however, it is no longer a protective mechanism, and it becomes a disease in itself. This purpose of this chapter is to provide an overview of the assessment and management of chronic, nonmalignant pain. Common chronic painful conditions include spinal pain with or without radiculopathy, complex regional pain syndrome, fibromyalgia syndrome, spondyloarthropathies, myofascial pain syndrome, temporomandibular joint dysfunction, painful peripheral neuropathy and postherpetic neuralgia.

PATIENT ASSESSMENT

Assessing patient-reported outcomes is important in the provision of optimal care for persons with persistent pain. The patients' input is a critical part of the decision making process as it incorporates insight not provided by healthcare providers or other proxies. These data, commonly referred to as patient-reported outcomes, include issues such as the patient's global condition and functional status, symptoms, health-related quality of life (HRQL), and satisfaction with care.[31] The purpose of this discussion is to address some common issues in pain evaluation and treatment, and to describe several tools used to assess outcomes in persons with persistent pain.

It is important to remember several limitations of outcomes research impacting this topic. First, questionnaires and surveys are often designed and tested for use in one population, but then used in others. This is not necessarily wrong, but it is important to assess the validity and reliability of the instrument prior to using it in the new population. Second, HRQL and quality of life may be incorrectly used interchangeably. Quality of life is a broad construct including dimensions reflecting individual preferences, including health, work, housing, and family, among others.[31] In comparison, HRQL reflects concepts such as health status, satisfaction, and well-being as a function of health. The Short-Form 36-item Health Survey (SF-36) is a well-known example of a generic HRQL questionnaire.[32] Third, patient satisfaction alone is a crude measure of health care quality; it is best used in combination with other data.[10]

Many generic and specific HRQL instruments exist, and have been used to assess outcomes in persons with pain.

INSTRUMENTS

Visual Analog Scales

A Visual Analog Scale (VAS) is a straight line with labels at the ends expressing extremes of pain, such as "no pain" and "pain as bad as it could be." The person is asked to indicate where their pain lies between those two endpoints, and intensity is measured from the "no pain" end to the person's mark.[33] VASs are valid and are thought to have ratio–scale properties for groups of people.[34,35] They are easy to use and interpret, but they measure only one dimension of the pain experience, require some level of dexterity, and appear to be more difficult to understand than other measures.[10,34]

Numeric Rating Scales

These scales are analogous to a VAS, and may be written or verbal. The person is asked to rate their pain on a 0-to-10 scale, where 0 is no pain, and 10 is the worst possible pain. Numeric rating scales (NRSs) are valid, but may not have ratio–scale properties.[36,37] Thus, a change from an intensity of 9 to 6 cannot necessarily be interpreted as a one-third decrease. Nevertheless, NRSs are valid, easy to administer and interpret, do not need to be written, and generally considered preferable to the VAS unless the clinician or researcher requires a scale with ratio properties.[33]

McGill Pain Questionnaire

The McGill Pain Questionnaire provides estimates of the sensory, affective, and descriptive qualities of the person's pain through three scores.[38,39] First, the person rates their present pain intensity on a 5-point scale. Second, the person chooses words that describe the sensory and affective qualities of their pain from among twenty groups of qualitatively similar words. The pain rating intensity score based on the number of words chosen and the intensity of the pain these words describe. For example, one group includes "jumping, flashing, or shooting." The patient might choose jumping, flashing, or shooting, and receive 1, 2, or 3 points, respectively, or no points if no words in this group are selected. Scores are generated for sensory, evaluative, and miscellaneous word group, as well as an overall total. The McGill Pain Questionnaire has been extensively validated, although the present pain intensity score does not necessarily echo the pain rating intensity or the number of words chosen scores.[38]

Brief Pain Inventory

The Brief Pain Inventory (BPI) includes measures of pain intensity, location, and the effect on function.[40] This instrument was originally designed for use in cancer patients, but has since been validated in persons with other painful conditions.[41,42] Pain intensity is assessed at present, at its peak, average, and least intensity over the past day or week using NRSs. The consequences of pain are assessed by questions on the effects of pain on mood, walking, and other physical activity, work, social activity, relations with others, and sleep. The BPI and its shortened version, the BPI-short form (BPI-SF), are valid and reliable.[43]

SF-36

The SF-36 measures the effects of medical conditions on eight important health-related domains. These are not specific to age, treatment or disease: physical functioning, functioning related to physical health, bodily pain, general health, vitality, social functioning, functioning related to emotional health, and mental health. The SF-36 has been extensively used in health outcomes research and has been validated in populations with a wide variety of medical conditions.[44,45] While the SF-36 is one of the most commonly used HRQL instruments, it assumes a higher level of function than that of many patients with chronic pain.[46,47] The SF-36 is available in shortened versions, the SF-12, and the SF-8.[48,49]

Treatment Outcomes in Pain Survey

The Treatment Outcomes in Pain Survey (TOPS) is a validated disease-specific questionnaire designed to provide more information about the effect of chronic nonmalignant pain on HRQL and functioning.[46,47] It is an "augmented SF-36" and assesses outcomes in persons treated in outpatient multidisciplinary pain centers. The main advantage of the TOPS is that it is sensitive and valid for use in persons with persistent pain. The disadvantage is that it is relatively long, Asking the person to complete the TOPS before coming to clinic or before they see their healthcare provider helps address that issue.

DIAGNOSTIC TESTING

There is no specific laboratory or diagnostic test beyond the patient's report to confirm pain.[50] Tests to determine the etiology of pain and define management should be based on the history and examination.[50–53] Tests to consider include:

1. Radiological studies (plain radiographs, computed tomography, magnetic resonance imaging, and/or nuclear medicine studies)
2. Electrodiagnostic studies (electromyography, nerve conduction studies)
3. Diagnostic nerve blocks
4. Psychological testing
5. Laboratory testing
6. Functional assessment (patient self report or observation of mobility, self-care, physical performance; patient self report of vocational, social, familial, sexual function)

PATHOPHYSIOLOGY

Pain is a complex sensation, intricately related to emotion and cognition, which is intrinsically unpleasant. It is provoked by tissue damage leading to cellular breakdown and release of biochemical substances that stimulate autonomic responses, and psychological and behavioral reactions.[54] The pathophysiology of nociceptive and neuropathic pain is described in the following sections.

NOCICEPTIVE PAIN

Nociception can be described in terms of transduction, transmission, perception and modulation.[55] Transduction is the conversion of noxious thermal, mechanical, or chemical stimulus into electrical activity in the peripheral terminals of sensory nerve fibers.[55,56] The action potentials pass from the peripheral nerve terminal along axons to the central nervous system (CNS).[54] Transmission is the synaptic transfer and modulation of input from one neuron to another. Perception is the conscious experience that occurs in higher cortical structures.[50] The brain can accommodate only a limited number of pain signals, and so pain modulation occurs via endorphins and others systems.[55,50]

Nociceptors are free nerve endings that distinguish between noxious and nonnoxious stimuli.[50] Noxious stimuli may be the release of bradykinins, potassium, serotonin, and histamine following tissue injury.[50] Damage to tissue may also stimulate release of prostaglandins, leukotrienes, and substance P; these stimuli sensitize the nociceptors but do not stimulate them directly.[56] There are silent nociceptors that are silent during normal nociception, but are activated in response to neurogenic inflammation.[54,56] Nociceptive pain results from thermal, chemical, or mechanical stimulation of nociceptors in tissues which transmit electrical signals along intact, functional nerves from the periphery through the spinal cord, brain stem, and thalamus to the cerebral cortex where the sensation of pain is perceived.[54]

Tissues are innervated by slow, small diameter, unmyelinated type C fibers and fast, large diameter, myelinated type A-δ fibers that transmit impulses via action potentials generated at nociceptors.[50,54] Type C fibers are responsible for dull, aching, poorly localized pain, whereas type A-δ fibers are responsible for fast, sharp, well-localized pain. These fibers synapse in the dorsal horn of the spinal cord and release a myriad of neurotransmitters including glutamate, substance P, and calcitonin gene-related peptide.[50] These neurotransmitters are responsible for stimulating continued transmission of the pain signal to ascending pathways in the spinal cord, through the thalamus to higher cortical regions. A-δ fibers also become chemosensitive during inflammation and affect CNS pain pathways.[54] Peripheral nerve fibers demonstrate plasticity that can be induced within seconds or delayed hours to days depending on electrophysiologic properties, growth factors, cytokines, or other tissue factors.[54]

The endogenous opiate system modulates pain perception in the CNS by release of endorphins (enkephalins, dynorphins, and β-endorphins) that bind to μ-, δ-, and κ-opioid receptors in the CNS.[50–54] Endorphins inhibit the transmission of pain impulses or alter pain perception within the CNS.[50] Stimulation of the N-methyl-D-aspartate receptor in the dorsal horn decreases μ receptor response to opioids, hence drugs that antagonize N-methyl-D-aspartate receptors may enhance the response to opioids.[50]

Pain can be modulated at several levels. The brain can only process a limited number of signals allowing nonnoxious input to alter the perception of pain.[50] This can be accomplished via topical medications providing a counterirritant effect, mild stimulation of type A-δ fibers causing a reduction in transmission along type C fibers, or by cognitive behavioral techniques including relaxation, distraction, and guided mental imagery. This ability to diffuse the pain signal may explain why nonpharmacologic methods such as acupuncture, transcutaneous electrical stimulation, and cognitive behavioral therapy are effective for some patients.[50,55]

NEUROPATHIC PAIN

Neuropathic pain may be initiated by a relatively minor physical insult. The level of pain does not necessarily correlate with the degree of nerve damage nor the level of functional preservation.[57] Patients may experience negative signs such as sensory deficits, weakness, and reflex changes, positive signs including hyperalgesia and allodynia, or paresthesias and dysesthesias.[57] Infection, trauma, metabolic abnormalities, chemotherapy, irradiation, tumor infiltration, surgery, neurotoxins, nerve compression, and inflammation are some of the underlying causes of neuropathic pain.[54,57] It is generally classified as central or peripheral, based on the location of the primary lesion. Common neuropathic pain syndromes are listed in Table 18-2.

There may be neurophysiologic and neuroanatomic changes that contribute to the development of peripheral neuropathic pain, including abnormal nerve regeneration and neuroma formation.[54,57] Neuroma and abnormal nerve endings may generate spontaneous, abnormal activity. Ectopic neuronal activity may cause peripheral neuropathic pain directly via continuous abnormal afferent stimulation (e.g., paresthesias in response to continuous discharge in C fibers), through

Table 18-2. Common Neuropathic Pain Syndromes [54,55,57]

Central Neuropathic Pain Syndromes	Peripheral Neuropathic Pain Syndromes
Compressive myelopathy from spinal stenosis	Painful diabetic neuropathy
HIV myelopathy	HIV-associated neuropathy
Postischemic myelopathy	Phantom limb pain
Poststroke pain	Trigeminal neuralgia
Posttraumatic spinal cord injury pain	Nerve injury due to trauma (brachial plexopathy)
Syringomyelia	Complex regional pain syndrome
Phantom limb pain	Cancer related nerve infiltration or compression
Pain related to multiple sclerosis or Parkinson disease	Chemotherapy induced neuropathy
Postherpetic neuralgia*	Postherpetic neuralgia*

*Postherpetic neuralgia initially damages the peripheral nervous system, but damage to the dorsal root ganglion can result in anatomic changes to the dorsal horn of the CNS, causing a mixed central and peripheral neuropathy.

hypersensitive neurons that respond with a painful sensation in response to a mechanical or chemical stimulation that would normally be nonpainful, or via central sensitization.[57] Sensitization of central neurons occurs after brief and intense or sustained, low-level nociceptor input; once sensitized, the central neurons perceive innocuous mechanoreceptor stimulation from the area surrounding the nerve injury as painful.[54,57] Central sensitization contributes to hyper-responsive conditions of neuropathic pain, fibromyalgia, and gastrointestinal pain. Central sensitization may be mediated through the release of various neurotransmitters including substance P, glutamate, calcitonin gene-related peptide, γ-amniobutyric acid (GABA) and neurokinin K, via activation of the N-methyl-D-aspartate receptor, increased calcium flux, and prostaglandin synthesis.[57]

Some of the older anticonvulsants such as carbazepime and phenytoin, and local anesthetics including lidocaine, block sodium channels at concentrations lower than necessary to inhibit normal action potentials in nerves. These agents relieve pain by blocking abnormal, ectopic discharge generated by damaged, dysfunctional primary sensory neurons and their axons.[54] The mechanism of action of relief of pain of the newer anticonvulsants, including gabapentin and pregabalin, remains elusive. It is likely related to central neuronal inhibition of release of excitatory amino acids, blockade of neural calcium channels and/or augmentation of CNS inhibitory pathways by increasing GABA-ergic transmission.[54]

MANAGEMENT

PHARMACOTHERAPY

Medications are a key component in a comprehensive treatment plan for persistent pain, and may be used in combination with interventional, surgical, psychological and rehabilitation treatment modalities.[53] Pharmacotherapy for chronic pain may be targeted at pain itself, or at comorbid conditions. Anxiety, depression, and insomnia may result from and contribute to chronic pain and treatment of these comorbidities may help alleviate pain. Choice of therapy depends on the type; nociceptive, inflammatory, or neuropathic, as well as the severity of the pain. Key points described in guidelines for the management of chronic pain include the following[53,54]:

1. Give an adequate therapeutic trial of a medication specific to the anticipated time to note beneficial effects for that drug; time periods to assess medication effectiveness may be found in Tables 18-3, 18-5, and 18-6.

2. Give adequate doses and titrate to provide pain relief with manageable adverse effects.
3. Anticipate and manage adverse reactions.
4. Utilize combination therapy with complementary mechanisms of action.
5. Taper and discontinue ineffective medications and try a different strategy, either a new class of drugs, or nondrug alternatives.

Nonopioid Analgesics
Acetaminophen. Acetaminophen appears to act as a prostaglandin synthesis inhibitor, with more pronounced activity centrally than peripherally, and little anti-inflammatory activity.[58] It is used to treat mild to moderate pain and can be given as needed or around the clock. It has well established safety, efficacy, low cost, and few adverse effects or clinically significant drug interactions, making it a common first line agent for chronic pain.[59] It has few adverse effects when given in the recommended therapeutic dose to a maximum of 4000 mg/day, although toxic doses (more than 10–15 g) may cause hepatotoxicity, nephrotoxicity and thrombocytopenia.[58] Alcoholics or those with significant hepatic dysfunction may be at increased risk for toxicity. Periodic monitoring should include transaminases, alkaline phosphatase, blood urea nitrogen, and creatinine.[53]

Nonsteroidal Anti-Inflammatory Drugs. Inflammation occurs in response to tissue injury and causes membrane phospholipid conversion to arachidonic acid via the phospholipase A_2 enzyme.[58] Arachidonic acid is converted to endoperoxides by the cyclooxygenase (COX) enzyme. These endoperoxides include prostaglandins, prostacyclins and thromboxane A_2. Prostaglandin E_2 is the main eicosanoid that contributes to inflammation and pain and it acts to sensitize nociceptors to other stimuli.[58] Nonsteroidal anti-inflammatory drugs (NSAIDs) act both centrally and peripherally to relieve pain by inhibition of prostaglandin synthesis via the COX enzymes.[50,58] There are three isoenzymes of COX, COX-1, COX-2, and COX-3. COX-1 is a constitutive enzyme involved in the homeostasis of the normal physiology of the gastric mucosa, kidney, platelets, and the endothelium.[58] COX-2 is inducible and produces prostaglandins in response to inflammation.[58] Pain may be from inflammation related to direct tissue injury or the result of mediators released in response to pain. For example, central sensitization occurs following injury and results in upregulation of gene expression of COX-2, contributing to generalized aches and pains, loss of appetite, and changes in mood and sleep cycle.[55] NSAIDs may thus be useful even if the injury is not inflammatory in nature.[55]

Table 18-3. FDA Approved Nonopioid Analgesics in Adult Pain (excludes those only approved for osteoarthritis or rheumatoid arthritis)[50, 58, 60, 63]

Drug Class	Oral Dosing Regimen (mg)	Maximum Adult Daily Dose (mg)	Analgesic onset (h)	Analgesia duration (h)	Comments
Para-aminophenol					✓ Avoid in patients with a history of liver dysfunction or alcoholism
Acetaminophen	300–325 (q4–6h)	4000	0.5–1	3–6	✓ NSAIDs are associated with increased risk of cardiovascular events including stroke, myocardial infarction, and hypertension
Salicylate					✓ Use caution in patients with fluid retention, heart failure, hypertension, or other cardiovascular risk factors
Acetylsalicylic acid (aspirin)	325–650 (q4h)	4000	0.5	3–6	✓ NSAIDs may compromise renal function, patients more susceptible include those with impaired renal function, dehydration, heart failure, liver dysfunction, those taking ACE inhibitors, and the elderly
Choline magnesium trisalicylate (Trisilate)	500–1500 (q8–12h)	4500	2	4	✓ NSAIDs may increase risk of gastrointestinal bleeding, ulceration, and perforation; use in caution in patients with a history of bleeding or ulcers, concurrent aspirin, anticoagulants, corticosteroids, use of alcohol, smoking, and the elderly
Diflunisal	500–1000 initially, then 250–500 (q8–12h)	1500	1	8–12	✓ Use the lowest effective dose for the shortest duration of time consistent with patient goals to reduce risk of cardiovascular and gastro-intestinal events.
Magnesium Salicylate	650 (q4h) or 1090 (q8h)	4800	NA	4	✓ NSAIDs may cause serious skin reactions including Stevens-Johnson syndrome, toxic epidermal necrolysis
Sodium salicylate	325–650 (q3–4h)	5400	NA	4	✓ Anaphylaxis may occur, even with out prior exposure; patients with "aspirin triad" (bronchial asthma, aspirin intolerance, rhinitis) may be at increased risk
Salsalate	500 (q4h)	3000	NA	NA	
Fenamate					
Meclofenamate (Meclomen)	50–100 (q4–6h)	400	NA	4–6	
Mefenamic acid (Ponstel)	500 initially, then 250 (q6h)	1000–1250 (maximum 7 d)	NA	6	
Pyranocarboxylic acid					
Etodolac	200–400 (q6–8h)	1000	0.5–1	6–8	
Acetic acid					
Diclofenac potassium (Cataflam, Voltaren, Arthrotec)	100 initially, then 50 (q8h)	150	0.5	6–8	
Propionic acid					
Ibuprofen (Advil, Motrin, others)	200–400* (q4–6h)	*1200 / 3200	0.5	4–6	
Fenoprofen (Nalfon)	200 (q4–6h)	3200	0.25–0.5	4–6	
Ketoprofen	12.5–25* (q4–6 h) or 25—75 (q6–8 h)	*75 / 300	1	4–8	
Naproxen (Naprosyn, others)	200* (q12 h) / 500† initially, then 250 (q6–8h)	*600 / †1250	1	Up to 12	
Naproxen sodium (Anaprox, Aleve)	440* initially, then 220 (q8–12h) / 500–1000‡ (q12–24h)	*660 / ‡1500	0.5–1	Up to 12	
Pyrrolizine carboxylic acid					
Ketorolac (Toradol)	20 initially, then 10 (q4–6h)	40 (maximum 5 d)	0.5–1	4–6	
COX-2 inhibitor					
Celecoxib (Celebrex)	400 initially, then 200 (q12h)	400	1	12–24	

*Over-the-counter.
†Dose expressed as naproxen base; 200 mg naproxen base = 220 mg naproxen sodium.
‡Delayed release or controlled release formulations available.
NA, not available.

NSAIDs are most effective at relieving mild to moderate somatic pain that is nociceptive or inflammatory and tend to be less effective for visceral or neuropathic pain.[58] They are the drug of choice for moderate to severe bone pain associated with metastatic malignancy.[60] NSAIDs have uricosuric effects and are first line therapy to treat acute attacks of gout.[58] The choice of NSAID often depends on availability, cost, pharmacokinetics, and adverse effect profile as clinical trials have not consistently favored one agent over another for efficacy.[50] Table 18-3 is a useful reference for selection of nonopioid analgesics.

Gastrointestinal ulceration, bleeding, gastritis, esophagitis and perforation remain the most common morbidity of NSAIDs and are the major limitations to their use.[58] There is a fourfold higher risk for gastrointestinal bleeding with a nonselective NSAID compared to nonusers.[61] Risk factors for ulceration include increasing age, prior history of gastrointestinal bleeding, and aspirin, warfarin, or corticosteroid use.[62] NSAIDs cause direct gastric mucosal irritation in addition to inhibiting the production of protective prostaglandins within the gastrointestinal tract. Chronic NSAID use may lead to iron deficiency anemia from gastrointestinal tract blood loss.[58] Two strategies are recommended to prevent gastrointestinal complications in patients at risk; utilizing a COX-2 selective inhibitor or combining a traditional NSAID with a proton pump inhibitor.[62] Data suggests the two strategies are similar with respect to ulcer prevention, however a recent meta-analysis suggests an NSAID combined with a proton pump inhibitor provides a greater absolute reduction in dyspepsia.[62] Misoprostal reduces the risk of serious gastrointestinal complications as well, but its use may be limited by abdominal pain and diarrhea.

COX-2 selective inhibitors, such as celecoxib and valdecoxib, as well as nonselective NSAIDs, may increase the risk of cardiovascular events including myocardial infarction, stroke, and cardiovascular death.[60] NSAIDs may cause mild sodium retention in 10% to 25% of patients, and tends to be more severe in patients with edema caused by congestive heart failure, cirrhosis of the liver, or nephrotic syndrome.[58] NSAIDs also inhibit renal prostaglandins responsible for renal vasodilation, in states of hypoperfusion they may contribute to the development of renal failure.[58] NSAIDs can also cause CNS side effects including headache, dizziness, and confusion.

NSAIDs interfere with platelet function by inhibiting the production of thromboxane A_2.[58] Aspirin's antiplatelet effect is irreversible for the life of the platelet. Other NSAIDs have reversible activity on platelets, and the platelets return to normal function as the level of COX-1 inhibition decreases. COX-2 selective agents do not affect platelet function or alter bleeding time.[53]

Aspirin sensitivity may cause urticaria and angioedema, or a triad of bronchospasm, severe rhinitis, and nasal polyps, which is more common in asthmatic patients. There is a cross-sensitivity with potent NSAIDs and aspirin.[58]

Patients on chronic NSAID therapy should have periodic monitoring including abdominal examination, hemoglobin, stool occult blood, blood urea nitrogen, and creatinine.[53]

Opioids

Pure opioid agonists are full agonists at the μ receptor; these agents include morphine, hydromorphone, codeine, oxycodone, hydrocodone, fentanyl, meperidine, propoxyphene and methadone. Analgesia has no ceiling with these agents, and the maximum dose is determined by intolerable adverse effects.[50] Opioids may be used for pain of any type or duration although they are most effective for nociceptive pain. The lack of clinical evidence on efficacy and risks of opioids for nonmalignant persistent pain has prompted several groups (American Pain Society, American Academy of Pain Medicine, American Society of Addiction Medicine, and American Society of Interventional Pain Physicians) to advocate cautious use in selected, carefully monitored patients.[54,64] The American Society of Interventional Pain Physicians notes that the populations studied were heterogeneous, and studies were short term, but recommend use in "well selected patients with long-lasting or recurrent pain that is severe enough to reduce their quality of life, and for whom no other more effective and less risky therapies are available." They believe opioid analgesics may "reduce the intensity of pain, increase functioning, and improve quality of life for prolonged periods."[64] They recommend periodic review of the "4 As," Analgesia, Activity, Aberrant behavior, and Adverse effects. Based on this assessment, therapy may be continued or, for patients in whom there is no relief of pain or intolerable adverse effects, it may be discontinued. Table 18-4 is an algorithm for management of persistent pain with opioids. Patients should be informed of the risks, including development of tolerance or dependence, and consideration given to use of a controlled substance agreement to establish clear patient responsibilities when prescribing controlled substances.[54]

Table 18-5 provides common initial dosing regimens for opioids, anticipated duration of action for the immediate release formulations, and a conversion for "equianalgesic" dosing. Note that this chart should be used as guide because there is incomplete cross tolerance among opioids and patients metabolize drug differently as a result of drug interactions and genetic

Table 18-4. Ten Step Approach for Long-Term Opioid Therapy in Persistent Pain[54,64]

STEP I	Comprehensive initial evaluation
	History of present illness
	Medical and psychiatric comorbidites including substance abuse and addiction
	Social aspects and family history
STEP II	Establish diagnosis
	X-rays, MRI, CT, neurophysiological studies
	Psychological evaluation
	Precision diagnostic intervention
STEP III	Establish medical necessity (lack of progress or a supplemental therapy)
	Physical diagnosis
	Therapeutic interventional pain management
	Physical modalities
	Behavior therapy
STEP IV	Assess risk-benefit ratio
	Treatment is beneficial
	Type of pain is likely to respond to opioid analgesia
	Opioids have an equal or better therapeutic index than alternative therapies
	The patient is likely to be responsible using the drug
STEP V	Establish treatment goals
	Diminished pain severity
	Improved quality of life
	Analgesic gains should enable improved physical, psychological, occupational and social functioning
STEP VI	Obtain informed consent and agreement
STEP VII	Initial dose adjustment phase (up to 8–12 weeks)
	Start low dose
	Utilize opioids, NSAIDs, and adjuvants
	Discontinue due to
	Lack of analgesia
	Side effects
	Lack of functional improvement
STEP VIII	Stable phase (stable—moderate doses)
	Monthly refills
	Assess for four A's
	Analgesia
	Activity
	Aberrant behavior
	Adverse effect
	Manage side effects
STEP IX	Adherence monitoring
	Prescription monitoring programs
	Random drug screens
	Pill counts
STEP X	Outcomes
	Successful—continue
	Stable doses
	Analgesia, activity
	No abuse, side effects
	Failed—discontinue
	Dose escalation
	No analgesia
	No activity
	Abuse side effects
	Noncompliance

polymorphisms. It is recommended to calculate an equivalent 24-hour dose, divide by the dosing schedule, then "under dose" and subsequently titrate to effect.[64] Patients should be given a long-acting agent for continuous pain relief and a short acting agent for breakthrough pain.[59] Start with a low dose in opioid naïve patients, assess response and then increase by 25% to 50% for mild to moderate pain, and 50% to 100% for severe, persistent pain.[53]

Adverse effects include constipation, nausea, urinary retention, confusion, sedation, pruritis, respiratory depression, and syndrome of inappropriate antidiuretic hormone.[50] Patients often develop tolerance to these effects except for constipation and syndrome of inappropriate antidiuretic hormone. Patients should begin a bowel regimen when initiating opioid therapy including a stool softener (docusate) and a stimulant laxative (senna, bisacodyl) with dose titration to achieve a bowel movement at least every other day.[54,59]

Tolerance to opioids occurs when a higher dose of an opioid is needed to achieve the same effect.[53] If tolerance occurs, consider increasing the dose of the medication. If this is unsuccessful consider switching to another opioid as there may be incomplete cross tolerance.[53,59] Physical dependence is seen when patients are maintained on opioids and experience a "withdrawal syndrome" when the medication is abruptly discontinued. When discontinuing opioid therapy, taper the dose slowly to avoid withdrawal symptoms. Physical dependence is expected with chronic opioid therapy and is not synonymous with addiction. Addiction is a compulsive disorder in which an individual becomes preoccupied with obtaining and using a substance, the continued use of which results in a decreased quality of life.[53,59] The risk of addiction is low in patients who have no history of alcohol or substance abuse but all patients should be followed for aberrant behavior suggestive of opioid addiction. These include adverse consequences of opioid use, impaired control over medication use, and craving or preoccupation with opioids. In patients with a history of substance abuse, providing the patient with a controlled substance contract prior to prescribing the medication will help ensure the patient has a clear understanding of their responsibilities.[64]

Adjuvant Analgesics for Neuropathic Pain

A variety of agents have demonstrated efficacy against various types of neuropathic pain including anticonvulsants, antidepressants, topical lidocaine, opioids and tramadol but few are U.S. Food and Drug Administration (FDA) approved for specific types of neuropathic pain.[57] Acetaminophen and NSAIDs are generally less effective for neuropathic pain. Anticonvulsants, antidepressants, and local anesthestics typically reduce neuropathic pain by

Table 18-5. Opioid Analgesics [50,60,63]

Generic Name	Duration of Effect—Immediate Release (h)	Initial Dosing Regimen	Equianalgesic Dose (mg)	Comments
μ-Opioid receptor agonist				
Morphine	4–5	*Immediate release*		Hepatic and renal dysfunction may prolong effects
		IV: 10 mg IV q3–4h	10	
		PO: 15–30 mg q3–5h	30	
		Controlled release		
		MS Contin 15–30 mg q1 h		
		Oramorph SR 15–30 mg q 12h		
		Kadian 20 mg q24h		
		Avinza 30 mg q24h		
Hydromorphone	4–5	*Immediate release*	1.5	Useful agent for patients with renal dysfunction
		IV: 1.5 mg q3–4h	7.5	
		PO: 2–8 mg q3–4h		
Codeine	4–6	*Controlled release*		Available in combination with acetaminophen or aspirin
		PO: 12 mg q12h		
		PO: 30–60 mg q3–4h	NA	
Oxycodone	3–6	*Immediate release*		Available in combination with acetaminophen
		PO: 10–30 mg q4h		
		Controlled release	20–30	
		PO: 10 mg q12h		
Hydrocodone	4–8	*PO: 5–10 mg q4–6h	NA	Available in combination with acetaminophen and ibuprofen
Fentanyl	24–48	Transdermal: 25 mcg/h q72h	12.5–25 mcg/h	It takes 12–24 h to observe optimal analgesia
Meperidine	2–4	Not recommended for chronic pain	75–300	Not recommended for chronic pain
Methadone	4–8	IV: 2.5–10 mg q3–4h	Variable	Antagonist activity at the NDMA receptor which may contribute to neuropathic pain relief
	†22–48	PO: 5–20 mg q4–8h	Variable	
Propoxyphene	3–4	PO*: 65 mg q4h	NA similar to codeine	Weak analgesic. Avoid using in older adults
μ-Opioid receptor partial agonist				
Tramadol	9	PO*: 50–100 mg q6h	NA similar to codeine	Avoid use with seizure history. Dose reduce in older adults and patients with renal dysfunction
		Maximum dose: 400 mg/d		

*Starting dose only (equianalgesia not established).
†Repeated doses.
NA, not available.

30% to 50% in those patients that experience relief. No single agent is effective for all patients or all symptoms, likely reflective of the incompletely understood pathophysiology of the different components of neuropathic pain. It is advisable to try a different agent with a different mechanism of action, or utilize combination therapy with an opioid if a patient does not experience complete relief. Table 18-6 provides key information for prescribing the antidepressants and anticonvulsants with the most evidence to support their use in neuropathic pain.[57,63,66–69]

Antidepressants. Tricyclic antidepressants (TCAs) provide analgesia independent from their antidepressant activity at lower doses than those needed to treat depression.[57] TCAs inhibit both norepineprhine and serotonin and this likely contributes to analgesia. There have been several randomized controlled trials demonstrating the efficacy of TCAs in postherpetic neuralgia and diabetic peripheral neuropathy as well as a metanalysis corroborating the results. TCAs should be the initial therapy for patients with neuropathic pain and

Table 18-6. Selected Adjuvant Analgesics for Neuropathic Pain[57,63,65–69]

Drug Class	Number Needed to Treat and/or FDA Approval	Initial Dose (mg)	Titration (mg)	Maximum Daily Dose (mg)	Duration of Adequate Trial	Comments
TCA Amitriptyline Desipramine Nortriptyline	2 for neuropathic pain 1.3 for DPN 2.2 for PHN	10–25 (q HS)	10–25 per d (every 3–5 d)	75–150 per d	6–8 weeks with at least 1–2 weeks at maximum tolerated dose	✓ May be useful in concomitant insomnia or depression ✓ Sedation, weight gain, and anticholingeric effects are common ✓ Avoid in patient with cardiac conduction abnormalities, recent cardiac events, heart block, ischemic heart disease ✓ Avoid use in narrow angle glaucoma, high risk for suicide, and elderly patients ✓ Desipramine and nortriptyline have fewer anticholinergic effects than amitriptyline
Serotonin/ Norepinephrine reuptake inhibitor Duloxetine	FDA approval in DPN	60 daily	May start with lower doses in elderly patients or renal impairment	60 per d bid in fibromyalgia)	2–3 weeks	✓ Avoid use if history of substantial alcohol use or liver dysfunction ✓ May cause urinary hesitancy ✓ Avoid use if CrCL<30 mL/min
Anticonvulsant Gabapentin	4.3 for chronic pain 2.9 for DPN 3.9 for PHN FDA approval in PHN	100–300 (q HS) or 100–300 (tid)	100–300 tid (every 1–7 d as tolerated)	1800–3600 per d	3–8 weeks for titration plus 1–2 weeks at maximum tolerated dose	✓ Dizziness, somnolence, gastrointestinal complaints are common adverse events ✓ May exacerbate cognitive impairment in elderly patients ✓ Reduce dose if CrCL <60 mL/min ✓ Doses over 1800 mg/d have not shown benefit for PHN
Pregabalin	FDA approval in DPN and PHN	50 (tid) or 75 (bid)	100 per d(tid after 1 week)	300 per d	2–4 weeks at maximum tolerated dose	✓ Reduce if CrCL <60 c/min ✓ Dizziness, somnolence, edema and weight gain are common adverse events.
Carbamazepine	1.8 FDA approval in trigeminal neuralgia	100 (bid)	100 per d (q7d)	1200 (in divided doses)	NA	✓ Sedation, ataxia, fatigue, vertigo, blurred vision are dose related adverse effects ✓ Transient leukopenia, rare aplastic anemia ✓ Rash ✓ Monitor liver function tests, complete blood count, and serum drug concentration
Phenytoin	2.1 for DPN	150 daily	50 per d q (1–2 weeks)	300–400 per d	NA	✓ Sedation, ataxia, nystagmus, emesis, blurred vision are dose related adverse effects ✓ Transient leukopenia, thrombocytopenia, agranulocytosis ✓ Rash ✓ Monitor liver function tests, complete blood count, and serum drug concentration

TCA, tricyclic antidepressant; DPN, diabetic peripheral neuropathy; PHN, postherpetic neuralgia; NA, not available.

coexisting insomnia or depression. A baseline electrocardiogram is recommended in patients at risk for cardiac conduction abnormalities because TCAs predispose patients to arrhythmias, heart block, and postural hypotension.[57] TCAs should be avoided in patients with suicidal thoughts as they may be fatal in overdose.[63] TCAs are generally initiated at lower doses and titrated up to minimize adverse effects including sedation and orthostatic hypotension. Nortriptyline and desipramine may be preferred over amitriptyline because of fewer anticholinergic adverse effects.[55] TCAs are generally the least expensive option to treat peripheral neuropathy.

Selective serotonin reuptake inhibitors (SSRIs) have not been shown to be as effective as drugs with norepinephrine reuptake inhibition including duloxetine, venlafaxine, and TCAs. Among the SSRIs, only paroxetine and citalopram have been shown to provide benefit.[57] Although SSRIs may be better tolerated than TCAs, they should be considered a second line option to antidepressants with norepinephrine reuptake inhibition.

Anticonvulsants. Anticonvulsants are commonly used for neuropathic pain, especially the newer agents because of better side effect profiles and no need for serum drug monitoring. Gabapentin is a structural analog of GABA, but does not influence synthesis, uptake or binding of GABA; rather it appears to have activity at voltage-gated calcium channels.[63] It has been shown to significantly reduce mean daily pain scores in both postherpetic neuralgia and diabetic peripheral neuropathy.[57] The most common side effect is sedation; titrating the dose over 3 to 8 weeks will allow for tolerance to develop. Pregabalin, another structural analog of GABA, has also been shown to be effective in postherpetic neuralgia and diabetic neuropathy and may be easier to titrate than gabapentin because of a more favorable pharmacokinetic profile.[55] Carbamazepine was originally proven effective in trigeminal neuralgia and has demonstrated efficacy for diabetic neuropathy, but has more adverse effects than newer anticonvulsants. Dose-related side effects include fatigue, sedation, ataxia, vertigo, blurred vision, nausea, and vomiting. Hematologic monitoring is recommended as it rarely causes bone marrow suppression and irreversible aplastic anemia.[55] Oxcarbazepine, sodium valproate, topiramate, levetiracetam, and zonisamide have limited data supporting use in neuropathic pain.[57]

Topical Therapy. Topical agents include capsaicin and the topical lidocaine patch. They are often used in combination with other oral agents.[57] Both work locally at the site of application with minimal systemic absorption, and should only be applied to intact skin. Lidocaine appears to act by inhibition of voltage-gated sodium channels.[57] In postherpetic neuralgia, topical lidocaine is most effective in the earlier phase of the disease when peripheral nociceptors are sensitized. As the disease progresses and these receptors are lost, pain is caused by central mechanisms, and treatments that act centrally are more effective. Topical lidocaine works quickly without need for titration, and there is minimal risk for drug interactions. It is currently FDA approved for application for 12 hours, then removed for 12 hours. This provides inadequate relief for some patients; recent studies have explored alternate dosing regimens and found no increase in adverse systemic effects.[57]

Capsaicin is thought to increase the pain threshold by locally depleting substance P from the membranes of type C nociceptive fibers.[57] This occurs with repeated application and capsaicin must be applied four times daily for several weeks before benefit is observed. Patients may experience significant burning at the site of application, thus many patients will not continue therapy long enough to derive benefit. The burning subsides with continued application, and usually correlates with the onset of efficacy.[57] Patients should wash their hands following application to prevent application to other areas of the body. Clinical trials in postherpetic neuralgia and diabetic peripheral neuropathy have shown mixed results, although anecdotally it has been effective for selected patients.[57]

Opioids. Opioids are not first line therapy for neuropathic pain, but they can be titrated quickly, and can help control severe pain.[55,57] Morphine has been studied in combination with gabapentin. This results in reduction of pain and improved daily functioning with lower doses of each medication and a lower rate of adverse effects.[65] Methadone is beneficial in some patients and has activity at the N-methyl-D-aspartate receptor which contributes to neuropathic pain relief. Controlled release oxycodone and tramadol also have shown benefit.[55]

Other. Baclofen may be helpful in lancinating, paroxysmal neuropathic pain and painful spasticity. There are case reports of efficacy in neuropathic pain and fibromyalgia with tizanidine, another antispasticity agent.[55]

INTERVENTIONAL THERAPY

Interventional techniques should be used in conjunction with other modalities, and may be useful in diagnosing the source of pain as well as in pain management.[53] Some effective techniques include neural blockade, neuroaugmentation or provision of intraspinal drug delivery. The latter may provide analgesia at a lower dose, and therefore with fewer systemic side effects.[53,71]

Neural Blockade

Diagnostic blocks may be done to determine the anatomic source of pain, and to differentiate somatic from visceral pain, local from referred pain, and peripheral from central pain. They may also help determine whether a painful deformity is mechanically fixed or a result of neurally-mediated muscle spasm.[53] Nerve blocks using local anesthetics and steroids can be therapeutic in specific pain syndromes including radicular pain, rotator cuff injury, tendonitis, and bursitis.

Neuroaugmentation

Implanted nerve stimulators are generally most effective for the treatment of peripheral neuropathic pain syndromes.[53] Transcutaneous electrical nerve stimulation (TENS) should be considered as an early management option because of low complexity and low risk.[52] Peripheral stimulation may benefit those with painful peripheral neuropathies such as upper or lower limb mononeuropathies or facial neuralgic conditions. It should be reserved for those who have responded to a diagnostic sequence of local neural blockade and a stimulation trial.[52] Spinal cord stimulation may improve neuropathic pain originating at cervical, thoracic, or lumbrosacral spinal nerve roots or cord, but should be considered only for those who fail oral medications.[52]

NONPHARMACOLOGIC

Rehabilitation

Pain rehabilitation is a useful and cost-effective part of comprehensive pain therapy encompassing pharmacological, psychological, surgical, and interventional approaches as appropriate for the patient.[53] The goals of pain rehabilitation include restoring function, alleviating pain, and improving pain management skills for patients with persistent pain. Adjuvant pain rehabilitation options include physical and/or occupational therapy, exercise programs directed toward the specific pain condition, ergonomic modifications, and vocational rehabilitation.

Cognitive Behavioral Therapy

Pain medications do not reverse tissue damage and the pain will return if medication is discontinued in patients with persistent pain. In addition, a patient's perception of pain may persist despite pharmacologic treatment. Thus, psychological therapy, including cognitive and behavioral treatments may contribute. Individual cognitive behavioral psychotherapy is insight-based with emphasis on cognitive strategies for life planning, pacing of activities, and acceptance of physical limitations and their emotional consequences.[53] It produces significant improvements in pain experience, mood/affect, cognitive coping and appraisal, pain behavior, activity level, and social role function compared to a waiting list control. Psychological therapy produces improvements in pain experience, positive coping and social role function compared with other treatments.[70]

SPECIAL POPULATION

Elderly Patients

Patients 65 years and older commonly report pain. Comorbid illnesses may cloud the determination of pain etiology, and use of other medication increases the risk of adverse effects and drug interactions. Cognitive impairment may necessitate use of simplified pain scales or reliance on nonverbal cues to suggest pain. Verbal descriptor scales, numeric scales and faces scales have demonstrated reliability and validity in older adults.[71] Behaviors suggestive of pain in those who have difficulty communicating include bracing, rubbing, guarding, agitation, delirium, altered mobility/activity and facial expressions.[71] These behaviors should be evaluated with respect to established baseline behaviors when possible.

Pharmacotherapy is commonly used for persistent pain in older patients, although clinical trials often exclude patients 65 years and older.[72] In general, older patients have decreased hepatic and renal function and are prone to increased drug concentrations and accumulation of drug. To manage chronic pain, practitioners should "start low and go slow." The American Geriatrics Society Panel on Persistent Pain in Older Persons has recommended some practice adjustments when caring for older patients.[72] Acetaminophen, scheduled around the clock, is a suitable choice for mild to moderate pain in older persons. Those with multiple comorbidities have an unacceptably high rate of life-threatening gastrointestinal bleeding with long-term use of nonselective NSAIDs. Nephrotoxicity may result if the patient becomes dehydrated or is taking interacting medications such as angiotensin converting enzyme (ACE) inhibitors. For bone pain or similar conditions, practitioners may use a nonselective NSAID with a gastrointestinal protective medication such as a proton-pump inhibitor or histamine$_2$ antagonist, or a nonacetlyated salicylate, or a COX-2 inhibitor. Propoxyphene has similar efficacy to aspirin and acetaminophen but should be avoided in elderly patients because of drug accumulation, neuroexcitatory effects, ataxia and dizziness.[72] When initiating opioid therapy, the clinician should be especially vigilant seeking and managing adverse events, and titrating medication carefully. Meperidine should be avoided in elderly patients. TCAs should be used cautiously, because of anticholinergic adverse effects including urinary retention, constipation, blurred vision, and orthostasis which can contribute to falls.[72] Gabapentin, when slowly titrated to allow tolerance to develop to dizziness and sedation, may have fewer adverse effects and similar efficacy for management of neuropathic pain. Nonpharmacologic strategies should be strongly considered in elderly patients because of safety, and can be adapted to their level of physical and cognitive function.[72]

EVIDENCE-BASED SUMMARY

- The goal of chronic pain management is to decrease pain when possible and improve function for the patient with persistent pain
- Patient goals should be "*SMART*"—*S*pecific, *M*easurable, *A*chievable, *R*ealistic, and *T*imebased
- Perform a comprehensive pain assessment of all patients with persistent pain and use the patient's self-report as the basis for the assessment
- Utilize a valid measurement tool to assess pain at regular intervals to determine efficacy of pain management strategy
- A referral to a specialized pain center may be indicated for diagnostic assistance, treatment planning for initial and long-term pain management, advice on optimal pharmacotherapy, or utilization of management strategies that require specific expertise or training (e.g., methadone or epidural opioid pump).
- Taper and discontinue ineffective medications and try a different strategy, either a new class of drugs, or nondrug alternatives
- Utilize combination therapy with complementary mechanisms of action if monotherapy is ineffective or poorly tolerated
- Consider a multimodality approach that employs both pharmacologic and nonpharmacologic strategies

Nociceptive Pain
- Give adequate doses of medication and titrate to provide pain relief with manageable adverse effects
- Anticipate and manage side effects

Neuropathic Pain
- A TCA is the preferred agent in patients with concomitant insomnia or depression
- An antiepileptic agent, such as gabapentin or pregabalin, are preferable in patients with contraindications or intolerance to a TCA
- Medications should be titrated to an appropriate dose to provide analgesia and given an adequate trail to determine response

REFERENCES

1. Middleton KR, Hing E. *National Hospital Ambulatory Medical Care Survey: 2003 Outpatient Department Summary. Advance Data from Vital and Health Statistics*, Vol. 366. Hyattsville, MD: National Center for Health Statistics; 2005.
2. Gureje O, Von Korff M, Simon GE, et al. Persistent pain and well-being. A world health organization study in primary care. *JAMA.* 1998;280:147–151.
3. Breivik H, Collett B, Ventafridda V, at al. Survey of chronic pain in Europe: Prevalence, impact on daily life, and treatment. *Eur J Pain.* 2006;10:287–333.
4. Donovan M, Dillon P, McGuire L. Incidence and characteristics of pain in a sample of medical-surgical inpatients. *Pain.* 1987;30:69–78.
5. Good M, Stanton-Hicks M, Grass JA, et al. Pain outcomes after intestinal surgery. *Outcomes Manag Nurs Pract.* 2001;5:41–46.
6. Cleeland CS, Gonin R, Hatfield AK, et al. Pain and its treatment in outpatients with metastatic cancer. *N Engl J Med.* 1994;330:592–596.
7. Marks RM, Sachar EJ. Undertreatment of medical inpatients with narcotic analgesics. *Ann Intern Med.* 1973; 78:173–181.
8. Sriwatanakul K, Weis OF, Alloza JL, et al. Analysis of narcotic analgesic usage in the treatment of postoperative pain. *JAMA.* 1983;250:926–929.
9. Warfield CA, Kahn CH. Acute pain management: Programs in US hospitals and experiences and attitudes among US adults. *Anesthesiology.* 1995;83:1090–1094.
10. Miaskowski C, Nichols R, Brody R, et al. Assessment of patient satisfaction utilizing the American Pain Society's Quality Assurance Standards on acute and cancer-related pain. *J Pain Symptom Manage.* 1994;9:5–11.
11. The SUPPORT Principal Investigators. A controlled trial to improve care for seriously ill hospitalized patients. The study to understand prognoses and preferences for outcomes and risks of treatments (SUPPORT). *JAMA.* 1995; 274:1591–1598.
12. Wolfe J, Grier HE, Klar N, et al. Symptoms and suffering at the end of life in children with cancer. *N Engl J Med.* 2000;342:326–333.
13. Kehlet H. Surgical stress: The role of pain and analgesia. *Br J Anaesth.* 1989;63:189–195.
14. Gottschalk A, Smith DS, Jobes DR, et al. Preemptive epidural analgesia and recovery from radical prostatectomy. A randomized controlled trial. *JAMA.* 1998;279: 1076–1082.
15. Kiecolt-Glaser JK, Page GG, Marucha PT, et al. Psychological influences on surgical recovery: Perspectives from psychoneuroimmunology. *Am Psychol.* 1998;53:1209–1218.
16. Coley KC, Williams BA, DaPos SV, et al. Retrospective evaluation of unanticipated admissions and readmissions after same day surgery and associated costs. *J Clin Anesth.* 2002;14:349–353.
17. Cepeda MS, African JM, Polo R, et al. What decline in pain intensity is meaningful to patients with acute pain? *Pain.* 2003;105(1–2):151–157.

18. Bonica JJ. Importance of effective pain control. *Acta Anaesthesiol Scand.* 1987;31(Suppl 85):1–16.

19. Carr DB, Goudas L. Acute pain. *Lancet.* 1999;353: 2051–2058.

20. Kehlet H, Holte K. Effect of postoperative analgesia on surgical outcome. *Br J Anaesth.* 2001;87:62–72.

21. Strassels SA, Chen C, Carr DB. Postoperative analgesia: Economics, resource use, and patient satisfaction in an Urban teaching hospital. *Anesth Analg.* 2002;94:130–137.

22. Perkins FM, Kehlet H. Chronic pain as an outcome of surgery – a review of predictive factors. *Anesthesiology.* 2000; 93:1123–1133.

23. Stewart WF, Ricci JA, Chee E, et al. Lost productive time and cost due to common pain conditions in the US workforce. *JAMA.* 2003;290:2443–2454.

24. Berger A, Dukes EM, Oster G. Clinical characteristics and economic costs of patients with painful neuropathic disorders. *J Pain.* 2004;5:143–149.

25. Gordois A, Scuffham P, Shearer A, et al. The health care costs of diabetic peripheral neuropathy in the US. *Diabetes Care.* 2003;26:1790–1795.

26. IASP Task Force on Taxonomy. Part III: Pain Terms, A Current List with Definitions and Notes on Usage. In: Merskey H, Bogduk N, eds. *Classification of Chronic Pain,* 2nd ed. Seattle, WA: IASP Press; 1994:209.

27. Pasero C, Paice JA, McCaffery M. Basic mechanisms underlying the causes and effects of pain. In: McCaffery M, Pasero C, eds. *Pain: Clinical Manual,* 2nd ed. St. Louis, MO: Mosby; 1999.

28. Fishman S, Berger L. *The War on Pain.* New York, NY: HarperCollins; 2000.

29. Ready LB, Edwards WT, eds. *Management of Acute Pain: A Practical Guide.* Seattle, WA: IASP; 1992.

30. Carr DB, Goudas L. Acute pain. *Lancet.* 1999;353: 2051–2058.

31. Berger ML, Bingefors K, Hedblom EC, et al., eds. *Health Care, Cost, Quality, and Outcomes. ISPOR Book of Terms.* Lawrenceville, NJ: International Society for Pharmacoeconomics and Outcomes Research; 2003:129.

32. Ware JE, Sherbourne CD. The MOS 36-item short-form health survey (SF-36). I. Conceptual framework and item selection. *Med Care.* 1992;30:473–483.

33. Jensen MP, Karoly P. Self-report scales and procedures for assessing pain in adults. In: Turk DC, Melzack R, eds. *Handbook of Pain Assessment,* 2nd ed. New York, NY: Guilford Press; 2001:15–34.

34. Paice JA, Cohen FL. Validity of a verbally-administered numeric rating scale to measure cancer pain intensity. *Cancer Nurs.* 1997;20:88–93.

35. Price DD, Harkins SW. Combined use of experimental pain and visual analog scales in providing standardized measurement of clinical pain. *Clin J Pain.* 1987;3:1–8.

36. Jensen MP, Karoly P, Braver S. The measurement of clinical pain intensity: A comparison of six methods. *Pain.* 1986;27:117–126.

37. Price DD, Bush FM, Long S, et al. A comparison of pain measurement characteristics of mechanical visual analog and simple numerical rating scales. *Pain.* 1994;56: 217–226.

38. Melzack R. The McGill Pain Questionnaire: Major properties and scoring methods. *Pain.* 1975;1:277–299.

39. Melzack R, Katz J. The McGill Pain Questionnaire: Appraisal and current status. In: Turk DC, Melzack R, eds. *Handbook of Pain Assessment,* 2nd ed. New York, NY: Guilford Press; 2001:35–52.

40. Daut RL, Cleeland CS, Flanery RC. Development of the Wisconsin Brief Pain Questionnaire to assess pain in cancer and other diseases. *Pain.* 1983;17:197–210.

41. Mendoza TR, Chen C, Brugger A, et al. The utility and validity of the modified brief pain inventory in a multiple-dose postoperative analgesic trial. *Clin J Pain.* 2004;20: 357–362.

42. Keller S, Bann CM, Dodd SL, et al. Validity of the brief pain inventory for use in documenting the outcomes of patients with noncancer pain. *Clin J Pain.* 2004;20:309–318.

43. Daut RL, Cleeland CS. The prevalence and severity of pain in cancer. *Cancer.* 1982;50:1913–1918.

44. Ware JE, Jr., Snow KK, Kosinski M, et al. *SF-36 Health Survey Manual and Interpretation Guide.* Boston, MA: Medical Outcomes Trust; 1993.

45. McHorney CA, Ware JE, Jr., Raczek AE. The MOS 36-item short-form health survey (SF-36): II, psychometric and clinical tests of validity in measuring physical and mental health constructs. *Med Care.* 1993;31:247–263.

46. Rogers WH, Wittink HM, Ashburn MA, et al. Using the "TOPS", an outcomes instrument for multidisciplinary outpatient pain treatment. *Pain Med.* 2000;1:55–67.

47. Rogers WH, Wittink H, Wagner A, et al. Assessing individual outcomes during outpatient multidisciplinary chronic pain treatment by means of an augmented SF-36. *Pain Med.* 2000;1:44–54.

48. Ware J, Jr., Kosinski M, Keller SD. A 12-Item Short-Form Health Survey: Construction of scales and preliminary tests of reliability and validity. *Med Care.* 1996;34:220–233.

49. The SF-8 Health Survey. Available at: http://www.sf-36.org/tools/sf8.shtml. Accessed May 19, 2006.

50. Bauman TJ. Pain management. In: Dipiro JT, Talbert RL, Yee GC, eds et al. *Pharmacotherapy: A Pathophysiologic Approach,* 6th ed. New York, NY: McGraw-Hill; 2005:1089.

51. Institute for Clinical Systems Improvement (ICSI). *Assessment and Management of Chronic Pain.* Bloomington, MN: Institute for Clinical Systems Improvement; 2005.

52. Wilson PR, Caplan RA, Connis RT, et al. Practice Guidelines for chronic pain management: A report by the American society of anesthesiologists task force on pain management, chronic pain section. *Anesthesiology.* 1997; 86:995–1004.

53. Wisconsin Medical Society Task Force on Pain Management. Guidelines for the assessment and management of chronic pain. *Wis Med J.* 2004;103:14–42.

54. Byers MR, Bonica JJ. Peripheral pain mechanisms and nociceptor plasticity. In: Loeser JD, Butler SH, Chapman CR, eds et al. *Bonica's Management of Pain,* 3rd ed. Philadelphia, PA, Lippincott; 2001:26.

55. Pain Management: The Online Series. Release date, December 2005, expiration date, December 2006. American Medical Association. Available at: http://www.ama-cmeonline.com/. Accessed May 15, 2006.

56. Woolf CJ. Pain: Moving from symptoms control toward mechanism-specific pharmacologic management. *Ann Intern Med.* 2004;140:441–451.

57. Stacey BR. Management of peripheral neuropathic pain. *Am J phys Med Rehabil.* 2005;84:S4–S16.

58. Miyoshi HR. Systemic nonopioid analgesics. In: Loeser JD, Butler SH, Chapman CR, eds et al. *Bonica's Management of Pain*, 3rd ed. Philadelphia, PA: Lippincott; 2001: 1668.

59. Whelton A. Appropriate analgesia: An evidence-based evaluation of the role of acetaminophen in pain management. *Am J Ther.* 2005;12:43–45.

60. Miaskowski C, Cleary J, Burney R, et at. *Guideline for the Management of Cancer Pain in Adults and Children. APS Clinical Practice Guidelines Series*, Vol. 3. Glenview, IL: American Pain Society; 2005.

61. Arthritis Advisory Committee and Drug Safety and Risk Management Advisory Committee. Celecoxib and valdecoxib cardiovascular safety. FDA Advisory Committee briefing document. Available at: http://www.fda .gov/ohrms/dockets/ac/05/slides/2005-4090S1_10_ Pfizer-Valdecoxib-Parecoxib_files/frame.htm. Accessed May 18, 2006.

62. Spiegel B, Farid M, Dulari G, et al. Comparing rates of dyspepsia with coxibs vs. NSAID + PPI: A meta-analysis. *Am J Med.* 2006;119:448.e27–448.e36.

63. Lacy CF, Armstrong LL, Goldman MP et al., eds. *Lexi-Drugs for Palm OS*. Lexi-Comp, Inc. Available at: http:// www.lexi.com. Updated May 16, 2006.

64. Trescot AM, Boswell, MV, Atluri SL, et al. Opioid guidelines in the management of chronic non-cancer pain. *Pain Physician.* 2006;9:1–40.

65. Saarto T, Wiffen PJ. Antidepressants for neuropathic pain. *Cochrane Database Syst Rev.* 2005;3:CD005454.

66. Wiffen P, Collins S, Mcquay H, et al. Anticonvulsant drugs for acute and chronic pain. *Cochrane Database Syst Rev.* 2005;3:CD001133.

67. Wiffen PJ, McQuay HJ, Moore RA. Carbamazepine for acute and chronic pain. *Cochrane Database Syst Rev.* 2005; 3:CD005451.

68. Wiffen PJ, McQuay HJ, Edwards JE, Moore RA. Gabapentin for acute and chronic pain. *Cochrane Database Syst Rev.* 2005;3:CD005452.

69. Gilron I, Bailey JM, Tu D, et al. Morphine, Gabapentin, or their combination for neuropathic pain. *NJEM.* 2005;352: 1324–1334.

70. Boswell MV, Shah RV, Everett CR, et al. Interventional techniques in the management of chronic spinal pain: Evidence based practice guidelines. *Pain Physician.* 2005: 8:1–47.

71. Morley S, Eccleston C, Williams A. Systematic review and meta-analysis of randomized controlled trials of cognitive behavior therapy and behaviour therapy for chronic pain in adults, excluding headache. *Pain.* 1999;80:1–13.

72. Charlton JE, ed. *Core Curriculum for Professional Education in Pain*. Seattle, WA: IASP Press; 2005.

73. American Geriatrics Society Panel on Persistent Pain in Older Persons. The management of persistent pain in older persons. *J Am Geriat Soc.* 2002:50:S205–S224.

Chapter 19

Headache Disorders

Deborah S. Minor and Dena Jackson

SEARCH STRATEGY

A systematic search of the medical literature was performed in November 2004 and January 2007. The search, limited to human subjects and English language journals, included the National Guideline Clearinghouse, PubMed, and UpToDate®.

Headache is one of the most common complaints encountered by health care practitioners. Headache may be symptomatic of a distinct pathologic process (secondary headache) or may occur without an underlying cause (primary headache). Most recurrent headaches are the result of a benign chronic headache disorder but headache may also be associated with a serious underlying medical condition.[1] The primary headache disorders are migraine, tension-type, and cluster headache. The differential for secondary headache is quite long but may include infection, cerebral hemorrhage, or mass lesions. A complete headache history and physical examination are essential for accurate headache diagnosis. Primary care providers should be able to diagnose these conditions and provide appropriate therapeutic interventions. This chapter will focus on the diagnosis and management of the primary headache disorders.

CLINICAL PRESENTATION

The presentation of migraine can vary and is usually divided into several phases (premonitory, aura, headache, and resolution). Premonitory symptoms are experienced by 20% to 60% of patients, usually a few hours or days before headache onset.[2,3] Symptoms vary widely among migraine patients, but are generally consistent among individuals. Common neurologic symptoms include phonophobia, photophobia, hyperosmia, and difficulty in concentrating. Psychological symptoms include anxiety, depression, euphoria, irritability, drowsiness, hyperactivity, and restlessness. Constitutional symptoms include stiff neck, yawning, thirst, food cravings, and anorexia.[4]

The migraine aura is a complex of positive and negative focal neurologic symptoms that precede, accompany, or, rarely, follow an attack. Aura is experienced by approximately 31% of migraine patients and is most often visual. Other aura symptoms include paresthesias involving the arms or face, dysphasia, or aphasia.[2,4]

Migraines may occur at any time of the day or night but commonly occur early in the morning. The onset is gradual and the pain reaches a peak in a few minutes or hours. If left untreated, migraines typically last between 4 and 72 hours. The pain is most often unilateral, frontotemporal, and throbbing or pulsating. However, it, may be bilateral at onset or become generalized during the attack. Gastrointestinal symptoms are common and include nausea, emesis, anorexia, food cravings, constipation, diarrhea, and abdominal cramping.

Presentation of tension-type headache differs from that of migraine in that premonitory symptoms and aura are absent. The pain is commonly bilateral and is described as a dull, nonpulsatile tightness or pressure. The classical description is that of pain having a "hatband" pattern. Associated symptoms are generally absent although mild photophobia and phonophobia may be reported.[2,4]

Attacks of cluster headaches, as the name suggests, occur in cluster periods, lasting from 2 weeks to 3 months in most patients, followed by pain-free or remission intervals. They occur most often at night and appear to be more common in the spring and fall. Pain peaks quickly, is excruciating and penetrating though generally not throbbing, and is located unilaterally in orbital, supraorbital, or temporal locations. There can be autonomic features on the side of the pain including conjunctival injection, lacrimation, and nasal stuffiness or rhinorrhea. Ipsilateral scalp and facial tenderness, ptosis, miosis, and periorbital edema are also described. During the cluster period, attacks may occur once in 2 days up to 8 times per day.[2,4,5]

PHYSICAL FINDINGS

Physical findings may be absent in individuals presenting with primary headaches. Secondary headaches or those caused by organic disease can generally be identified or excluded on the basis of the history as well as general medical and detailed neurological examinations. In the headache evaluation, diagnostic alarms should be identified. These include acute onset of the "first" or "worst" headache ever, accelerating pattern of headache following subacute onset, onset of headache after the age of 50 years, headache associated with systemic illness (fever, nausea, vomiting, stiff neck, rash), headache with focal neurologic symptoms or papilledema, or new onset headache in a patient with cancer or HIV infection. The presence of any of these should be considered a diagnostic alarm and prompt further evaluation for the underlying etiology.

DIAGNOSTIC EVALUATION

A headache history is most important in establishing the diagnosis of migraine, cluster, or tension-type headache. The detailed headache history and physical examination findings generally dictate any further diagnostic evaluation. If secondary headache is suspected, appropriate diagnostic testing for the suspected organic disease may be pursued. Evaluation may include laboratory or imaging studies. In selected circumstances, serum chemistries, urine toxicology profiles, thyroid function, Lyme studies, complete blood count, antinuclear antibody, erythrocyte sedimentation rate, and antiphospholipid antibody titers may be considered.

The use of neuroimaging with computed tomography or magnetic resonance imaging is generally not indicated in migraine patients with normal neurologic examination findings, but should be considered in patients with unexplained abnormalities in neurological examination or with an atypical headache history.[6] Because migraines usually begin by the second or third decade of life, headaches beginning after the age of 50 years suggest an organic etiology such as a mass lesion, cerebrovascular disease, or temporal arteritis. Atypical features that might prompt imaging include an unstable pattern, new onset daily headache, or the absence of associated triggers. Although aura is typical, its absence should not be the sole trigger for imaging.

Table 19-1. International Headache Society Diagnostic Criteria for Migraine

Migraine without aura
At least 5 attacks
Headache attack lasts 4–72 h (untreated or unsuccessfully treated)
Headache has at least 2 of the following characteristics:
Unilateral location
Pulsating quality
Moderate or severe intensity
Aggravation by or avoidance of routine physical activity (i.e., walking or climbing stairs)
During headache at least one of the following occur:
Nausea, vomiting, or both
Photophobia and phonophobia
Not attributed to another disorder
Migraine with Aura (Classic Migraine)
At least 2 attacks
Migraine aura fulfills criteria for typical aura, hemiplegic aura, or basilar-type aura.
Not attributed to another disorder
Typical Aura
Fully reversible visual, sensory, or speech symptoms (or any combination) but no motor weakness
Homonymous or bilateral visual symptoms including positive features (e.g., flickering lights, spots, lines) or negative features (e.g., loss of vision), or unilateral sensory symptoms including positive features (e.g., visual loss, pins and needles) or negative features (e.g., numbness), or any combination
During typical aura one of following occurs:
At least one symptom develops gradually over a minimum of 5 min, or different symptoms occur in succession, or both
Each symptom lasts for at least 5 min and for no longer than 60 min
Headache that meets criteria for migraine without aura begins during the aura or follows aura within 60 min

Adapted from: Headache Classification Committee of the International Headache Society. The International Classification of Headache Disorders, 2nd ed. *Cephalalgia.* 2004;24(1):1–151.

The International Headache Society has recently updated the diagnostic criteria for migraine with and without aura (Table 19-1). Specific diagnostic criteria are provided within the International Headache Society classification system for tension-type and cluster headaches.[2]

RISK STRATIFICATION

A thorough headache history should always be obtained, including age at onset, attack frequency and timing, duration of attacks, precipitating or aggravating factors, ameliorating factors, description of neurologic symptoms, characteristics of the pain (quality, intensity, location, and radiation), associated signs and symptoms, treatment history, family and social history, and the impact of headaches on daily life.

Pharmacotherapeutic management of headache may be acute (e.g., symptomatic or abortive) or preventive (e.g., prophylactic) (Tables 19-2 and 19-3).

Table 19-2. Acute Migraine Therapies*

Medications	Dosage	Comments
Analgesics		
Acetaminophen	1000 mg at onset; repeat every 4–6 h as needed 2 tablets at onset and every 6 h	Maximum daily dose is 4 g
Acetaminophen 250 mg/aspirin 250 mg/ caffeine 65 mg		Available over-the-counter as Excedrin Migraine
Aspirin or acetaminophen with butalbital, caffeine	1–2 tablets every 4–6 h	Limit dose to 4 tablets/d and usage to 2 d/wk
Isometheptene 65 mg/dichloralphenazone 100 mg/acetaminophen 325 mg (Midrin)	2 capsules at onset; repeat 1 capsule every hour as needed	Maximum of 6 capsules/d and 20 capsules/mo
Nonsteroidal Anti-Inflammatory Drugs		
Aspirin	500–1000 mg every 4–6 h	Maximum daily dose is 4 g
Ibuprofen	200–800 mg every 6 h	Avoid doses >2.4 g/d
Naproxen sodium	550–825 mg at onset; may repeat 220 mg in 3–4 h	Avoid doses >1.375 g/d
Diclofenac potassium	50–100 mg at onset; may repeat 50 mg in 8 h	Avoid doses >150 mg/d
Ergotamine Tartrate		
Oral tablet (1 mg) with caffeine 100 mg	2 mg at onset; then 1–2 mg every 30 min as needed	Maximum dose is 6 mg/d or 10 mg/week; consider pretreatment with an antiemetic
Sublingual tablet (2 mg)		
Rectal suppository (2 mg) with caffeine 100 mg	Insert 1/2 to 1 suppository at onset; repeat after 1 h as needed	Maximum dose is 4 mg/d or 10 mg/wk; consider pretreatment with an antiemetic
Dihydroergotamine		
Injection 1 mg/mL	0.25–1 mg at onset IM or SC; repeat every hour as needed	Maximum dose is 3 mg/d; or 6 mg/wk
Nasal spray	1 spray (0.5 mg) in each nostril at onset; repeat sequence 15 min later (total dose is 2 mg or 4 sprays)	Maximum dose is 3 mg/d; Prime sprayer 4 times before using; do not tilt head back or inhale through nose while spraying; discard open ampules after 8 h
Serotonin Agonists (Triptans)		
Sumatriptan		
Injection	6 mg SC at onset; may repeat after 1 h if needed	Maximum daily dose is 12 mg
Oral tablets	25, 50, or 100 mg at onset; may repeat after 2 h if needed	Optimal dose is 50–100 mg, maximum daily dose is 200 mg
Nasal spray	5, 10, or 20 mg at onset; may repeat after 2 h if needed	Optimal dose is 20 mg; maximum daily dose is 40 mg; single-dose device delivering 5 or 20 mg; administer 1 spray in 1 nostril
Zolmitriptan	2.5 or 5 mg at onset as regular or orally disintegrating tablet; may repeat after 2 h if needed	Optimal dose is 2.5 mg, maximum dose is 10 mg/d, do not divide ODT dosage form
Nasal spray	5 mg at onset; may repeat after 2 h if needed	Maximum dose is 10 mg/d
Naratriptan	1 mg or 2.5 mg tablet at onset; may repeat after 4 h if needed	Optimal dose is 2.5 mg, maximum daily dose is 5 mg

(continued)

Table 19-2. Acute Migraine Therapies* *(Continued)*

Medications	Dosage	Comments
Serotonin Agonists (Triptans)		
Rizatriptan	5 or 10 mg at onset as regular or orally disintegrating tablet; may repeat after 2 h if needed	Optimal dose is 10 mg; maximum daily dose is 30 mg; onset of effect is similar with standard and orally disintegrating tablets; use 5 mg dose (15 mg/d max) in patients receiving propranolol
Almotriptan	6.25 or 12.5 mg at onset; may repeat after 2 h if needed	Optimal dose is 12.5 mg Maximum daily dose is 25 mg
Frovatriptan	2.5 or 5 mg at onset; may repeat in 2 h if needed	Optimal dose 2.5–5 mg, maximum daily dose is 7.5 mg (3 tablets)
Eletriptan	20 or 40 mg at onset; may repeat after 2 h if needed	Maximum single dose is 40 mg Maximum daily dose is 80 mg
Miscellaneous		
Butorphanol nasal spray	1 spray in 1 nostril (1 mg) at onset; repeat in 1 h if needed	Limit to 4 sprays/d; consider use only when nonopioid therapies are ineffective or not tolerated
Metoclopramide	10 mg IV at onset	Useful for acute relief in the office or emergency department setting
Prochlorperazine	10 mg IV or IM at onset	Useful for acute relief in the office or emergency department setting

*Limit use of symptomatic medications to 2 d/wk when possible to avoid medication-misuse headache.
IM, intramuscularly; SC, subcutaneously; IV, intravenously; ODT, orally disintegrating tablets.
Adapted from: Silberstein SD. Migraine. *Lancet.* 2004;363:381–391; Bigal ME, Lipton RB, Krymchantowski AV. The medical management of migraine. *Am J Ther.* 2004;11(2):130–140; Evans RW, Bigal ME, Grosberg B, Lipton RB. Target doses and titration schedules for migraine preventive medications. *Headache.* 2006;46:160–164.

Pharmacotherapy should be individualized based on drug efficacy, individual patient response, tolerability, comorbid conditions, and the clinical presentation and medical history. Abortive or acute therapies can be specific (e.g., ergots and triptans) or nonspecific (e.g., analgesics, antiemetics, nonsteroidal anti-inflammatory drugs [NSAIDs], corticosteroids) for the headache, and are most effective at relieving pain and associated symptoms when administered at the onset of headache.[3] A stratified-care approach, in which the selection of initial treatment is based on headache-related disability and symptom severity, is preferred.[6] Because severity varies in individuals, patients may be advised to use nonspecific agents for mild-to-moderate headache, while reserving specific medications for more severe attacks.

Preventive therapy should be considered for recurring headaches with significant disability; attacks requiring symptomatic medication more than twice per week; symptomatic therapies that are ineffective, contraindicated, or produce serious side effects; and uncommon headache variants causing profound disruption and(or) risk of neurologic injury. Efficacy of a prescribed prophylactic regimen should be reassessed periodically, and gradually reduced and discontinued after a prolonged headache-free interval.

Patients should be monitored for frequency, intensity, and duration of headaches, as well as for any change in the headache pattern. Careful monitoring is essential to initiate the most appropriate pharmacotherapy, document therapeutic successes and failures, identify medication contraindications, and prevent or minimize adverse events. The use of prescription and over-the-counter medications should be monitored to identify potential medication-misuse headache. Strict adherence to dosing guidelines should be stressed to minimize potential toxicity. Patterns of abortive medication use can be documented to establish the need

Table 19-3. Prophylactic Migraine Therapies

Medication	Dose
β-Adrenergic Antagonists	
Atenolol	25–100 mg/d
Metoprolol*	50–300 mg/d in divided doses
Nadolol	80–240 mg/d
Propranolol*,†	80–240 mg/d in divided doses
Timolol†	20–60 mg/d in divided doses
Antidepressants	
Amitriptyline	25–150 mg at bedtime
Doxepin	10–200 mg at bedtime
Imipramine	10–200 mg at bedtime
Nortriptyline	10–150 mg at bedtime
Protriptyline	5–30 mg at bedtime
Fluoxetine	10–80 mg/d
Venlafaxine*	37.5–225 mg/d
Phenelzine‡	15–60 mg/d in divided doses
Anticonvulsants	
Gabapentin	1800–2400 mg/d in divided doses
Topiramate†	25–200 mg/d in divided doses
Valproic acid	500–1500 mg/d in divided doses
Divalproex sodium†	
Verapamil*	240–360 mg/d in divided doses
Methysergide†,‡	2–8 mg/d in divided doses with food
Nonsteroidal Anti-Inflammatory Drugs‡	
Aspirin	1300 mg/d in divided doses
Ketoprofen*	150 mg/d in divided doses
Naproxen sodium*	350–1100 mg/d in divided doses
Vitamin B₂	400 mg/d

*Sustained-release formulation available.
†Approved by the U.S. Food and Drug Administration for prevention of migraine.
‡Daily or prolonged use limited by potential toxicity.
Adapted from: Silberstein SD. Migraine. *Lancet.* 2004;363:381–391; Ferrari MD, Roon KI, Lipton RB, Goadsby PJ. Oral triptans (serotonin 5_HT1B/1D agonists) in acute migraine treatment: A meta-analysis of 53 trials. *Lancet.* 2001;358:1558–1575; Evans RW, Bigal ME, Grosberg B, Lipton RB. Target doses and titration schedules for migraine preventive medications. *Headache.* 2006;46:160–164; Jensen R, Olesen J. Tension-type headache: An update on mechanisms and treatment. *Curr Opin Neurol.* 2000;13:285–289.

for prophylactic therapy. Prophylactic therapies should also be monitored closely for adverse reactions, abortive therapy needs, adequate dosing, and compliance.

MANAGEMENT

MIGRAINE HEADACHES

Nonpharmacologic and pharmacologic interventions are available for the management of migraine headaches. Drug therapy is the mainstay of treatment for most patients and is stratified according to the individual presentation, in both acute care and prevention (Figs. 19-1 and 19-2).

Nonpharmacologic Therapy

Nonpharmacologic therapy of acute migraine headache is limited, but may include application of ice to the head and periods of rest or sleep, usually in a dark, quiet environment. Prevention should begin with the identification and avoidance of factors that consistently provoke migraine attacks in the susceptible individual including food, environmental, behavioral or physiologic triggers or medications. Patients may also benefit from adherence to a wellness program including regular sleep, exercise, and eating habits, smoking cessation, and limited caffeine intake. Behavioral interventions such as relaxation therapy, biofeedback, and cognitive therapy are preventive treatment options for patients who prefer a nondrug therapy or when symptomatic therapies are poorly tolerated, contraindicated, or ineffective.[6]

Acute Migraine Therapy

Acute migraine treatment may involve the use of nonspecific or specific drugs, such as triptans or ergot alkaloids. Most experts recommend limiting the use of acute migraine therapies to *2 days per week* in order to avoid the development of medication misuse or rebound headache.[2,6,7] The syndrome appears to evolve as a self-sustaining, headache–medication cycle in which the headache returns as the medication effect wears off, leading to the consumption of more drugs for relief. The headache history often reflects the gradual onset of an atypical daily or near-daily headache with superimposed episodic migraine attacks. Medication overuse is one of the most common causes of chronic daily headache.[4] Agents most commonly implicated in this syndrome include simple and combination analgesics, opiates, ergotamine tartrate, and triptans.[6]

Analgesics and NSAIDs. Simple analgesics and NSAIDs are effective medications for many migraine attacks. They are a reasonable first-line choice for mild-to-moderate migraine attacks or even severe attacks in those who have previously demonstrated a beneficial response.[6] Of the NSAIDs, aspirin, ibuprofen, naproxen sodium, tolfenamic acid, and the combination of acetaminophen plus aspirin and caffeine have demonstrated the most consistent efficacy.[3–8] Acetaminophen alone is not generally recommended for migraine because of the lack of scientific support.[3,6,7]

Acute NSAID therapy is associated with gastrointestinal (e.g., dyspepsia, nausea, vomiting, diarrhea) and central nervous system side effects (e.g., somnolence, dizziness). NSAIDs should be used cautiously in patients with previous ulcer disease, renal disease, or hypersensitivity to aspirin.[7]

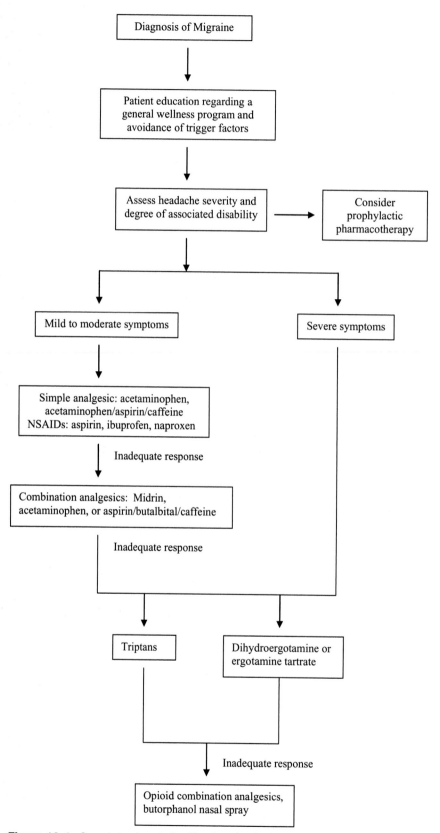

Figure 19-1. Sample treatment algorithm for migraine headaches.

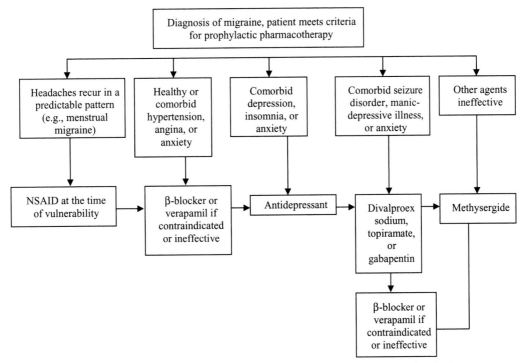

Figure 19-2. Sample treatment algorithm for prophylactic management of migraine headaches.

Though prescription products of aspirin or acetaminophen combined with a short-acting barbiturate (butalbital) are frequently used in the treatment of migraine, no rigorous studies support their efficacy. The use of butalbital-containing products should be limited because of concerns about overuse, headache caused by medication overuse, and withdrawal.[3,6,7] Midrin, a combination of acetaminophen, isometheptene mucate (a sympathomimetic amine), and dichloralphenazone (a chloral hydrate derivative), has demonstrated modest benefits in placebo-controlled studies and is generally viewed as an alternative for patients with mild-to-moderate migraine attacks.[6,7] Of note, combination analgesics appear to pose a greater risk of medication-overuse headache than aspirin or acetaminophen alone.

Opiate Analgesics. Narcotic analgesic drugs (e.g., meperidine, butorphanol, oxycodone, hydromorphone) are effective, but should generally be reserved for patients with moderate-to-severe infrequent headaches in whom conventional therapies are contraindicated or be given as "rescue medication" after patients have failed to respond to conventional therapies.[3] The intranasal formulation of butorphanol, a synthetically derived opioid agonist–antagonist, is an alternative to frequent office or emergency department visits. Butorphanol use should be closely supervised because of the established risk of overuse and dependence.[6,7]

Antiemetics. Adjunctive antiemetic therapy is useful for the nausea and vomiting associated with migraines and acute migraine medications. A single dose of an antiemetic, such as metoclopramide, chlorpromazine, or prochlorperazine, administered 15 to 30 minutes before ingestion of oral abortive migraine medications, is often sufficient. Suppository preparations are available when nausea and vomiting are particularly prominent. Metoclopramide is also useful to reverse gastroparesis and improve gastrointestinal absorption during severe attacks.[6,7]

In addition to the antiemetic effects, dopamine antagonists have been used successfully as monotherapy for the treatment of intractable headache, and offer an alternative to narcotic analgesics. Intravenous or intramuscular prochlorperazine and intravenous metoclopramide provide more effective pain relief than placebo. The precise mechanism of action is unknown.[7]

Miscellaneous Nonspecific Medications. Corticosteroids may be an effective rescue therapy for status migrainosus (severe, continuous migraine lasting up to 1 week).[6] Short courses of oral or parenteral prednisone, dexamethasone, and hydrocortisone may be useful in the management of refractory headache persisting for several days.[7]

Limited studies suggest a role for intranasal lidocaine in the treatment of acute migraine headache.[7] Intranasal lidocaine provides rapid pain relief, but headache recurrence is common. Adverse effects are generally limited to local irritation of the nose or eye, unpleasant taste, and numbness of the throat.

Ergot Alkaloids and Derivatives. Ergotamine tartrate and dihydroergotamine are useful and may be considered for the treatment of moderate-to-severe migraine attacks.[6] These drugs are nonselective 5-hydroxytryptamine-1 (5-HT1) receptor agonists that constrict intracranial blood vessels and inhibit the development of neurogenic inflammation in the trigeminovascular system; central inhibition of the trigeminovascular pathway as well as activity at adrenergic and dopaminergic receptors are also reported.

Ergotamine tartrate and dihydroergotamine are available in various dosage forms. Some patients respond preferentially to a particular dosage form, such as rectal dosing. Despite widespread clinical use since 1925, evidence supporting the efficacy of ergotamine tartrate is inconsistent.[3,7]

Nausea and vomiting are among the most common adverse effects of the ergotamine derivatives. Vasoconstriction also occurs with therapeutic doses. Ergotamine is more likely to cause these effects than dihydroergotamine. Pretreatment with an antiemetic agent should be considered with ergotamine and intravenous dihydroergotamine. Other common side effects include abdominal pain, weakness, fatigue, paresthesias, muscle pain, diarrhea, and chest tightness. Occasionally, severe peripheral ischemia (ergotism) may occur including cold, numb, painful extremities; continuous paresthesias; diminished peripheral pulses; and claudication. Gangrenous extremities, myocardial infarction, hepatic necrosis, and bowel and brain ischemia have been rarely reported.[4] Triptans should not be used within 24 hours of ergot derivatives. Ergotamine derivatives are contraindicated in patients with renal or hepatic failure; coronary, cerebral, or peripheral vascular diseases; uncontrolled hypertension; sepsis; and in women who are pregnant or nursing.[1] Dihydroergotamine does not appear to cause rebound headache; however, dosage restrictions for ergotamine tartrate should be strictly observed to prevent this complication.[4]

Serotonin Receptor Agonists (Triptans). The triptans represent a significant advance in migraine pharmacotherapy. These drugs are selective agonists of the 5-HT$_{1B}$ and 5-HT$_{1D}$ receptors. Migraine relief results from vasoconstriction of pain-producing intracranial blood vessels through stimulation of vascular 5-HT$_{1B}$ receptors, inhibition of vasoactive neuropeptide release from trigeminal perivascular nerves through stimulation of presynaptic 5-HT$_{1D}$ receptors, and interruption of pain-signal transmission within the brainstem trigeminal

nuclei through stimulation of 5-HT$_{1D}$ receptors. The triptans are appropriate as first-line therapy for patients with moderate-to-severe migraine, or as rescue therapy when nonspecific medications are ineffective.

Sumatriptan, the first triptan, is the most extensively studied antimigraine therapy and is available in the most dosage forms. Subcutaneous sumatriptan has the most rapid onset (10 minutes) and is the most effective of the triptans.[3] Intranasal sumatriptan and zolmitriptan usually provide a faster onset of effect (15 minutes) than the oral formulations, and produce similar rates of response.

The newer or second-generation triptans offer improved pharmacokinetic and pharmacodynamic profiles compared to oral sumatriptan. These agents have higher oral bioavailability and longer half-lives, which could theoretically improve within-patient treatment consistency and reduce headache recurrence.

Placebo-controlled studies with each of the second-generation agents reveal somewhat comparable 2-hour response rates. Direct comparative clinical trials are available for only a few of the triptans. A recent meta-analysis summarized the efficacy and tolerability of the oral triptans across both published and unpublished studies.[8] At all marketed doses, the oral triptans are effective and well tolerated. Sumatriptan (100 mg) resulted in a 59% 2-hour headache response; 29% were pain free at 2 hours; 20% had sustained pain relief; and 67% had consistent relief. Compared with sumatriptan (100 mg), rizatriptan (10 mg) showed better efficacy and consistency and similar tolerability; eletriptan (80 mg) showed better efficacy, similar consistency, but lower tolerability; almotriptan (12.5 mg) showed similar efficacy at 2 hours but better consistency and tolerability; naratriptan (2.5 mg) and eletriptan (20 mg) showed lower efficacy and better tolerability; zolmitriptan (2.5 and 5 mg), eletriptan (40 mg), and rizatriptan (5 mg) all showed similar results. Available data suggest lower efficacy for frovatriptan.[8]

Clinical response to the triptans can vary considerably among individual patients. Individual responses cannot be predicted, and if one triptan fails, a patient may be successfully treated with another. After an effective agent and dose have been identified, subsequent treatments should begin with that same regimen.[3,8]

Side effects to the triptans are common, but usually mild-to-moderate and of short duration. Adverse effects include paresthesias, fatigue, dizziness, flushing, warm sensations, and somnolence. Minor injection-site reactions are reported with the subcutaneous route and taste perversion and nasal discomfort with the intranasal route. "Chest symptoms," including tightness, pressure, heaviness, or pain in the chest, neck, or throat are relatively common. All triptans are partial agonists of human 5-HT coronary artery receptors and produce modest coronary artery vasoconstriction. This physiologic effect is hemodynamically insignificant in patients with healthy coronary arteries and poses minimal risk in appropriately selected patients.[9]

The triptans are contraindicated in patients with a history of ischemic heart disease, uncontrolled hypertension, and cerebrovascular disease. Patients at risk for unrecognized coronary artery disease (e.g., postmenopausal women, men over 40 years of age, and patients with multiple risk factors) should receive a cardiovascular assessment prior to triptan use and have their initial dose administered under medical supervision. Triptans are also contraindicated in patients with hemiplegic and basilar migraine. The triptans should not be given within 24 hours of the ergotamine derivatives. Administration of sumatriptan, rizatriptan, and zolmitriptan within 2 weeks of therapy with monoamine oxidase inhibitors is not recommended. Concomitant therapy with the selective serotonin reuptake inhibitors should be carefully monitored because of isolated reports of serotonin syndrome in sumatriptan-treated patients.[6,7]

Preventive Migraine Therapy

Preventive migraine therapies are administered on a daily basis to reduce the frequency, severity, and duration of attacks, and to improve responsiveness to symptomatic migraine therapies.[6] Preventive therapy may also be administered preemptively or intermittently when headaches recur in a predictable pattern (e.g., exercise-induced migraine, menstrual migraine). The efficacy of the various agents appears to be similar; however, the quality of published data is limited for many commonly used drugs. Only propranolol, timolol, topiramate, and valproic acid are currently approved by the U.S. Food and Drug Administration for this indication. The selection of an agent is typically based on its side-effect profile and the patient's comorbid conditions. A full therapeutic trial of 2 to 6 months is necessary to judge the efficacy of the drug. Therapy should be initiated at low doses and advanced slowly until a therapeutic effect is achieved or side effects become intolerable. Drug doses for migraine prophylaxis are often lower than those used for other indications.[4] Prophylactic treatment is usually continued for at least 3 to 6 months after the frequency and severity of headaches has diminished, and then gradually tapered and discontinued. Many migraine patients experience fewer and less severe attacks for lengthy periods following discontinuation of prophylactic medications or when tapering to a lower dose.

β-Blockers. Propranolol, nadolol, timolol, atenolol, and metoprolol have proven efficacy in reducing the frequency of migraine attacks.[3] The precise mechanism is unknown; the migraine threshold may be raised by modulation of adrenergic or serotonergic neurotransmission in cortical or subcortical pathways. Selection of a β-blocker is based on β selectivity, convenience of the formulation, and tolerability. β-Blockers are particularly useful in patients with comorbid anxiety, hypertension, or angina. Potential side effects of β-blockers include drowsiness, fatigue, sleep disturbances, vivid dreams, memory disturbance, depression, impotence, bradycardia, and hypotension. They should be used with caution in patients with congestive heart failure, peripheral vascular disease, atrioventricular conduction disturbances, asthma, depression, and diabetes.

Antidepressants. The beneficial effects of antidepressants in migraine are independent of their antidepressant activity, and may be related to downregulation of central 5-HT$_2$ and adrenergic receptors.[10] Amitriptyline is the most widely studied antidepressant for migraine prophylaxis. Use of other antidepressants is based primarily on clinical and anecdotal experience. Other tricyclic antidepressants that have been used successfully include doxepin, nortriptyline, protriptyline, and imipramine.[6,10] Anticholinergic side effects are common and limit the use of these agents in patients with benign prostatic hyperplasia and glaucoma. Increased appetite and weight gain may occur. Orthostatic hypotension and cardiac toxicity (slowed atrioventricular conduction) are also occasionally reported. Nortriptyline and protriptyline may be advantageous in patients who are particularly intolerant of the anticholinergic and sedative side effects of amitriptyline.

The selective serotonin reuptake inhibitors have not been extensively studied for migraine prophylaxis and are considered to be less effective than tricyclic antidepressants. These agents should not be considered as first- or second-line medications; however, they are useful in patients with comorbid depression or anxiety disorders.[4,10] Recent studies have demonstrated the benefits of venlafaxine, an inhibitor of serotonin and norepinephrine reuptake in migraine prophylaxis.[11]

Monoamine oxidase inhibitors, such as phenelzine, have been used in the management of refractory headache, but their use is limited because of their complex adverse effect profiles.

Anticonvulsants. Anticonvulsant medications are increasingly recommended for the prevention of migraine headaches. These seem to have multiple mechanisms of action, including enhancement of gamma aminobutyric acid mediated inhibition, modulation of the excitatory neurotransmitter glutamate, and inhibition of sodium- and calcium-ion-channel activity. Anticonvulsants are particularly useful in those with comorbid seizure, anxiety, or bipolar disorders.[4] The efficacy of valproic acid and divalproex sodium (a 1:1 molar combination of valproate sodium and valproic acid) has been demonstrated in multiple placebo-controlled studies.[10] Nausea, vomiting, alopecia, tremor, asthenia, somnolence, and weight gain are the most common adverse effects.[3,10] The extended-release formulation of divalproex sodium is administered once daily and is better tolerated than the enteric-coated formulation. Hepatotoxicity is the most serious side effect of valproate therapy, though irreversible hepatic dysfunction is extremely rare in adults. Baseline liver function tests should be obtained, but routine follow-up studies are not necessary in asymptomatic adults on monotherapy. Patient evaluation is recommended every 1 to 2 months during the first 6 to 9 months of therapy. Valproate is contraindicated in pregnant women and patients with a history of pancreatitis or chronic liver disease.

Topiramate has recently received the approval of the U.S. Food and Drug Administration for migraine prophylaxis. With chronic use, topiramate is associated with weight loss. This may offer a distinct advantage, since weight gain is a common reason for discontinuation of migraine prevention therapy. Adverse events associated with topiramate include paresthesia, fatigue, anorexia, diarrhea, weight loss, memory difficulty, and nausea. The initial dose of topiramate should be much lower than the targeted dose to minimize adverse effects. Kidney stones, acute myopia, acute angle-closure glaucoma, and oligohidrosis have been infrequently reported with topiramate use.[11]

Gabapentin may also be an effective agent for migraine prevention, based on the results of a recent trial.[3] Dizziness and drowsiness were the most common adverse events associated with the use of gabapentin.

Calcium-Channel Blockers. The use of calcium-channel blockers for migraine prevention should be considered when other drugs with established clinical benefit are ineffective or contraindicated. Verapamil is the most widely used calcium-channel blocker for preventive treatment; however, only modest benefits have been seen in two placebo-controlled studies.[4] It is perhaps most useful in patients with comorbid hypertension or with contraindications to β-blockers. The most common side effect of verapamil is constipation. Evaluations of nifedipine, nimodipine, diltiazem, and nicardipine have yielded equivocal results.[10]

Methysergide. The semisynthetic ergot alkaloid, methysergide, is a potent 5-HT$_2$ receptor antagonist that appears to stabilize serotonergic neurotransmission in the trigeminovascular system, preventing migraine by blocking the development of neurogenic inflammation. Its utility is limited by the rare development of retroperitoneal, endocardial, and pulmonary fibrosis during long-term administration.[4] Consequently, a medication-free interval of 4 weeks is recommended following each 6-month treatment period along with periodic assessment.[12] In addition to gastrointestinal intolerance, muscle aching, leg cramps, claudication, weight gain, and hallucinations are also reported. Methysergide is reserved for patients with refractory headaches that do not respond to other preventive therapies.

Nonsteroidal Anti-Inflammatory Drugs. NSAIDs are modestly effective for reducing the frequency, severity, and duration of migraine attacks; however, potential gastrointestinal and renal toxicity may limit the daily or prolonged use of these agents.[10] Consequently, NSAIDs have been used intermittently to prevent headaches that recur in a predictable pattern, such as menstrual migraine. NSAIDs should be initiated 1 to 2 days prior to the expected onset of headache and continued during the period of vulnerability.[4]

Miscellaneous Preventive Agents. A limited number of double-blind, placebo-controlled studies have demonstrated the efficacy of several other agents in migraine prophylaxis. These include riboflavin (vitamin B$_2$), 400 mg daily, localized injections of botulinum toxin type A, petasites extract, 75 mg twice daily (from the plant *Petasites hybridus*), and coenzyme Q10.[4] Further study is needed to determine the clinical utility and comparative efficacy of these agents for the prophylactic management of migraine.

TENSION-TYPE HEADACHES

The vast majority of people suffering from episodic tension-type headache self-medicate with over-the-counter medications and do not consult a health care professional. While pharmacologic and nonpharmacologic treatments are available, simple analgesics and NSAIDs are the mainstay of acute therapy. Most agents used for tension-type headache have not been studied in controlled clinical trials.[13]

Nonpharmacologic Therapy
Psychophysiological therapy and physical therapy have been utilized in the management of tension-type headache. Psychophysiological therapy may consist of reassurance and counseling, stress management, relaxation training, and biofeedback. Relaxation training and biofeedback training (alone or in combination) can result in a 50% reduction in headache activity.

Evidence supporting physical therapeutic options, such as heat or cold packs, ultrasound, electrical nerve stimulation, stretching, exercise, massage, acupuncture, manipulations, ergonomic instructions, and trigger-point injections or occipital nerve blocks, is somewhat inconsistent. However, patients may benefit from selected modalities during an acute episode of tension-type headache.[4]

Pharmacologic Therapy

Simple analgesics (alone or in combination with caffeine) and NSAIDs are effective for the acute treatment of mild-to-moderate tension-type headache. Acetaminophen, aspirin, ibuprofen, naproxen, ketoprofen, indomethacin, and ketorolac have demonstrated efficacy in placebo-controlled and comparative studies.[4] Failure of over-the-counter agents may warrant therapy with prescription drugs. High-dose NSAIDs or the combination of aspirin or acetaminophen with butalbital or, rarely, codeine are effective options. Use of butalbital and codeine combinations should be avoided, when possible, because of the high potential for overuse and dependency. As with migraine headache, acute medication should be taken for no more than 2 days per week to prevent the development of chronic tension-type headache.[4,14] Preventive treatment should be considered if headache frequency (more than two per week), duration (more than 3 to 4 hours), or severity results in medication overuse or substantial disability. The principles of preventive treatment for tension-type headache are similar to those of migraine headache. Tricyclic antidepressants are most often prescribed for prophylaxis; however, other drugs can also be selected after consideration of comorbid medical conditions and respective side-effect profiles.[4] The use of botulinum toxin has not consistently demonstrated clinical efficacy in the prophylaxis of chronic tension-type headaches.[12]

CLUSTER HEADACHES

As in migraine, therapy for cluster headaches involves both abortive and prophylactic therapies. Abortive therapy is directed at managing the acute attack. Prophylactic therapies are started early in the cluster period in an attempt to induce remission and may be transitional using, agents not suitable for long-term or chronic use. Patients with chronic cluster headache may require prophylactic medications indefinitely.

Acute Cluster Therapy

Oxygen. The standard acute treatment of cluster headache is inhalation of 100% oxygen by nonbreather facial mask at a rate of 7 to 10 L/min for 15 to 25 minutes.[4,5] Repeat administration may be necessary because of recurrence, as oxygen appears to merely delay, rather than abort, the attack in some patients.[5] No side effects have been reported with the use of oxygen but caution should be used for those who smoke or have chronic obstructive pulmonary disease.

Triptans. The quick onset of subcutaneous and intranasal triptans make them safe and effective abortive agents for cluster headaches. Subcutaneous sumatriptan (6 mg) is the most effective agent. Nasal sprays are less effective but may be better tolerated in some patients. Adverse events reported in cluster headache patients are similar to those seen in migraine patients. Orally administered triptans have limited use in cluster attacks because of their relatively slow onset of action; oral zolmitriptan (10 mg), however, was beneficial in patients with episodic cluster headache at 30 minutes.[5]

Ergot Alkaloids and Derivatives. All forms of ergotamine have been used in cluster headaches although, in general, their role has been supplanted by the triptans. Intravenous dihydroergotamine results in the quickest response and repeated administration for 3 to 7 days can break the cycle of frequent cluster headache attacks.[5] Ergotamine tartrate has also provided effective relief of cluster headache attacks when administered sublingually or rectally; however, the pharmacokinetics of these preparations frequently limit their clinical utility.[4,5] Dosing guidelines are similar to those for migraine headache therapy.

Corticosteroids. Corticosteroids are useful for inducing remission.[4,5] Therapy is initiated with 40 to 60 mg/day of prednisone and tapered over approximately 3 weeks. Relief appears within 1 to 2 days of initiating therapy. To avoid steroid-induced complications, long-term use is not recommended. Headaches may recur when therapy is tapered or discontinued.

Preventive Cluster Therapy

Verapamil. Verapamil is the agent of choice for the prevention of cluster headaches.[4] The beneficial effects of verapamil often appear after 1 week of therapy. A typical suggested dosage range is from 360 to 720 mg/day.

Lithium. Lithium carbonate is effective for episodic and chronic cluster headache attacks, and can be used in combination with verapamil. A positive response is seen in up to 78% of patients with chronic cluster headache, and in up to 63% of patients with episodic cluster headache.[4] The usual dose is 600 to 1200 mg/day, with a suggested starting dose of 300 mg twice daily. Optimal plasma lithium levels for prevention of cluster headache have not been established, but trough values should not be more than 1.0 mEq/L.[4,5]

Initial side effects are mild and include tremor, lethargy, nausea, diarrhea, and abdominal discomfort. Thyroid and renal function must be monitored during lithium therapy. Lithium should be administered with caution to patients with significant renal or cardiovascular disease, dehydration, pregnancy, or concomitant diuretic or NSAID use.

Ergotamine. Ergotamine can be an efficacious agent for prophylactic as well as abortive therapy of cluster headaches.[4] A 2-mg bedtime dose is often beneficial for the prevention of nocturnal headache attacks. Daily use of 1 to 2 mg of ergotamine alone or in combination with verapamil or lithium may provide effective headache prophylaxis in patients refractory to other agents with little risk of ergotism or rebound headache.[4,5]

Methysergide. In patients unresponsive to other therapies, methysergide, 4 to 8 mg/day in divided doses, is usually effective in shortening the course of cluster headaches. Response to treatment usually occurs within 1 week. Response rates in patients with episodic cluster headache approach 70%, but chronic cluster headache patients receive less benefit.[5] Precautions regarding methysergide use were described earlier in this chapter.

Miscellaneous Agents. Other therapies that have been used in the acute management of cluster headache include intranasal lidocaine, cocaine, capsaicin, and civamide. Limited studies also support the use of divalproex sodium, topiramate, nifedipine, nimodipine, melatonin, and baclofen for cluster prophylaxis. Neurosurgical intervention may be necessary for patients with chronic cluster headache that is resistant to all medical therapies.[4,5]

EVIDENCE-BASED SUMMARY

- A careful workup, including patient history, physical examination, and appropriate laboratory tests, should identify most headache patients with major disease. A variety of strategies can be helpful for managing migraine, tension-type, and cluster headaches. Management of primary headache disorders is directed at suppressing acute attacks and preventing recurrences.
- Acute headache therapies should provide consistent, rapid relief, and enable the patient to resume his or her normal activities at home, school, or work.
- A stratified care approach, in which the selection of initial treatment is based on headache-related disability and symptom severity, is the preferred treatment strategy.
- Strict adherence to maximum daily and weekly doses of headache medications is essential.
- Preventive therapy should be considered in the setting of recurring headaches that produce significant disability; frequent attacks requiring symptomatic medication more than twice per week; symptomatic therapies that are ineffective, contraindicated, or produce serious side effects; and uncommon migraine or other headache variants that cause profound disruption and/or risk of neurologic injury.
- The selection of an agent for headache prophylaxis should be based on efficacy, individual patient response, tolerability, convenience of the drug formulation, and comorbid conditions of the patient.
- Each prophylactic medication should be given an adequate therapeutic trial to judge its efficacy, usually at least 2 to 3 months.
- A general wellness program and avoidance of triggers should be included in the headache management plan.
- After an effective abortive agent and dose have been identified, subsequent treatments should begin with that same regimen.

REFERENCES

1. Silberstein SD, Lipton, RB, Dalessio DJ. Overview, diagnosis, and classification of headache. In: Silberstein SD, Lipton RB, Dalessio DJ, eds. *Wolff's Headache and Other Head Pain.* 7th ed. New York, NY: Oxford University Press; 2001:6–26.
2. Headache Classification Committee of the International Headache Society. The International Classification of Headache Disorders, 2nd ed. *Cephalalgia.* 2004;24(1): 1–151.
3. Silberstein SD. Migraine. *Lancet.* 2004;363:381–391.
4. Silberstein SD, Lipton RB, Goadsby PJ. *Headache in Clinical Practice.* London, UK: Martin Dunitz; 2002:21–33, 69–128.
5. McGeeney BE. Cluster headache pharmacotherapy. *Am J Ther.* 2005;12(4):351–358.
6. Silberstein SD. Practice parameter: Evidence-based guidelines for migraine headache (an evidence-based review). *Neurology.* 2000;55:754–763.
7. Matchar DB, Young WB, Rosenberg JA, et al. Evidence-based guidelines for migraine headache in the primary care setting: Pharmacological management of acute attacks. The US Headache Consortium. 2000. Available at

www.aan.com/professionals/practice/guidelines. Accessed November 20, 2005.

8. Ferrari MD, Roon KI, Lipton RB, Goadsby PJ. Oral triptans (serotonin 5_HT1B/1D agonists) in acute migraine treatment: A meta-analysis of 53 trials. *Lancet.* 2001;358:1558–1575.

9. Bigal ME, Lipton RB, Krymchantowski AV. The medical management of migraine. *Am J Ther.* 2004;11(2):130–140.

10. Silberstein SD, Goadsby PJ. Migraine: Preventive treatment. *Cephalalgia.* 2002;22:491–512.

11. Evans RW, Bigal ME, Grosberg B, Lipton RB. Target doses and titration schedules for migraine preventive medications. *Headache.* 2006;46:160–164.

12. Schulte-Mattler WJ, Krack P, BoNTTH Study Group. Treatment of chronic tension-type headache with botulinum toxin A: A randomized, double-blind, placebo-controlled multicenter study. *Pain.* 2004;109(1, 2):110–114.

13. Jensen R, Olesen J. Tension-type headache: An update on mechanisms and treatment. *Curr Opin Neurol.* 2000;13:285–289.

14. Solomon S, Newman LC. Episodic tension-type headaches. In: Silberstein SD, Lipton RB, Dalessio DJ, eds. *Wolff's Headache and Other Head Pain.* 7th ed. New York, NY: Oxford University Press; 2001:238–246.

PART 5

Psychiatric Disorders

CHAPTERS

Chapter 20

Pharmacotherapy for Alzheimer's Disease

Robb McIlvried

SEARCH STRATEGY

A systematic medline search of the medical literature was performed using Ovid in January 2008. Subject headings included Alzheimer's, Drug therapy, acetylcholinesterase inhibitors, memantine, and dementia.

BACKGROUND

In 1901, Alois Alzheimer encountered a 51-year-old woman admitted to a psychiatric hospital in Frankfurt, Germany. Alzheimer observed and recorded the features that we now recognize as symptoms of the disease that bears his name, "… a rapidly increasing loss of memory. At times she would think someone wanted to kill her and would begin shrieking loudly. She could not find her way around in her own apartment." More recently, the death of President Ronald Reagan related to Alzheimer's disease (AD) raised awareness of the condition and provoked calls for more research into prevention, treatment, and cure.

AD is the most common form of dementia. It is estimated that more than 4 million Americans are affected by AD, and this number is expected to increase to approximately 14 million by the year 2050.[1] The incidence increases with age. AD affects one-tenth of the population older than 65 years and almost half of the population older than 85 years.[2] As the population ages, the number of patients with AD will increase, and with it the burden of caring for these patients. Finding effective treatment for AD is increasingly important.

AD costs the American economy more than $100 billion annually. It is one of the leading causes of institutionalization of older Americans. Direct and indirect costs to family members caring for a loved one with AD can be devastating. If effective treatment could reduce the cost of caring for someone with AD, the economic impact could be quite dramatic.

CLINICAL PRESENTATION

AD is the most common cause of the clinical syndrome of dementia. By definition, dementia presents with impairment of memory as well as aphasia, apraxia, and agnosia.[3] There is also frequently impairment of executive functioning, a higher level of cognitive functioning responsible for planning and organizing complex tasks. Social impairment, including social withdrawal or inappropriate behaviors, is usually evident.

Typically, although not exclusively, the patient is unaware of any impairment. Most commonly, a family member will notify the physician of a concern. Often signs of cognitive impairment are mild and overlooked or unnoticed until a serious event, such as an auto accident or financial indiscretion, alerts family members to a problem. The primary care physician is usually the first health care professional to be involved.

Diagnosis of early dementia can be difficult as the symptoms may be mild and attributed to normal aging. Early signs of AD can include repetitiveness or perseveration, changes in mood or personality, loss of initiative, and difficulty with complex tasks. These impairments can lead to social withdrawal and isolation and must be distinguished from depression. Early diagnosis is important because early treatment may more effectively slow the progression of the condition. Additionally, this is the best time to discuss advance care planning, such as living wills, power of attorney, or future living arrangements. The diagnosis of AD becomes more evident as the disease progresses. Symptoms of later stages include disorientation, aggression or agitation, paranoid and delusional thoughts, hallucinations, and severe memory impairment. Eventually, AD will progress to loss of motor function, incontinence, and complete aphasia.

DIAGNOSIS

Dementia must be distinguished from delirium. Delirium is a potentially reversible, transient condition that can present with impaired cognition. Delirium typically presents acutely, whereas dementia presents insidiously. Delirium is associated with altered levels of consciousness and is usually secondary to an underlying medical condition. The underlying condition may not be easily identified and the delirium can persist as long as the precipitating factor is untreated, and perhaps even longer. Dementia should also be distinguished from depression, which may present with predominantly cognitive features in older patients.

The term "reversible dementia" is used to describe conditions that are potentially treatable, but can cause a progressive loss of cognition. However, treatment of the underlying condition does not always lead to improvement in cognition. Most will eventually develop overt dementia. Conditions that cause potentially "reversible" dementia include hypothyroidism, vitamin B_{12} deficiency, neurosyphilis, and normal pressure hydrocephalus. These conditions can be ruled out by history and physical, laboratory studies, and imaging.

Once dementia has been diagnosed and treatable conditions ruled out, the underlying cause of the dementia should be considered. Dementia of the Alzheimer type is the most common cause, followed by multi-infarct dementia and dementia with Lewy bodies. Distinction between the types of dementia is often difficult clinically and may not be vital to treatment decisions. Evidence suggests that common treatments used for Alzheimer's disease may also be effective in dementia with Lewy bodies or multi-infarct dementia. However, it is clinically useful to recognize dementia with Lewy bodies as the behavioral symptoms of this condition respond poorly to antipsychotics. Diagnosis is made from the history, usually obtained from family members or caregivers, and from cognitive testing. In the primary care setting, the Mini Mental State Examination (MMSE) and clock drawing test are two of the more commonly used tests. These are easy to administer and can be done during a typical office encounter. The MMSE measures several domains of cognition including memory, orientation, praxis, and attention. The clock drawing task is primarily a test of executive function. Physical examination is useful to evaluate for neurodegenerative conditions such as Parkinson's disease.

Neuroimaging is generally recommended as part of the evaluation, although the diagnosis is usually quite evident-based on the history and physical alone. Imaging is primarily useful for evaluating for normal pressure hydrocephalus, chronic subdural hematoma or mass lesion. Usually, a noncontrast computerized tomography is adequate. Complete blood count, vitamin B_{12} levels, thyroid stimulating hormone, calcium and electrolytes are generally recommended. A rapid plasma reagin is also frequently included, although there is some debate on the continued utility of this test. Newer technologies such as positron emission tomography scanning and the apolipoprotein E4 allele carrier status are generally not helpful in the routine evaluation of dementia. In cases where the diagnosis is in question, there are neurologic deficits, or at family's request, a neurology consultation should be obtained.

TREATMENT

NONPHARMACOLOGIC INTERVENTIONS

Breaking the News

Informing a patient or a family of the diagnosis of AD is a very difficult and important task. Frequently this is done inadequately causing unnecessary stress and negative emotions. As in breaking any bad news, it is best done in a quiet, comfortable room with adequate time for questions and concerns. A brief office visit addressing several other medical issues is not adequate. The patient should be given assistance finding more information and accessing community resources. Although there is some controversy, it is generally accepted that a cognitively impaired patient should be informed that he or she has Alzheimer's dementia. Patients with very advanced dementia are unlikely to truly understand the diagnosis and are unlikely to be harmed by being informed. Less impaired patients deserve to be informed so they may make decisions to the extent of their ability.

Early diagnosis is vital to allow patients to plan for the future. At the time of diagnosis it is helpful to suggest advance care planning including a living will, power of Attorney and consideration of higher levels of care, such as assisted living, personal care or nursing home placement. The earlier the diagnosis, the more likely the patient will be able to participate in these decisions.

Safety

Perhaps the most important issue for someone newly diagnosed with dementia is safety. As a result of impaired judgment and cognition, a person with AD is at risk for injury caused by falls, motor vehicle accidents, household accidents, wandering, or fires. A physical or occupational therapist or the family should do a home safety evaluation, including checking for loose floorboards or steps, exposed electrical cords, loose throw rugs, clutter and other fall hazards, and functioning smoke detectors. If there is a risk the patient may leave the stove on, it should be disconnected. Prescription medications and household cleaners should be removed to prevent accidental poisoning. Firearms and power tools should be removed or stored in locked cabinets. The clinician should consider suspending driving privileges and suggest disabling the vehicle in cases where the patient may still drive.

PHARMACOTHERAPY

ASSESSMENT OF PHARMACOTHERAPY

The perfect drug for AD should possess the following features:

1. Improve memory and cognition.
2. Slow the progression of the disease.
3. Delay admission to nursing home.
4. Control inappropriate and disruptive behaviors.
5. Improve the ability to perform activities of daily living (ADL).
6. Decrease the burden to caregivers.

Although there is no perfect drug for AD it is helpful to consider these features when evaluating the currently available pharmacologic therapies.

One of the difficulties for clinicians in making treatment decisions is that the outcome measures used in studies are not common tools used in clinical practice. Whereas cardiac drug trials typically use endpoints of death or myocardial infarction, Alzheimer medication trails use a confusing alphabet soup of cognitive, behavioral and functional assessments, such as the Alzheimer's Disease Assessment Scale-cognitive subscale (ADAS-cog), Clinical Dementia Rating (CDR), Clinician's Interview Based Impression of Change plus Caregiver Input (CIBIC-plus), etc. This has led to concerns that the beneficial outcomes are not always clinically meaningful. Only a minority of studies use outcomes such as caregiver time and time to nursing home placement.

Another concern in AD trials is the lack of a gold standard diagnostic test. Although the diagnosis of AD is often obvious in a clinical setting, strict diagnostic criteria for research purposes can be problematic. As the only unequivocal test for AD is autopsy, subjects in Alzheimer's disease research are labeled as "probable" or "possible" Alzheimer. Despite, this, researchers attempt to use comparable populations, and the majority of the trials utilize the National Institute of Neurological and Communicative Disorders and Stroke-Alzheimer's disease and Related Disorders Association criteria of probable or possible AD.[4]

The domains of function assessed by the commonly used instruments include cognition, behavior, function, and global functioning. The U.S. Food and Drug Administration (FDA) requires that an AD medication show benefit over placebo in a performance-based assessment of cognitive function and a clinician's global assessment.[5] Table 20-1 outlines some of the more commonly used assessment methods in AD research.

PHARMACOTHERAPY OVERVIEW

Currently, there are only two classes of medications that are FDA approved for the treatment of AD, the acetylcholinesterase inhibitors (AchEI) and an N-methyl-D-aspartate receptor antagonist, memantine. Many other agents have been evaluated with variable results, including nonsteroidal anti-inflammatory agents, herbal preparations, estrogen, and antioxidants. Anticonvulsants and antipsychotics and others are frequently used to control symptoms associated with Alzheimer's dementia such as the hallucinations, agitation, and aggression.

ACETYLCHOLINESTERASE INHIBITORS

The first class of medications approved by the FDA for treatment of AD is the Acetylcholinesterase inhibitors. These medications include tacrine, donepezil, rivastigmine, and galantamine. These medications appear to act by binding to and inactivating the cholinesterase enzymes thus preventing degradation of acetylcholine in the synapse.

The benefits of the AchEI are generally mild. Most studies' outcomes were scales of cognition and global change. Most studies also evaluated behavior and function, and benefits were found in all these domains. A meta-analysis of trials on all three approved agents showed that the number of subjects rated as improved was 9% in excess of placebo.[6] Another meta-analysis focused on the neuropsychiatric symptoms and functional impairment also found a modest benefit.[7] However, some authors feel that the benefit of these medicines is questionable, as result of methodologic flaws and the small size of the benefit.[8] See Table 20-2 for overview of selected trials of AchEI.

It is difficult to recommend any one agent over another in this class, as there is little data to suggest that any agent is more effective than the others. There is also little data to support the practice of switching from one medication in this class to another for a perceived lack of efficacy. Additionally, there is debate about the appropriate length of therapy. Given that AD is a chronic progressive illness with no cure, patients will

Table 20-1. Assessment Scales Commonly Used in AD Trials

Test	Type	Domains	Source	No. of Items	Range of Scores	Interpretation
ADAS-cog	Cognition	Memory, orientation, attention, reasoning, language, praxis	Patient examination	11	0–70	Higher score reflects worse function
MMSE	Cognition	Orientation, memory, language, praxis	Patient examination		0–30	Higher score reflects better function
SIB	Cognition	Social interaction, memory, orientation, language, attention, praxis	Patinet examination	51	0–100	
ADCS-CGIC	Global	Cognition, behavior, social functioning	Caregiver and patient interview	15	1–7	1 = very much improved, 2 = much improved, 3 = minimally improved, 4 = no change, 5 = minimally worse, 6 = much worse, 7 = very much worse
CIBIC/CIBIC+	Global		Patient interview, (caregiver interview-CIBIC+)			
CDR	Global	Memory, orientation, judgment, community activities, home and hobbies, personal care	Patient and informant interview		0–5	0 = no impairment, 0.5 = questionable, 1 = mild impairment, 2 + moderate, 3 = severe
GDS	Global				1–7	Higher scores worse
ADCS-ADL	Functional		Informant interview	27		
FAST	Functional		Caregiver interview	16		
PDS	Functional		Caregiver interview	29	0–100	
DAD	Functional	Basic ADL, Instrumental ADL	Caregiver information	40		
NPI	Behavioral		Caregiver interview	10	0–120	
ADAS-noncog	Behavioral	Mood, concentration, uncooperativeness, delusions, hallucinations, motor activities			0–50	Higher scores worse
BEHAVE-AD	Behavioral	Paranoia, hallucinations, activity disturbances, aggressiveness, sleep disturbances, mood disturbances, anxiety and phobias	Caregiver interview and subject observation	25	Mild, moderate, or severe	

inevitably worsen despite treatment. AchEI should be stopped when patients progress to the severe stages, as it is unlikely that they are receiving any clinical benefit at this point.

There is debate about whether the modest benefits achieved in the clinical trials merit the expense of these medications. If the medications can result in decreased caregiver time, delayed progression to severe disease, or delay of institutionalization, some of the expense may be offset. In moderately- to severely-demented subjects, there may be a modest cost savings for donepezil-treated patients when factoring in a cost of caregiver time.[9] However, this benefit has not been noted in similar studies, and the United Kingdom has considered withdrawing coverage for these medications.[10] However, even a small benefit may be worth a significant price if it improves a patient's daily interaction and communication with their loved one.

It is appropriate for a primary care physician to initiate treatment with these medications when the diagnosis is clear. It is important to titrate to the highest recommended dose, the dose shown to be most effective.

The primary side effects are gastrointestinal, caused by the cholinergic properties, including diarrhea, nausea, and vomiting. In clinical trials, the symptoms were most commonly seen at initiation and dose escalation. They were generally mild, and resolved with decreasing to the last-tolerated dose and did not require discontinuation of the drug. The side effects tend to be fairly similar across the class.

Tacrine

Tacrine was the first AchEI approved for use in Alzheimer's dementia, but it is rarely used today because of limitations and adverse events. It is a nonselective, reversible AchEI. The half-life is 2 to 4 hours necessitating multiple daily doses, which can be prohibitive in this population. Also, tacrine may cause significant elevations in serum aminotransferases, and other severe side effects.

Donepezil

Donepezil was approved for the treatment of AD in 1996. Donepezil is a reversible, selective anticholinesterase inhibitor. The half-life is much longer than tacrine, approximately 70 hours, and is approved for once daily dosing. Donepezil also has minimal peripheral anticholinesterase inhibitor activity and thus has fewer systemic side effects than tacrine. Donepezil is initiated at a dose of 5 mg daily. After 4 to 6 weeks the dose can be increased to 10 mg.

Most studies of donepezil in subjects with mild-to-moderate dementia showed benefit in the cognitive outcome measures, but the differences were small. For example, Rogers et al.[11] conducted a 15-week, double-blind placebo controlled study in 468 patients in 23 centers in the United States. Donepezil showed a mean difference of 3.1 points for the ADAS-cog at the endpoint. The investigators also found a mean difference of 0.4 points favoring donepezil on the CIBIC-plus and 1.3 points favoring donepezil on the MMSE. A 1-year placebo controlled preservation of function study showed that donepezil extended the mean time to clinically evident functional decline by 5 months.[12] In a meta-analysis of 16 trials, involving 4365 participants, the investigators found a statistically significant improvement in cognition at both 24 weeks and 52 weeks, as well as improvement in global clinical state, behavior, and ADL.[13]

There have been a few investigations of more impaired subjects. Feldman et al.[13] conducted a 24-week, randomized, double-blind study of donepezil in moderate-to-severe AD, mean MMSE of 5 to 17. The subjects were all community dwelling or residing in an assisted living setting. Subjects were excluded if they required skilled nursing facility placement. Donepezil showed benefit over placebo in the primary outcome measure CIBIC-plus at all visits up to week 24 and on the week-24 visit using last observation carried forward analysis. There were also benefits seen in measures of behavior, cognition, and function. Tariot et al.[14] evaluated donepezil in a more impaired group of subjects with AD, mean MMSE 14, who resided in a nursing home. In this study, the primary efficacy variable was the Neuropsychiatric Inventory-Nursing Home (NPI-NH) version and there was no difference between donepezil and placebo. However, both groups did show improvement from baseline, probably because of other medications and nonpharmacologic interventions, which may have contributed to the lack of drug placebo difference in this study. Although there was no effect seen on the primary outcome variable, differences in the CDR, and MMSE favored donepezil.

Rivastigmine

Rivastigmine is a selective inhibitor of acetylcholinesterase. The half-life of Rivastigmine is 1.5 hours and it is dosed twice daily. The initial dose of rivastigmine is 1.5 mg bid and increased at 2-week intervals by 3 mg/d to a maximum of 12 mg/d. As with other AchEI the side effects are gastrointestinal and typically occur at initiation and dose escalation. Rosler et al.[17] conducted a study in 725 subjects with mild-to-moderately severe AD (MMSE 10–26) over 26 weeks. The investigators found that cognitive function deteriorated in the placebo group, but improved in the groups on the higher dose (6–12 mg/d). Significantly, more patients in the high-dose group showed improvement of 4 points or more on the ADAS-cog, 24% versus 16% for the placebo group. A meta-analysis of seven studies involving 3370 participants showed that rivastigmine at 6 to 12 mg daily was associated with a 2.1 point improvement on ADAS-cog compared to placebo.[21] A 2.2-point improvement on the PDS at 26 weeks was also found. Smaller doses of rivastigmine were associated with significant differences in cognition, but not in other outcome measures.

Galantamine

Galantamine is a selective reversible inhibitor of acetylcholinesterase and an allosteric modulator at nicotinic cholinergic receptors. The initial dose is 4 mg twice daily and can be increased by 8 mg/d divided bid every 4 weeks. The maximum dose is 24 mg/d, and 16 mg/d in patients with hepatic or renal. Raskind et al.[22] conducted a 6-month, multicenter, double blind, placebo controlled trial in 636 patients at 33 centers in the United States. In patients with mild-to-moderate AD, MMSE score of 11 to 24, there was a 3.9-point difference in the ADAS-cog score in

Table 20-2. Selected trials of AchEI for Treatment of AD

Author	Duration	Subjects	No	Treatment	Primary Outcome	Secondary Outcome	Results	Comments
Rogers et al.[11]	12 wks	Probable AD, mild-to-moderate, MMSE 12–26	468 / 10 mg	Placebo, donepezil 5 mg, donepezil 10 mg	ADAS-cog, CIBIC+	MMSE	Better outcome on on ADAS-cog, CIBIC+, MMSE, higher proportion showing improvement	
Mohs et al.[12]	1 yr	Probable AD, mild-to-moderate, MMSE 12–20	431	Placebo, donepezil 10 mg	ADFACS, MMSE, CDR*		Donepezil extended median time to clinically evident decline by 5 months	
Winblad et al.[15]	1 yr	Possible or probable AD, mild-to-moderate, MMSE 10–26	286	Placebo, donepezil 10 mg	GBS	MMSE, PDS, NPI, GDS	Stabilization in donepezil group decline in placebo	
Feldman et al.[13]	24 wks	Possible or possible AD, moderate-to-severe MMSE 5–17	290	Placebo, donepezil 10 mg	CIBIC+	sMMSE, SIB, DAD, IADL+, NPI, PSMS < FRS	Better outcome on measures of function, cognition, and behavior for donepezil group	Subject more impaired than in most AD trials
Tariot et al.[16]	24 wks	Possible or probable AD, NH residents, MMSE 5–206	208	Placebo, donepezil 10 mg	NPI-NH	MMSE, CDR-SB, PSMS	No difference on NPI-NH, benefit on MMSE and CDR	Subjects were in NH
Rosler et al.[17]	26 wks	Probable AD, mild-to-moderate MMSE 10–26	725	Placebo, Rivastigmine 1–4 mg/d, rivastigmine 6–12 mg/d	ADAS-cog, CIBIC+, PDS	GDS, MMSE	Mean deterioration in placebo with slight improvement in rivastigmine, greater proportion improving in the rivastigmine group	
Wilcock et al.[18]	6 mo	Probable AD, mild-to-moderate MMSE 11–24	653	Placebo, galantamine 24 mg/d, galantamine 32 mg/d	ADAS-cog, CIBIC+	DAD	Galantamine showed better outcome on ADAS-cog, CIBIC+, and DAD	
Tariot et al.[19]	5 mo	Probable AD, mild-to-moderate MMSE 10–22	978	Placebo, galantamine 16 mg/d, galantamine 24 mg/d	ADAS-cog, CIBIC+	ADCS/ADL, NPI	Better outcome in ADAS-cog, CIBIC+, and proportion of responders	
Wilkinson et al.[20]	12 wks	Probable AD, mild-to-moderate MMSE 13–24	285	Placebo, galantamine 18 mg/d, 24 mg/d, galantamine 32 mg/d	ADAS-cog	CGIC, PDS	Significant differences favoring galantamine on ADAS-copg and CGIC	

*Analysis done using predetermined criteria for clinically evident decline using these scales.

favor of the galantamine group and a significant improvement in outcome on the CIBIC-plus. Tariot et al.[19] conducted a 5-month randomized, placebo controlled trial of galantamine that showed a difference of 3.6 points on the ADAS-cog in favor of galantamine 24 mg/d. This study also showed a better outcome in ADL, CIBIC+, and behavioral symptoms. In a 6-month, randomized, double blind, placebo-controlled study involving 653 patients in Europe and Canada, galantamine showed better outcome compared to placebo on the ADAS-cog.[18] The mean treatment effect was 3.1 points. In addition, subjects in the galantamine group were found to have significantly better scores on the CIBIC+ compared to placebo. A meta-analysis found statistically significant consistent positive effects for galantamine with doses of greater than 8 mg/d.[23] The magnitude of the effect was felt to be similar to other cholinesterase inhibitors.

MEMANTINE

In 2003, the FDA approved a new medication for the treatment of AD, memantine. Memantine is an uncompetitive, N-methyl-D-aspartate receptor antagonist. This medication is postulated to block the glutamatergic overstimulation that may result in neurotoxicity. This neurotoxicity, called excitotoxicity, may play a role in AD. Memantine is initiated at a dose of 5 mg daily and increased by 5 mg/d every week to a maximum dose of 20 mg/d divided twice daily.

Unlike the cholinesterase inhibitors, memantine has been studied in more severely impaired subjects. In fact, memantine is currently only approved for the treatment of moderately severe to severe AD. Reisberg et al.[24] conducted a randomized, placebo-controlled, trial of memantine in 252 patients in 32 centers in the United States. The subjects had MMSE scores ranging from 3 to 14 and a stage 5 or 6 on the Global Deterioration Scale. The primary outcome variables were the CIBIC+ and the Alzheimer's Disease Cooperative Study Group-Activities of Daily Living modified for severe dementia (ADCS-ADLsev). The mean difference between the two groups in the CIBIC+ was 0.3 favoring the memantine group ($p = 0.03$ analysis of observed cases, $p = 0.06$ analysis with lost observation carried forward). There was significantly less deterioration in the memantine group compared to placebo group based on the ADCS-ADLsev with a mean difference of 2.1 ($p = 0.02$) in the last observation carried forward and 3.4 ($p = 0.003$) in the observed case analysis. No differences were seen in the MMSE, GDS, or NPI. Perhaps the most beneficial effect seen with memantine was a reduction in caregivers time, a mean difference of 45.8 hours (95% CI 10.37–81.27) over 28 weeks. A meta-analysis of the available trials concluded that memantine caused a clinically noticeable reduction in deterioration over 28 weeks in patients with moderate-to-severe AD.[25]

COMBINATION THERAPY

Given the different classes of medicines for Alzheimer type dementia, there is interest in combination therapy. Tariot et al.[16] conducted a study evaluating the addition of memantine to patients already receiving donepezil. Four hundred and four subjects with moderate-to-severe dementia, MMSE 5 to 14, who had been on donepezil for 6 months and at a stable dose for 3 months, were randomized to receive memantine or placebo. There was a statistically significant benefit of memantine on the primary efficacy variables the SIB and the ADCS-ADL and the secondary outcome variables, NPI, and CIBIC. The combination was well tolerated, with more patients discontinuing treatment in the placebo group. The most common adverse events in the memantine group were confusion and headache. Although the results of this trial are promising, whether the same results would be seen in patients with less severe dementia or with other AchEI is unknown.

ANTIOXIDANTS

It has been theorized that the neuronal damage in AD may be related to oxidative stress and the accumulation of free radicals. This has led to speculation that anti-oxidants may slow the progression of disease. Sano et al.[26] conducted a trial of selegiline and α-tocopherol (vitamin E) as treatment for AD. This was a randomized, placebo-controlled double blind trial of 341 patients with moderate dementia over 2 years. The primary outcome was the time to death, institutionalization, loss of ability to perform ADL, or severe dementia (CDR of 3). In the initial unadjusted analysis there was no difference in any of the outcome measures. However, the baseline MMSE was higher in the placebo group, and when this was used as a covariate, there were significant delays in the primary outcome for both the selegiline and the vitamin E groups and the combination group. However, there were no added benefits seen in the combination group than in either therapy alone. Given the higher rate of adverse effects with selegiline, this medication is not widely used for AD. The dose of vitamin E used in this trial, 2000 IU per day, is much higher than is typically used for other indications for vitamin E therapy and whether lower doses would show the same results is unclear. This study by Sano et al.[26] is to date the only one with acceptable methodology and given the questions in interpreting these results, it is difficult to recommend vitamin E for treatment of AD.[27] A further concern is that some data suggest a potential harm from the use of high-dose vitamin E.[28]

ALTERNATIVE AND HERBAL THERAPIES

Ginkgo Biloba

Given the limitations of the FDA-approved therapies, it is not surprising that many of those afflicted with or caring for someone with AD seek alternative or complementary therapies. Perhaps the most commonly used herbal preparation is ginkgo biloba. Many claim that this plant extract has effects on cognition and memory. However, a randomized controlled trial of nondemented older subjects did not show any improvement on neuropsychological tests of learning, memory, attention, and concentration.[29] The extract of ginkgo biloba, is widely used in Europe for improved cognition and is approved in Germany for the treatment of dementia. A 52-week trial in 309 patients with AD or multi-infarct dementia showed a 1.4 point difference in ADAS-cog favoring extract of ginkgo biloba.[30] A meta-analysis of 33 trials of ginkgo found promising evidence of improvement in cognition and function.[31] However, the authors expressed concern that many of the trials were small, few used an intention to treat analysis, and the more recent studies showed inconsistent results. Larger trials with improved methodology are necessary to better evaluate the efficacy of ginkgo biloba.

ESTROGEN

The role of estrogen in AD has been debated and there is some biological plausibility for a beneficial effect on cognition. Epidemiologic data also suggest a beneficial effect of hormone replacement therapy (HRT) on cognition. However, in an evaluation of the effects of HRT on tests of cognitive function in healthy older women in the Nurses Health Study only tests of verbal fluency showed improvement while overall cognitive function seemed to be no different in women who took HRT.[32] The Study of Osteoporotic Fractures found that endogenous estrogen levels were not associated with improved cognitive performance or likelihood of cognitive decline.[33] The Women's Health Initiative Memory Study, a randomized double-blind, placebo controlled trial of 4532 postmenopausal women, showed that estrogen and progesterone replacement therapy may be associated with an increased risk of developing AD.[34] As there is conflicting evidence about the use of estrogen as far as prevention of dementia and preservation of cognition, there is also conflicting data about the use of estrogen for the treatment of AD. In a small study involving only 20 women with mild-to-moderate

dementia, high-dose estrogen improved attention and memory.[35] However, a larger study of 50 women with mild-to-moderate dementia found no improvement in cognition, dementia severity, or behavior over 12 weeks.[36] In larger study involving 120 participants in the AD Cooperative Study with mild-to-moderate AD (MMSE 12–28), found no difference on the primary outcome variable, the CGIC, between estrogen and placebo.[37] Given data from the Women's Health Initiative Study suggesting increased risk of stroke with HRT and the lack of data suggesting a benefit in treatment of AD, it is not recommended to use HRT to treat AD.[38,39]

Anti-Inflammatory Agents

Evidence suggests there may be an inflammatory contribution to the development of AD. Thus, it is plausible that nonsteroidal anti-inflammatory drugs may treat or prevent Alzheimer. There is evidence from case control trials that nonsteroidal anti-inflammatory drugs may have an effect in preventing dementia.[39,40] Several different agents have been evaluated. A small trial of indomethacin suggested some benefit in cognition but more than 20% of patients had adverse effects leading to discontinuation of the trial.[41] Rofecoxib was not found to be superior to placebo in 692 patients with mild-to-moderate AD over 12 months in measures of cognition or global impression of disease severity.[42] Rofecoxib and naproxen showed no benefit for the treatment of mild-to-moderate AD.[43] Given the risk of gastrointestinal bleeding with nonselective cyclooxygenase inhibitors and the more recent concerns regarding the Cox-2 inhibitors, these agents should not be used for the treatment of AD.[44]

TREATMENT OF BEHAVIORAL ASPECTS OF AD

One of the most distressing aspects of dementia for families and caregivers is agitation and disruptive behaviors, which frequently leads to institutionalization. It is also a frequent source of frustration on the part of the clinician. There are several agents that are used for the treatment of the behaviors associated with AD, including antidepressants, mood stabilizers, antipsychotics, anticonvulsants, the AchEI, and memantine.

ANTIPSYCHOTICS

The most commonly used medications for controlling agitation, psychosis, and behaviors in dementia are the antipsychotics. The older antipsychotics have been used for treatment of psychosis in dementia, but the side effects, such as the extrapyramidal symptoms, are often limiting. A randomized, double blind placebo controlled trial of haloperidol for psychosis and disruptive behaviors in 71 subjects with AD showed no difference with 0.5–0.75 mg/d compared to placebo.[45] Patients on 2–3 mg/d had a higher response rate with a reduction of psychosis and disruptive behaviors, but a 20% increase in extrapyramidal effects. The authors recommended starting at 1 mg/d with gradual dose titration to 2–3 mg/d. Another trial showed no difference between haloperidol, trazodone, behavioral management techniques (BMT), or placebo.[46] Haloperidol was initiated at 0.5 mg/d and increased until the subject improved, significant adverse events were noted or to a maximum of 3 mg/d. The mean dose of haloperidol was lower in this trial, 1.8 mg/d, and fewer side effects were seen. An analysis of the available trials of haloperidol for agitation concluded that haloperidol decreased aggression but did not decrease agitation and increased some adverse events.[47]

The second generation antipsychotics are less likely than the older agents to have extrapyramidal side effects and are frequently used in the management of behavioral symptoms in AD; however these agents are not FDA approved for this purpose. Risperidone, olanzapine, and aripiprazole have shown modest benefits; however these trials also showed a large placebo response and the differences were modest over placebo.[48–50] The FDA has issued a health advisory reporting increased mortality in elderly patients with dementia-related behavioral disorders treated with these agents.[51] There are also concerns that these agents may promote a decline in cognition. One study showed no benefit in behaviors from quetiapine or rivastigmine compared to placebo, and quetiapine was associated with greater cognitive decline.[52] These medications have significant side effects, including falls, hyperglycemia, and stroke.

These agents are probably overprescribed in the nursing home population. However, this class still probably represents one of the more effective and well-studied class of medications for the treatment of agitation in Alzheimer's dementia. Primary care physicians who prescribe these medicines should start with low doses, increase carefully, monitor closely, and consult a specialist in difficult cases.

MOOD STABILIZERS

The mood stabilizers carbamazepine and valproate are commonly used for the management of behaviors in AD. Carbamazepine provided some benefit in managing agitation in 51 nursing home patients.[53] However, some caution against their use because of side effects and limited supporting data.[54]

DISCUSSION OF TREATMENT OPTIONS

There are several important issues to discuss with capable patients and their family members. Family members and caregivers should be informed of the limitations of these medications. Those seeking a cure or even a reversal of the inevitable progressive decline in cognition will be disappointed. Therefore, it is important to discuss realistic outcomes. Financial considerations are a common barrier to medication compliance. Given the expense involved in caring for someone with AD including possibly nursing home care, incontinence supplies, and home health equipment, as well as medications for other comorbid conditions, the additional expense of a rather costly AD medication could be prohibitive. Some may feel that the modest benefits are not worth the additional expense. Discussion of some of the unanswered questions involved in treatment of AD should also be considered when initially prescribing the medication. These include a discussion of the uncertainty over the duration of therapy and whether to continue therapy when the patient has advanced to the severe stages.

EVIDENCE-BASED SUMMARY

- The acetycholinesterase inhibitors are FDA-approved for mild-to-moderate AD and show modest benefits on measures of cognition, function, and behavior.
- There is no definite benefit of one acetylcholinesterase over another.
- Memantine is FDA-approved for moderate-to-severe Alzheimer's dementia and shows benefit on measures of cognition, function, behavior, and caregiver time.
- There may be benefit in adding memantine to donepezil.
- The medications have not been shown to delay institutionalization and cost effectiveness is unproven.
- The primary adverse events for AchEI are gastrointestinal including diarrhea and nausea.
- There is little evidence to support using vitamin E.
- There is no evidence to support using estrogen or anti-inflammatories.
- There is little evidence supporting any class of medication in treating behavioral symptoms of AD, including agitation and aggression, but the atypical (second generation) antipsychotic medications can be used at low doses with caution.

REFERENCES

1. Hebert LE, Scherr PA, Bienias JL, et al. Alzheimer's disease in the US population: Prevalence estimates using the 2000 census. *Arch Neurol.* 2003;60(8):1119–1122.
2. Evans DA, Funkenstein HH, Albert MS, et al. Prevalence of Alzheimer's disease in a community population of older persons: Higher than previously reported. *JAMA.* 1989;262(18):2552–2556.
3. American Psychiatric Association. *Diagnostic and statistical manual of mental disorders,* 4th ed. Washington DC: American Psychiatric Press; 1994.
4. McKhann G, Drachman D, Folstein M, et al. Clinical diagnosis of Alzheimer's disease: Report of the NINCDS-ADRDA work group under the auspices of Department of Health and Human Services Task force on Alzheimer's disease. *Neurology.* 1984;34:939–944.
5. Food, Drug and Cosmetic Reports: *FDA Guidance on Alzheimer's Drug Clinical Utility Assessments.* Washington DC: FDC Reports; 1992.
6. Lanctot KL, Herrmann N, Yau KK, et al. Efficacy and safety of cholinesterase inhibitors in Alzheimer's disease: A meta-analysis. *CMAJ.* 2003;169:557–564.
7. Trinh NH, Hoblyn J, Mohanty S, et al. Efficacy of cholinesterace inhibitors in the treatment of neuropsychiatric symptoms and functional impairment in Alzheimer's disease: A meta-analysis. *JAMA.* 2003;289:210–216.
8. Kaduszkiewicz H, Zimmerman T, Beck-Bornholdt HP, et al. Cholinesterase inhibitors for patients with Alzheimer's disease: Systematic review of randomized clinical trials. *BMJ.* 2005;331:321–327.
9. Feldman H, Gauthier S, Hecker J, et al. Economic evaluation of donepezil in moderate to severe Alzheimer's disease. *Neurology.* 2004;63:644–650.
10. AD2000 Collaborative Group. Long-term donepezil treatment in 565 patients with Alzheimer's disease (AD2000): Randomized double-blind trial. *Lancet.* 2004;363:2105–2115.
11. Rogers SL, Doody RS, Mohs RC, et al. Donepezil improves cognition and global function in Alzheimer's Disease: A 15-week, double blind placebo controlled study. *Arch Int Med.* 1998;158:1021–1031.
12. Mohs RC, Doody RS, Morris JC, et al. A 1-year, placebo-controlled preservation of functional survival study of donepezil in AD patients. *Neurology.* 2001;57:481–488.
13. Feldman H, Gauthier S, Hecker J, et al. A 24-week, randomized, double-blind, study of donepezil in moderate to severe Alzheimer's disease. *Neurology.* 2001;57:613–620.
14. Tariot PN, Cummings JL, Katz IR, et al. A randomized, double-blind, placebo-controlled study of the efficacy and safety of donepezil in patients with Alzhemier's disease in the nursing home setting. *J Am Geriatr Soc.* 2001;49: 1590–1599.
15. Winblad B, Engedal K, Soininen H, et al. A 1-year, randomized, placebo-controlled study of donepezil in patients with mild to moderate AD. *Neurology.* 2001;57: 489–495.
16. Tariot PN, Farlow MR, Grossberg GT, et al. Memantine treatment in patients with moderate to severe Alzheimer's disease already receiving donepezil: A randomized controlled trial. *JAMA.* 2004;291:317–324.
17. Rosler M, Anand R, Cicin-Sain A, et al. Efficacy and safety of rivastigmine in patients with Alzheimer's disease: International randomized controlled trial. *BMJ.* 1999;318:1633–639.
18. Wilcock GK, Lillienfeld S, Gaens E, et al. Efficacy and safety of galantamine in patients with mild to moderate Alzheimer's disease: Multicentre randomized controlled trial. *BMJ.* 2000;321:1445–1449.
19. Tariot PN, Solomon PR, Morris JC, et al. A 5-month, randomized, placebo-controlled trial of galantamine in AD. *Neurology.* 2000;54:2269–2276.
20. Wilkinson D, Murray J, Galantamine Research Group. Galantamine: A randomized, double-blind, dose comparison in patients with Alzheimer's disease. *Int J Geriatr Psychiatry.* 2001;16:852–857.
21. Birks J, Grimley Evans J, Iakovidou V, Tsolaki M. Rivastigmine for Alzheimer's disease. *Cochrane Database Syst Rev.* 2000;(4):CD001191. doi: 10.1002/14651858.CD001191.
22. Raskind MA, Peskind ER, Wessel T, et al. Galantamine in AD. A 6-month randomized, placebo controlled trial with a 6 month extension. *Neurology.* 2000;54:2261–2268.
23. Loy C, Schneider L. Galantamine for Alzheimer's disease and mild cognitive impairment. *Cochrane Database Syst Rev.* 2006;(1):CD001747. doi: 10.1002/14651858.CD001747. pub3.
24. Reisberg B, Doody R, Stoffler A, et al. Memantine in Moderate-to-Severe Alzheimer's Disease. *N Engl J Med.* 2003;348: 1333–1341.
25. McSHane R, Areosa Sastre A, Minakaran N. Memantine for dementia. *Cochrane Database Syst Rev.* 2006;(2):CD003154. doi: 10.1002/14651858.CD003154.pub5.
26. Sano M, Ernesto C, Thomas RG, et al. A controlled trial of selegeline, alpha-tocopherol or both as treatment for Alzheimer's disease. *N Eng J Med.* 1997;336:1216–1222.
27. Isaac M, Quinn R, Tabet N. Vitamin E for Alzheimer's disease and mild cognitive impairment. *Cochrane Database Syst Rev.* 2000;(4):CD002854. doi: 10.1002/14651858.CD002854.
28. Miller ER, Pastor-Barriuso R, Dalal D, et al. Meta-analysis: High dose Vitamin E supplementation may increase all cause mortality. *Ann Intern Med.* 2005;142:37–46.
29. Solomon PR, Adams F, Silver A, et al. Ginkgo for memory enhancement. a randomized controlled trial. *JAMA.* 2002; 288:835–840.
30. Le Bars PL, Katz MM, Berman N, et al. A placebo controlled, double-blind, randomized trial of an extract of gingko biloba for dementia. *JAMA.* 1997;278:1327–1332.
31. Birks J, Grimley Evans J, Lee H. Gingko biloba for cognitive impairment and dementia. *Cochrane Database Syst Rev.* 2007;(2):CD003120. doi: 10.1002/14651858.CD003120. pub2.
32. Grodstein F, Chen J, Pollen D, et al. Postmenopausal hormone therapy and cognitive function in healthy older women. *J Amer Geriatr Soc.* 2000;48:746–752.
33. Yaffe K, Grady D, Pressman A, et al. Serum estrogen levels, cognitive performance, and risk of cognitive decline in older community women. *J Amer Geriatr Soc.* 1998;46: 816–821.

34. Shumaker SA, Legault C, Rapp SR, et al. Estrogen plus progestin and the incidence of dementia and mild cognitive impairment in postmenopausal women: The Women's Health Initiative Memory Study: A randomized controlled trial. *JAMA.* 2003;289:2651–2662.

35. Asthana S, Baker LD, Craft S, et al. High-dose estradiol improves cognition for women with AD. *Neurology.* 2001;57: 605–612.

36. Wang PN, Liao SQ, Liu RS, et al. Effects of estrogen on cognition, mood and cerebral blood flow in AD. *Neurology.* 2000;54:2061–2066.

37. Mulnard RA, Cotman CW, Kawas C, et al. Estrogen replacement therapy for treatment of mild to moderate Alzheimer's disease. *JAMA.* 2000;283:1007–1014.

38. Anderson GL, Limacher M, Assaf AR, et al. Effects of conjugated equine estrogen in postmenopausal women with hysterectomy: The Women's Health Initiative randomized controlled trial. *JAMA.* 2004;291:1701–1712.

39. Rossouw JE, Anderson GL, Prentice RL, et al. Risks and benefits of estrogen plus progestin in healthy postmenopausal women: Principal results from the Women's Health Initiative randomized controlled trial. *JAMA.* 2002;288:321–333.

40. Anthony JC, Breitner JCS, Zandi PP, et al. Reduced prevalence of AD in users of NSAIDs and H2 receptor antagonists. The Cache County Study. *Neurology.* 2000;54:2066–2071.

41. Beard CM, Waring SC, O'Brien PC, et al. Nonsteroidal anti-inflammatory drug use and Alzheimer's disease: A case-control study in Rochester, Minnesota, 1980–1984. *Mayo Clin Proc.* 1998;73:951–955.

42. Rogers J, Kirby LC, Hempelman SR, et al. Clinical trial of indomethacin in Alzheimer's disease. *Neurology.* 1993; 43:1609–1611.

43. Reines SA, Block GA, Morris JC, et al. Rofecoxib: No effect on Alzheimer's disease in a 1-year, randomized, blinded, controlled study. *Neurology.* 2004;62:66–71.

44. Aisen PS, Schafer KA, Grundman M, et al. Effects of rofecoxib or naproxen vs placebo on Alzheimer's disease progression: A randomized controlled trial. *JAMA.* 2003; 289:2819–2826.

45. Bresalier RS, Sandler RS, Quan H, et al. Cardiovascular events associated with rofecoxib in a colorectal adenoma chemoprevention trial. *N Engl J Med.* 2002;352:1092–1102.

46. Devanand DP, Marder K, Michaels KS, et al. A randomized placebo controlled dose-comparison trial of haloperidol for psychosis and disruptive behaviors in Alzheimer's disease. *Am J Psychiatry.* 1998;155:1512–1520.

47. Teri L, Logsdon RG, Peskind E, et al. Treatment of agitation in AD: A randomized placebo-controlled clinical trial. *Neurology.* 2000;55:1271–1278.

48. Lonergan E, Luxemberg J, Colford J, Birks J. Haloperidol for agitation in dementia. *Cochrane Database Syst Rev.* 2002;(2):CD002852. doi: 10.1002/14651858.CD002852.

49. Street JS, Clark WS, Gannon KS, et al. Olanzapine treatment of psychotic and behavioral symptoms in patients with Alzheimer's disease in nursing care facilities: A double-blind, randomized, placebo-controlled trial. *Arch Gen Psychiatry.* 2000;57:968–976.

50. De Deyn P, Jeste DV, Swanink R, et al. Aripiprazole for the treatment of psychosis in patients with Alzheimer's disease: A randomized, placebo-controlled study. *J Clin Psychopharmacol.* 2005;25:463–467.

51. FDA Public Health Advisory. Deaths with antipsychotics in elderly patients with behavioral disturbances. www.fda.gov/CDER/drug/advisory/antipsychotics.htm. Accessed April 11, 2005.

52. Ballard C, Margallo-Lana M, Juszczak E, et al. Quetiapine and rivastigmine and cognitive decline in Alzheimer's disease: Randomized double blind placebo controlled trial. *BMJ.* 2005;330:874.

53. Tariot P, Erb R, Podgorski CA, et al. Efficacy and tolerability of carbamazepine for agitation and aggression in dementia. *Am J Psychiatry.* 1998;155:54–61.

54. Sink KM, Holden KF, Yaffe K. Pharmacologic treatment of neuropsychiatric symptoms of dementia: A review of the evidence. *JAMA.* 2005;293:596–608.

Chapter 21

Depression

Cynthia A. Mascarenas and Troy A. Moore

SEARCH STRATEGY

This chapter was developed by searching the National Guideline Clearinghouse for all available treatment guidelines for depression. These guidelines were narrowed down to those focused on depression in the primary care setting. Epidemiologic information about depression was obtained from the National Institute of Mental Health and the World Health Organization. Additional evidence-based information from each section was obtained through Medline searches using the words, "depression" or "depressive disorder," "antidepressants," and "primary care."

INTRODUCTION

Depression is a whole body illness that can affect one's mood, thoughts, and physical well-being. Depressive symptoms may last weeks, months, or even years if left untreated.[1] The lifetime prevalence for major depressive disorder (MDD) ranges from 10% to 25% for women and 5% to 12% for men.[2] Statistics from the National Institute of Mental Health show that depression is a widespread illness affecting approximately 18.8 million Americans in any given year.[3] It is estimated that 32 to 35 million American adults will suffer from MDD in their lifetime.[4] Nearly one in six individuals with severe, untreated depression will commit suicide.[1]

In 2004, the World Health Organization (WHO) reported that 11.9% of disability is caused by unipolar depressive disorders; these disorders are the leading source of years with disability.[5] Depression causes more disability than hypertension, diabetes, cardiovascular disease, or low back pain[1] It is estimated that the annual direct cost of depression in the United States is $ 26 million.[4] Workers with depression cost employers in excess of $30 billion per year in lost productivity.[1] By the year 2020,

depression is projected to reach second place on disability adjusted life years calculated for all ages by the WHO.[5]

Depression is one of the top five conditions seen by primary care physicians. In fact, depressive disorders are one of the most common reasons for primary care visits. Fifty to sixty percent of all antidepressant therapy prescriptions are generated by primary care physicians.[6] Despite its recognition as a major health concern, depression is often under-recognized and left untreated. The WHO reported that fewer than 25% of all individuals with depression receive care.[5] Many patients are reluctant to seek treatment for fear of the stigma of having a mental disorder or are unaware of the gravity of the illness.

CLINICAL PRESENTATION

Individuals with a depressive disorder present with varying symptoms, the most evident being depressed mood. Patients may report loss of interest in activities, including sex. Patients may also report sleep disturbances, alterations in appetite, or significant changes in weight. Concentration may be impaired or patients may complain of distractibility. Hopelessness, helplessness, or feelings of excessive guilt may be present. Patients can feel fatigued, worn down, or exhausted even with little to no exertion. Movements may be either visibly slowed or increased. In addition, rate of speech may be decreased, as well as volume.

Healthcare providers must also be cognizant of non-specific signs and symptoms, including vague somatic complaints, which may be related to a depressive disorder. Often the etiology of these complaints cannot be determined. Symptoms such as headaches, gastrointestinal ailments, or bone or muscle aches that do not respond to appropriate medical treatment suggest a possible depressive disorder. Patients with persisting conditions despite adequate treatment should be evaluated for depression.

Current psychosocial stressors can affect mood and must also be examined. These include financial concerns, issues with marital or familial relationships, medical conditions, and work stressors. Patients with predominant psychosocial issues may be candidates for psychotherapy.

Patients with comorbid medical conditions, such as diabetes, cancer, myocardial infarction, and stroke need to be monitored for depression. It is estimated that 20% to 25% of patients with these conditions will suffer from a depressive episode.[2] Depression with comorbid medical conditions increases the complexity of the management of both conditions and makes the prognosis less favorable.[2]

SCREENING INSTRUMENTS

Because depression is often missed, routine screening for the disorder is recommended.[7] The optimal interval between screening is unknown, but recurrent screening may be most beneficial in patients with a history of depression, other psychological comorbidities, substance abuse, chronic pain, or somatic symptoms.[7] At a minimum, all patients should be routinely assessed for depressed mood and loss of interest or pleasure.[8,9]

There are a variety of tools available for use in the primary care setting. The Primary Care Evaluation of Mental Disorders (Prime-MD): 2 Item and the Brief Patient Health Questionnaire (BPHQ) each use simple yes or no questions (Table 21-1). If a patient answers yes to either of these questions, a more detailed interview should be performed. The 2-item questionnaires offer equal sensitivity but with less precision compared to extensive screening tools.

Table 21-1. Depression Screening Questions

Prime-MD: 2 Item Depression Screening[8]
  In the past month, have you often been bothered by feeling down, depressed, or hopeless?
  In the past month, have you often been bothered by little interest or pleasure in doing things?
BPHQ: 2 Item Depression Screening[9]
  In the past 2 weeks, have you often been bothered by feeling down, depressed, or hopeless?
  In the past 2 weeks, have you often been bothered by little interest or pleasure in doing things?

Other instruments are available but take longer to complete. Depression-specific tools such as the Beck Depression Inventory, Quick Inventory of Depressive Symptoms Self Report, the Center for Epidemiological Studies-Depression Scale, Zung Depression Scale, and Hamilton Depression Rating Scales are useful for more extensive assessment of symptoms. However, each of these tools also offers shorter, more time efficient versions that may be used in primary care settings. These instruments are available for administration by a clinician or self administration by the patient.

DIAGNOSIS

DIAGNOSTIC CRITERIA

The diagnosis of a depressive disorder is formulated utilizing the specific criteria set forth in the *Diagnostic and Statistical Manual of Mental Disorders, Fourth Edition, Text Revision* which include depressed mood, sleep or appetite disturbances, impaired concentration, anergia, and suicidal or homicidal ideation (Table 21-2). For a depressive episode, the specific symptoms must be present for at least 2 weeks, for most of the day, nearly every day, during that period. Additionally, the presence of symptoms must cause clinically significant distress or impair functioning in at least one domain: home, work, or social interactions. Diagnostic criteria for depression may be remembered utilizing the mnemonic of Sleep, Interest, Guilt, Energy, Concentration, Appetite, Psychomotor Activity, Suicidal Ideation (SIGECAPS) (Table 21-3). Careful evaluation must be

Table 21-2. Diagnostic Criteria for MDD[2]

Criteria	Symptoms
At least 5 symptoms with at least one being depressed mood and/or loss of interest/pleasure	Depressed mood
	Diminished or loss of interest/pleasure
	Weight or appetite disturbances
Symptoms cause distress or impair function	Insomnia or hypersomnia
	Restlessness or being slowed down
Symptoms are not due to general medical condition	Fatigue or loss of energy
Symptoms are not a reaction to a death	Feelings of worthless/guilt
Symptoms do not occur in the context of schizophrenia, schizophreniform disorder, delusional disorder, or psychotic disorder NOS	Decreased ability to think or concentrate
	Thoughts of death/suicide

Source: APA. Man of Mental Dis, 4/e. DC: APPress/2000.

Table 21-3. SIGECAPS Mnemonic

SIGECAPS Mnemonic:
In the past 2 weeks have you experienced . . .
  *S*leep disturbance (insomnia/hypersomnia)
  Loss of *I*nterest or pleasure
  *G*uilt (hopelessness, worthlessness or regret)
  *E*nergy deficit
  *C*oncentration impairment
  *A*ppetite or weight changes
  *P*sychomotor agitation or retardation
  *S*uicidal or homicidal ideation

performed to rule out medical causes (including neurological conditions and hormonal dysregulation).

PHYSICAL FINDINGS

No specific findings upon physical examination can be used to diagnose a depressive disorder. Likewise, laboratories cannot be used to "rule in" depression. However, these can be utilized to rule out medical causes of the patient's symptoms, such as hypothyroidism.

DIAGNOSTIC EVALUATION

A complete psychiatric evaluation should be performed, including a detailed history of present illness and description of current symptoms. A thorough psychiatric history must be obtained, including prior treatment and response, psychiatric hospitalizations, suicide attempts, and possible symptoms of mania. The practitioner should also detail substance abuse history, social history, and developmental history. Taking a family history of psychiatric illness is also necessary. A comprehensive review of medications is required. Physical examination, mental status examination, and laboratories including CBC, thyroid function, and serum chemistries should be performed.

SUICIDALITY

Assessment of the patient's risk for suicide is imperative. Determination of the presence or absence of suicidal or homicidal ideation, as well as measure of intent and extent of preparation is crucial. The clinician must determine the availability and means for a suicide attempt and make a clinical judgment on the lethality of those means. History of prior attempts should also be elucidated, as well as family history of suicide and recent exposure to suicide.[10] Patients with suicidal or homicidal ideation, intentions, or plans require close monitoring and should be referred to a psychiatrist. Factors that may increase a patient's risk for suicide

include the presence of psychotic symptoms, severe anxiety, panic attacks, and substance or alcohol abuse.

PSYCHIATRY CONSULT

Patients with depression should be referred to a psychiatrist if the patient is deemed at risk for suicide, or if psychotic features are present. Additionally, a consult should be submitted if the patient requires psychiatric hospitalization. A consultation is recommended if the patient fails an adequate trial of antidepressant medication of at least 6 weeks' duration or if the patient has a need for psychotherapy in addition to medication. Patients with a history of manic symptoms (i.e., decreased need for sleep, pressured speech, grandiosity, flight of ideas, or distractibility) should be referred to a psychiatrist for evaluation and treatment. Significant comorbidity, either medical or psychiatric, is also reason for referral to a psychiatrist. For "special populations" such as patients with substance abuse and psychiatric comorbidities, especially bipolar disorder, consider involving a substance abuse or mental health specialist.

MANAGEMENT

Depression can be treated with pharmacotherapy, psychotherapy, or a combination of both depending on severity of illness. Electroconvulsive therapy (ECT) can be used for those patients refractory to other treatments. No antidepressant agent or class has been shown to be more effective than the others. Therefore, selection of an antidepressant medication is based on potential side effects, prior response, comorbid medical conditions, patient preference, and medication cost. In most patients, SSRIs, bupropion, mirtazapine, venlafaxine, desipramine, and nortriptyline are appropriate agents.[10,11]

Patients initiated on antidepressant medication should be informed of potential side effects and monitored carefully to assess treatment response, emergence of adverse effects, clinical condition, and safety. Frequency of monitoring should be dependent on the severity of illness, cooperation with therapy, presence of social supports, and comorbid medical conditions. Follow-up should occur often enough to evaluate suicidality and encourage compliance with treatment.[10]

DURATION OF TREATMENT

Treatment for depression is divided into three phases (Fig. 21-1). The first, the "acute phase," includes the first 3 months of treatment. During this phase, strict monitoring of the patient's severity of illness including suicidality, medication compliance, side effects, and safety is required. The American Psychiatric Association

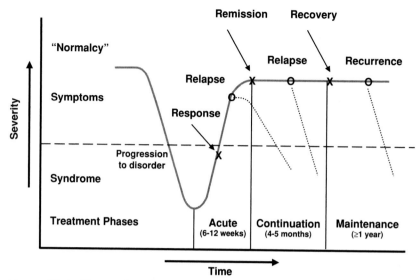

Figure 21-1. Phases of treatment for depression. (Adapted from Kupfer DJ. Long-term treatment of depression. *J Clin Psychiatry*. 1991;52(Suppl):28–34.)

recommends weekly visits during this period for less-severe cases, up to multiple times per week for more-severe cases of depression. The goal of treatment should be remission of the patient's depression symptoms, defined as minimal to no signs of depression remain. Response is defined as a significant level of improvement or 50% decrease in severity. By the sixth to eighth week of treatment, there should be a least a moderate improvement in depressive symptoms. If a moderate reduction in symptoms is not achieved by week 8, a dosage increase or medication change should be implemented.

The second phase, or "continuation phase," is the 16 to 20 weeks following remission. Patients on pharmacotherapy for depression should remain on their medication at the same dose during this phase to prevent relapse of the depressive episode. There is no data to support the reduction in antidepressant dosage during the continuation phase.

The third phase is the "maintenance phase." During this period, patients are treated to prevent recurrence of the disorder. Without long-term antidepressant therapy, relapse and recurrence occur in 50% to 80% of patients.[11] A multitude of factors must be addressed while considering maintenance treatment. First, the risk of recurrence for the patient can be evaluated by examining the number of prior episodes, the presence of comorbid conditions, and residual symptoms present between episodes.[10] The severity of episodes, such as suicidality, psychotic features, or severe functional impairments, should also be taken into account.[10] The patient's tolerability with the current medication regimen should be considered. Lastly,

the patient's willingness to continue the medication must be assessed. All these factors must be weighted together to determine if the patient should receive maintenance treatment.

The Institute for Clinical Systems Improvement guidelines suggest that patients with first-episode depression should be treated for 6 to 12 months; patients with a second episode should be treated for 3 years.[11] Those with a second episode with complicating factors (preexisting dysthymia, inability to reach full remission, or recurrence with dose lowering or discontinuation) should receive lifelong treatment.[11] Patients with three or more episodes of depression should be treated lifelong with antidepressant therapy.[11,12]

PHARMACOTHERAPY

There are many pharmacotherapeutic options for depression. Each class of antidepressant medications are briefly discussed in this section. Starting and target doses of each medication are listed in Table 21-4.

Selective Serotonin Reuptake Inhibitors

The selective serotonin reuptake inhibitors (SSRIs) are considered first-line treatment for depression, because of efficacy, tolerability, and safety in overdose. In addition, both the quality and quantity of clinical data supporting their use has lead to their widespread use. The SSRIs act by selectively binding to the serotonin transporter preventing the reuptake of serotonin. These agents are equally efficacious in treating depression, but differ in side effect burden and drug

Table 21-4. Commonly Used Antidepressant Medications (list is representative, not Comprehensive)

Generic Name	Starting Dose (mg/d)*	Usual Dose (mg/d)‡	Cost/30-Day Prescription§
SSRIs†			
Citalopram	20	20–60‡	$44.99–134.97
Escitalopram	10	10–20‡	$72.99–74.99
Fluoxetine	20	20–60‡	$24.99–74.97
Paroxetine	20	20–60‡	$57.99–173.97
Sertraline	50	50–200‡	$86.99–173.98
Dopamine-norepinephrine reuptake inhibitors†			
Bupropion, immediate release	200	200–450	$47.40–107.98
Bupropion, sustained release	150	150–400	$86.99–173.98
Bupropion, extended release	150	150–450	$113.99–148.99
Serotonin-norepinephrine reuptake inhibitors†			
Venlafaxine	37.5	75–375	$71.50–220.49
Venlafaxine, extended release	37.5	75–225	$99.99–229.98
Duloxetine	30	40–60	$109.99–200.99
Norepinephrine-serotonin modulator			
Mirtazapine	15	15–45	$75.99–$79.99
Serotonin modulators			
Nefazodone	50	150–300	$66.99–67.99
Trazodone	50	75–300	$9.99–40.98
Tricyclic and tetracyclic			
Tertiary amine tricyclics			
Amitriptyline	25–50	100–300	$7.99–17.99
Clomipramine	25	100–250	$37.20–103.98
Doxepin	25–50	100–300	$12.99–49.99
Imipramine	25–50	100–300	$20.40–61.20
Secondary amine tricyclics			
Desipramine†	25–50	100–300	$19.99–92.39
Nortriptyline†	25	50–200	$18.99–58.49
Tetracyclics			
Amoxapine	50	100–400	$38.10–152.40
Maprotiline	50	100–225	$29.94–76.50
MAOIs			
Phenelzine	15	15–90	$19.20–115.20
Tranylcypromine	10	30–60	$101.70–203.40

*Lower starting doses are recommended for elderly patients and for patients with panic disorder, significant anxiety or hepatic disease, and general comorbidity.
†These medications are likely to be optimal medications in terms of the patient's acceptance of side effects, safety, and quantity of clinical trial data.
‡Dose varies with diagnosis
§Cost estimated from price of prescription from retail pharmacy

interaction profile. Additionally, the availability of generic products for citalopram, fluoxetine, and paroxetine allows for lower cost. Selection of an agent should be made after careful consideration of these three distinctions between medications rather than minimal differences in efficacy.

Second-Generation Antidepressants

The second-generation antidepressants include medications with dual reuptake inhibition and/or non-selective binding, such as bupropion, duloxetine, mirtazapine, nefazodone, trazodone, and venlafaxine. Each medication has its own distinct receptor binding profile and is unique in mechanism of action, side effect profile, and pharmacokinetic parameters. These medications are used as first- or secondline treatment for depression. Bupropion, mirtazapine, and venlafaxine are incorporated in most guidelines as first-line agents because of safety profiles similar to the SSRIs. Bupropion is a dual reuptake inhibitor of dopamine and norepinephrine. Mirtazapine is a potent serotonin-2 and serotonin-3 receptor antagonist, which also exhibits strong histamine-1 antagonist and α-2 blocking properties, as well as moderate α-1 antagonism. Venlafaxine is a potent inhibitor of serotonin and norepinephrine and a weak inhibitor of dopamine. Duloxetine is an equipotent inhibitor of serotonin and norepinephrine. Duloxetine is not included in most of the recent guidelines as a result of its recent release onto the market, but it would be assumed to be a first- or second-line agent unless some undue side effects present themselves.

Trazodone blocks serotonin reuptake, histamine-1, and α-1 receptors. Trazodone is typically reserved for second-line treatment because of the higher sedative properties seen with doses used for depression. Nefazodone is a serotonin and norepinephrine reuptake inhibitor with serotonin-2 and α-1 antagonism. Nefazodone is considered as a last-line agent in many guidelines as a result of the black box warning issued by the FDA for hepatic failure. The incidence of hepatic failure with nefazodone is one in every 250 000 to 300 000.

Tricyclic Antidepressants

Tricyclic antidepressants (TCAs) are typically first- to third-line agents for the treatment of depression because of increased side effects, risk of overdose, and drug interactions exhibited in comparison to SSRIs and second generation antidepressants. Some of the more commonly prescribed TCAs are amitriptyline, nortriptyline, imipramine, desipramine, and doxepin. The secondary amine TCAs such as desipramine are generally better tolerated and are less sedating than the tertiary amine compounds (amitriptyline and nortriptyline). As these agents are all available in generic form, the cost of these medications may be substantially less than other classes of antidepressants.

Monoamine Oxidase Inhibitors

Although more effective than TCAs in atypical depression, monoamine oxidase inhibitors (MAOIs) are typically last-line pharmacological agents because of their high side effect profiles, risk of overdose, drug–drug interactions, and drug–food interactions. These agents are usually restricted to patients who have failed all other pharmacological treatments. The MAOIs include tranylcypromine and phenelzine.

ELECTROCONVULSIVE THERAPY

ECT is a very effective treatment option for depression. ECT can be used in patients who have failed medication therapy either because of adverse side effects or lack of efficacy. Clinical data supports ECT in geriatric depression, depression with psychotic features, catatonia, and in patients with depression and Parkinsonism.[11] The use of ECT is often performed in patients with severe, refractory depression. Unfortunately, the number of institutions and psychiatrists performing the procedure are limited in many areas.

PSYCHOTHERAPY

Psychotherapy is an effective, viable option for the treatment of depression. Various treatment approaches have been found to be effective, such as cognitive–behavioral, interpersonal, and structured educational group therapy.[11] Psychotherapy should be considered in patients with depression involving psychological and psychosocial issues. Psychotherapy involves a consultation to a mental health care professional that provides this care.

EVIDENCE-BASED SUMMARY

- Common depressive symptoms include depressed mood, loss of interest or pleasure, appetite changes, sleep disturbances, decreased energy, impaired concentration, and thoughts of death or suicide.
- Various tools can be utilized to screen for depression including the Prime MD: 2 item and BPHQ 2 item depression screening questions
- No antidepressant agent or class has been shown to be more effective than the others. Therefore, selection of an antidepressant medication is based on potential side effects, prior response, comorbid medical conditions, patient preference, and medication cost.
- During the "acute phase" of a depressive episode, patients should be monitored closely for safety, tolerability, and suicidality.
- Patients with first-episode depression should be treated at minimum for 6 months after obtaining remission; those with 3 or more episodes should receive lifelong therapy.

REFERENCES

1. Strock M. *Plain Talk about Depression.* Bethesda, MD: National Institute of Mental Health; 2000.
2. American Psychiatric Association. *Diagnostic and Statistical Manual of Mental Disorders Text Revision,* 4th ed. Washington, DC: American Psychiatric Press; 2000:349–426.
3. Robins LN, Regier DA, eds. *Psychiatric Disorders in America, The Epidemiologic Catchment Area Study.* New York, NY: The Free Press; 1990.
4. National Committee for Quality Assurance. *The State of Health Care Quality: 2004.* Washington, DC: National Committee for Quality Assurance; 2004:22–23.
5. World Health Organization. Mental health disorders management. Depression. Available at: http://www.who.int/mental_health/management/depression/definition/en/index.html. Accessed February 23, 2005.
6. Simon G, Von Korff M, Wagner EH, et al. Patterns of antidepressant use in community practice. *Gen Hosp Psychiatry.* 1993;15:399–408.
7. U.S. Preventative Services Task Force. Screening for depression: recommendations and rationale. *Ann Intern Med.* 2002;136:760–764.
8. Spitzer RL, Kroenke K, Williams JB. Validation and utility of a self-report version of PRIME-MD: The PHQ primary care study. Primary Care Evaluation of Mental Disorders. Patient Health Questionnaire. *JAMA.* 1999;282:1737–1744.
9. Whooley MA, Avins AL, Miranda J, Browner WS. Case-finding instruments for depression. Two questions are as good as many. *J Gen Intern Med.* 1997;12:439–445.
10. American Psychiatric Association. *Practice Guideline for the Treatment of Patients with Major Depressive Disorder,* 2nd ed. Arlington, VA: American Psychiatric Association; 2000.
11. Institute for Clinical Systems Improvement. *Health Care Guideline: Major Depression in Adults in Primary Care.* Bloomington, IN: Institute for Clinical Systems Improvement; 2004.
12. Kupfer DJ. Long-term treatment of depression. *J Clin Psychiatry.* 1991;52(Suppl):28–34.

Chapter 22

Anxiety Disorders

Laura A. Morgan and Cynthia K. Kirkwood

SEARCH STRATEGY

A comprehensive search of the medical literature was performed from January 1999 to December 2005. The search, limited to human subjects and English language journals, included MEDLINE®, PubMed, and the Cochrane Database of Systematic Reviews.

Anxiety disorders are vastly prevalent and often coexist with depression. The lifetime prevalence of anxiety disorders is approximately 29%, affecting *one in four adults*.[1] Symptoms of anxiety are more common in patients who are frequent users of healthcare resources. The diagnosis of an anxiety disorder requires significant impairment in daily functioning. Less than a third of patients diagnosed with anxiety disorders in primary care receive adequate counseling or drug therapy.[2] Five anxiety disorders commonly encountered in practice will be discussed in this chapter: Generalized anxiety disorder, panic disorder, posttraumatic stress disorder, social anxiety disorder, and obsessive–compulsive disorder (OCD).

Anxiety disorders are diagnosed using specific criteria from the *Diagnostic and Statistical Manual of Mental Disorders*, Fourth Edition, Text Revision.[3] Medical and pharmacological etiologies for anxiety should be assessed before diagnosing an anxiety disorder. Common medical conditions associated with anxiety include coronary artery disease, angina, stroke, hyperthyroidism, and pheochromocytoma. Drug-induced causes include stimulants, corticosteroids, anticonvulsants, antidepressants, sympathomimetics, thyroid hormones, and alcohol or central nervous system depressant withdrawal. A thorough history, including alcohol and substance use, should be obtained.

GENERALIZED ANXIETY DISORDER

CLINICAL PRESENTATION

Generalized anxiety disorder is a chronic disorder characterized by persistent, uncontrollable worry and anxious feelings that are difficult to control. Life stressors can worsen symptoms, but treatment is necessary for remission to occur. The lifetime risk of generalized anxiety disorder is 5.7%.[1]

DIAGNOSTIC EVALUATION

Anxiety symptoms must exist nearly every day for a minimum of 6 months for a diagnosis of generalized anxiety disorder. At least three of the following symptoms must be present: Fatigue, irritability, sleep disturbance, restlessness or feeling on edge, muscle tension, and poor concentration.[1,4] Increased heart rate may be evident on physical examination.

MANAGEMENT

The two modes of treatment for generalized anxiety disorder are drug therapy and psychotherapy. Psychotherapy should be considered for all patients with generalized anxiety disorder.[4] Antidepressants (i.e., selective serotonin reuptake inhibitors [SSRIs], serotonin norepinephrine reuptake inhibitors [SNRIs], or tricyclic antidepressants [TCAs]) are first-line agents because of the high comorbidity of depression and the chronicity of generalized anxiety disorder.[5] The SNRIs, venlafaxine and duloxetine, and the SSRIs, escitalopram and paroxetine, have less adverse effects than TCAs, and are first-line agents indicated for use in generalized anxiety

Table 22-1. First- and Second-line Pharmacotherapy of Anxiety Disorders

Anxiety Disorder	First-Line Drugs	Second-Line Drugs	Alternatives
Generalized anxiety	SNRIs Paroxetine Escitalopram	Benzodiazepines Imipramine Buspirone	Hydroxyzine
Panic disorder	SSRIs Venlafaxine XR*	Imipramine Clomipramine Alprazolam Clonazepam	Phenelzine
Posttraumatic stress disorder	Paroxetine Sertaline	Phenelzine TCAs	
Social anxiety disorder	Paroxetine Sertraline Venlafaxine XR*	Citalopram Escitalopram Fluvoxamine Clonazepam	Buspirone Gabapentin Phenelzine
OCD	SSRIs	Clomipramine	

*XR,, extended release.
Adapted from: Kirkwood CK, Melton ST. Anxiety disorders I: Generalized anxiety, panic, and social anxiety disorders. In: Dipiro JT, Talbert RL, Yee GC, eds. *Pharmacotherapy: A Pathophysiologic Approach*, 6th ed. New York, NY: McGraw-Hill; 2005:1285; Kirkwood CK, Makela EH, Wells BG. Anxiety disorders II: Posttraumatic stress disorder and obsessive–compulsive disorder. In: Dipiro JT, Talbert RL, Yee GC, eds. *Pharmacotherapy: A Pathophysiologic Approach*, 6th ed. New York, NY: McGraw-Hill; 2005:1307; Cymbalta [package insert]. Indianapolis, IN: Eli Lilly & Company; 2007.

disorder (Table 22-1). The onset of anxiolytic effects of antidepressants is 2 to 4 weeks and optimal response may take 6 to 8 weeks or longer, but both the psychic and somatic symptoms are relieved.[4] Benzodiazepines reduce the somatic symptoms and can provide relief in acute situations.[4] Long-term use of benzodiazepines is associated with dependence, withdrawal, and lack of documented efficacy. Buspirone and hydroxyzine are alternatives with a lag-time of effect similar to antidepressants but lack dependence and abuse.[4,5] The duration of treatment is not well defined, 12 months or for life is suggested.

PANIC DISORDER

Panic disorder is a chronic, relapsing illness with a lifetime prevalence rate of 4.7%.[1] It is characterized by recurrent panic attacks (distinct periods of unprovoked fear and discomfort). Panic attacks can include a combination of somatic (e.g., palpitations, sweating, chills, paresthesias, tremors, shortness of breath, feeling of choking, chest pain, gastrointestinal distress, dizziness) and psychic symptoms (i.e., fear of losing control, derealization, depersonalization, fear of dying) that peak within 10 minutes.[3]

DIAGNOSTIC EVALUATION

Panic disorder is diagnosed when unexpected panic attacks recur and one attack is followed by anticipatory anxiety about having another attack, worrying about the implications of the attack, or a distinct change in behavior as a result of the attack (e.g., avoiding shopping because a panic attack occurred in the mall).[3,4] Panic disorder is often misdiagnosed as physical illness. Also, patients can present with agoraphobia. Individuals with severe symptoms may require hospitalization for stabilization.

MANAGEMENT

Pharmacotherapy and cognitive behavioral therapy (CBT) are effective in panic disorder. An acute panic attack can be relieved by benzodiazepines. The SSRIs, TCAs, or extended-release venlafaxine should be used for maintenance therapy to reduce panic symptoms and the frequency of attacks. The SSRIs are first-line agents—fluoxetine, paroxetine, and sertraline are approved for panic disorder. Venlafaxine extended-release was recently approved for panic disorder. TCAs and monoamine oxidase inhibitors (MAOIs) are also effective, but less well tolerated. The dose of antidepressants must be low initially and titrated gradually to avoid activating effects (e.g., insomnia, restlessness). Antidepressants require 6 to 8 weeks for response. High-potency benzodiazepines (i.e., alprazolam, clonazepam) are effective in panic disorder and provide a faster onset of effect; however, discontinuation can be problematic. An initial combination of a benzodiazepine for 4 to 6 weeks and an antidepressant can be used to stabilize symptoms.[4,5] The minimum duration of therapy is 12 to 18 months.[5]

POSTTRAUMATIC STRESS DISORDER

Posttraumatic stress disorder requires an exposure (i.e., witnessing, experiencing, or confronting) to a traumatic event (e.g., rape, motor vehicle accident, a death) that led to real or threatened injury or death, or a risk to the safety of the patient or others.[3] The individual must have reacted with extreme fear, horror, or helplessness. The lifetime prevalence rate of posttraumatic stress disorder is 6.8%.[1]

CLINICAL PRESENTATION

Patients with posttraumatic stress disorder report symptoms in three core areas: reexperiencing, avoidance, and hyperarousal. Symptoms of re-experiencing include recurrent images or thoughts of the event, dreams or flashbacks, feelings as if the event were reoccurring, or distress with reminders of the event. The inability to recall aspects of the trauma, restricted affect, and efforts to avoid thoughts or conversations about the event encompass avoidance behavior. Increased arousal includes hypervigilance, sleep disturbances, difficulty concentrating, and an exaggerated startle response.

DIAGNOSTIC EVALUATION

The duration of posttraumatic stress disorder symptoms exceeds 1 month. Patients must have one or more symptoms of experiencing, three or more avoidance behaviors, and at least two symptoms of hyperarousal to meet the criteria for posttraumatic stress disorder.[3]

MANAGEMENT

Treatment options for posttraumatic stress disorder include drug therapy and/or CBT. The SSRIs are first-line treatment for reduction of the core symptoms of posttraumatic stress disorder.[6,7] TCAs and MAOIs are also effective. Antidepressants require at least 8 weeks to assess efficacy in posttraumatic stress disorder. Benzodiazepines can reduce anxiety and improve sleep disturbances, but should not be used as monotherapy because of reports of worsened symptoms. Atypical antipsychotics, anticonvulsants, α_2-adrenergic agents, and β-adrenergic blockers are agents that can be used as adjuncts to manage symptoms of psychosis, mood instability, and autonomic symptoms.[6] CBT and eye movement desensitization and reprocessing therapy are nonpharmacologic approaches effective in posttraumatic stress disorder. The minimum duration of therapy is 12 months.[8]

SOCIAL ANXIETY DISORDER

CLINICAL PRESENTATION

Social anxiety disorder occurs in 12.1% of the population during their lifetime[1] and is characterized by a marked and persistent fear of one or more social or performance situations in which a person may be negatively evaluated or scrutinized. Individuals with social anxiety disorder fear most social situations (generalized type) or specific social situations such as public speaking (nongeneralized type). Exposure to feared situations results in physical symptoms of anxiety including palpitations, tremor, sweating, gastrointestinal discomfort, diarrhea, muscle tension or blushing (the principal physical indicator in social anxiety disorder). Individuals can also experience situational panic attacks.[3]

Patients with social anxiety disorder had fewer visits to primary care physicians than well controls and patients with other psychiatric disorders. They often avoid seeking general medical care because of fears of scrutiny by unfamiliar people while sitting in a crowded waiting room or talking to people in authority.[9]

DIAGNOSTIC EVALUATION

Social anxiety disorder is differentiated from other anxiety disorders by the rationale behind the fear—fear of anxiety symptoms is typical of panic disorder while fear of embarrassment characterizes social anxiety disorder. The following yes-or-no statements were found to be 89% sensitive in detecting social anxiety disorder: "Being embarrassed or looking stupid is among my worst fears"; "Fear of embarrassment causes me to avoid doing things or speaking to people"; "I avoid activities in which I am the center of attention."[10]

Adults with social anxiety disorder recognize their fear is excessive and unreasonable, and tend to avoid the situation rather than endure significant distress, while children may not. Social anxiety disorder usually presents in the mid-teens and continues throughout life. Symptoms must be present for at least 6 months to diagnose social anxiety disorder in persons less than 18 years of age.[3]

MANAGEMENT

The goals of treatment for social anxiety disorder are to reduce physical symptoms of anxiety and avoidance behaviors in the acute phase and improve social functioning and quality of life in the continuation phase. Because of the disabling nature of social anxiety disorder, it should be treated aggressively. Patients may be resistant to treatment for fear of what others might think or say about seeking help. Treatment should be continued for at least 1 year to maintain remission and reduce risk of relapse.[11]

Treatment of social anxiety disorder includes CBT and pharmacotherapy. Paroxetine, sertraline, and venlafaxine extended-release are approved for the treatment of generalized social anxiety disorder and are considered first-line agents. Onset of effect is delayed, 4 to 8 weeks, with maximum benefit after treatment for 12 weeks or longer. Fluvoxamine, but not fluoxetine, was effective in improving psychosocial disability and symptoms.[12] Initial doses of SSRIs and venlafaxine are similar to those used in the treatment of depression. If a patient has comorbid panic disorder the dose should be started at a quarter to half of the antidepressant dose to avoid exacerbating panic symptoms. Phenelzine is a last-line agent for social anxiety disorder.

Benzodiazepines are not considered first-line agents in social anxiety disorder. Providers often use benzodiazepines for short-term management of anxiety symptoms in the acute phase of treatment lasting approximately 1 month. Benzodiazepines may be used in combination with an antidepressant, CBT or both for initial symptom relief. Clonazepam demonstrated significant improvement in fear and phobic avoidance, fears of negative evaluation, and disability measures and was effective within 1 to 2 weeks for patients requiring rapid relief of symptoms. Alprazolam was not effective in social anxiety disorder.

Gabapentin was superior to placebo in a 14-week trial of 69 patients with social anxiety disorder. Effective doses ranged from 900 to 3600 mg/d and was seen 2 to 4 weeks after beginning treatment.[12,13] β-Blockers are used to manage performance anxiety and nongeneralized social anxiety disorder to minimize the symptoms of anxiety (e.g., palpitations, tremor, sweating) during performance-related situations. Propranolol 10 to 80 mg or atenolol 25 to 100 mg taken 30 to 60 minutes before a performance situation can reduce anxiety symptoms. A test dose should be taken before the event to assure β-blockade is sufficient and there are no adverse events. Daily β-blocker therapy is not effective for generalized social anxiety disorder.[12,13]

OBSESSIVE–COMPULSIVE DISORDER

CLINICAL PRESENTATION

OCD is characterized by recurrent obsessions and/or compulsions. An obsession is a persistent thought, idea, impulse or image that is intrusive and results in marked anxiety or distress. The most common obsessions include repeated doubts (e.g., wondering whether one left the stove turned on), repeated thoughts of contamination (e.g., preoccupation with germs, dirt, or chemicals), and a need to have items in a particular order. These fixations cause significant feelings of anxiety. Individuals may try to simply ignore or suppress obsessions. Compulsions are repetitive behaviors (e.g., hand washing, checking) or mental acts (e.g., counting, repeating words silently,

praying) performed in response to an obsession. Compulsive behavior is not pleasurable and patients feel driven to perform these acts to reduce anxiety or prevent some dreaded event or situation.[3] The lifetime prevalence of OCD is 1.6%.[1] On physical examination patients may exhibit dermatological conditions because of excessive washing with water or caustic cleaning agents.[3]

DIAGNOSTIC EVALUATION

OCD can be difficult to diagnose because of a patient's reluctance to volunteer information about their thoughts and rituals. Three screening questions can be used to determine whether diagnostic criteria are met: "Do you have repetitive thoughts that make you anxious and that you cannot get rid of regardless of how hard you try?," "Do you keep things extremely clean or wash your hands frequently?," and "Do you check things excessively?"[14] The obsessions and compulsions are severe enough to be time-consuming (occupy more than 1 h/d). Individuals must recognize that their thoughts and compulsions are a product of their own mind, excessive, and unreasonable. Patients can become very skilled in hiding their illness from family (e.g., denying symptoms, disguising rituals).

MANAGEMENT

The goals of treatment in OCD are to improve social functioning and quality of life through reducing the degree of anxiety and frequency of obsessive thoughts and time spent performing compulsive acts. CBT and pharmacotherapy are the most effective treatments for OCD.[14] Treatment of OCD may not completely resolve obsessions or compulsions but patients may feel better with only partial resolution of symptoms.

CBT is the first-line treatment in adolescents or adults with mild OCD. It can be used in combination with pharmacotherapy in moderate to severe cases of OCD. CBT consists of exposure and response prevention. Patients are exposed to feared objects/activities and asked to delay their ritualistic response for as long as possible. Initially patients are unable to perform these activities but over time they are able to resist rituals for longer periods. Less than 25% of patients have a relapse of symptoms after successful treatment with CBT.[14]

Drug therapy is reserved for patients with moderate to severe symptoms. Approximately 40% to 60% of patients respond to SSRIs with a mean improvement in symptoms of 20% to 40%. An SSRI may be added to patients with mild symptoms not responding to CBT alone. Effective doses of SSRIs for OCD exceed those used in the treatment of major depression. An adequate trial of an agent for OCD is considered 10 to 12 weeks of therapy at target doses.[14]

The SSRIs fluoxetine, paroxetine, fluvoxamine, and sertraline and the TCA clomipramine are approved for OCD. A meta-analysis comparing data from trials of sertraline, fluoxetine, fluvoxamine, and clomipramine demonstrated clomipramine's superiority to SSRIs. The SSRIs are the drugs of choice in the treatment of OCD because they tend to be better tolerated. After 2 or 3 failed attempts with SSRIs, a trial of clomipramine is warranted.[15] Consider tapering drug therapy after 1 to 2 years of treatment. Patients with 2 to 4 severe relapses or 3 to 4 mild-to-moderate relapses may need long-term therapy.[16]

THERAPY OPTIONS

PSYCHOTHERAPY

The most common form of psychotherapy employed in anxiety disorders is CBT. It involves training patients to recognize their own internal or external cues associated with anxiety and alter maladaptive responses to reduce anxiety. CBT alone or in combination with pharmacotherapy is a standard of treatment for anxiety disorders. Access to CBT is often limited to those in large urban areas or academic teaching centers because of the lack of trained therapists and cost of treatment. CBT consists of exposure therapy, cognitive restructuring, relaxation techniques, and social skills training.

DRUG THERAPY

Selective Serotonin Reuptake Inhibitors

The SSRIs are the first-line of therapy for anxiety disorders because of the chronic nature of anxiety disorders, effectiveness in both anxiety and depressive disorders, tolerable side effect profile, lack of dependency and abuse potential, and safety in overdoses. Dosing for each agent appears in Table 22-2. The dosage must be tapered to prevent withdrawal symptoms upon discontinuation, except for fluoxetine.

Table 22-2. Doses of Drugs Used to Treat Anxiety Disorders

Class/Generic Name	Brand Name	Starting Dose (mg)	Dosage Range (mg/day)*
SSRIs			
Citalopram	Celexa	20, daily	20–40
Escitalopram[†]	Lexapro	10, daily	10–20
Fluoxetine[†,§]	Prozac	10–20, daily	20–60
Fluvoxamine[‡]	Luvox	50, daily	150–300
Paroxetine[†,‡,§,¶,**]	Paxil	20, daily	20–50
	Paxil CR[††]	25, daily	(panic disorder) 12.5–75 (social anxiety disorder) 12.5–75
Sertraline[‡,§,¶,**]	Zoloft	50, daily	50–200
SNRIs			
Duloxetine[†]	Cymbalta	30 or 60, daily	30–120
Venlafaxine[†,§,¶]	Effexor XR[††]	37.5 or 75, daily	75–225
Tricyclics			
Imipramine	Tofranil	25 or 50, daily	74–200
Clomipramine[‡]	Anafranil	25, daily	100–250
Azapirones			
Buspirone[†]	Buspar	7.5, twice daily	15–60
Diphenylmethane			
Hydroxyzine[†,‡‡]	Vistaril, Atarax	25 or 50, four times daily	200–400
Benzodiazepines			
Alprazolam[†,§]	Xanax, Niravam Xanax XR[††]	0.25–0.5, daily	1–4 (anxiety) 3–6 (panic)
Clonazepam[§]	Klonopin	0.25, twice daily	1–4

*Elderly patients are usually treated with approximately one-half of the dose listed.
[†]FDA-approved for generalized anxiety disorder.
[‡] FDA-approved for OCD.
[§]FDA-approved for panic disorder.
[¶]FDA-approved for social anxiety disorder.
[**]FDA-approved for posttraumatic stress disorder.
[††]Once daily dosing.
[‡‡]FDA-approved for anxiety and tension in children in divided daily doses of 50–100 mg.
Adapted from: Kirkwood CK, Melton ST. Anxiety disorders I: Generalized anxiety, panic, and social anxiety disorders. In: Dipiro JT, Talbert RL, Yee GC, eds. *Pharmacotherapy: A Pathophysiologic* Approach, 6th ed. New York, NY: McGraw-Hill; 2005:1285; Kirkwood CK, Makela EH, Wells BG. Anxiety disorders II: Posttraumatic stress disorder and obsessive–compulsive disorder. In: Dipiro JT, Talbert RL, Yee GC, eds. *Pharmacotherapy: A Pathophysiologic Approach*, 6th ed. New York, NY: McGraw-Hill; 2005:1307; Cymbalta Package Insert. Eli Lilly & Company, Indianapolis, IN, 2007.

Tricyclic Antidepressants

The adverse effects (i.e., anticholinergic, sedation, orthostatic hypotension, weight gain) of the TCAs and potential fatalities in overdose have limited widespread use of these agents for anxiety disorders. TCAs are usually used second line in patients who fail multiple attempts with SSRIs or venlafaxine (see Table 22-1).

Monoamine Oxidase Inhibitors

Phenelzine is effective for panic disorder and social anxiety disorder. However, because of dietary restrictions, potential drug–drug interactions, and adverse effects such as postural hypotension, insomnia, weight gain, sedation and hypertensive crisis, MAOIs are reserved for treatment-resistant patients.[13] To prevent hypertensive crisis patients should avoid tyramine-containing foods and sympathomimetic drugs. An appropriate washout period should be followed when switching a patient from another antidepressant to phenelzine.

Other Antidepressants

The SNRI venlafaxine is indicated for use in generalized anxiety disorder, panic disorder, and social anxiety disorder. The initial dose of venlafaxine extended-release in generalized anxiety disorder and social anxiety disorder is 75 mg/d given as a single dose. The dose may be titrated every 4 days to a maximum of 225 mg/d. The initial dose in panic disorder is 37.5 mg daily for 7 days and increased weekly to a maximum dose of 225 mg/d. Venlafaxine should be tapered slowly (37.5 mg/month) to reduce risk of relapse during discontinuation. Other antidepressants (e.g., mirtazapine, nefazodone) have limited data to support their use in anxiety disorders. Bupropion is not effective for anxiety disorders.

Benzodiazepines

Benzodiazepines are effective in reducing the somatic symptoms of anxiety, but do not manage the psychic symptoms. Limitations of benzodiazepine use include central nervous system side effects (e.g., drowsiness, memory impairment, psychomotor impairment), lack of efficacy in depression, abuse potential, and difficulty discontinuing therapy. Benzodiazepines should be reserved for patients with low risk for substance abuse, requiring rapid relief of symptoms, or nonresponse to other therapies. Patients should be educated not to decrease or discontinue benzodiazepines without consulting their provider. Benzodiazepines should be slowly tapered on discontinuation to avoid withdrawal effects.[12,13,17]

The starting dose of clonazepam in social anxiety disorder is 0.25 mg/d and may be titrated over several weeks to 3 mg/d as tolerated. The average daily dose in clinical trials was 2.5 mg/d. Adverse effects include dizziness, unsteadiness, difficulty concentrating, and sexual dysfunction.

Buspirone

Buspirone is a 5-HT_{1A} partial agonist that is effective in generalized anxiety disorder, with improved tolerability over benzodiazepines. It has a delayed onset of effect and is not effective in depression. Common adverse effects include nausea and headaches.

EVIDENCE-BASED SUMMARY

- Antidepressants are the first-line of therapy for the long-term management of anxiety disorders.
- Benzodiazepines can be used to manage acute anxiety symptoms for several weeks but should be avoided in patients with a history of substance abuse.
- Clomipramine should be considered after 2 or 3 failed trials with SSRIs in the management of OCD.
- At least 1 year of therapy is recommended for the management of anxiety disorders.
- Antidepressants and benzodiazepines should be tapered upon drug discontinuation to avoid withdrawal symptoms and prevent relapse.

REFERENCES

1. Kessler RC, Berglund P, Demler O, et al. Lifetime prevalence and age-of-onset distributions of DSM-IV disorders in the national comorbidity survey replication. *Arch Gen Psychiatry.* 2005;62:593–602.
2. Stein MB, Sherbourne CD, Craske MG, et al. Quality of care for primary care patients with anxiety disorders. *Am J Psychiatry.* 2004;161:2230–2237.
3. American Psychiatric Association. *Diagnostic and Statistical Manual of Mental Disorders,* 4th ed., Text Revision. Washington, DC: American Psychiatric Association; 2000:429.
4. Stein DJ. Algorithms for primary care: An evidence-based approach to the pharmacotherapy of depression and anxiety disorders. *Prim Psychiatry.* 2004;11:55–78.
5. Bandelow B, Zohar J, Hollander E, et al. World Federation of Societies of Biological Psychiatry (WFSBP) guidelines for the pharmacological treatment of anxiety, obsessive–compulsive disorder, and posttraumatic stress disorder (PTSD). *World J Biol Psychiatry.* 2002;3: 171–199.

6. American Psychiatric Association. Practice guideline for the treatment of patients with acute stress disorder and posttraumatic stress disorder. *Am J Psychiatry.* 2004;161 (suppl):1–96.

7. Stein DJ, Zungu-Dirwayi N, van der Linden GJH, Seedat S. Pharmacotherapy for post traumatic stress disorder (posttraumatic stress disorder). *Cochrane Database Syst Rev.* 2000;4:CD002795. DOI: 10.1002(14651858.CD00 2795.

8. Ballenger JC, Davidson JRT, Lecrubier Y, et al. Consensus statement update on posttraumatic stress disorder from the international consensus group on depression and anxiety. *J Clin Psychiatry.* 2004;65(Suppl 1):55–62.

9. Gross R Olfson M, Gameroff MJ, et al. Social anxiety disorder in primary care. *Gen Hosp Psychiatry.* 2005;3: 161– 168.

10. Bruce TJ, Saeed SA. Social anxiety disorder: A common, underrecognized mental disorder. *Am Fam Physician.* 1999;60:2311–2320, 2322.

11. Olfson M, Guardino M, Struening E, et al. Barriers to treatment of social anxiety. *Am J Psychiatry.* 2000;157: 521–527.

12. Blanco C, Raza MS, Schneier FR, et al. The evidence-based pharmacological treatment of social anxiety disorder. *Int J Neuropsychopharmacol.* 2003;6:427–442.

13. Van Ameringen M, Mancini C. Pharmacotherapy of social anxiety disorder at the turn of the millennium. *Psychiatr Clin North Am.* 2001;24:783–803.

14. Jenike MA. Obsessive–compulsive disorder. *N Engl J Med.* 2004;350:259–265.

15. Schruers K, Koning K, Luermans J, et al. Obsessive–compulsive disorder: A critical review of therapeutic perspectives. *Acta Psychiatr Scand.* 2005;111:261–271.

16. Fineberg NA, Gale TM. Evidence-based pharmacotherapy of obsessive–compulsive disorder. *Int J Neuropsychopharmacol.* 2005;8:107–129.

17. Kirkwood CK, Melton ST. Anxiety disorders I: Generalized anxiety, panic, and social anxiety disorders. In: Dipiro JT, Talbert RL, Yee GC, eds. *Pharmacotherapy: A Pathophysiologic Approach*, 6th ed. New York, NY: McGraw-Hill; 2005:1285.

Chapter 23

Obstructive Sleep Apnea Hypopnea Syndrome

Stephen S. Im and Michelle V. Conde

SEARCH STRATEGY

A comprehensive search of the medical literature was performed from January 1985 to June 2006. The search, limited to human subjects and English language journals, included MEDLINE®, PubMed, and the Cochrane Database of Systematic Reviews. Clinical practice parameters for obstructive sleep apnea submitted by the American Association of Sleep Medicine can be found at http://www.aasmnet.org

Obstructive sleep apnea/hypopnea syndrome (OSAHS) is a disease of repetitive episodes of nocturnal upper airway obstruction leading to sleep fragmentation, episodic oxyhemoglobin desaturations, and concomitant daytime hypersomnolence. The hypersomnia associated with OSAHS worsens intellectual capacity, motor coordination, and memory. Studies link this disease to increased motor vehicle accidents and suggest a causal link between OSAHS and cardiovascular disease. Despite increasing awareness of sleep disordered breathing, OSAHS continues to be under-diagnosed. Recognition and diagnosis of this disease is essential as treatment is associated with decreased cardiovascular mortality and improved cognitive function.

ETIOLOGY

A sleep apneic or hypopneic event is caused by pharyngeal narrowing or closure during sleep. In normal subjects, the negative inspiratory pressure of normal breathing tends to close the upper airway. Patency is maintained with activation of pharyngeal dilator mus-

cles. Neuromuscular tone in the upper airway musculature decreases with sleep.[1] Excessive adipose tissue, craniofacial abnormalities, and hypertrophic tonsils may result in a smaller upper airway diameter. In patients with a tendency to develop OSAHS, residual pharyngeal muscle activity during sleep may not adequately maintain airway patency. Snoring may cause significant trauma to the upper airway and uvula, leading to edema and further narrowing.[2] Sleep fragmentation occurs from arousals that are necessary to reestablish airway patency. These arousals contribute to daytime hypersomnolence.[3] The repeated obstructive respiratory events are associated with various cardiovascular effects related to increased sympathetic tone.[4]

EPIDEMIOLOGY

OSAHS is a common disorder. Up to 24% of men and 9% of women between 30 and 60 years of age will have significant sleep disordered breathing defined as more than five events (apneic and/or hypopneic) per hour. Four percent of men and 2% of women in this cohort will have OSAHS defined as a significant number of events with daytime symptoms of sleepiness.[5] The prevalence of OSAHS increases with age. Up to 50% of people above age 65 have sleep disordered breathing.[6] OSAHS is associated with common diseases. Sixty percent of middle-aged, obese men with a BMI ≥ 30 kg/m^2 will have sleep disordered breathing and 27% will have OSAHS.[7] Thirty percent of patients with essential hypertension and 37% of patients with diabetes have sleep apnea. Thirty to thirty-five percent of patients with coronary artery disease (CAD) have significant sleep apnea. OSAHS continues to be under-diagnosed.[8] As of 1997, one estimate suggests that 82% of men and 93% of women with moderate-to-severe OSAHS remain undiagnosed.[9]

MORBIDITY

CLINICAL MORBIDITY

In patients with apnea/hypopnea index (AHI) (the sum of apneas and hypopneas in 1 hour) greater than 11 events per hour, 50% use antihypertensive medications, 23% have cardiovascular disease, 3% have heart failure, 5% report a history of a cerebral vascular accident, and 15% have diabetes.[10] Immediate physiologic effects of repeated sleep apneic events include nocturnal oxygen desaturations, increased sympathetic tone, nocturnal, systemic, and pulmonary hypertension.[11] Compared to normal individuals, sleep apneic patients have an exaggerated sympathetic response to obstructive events. This altered sympathetic response appears to persist during wakefulness. Patients with moderate-to-severe OSAHS have increased resting heart rate, increased blood pressure variability, decreased heart rate variability, and increased sympathetic tone when compared with controls with similar blood pressures.[12] A large prospective study confirms that OSAHS is independently associated with hypertension, CAD, heart failure, and strokes.[10,13]

This study demonstrates statistically significant associations of the AHI and sleep time with oxygen saturations <90% with cardiovascular diseases when adjusted for other comorbid conditions including age, sex, and body mass index (BMI).[10] A number of cardiac arrhythmias can be seen with OSAHS. During the apneic event, common arrhythmias include sinus bradycardia, atrioventricular block, and ventricular ectopy. Use of a validated questionnaire suggests that up to 50% of patients with atrial fibrillation have OSAHS.[14] Patients with untreated OSAHS are twice as likely to revert back to atrial fibrillation after cardioversion. Use of continuous positive airway pressure (CPAP) decreases the risk of recurrence.[15] In the general population, sudden cardiac death occurs predominantly between 6 AM and noon. In patients with OSAHS, this peak occurs while asleep between midnight and 6 AM.[16] Increased AHI is also independently associated with insulin resistance and diabetes when adjusted for obesity. Desaturations ≥4% are associated with worsening glucose intolerance when adjusted for percent body fat, BMI, and AHI.[7,17] This glucose intolerance improves with CPAP treatment.[3]

NEUROCOGNITIVE MORBIDITY

Neurocognitive dysfunction is common with OSAHS. Deficiencies with intellectual capacity, mood, memory,

motor coordination, visual reaction times, and auditory learning are well documented when compared to normal controls.[1,18] When compared to other hypersomnolent groups, this impairment is not completely attributable to lack of sleep or the degree of sleepiness.[18]

The relationship of neurocognitive dysfunction caused by OSAHS and motor vehicle accidents has been extensively studied. Reports suggest that OSAHS confers a seven-fold increase in risk for motor vehicle accidents.[19] Treatment with CPAP ameliorates this increased risk.[20] Simulated driving tests show sleep apneic patients perform poorly compared to normal controls. These subjects perform similarly to legally intoxicated drivers.[21] These tests return to normal levels with CPAP treatment.[1] One survey shows 24% of commercial drivers have excessive sleepiness and 16% report a history of OSAHS. Those with severe sleepiness have increased multiple motor vehicle accidents.[22] Accidents associated with sleepiness carry higher mortality when compared to other causes. OSAHS is responsible for 810,000 collisions and 1400 fatalities annually at a cost of $15.9 billion.[21]

CLINICAL PRESENTATION

The best clinical predictors of OSAHS are male gender, BMI, neck girth, snoring, and witnessed apneas. All these correlate independently with an AHI of 15 or greater.[23] Risk factors for OSAHS include:[1]

- BMI >29 kg/m^2
- Male gender
- Thirty to sixty years of age
- Family history
- Alcohol and sedative use
- Hypothyroidism and acromegaly
- Craniofacial abnormalities

SYMPTOMS

The hallmark of OSAHS is daytime hypersomnolence. Up to 80% of patients referred to a sleep laboratory and diagnosed with OSAHS have hypersomnolence.[24] Excessive sleepiness may be less common in women and patients with congestive heart failure.[4,24] Some patients substitute excessive daytime sleepiness with complaints of depression, irritability, nonrestorative sleep, and problems with concentration or memory. The Epworth Score is a commonly utilized questionnaire that quantifies a patient's degree of sleepiness. The patient is asked to rate his likelihood of falling asleep with certain activities:

- Sitting and reading
- Watching television
- Sitting inactive in a public place

- Riding as a passenger in a car for an hour without a break
- Lying down to rest in the afternoon when circumstances permit
- Sitting and talking to someone
- Sitting quietly after lunch without alcohol
- In a car, while stopped for a few minutes in traffic

The patient assigns: 0, would never fall asleep; 1, slight chance of falling asleep; 2, moderate chance of falling asleep; 3, high chance of falling asleep. A score ≤6 is considered normal. A score ≥16 is considered a pathologic degree of sleepiness.[25] The Epworth scale is useful for quantifying the level of sleepiness but may not correlate well with the AHI.[3] Other symptoms include:[1]

- Snoring: 46% of partners sleep in separate room
- Witnessed apneas
- Restlessness and diaphoresis: 50%
- Choking or dyspnea: 18–31%
- Gastroesophageal reflux
- Nocturia: 28%
- Dry mouth
- Morning headaches: 50%

OSAHS can cause insomnia or worsen insomnia, which has numerous etiologies. In the patient presenting with chronic insomnia, a careful history should assess for a medication or substance cause, inadequate sleep hygiene, active psychosocial stressors, and an underlying psychiatric or medical condition.[26]

PHYSICAL EXAMINATION

The cardinal physical examination finding for OSAHS is obesity. A BMI ≥30 mg/kg^2 confers at least a 10-fold risk for OSAHS. The incidence of OSAHS is 20% to 40% in these patients versus 2% to 4% in the general population.[27] Upper body fat distribution as determined by waist-to-hip ratio is not independently associated with OSAHS.[23] Neck circumference >40 cm yields a specificity of 93% for OSAHS. Sensitivity, however, is only 61%.[1] Another physical examination finding is a small oral airway as determined by a modified Mallampati classification class of III or IV. The Mallampati classification is used by anesthesiologists to assess the size of the tongue in relation to the length of the palate when assessing airways for relative difficulties in endotracheal intubations. Other cranial facial abnormalities associated with OSAHS include high arched palate, long and thick uvula, enlarged tonsils, and severe septal deviation.[28]

DIAGNOSIS

The diagnosis of OSAHS cannot be made by history and physical examination alone. Multiple questionnaires have been developed and studied based on risk factors and symptoms. Sensitivity for patients with a high pretest probability of disease is approximately 30%. Specificity is 90%. This suggests that a diagnostic polysomnogram (PSG) is required to confirm a diagnosis of OSAHS. History and physical examination can reduce the likelihood of disease in patients with a low pretest probability.[24] Additionally, patients with systolic or diastolic heart failure, CAD, significant tachyarrhythmias or bradyarrhythmias, and history of stroke or transient ischemic attacks are at higher risk. Those with suggestive histories should undergo a diagnostic PSG.[29]

OVERNIGHT DIAGNOSTIC POLYSOMNOGRAM

The gold standard and recommended study for diagnosing OSA is a laboratory-based, full-night diagnostic PSG (Fig. 23-1). This test includes broad surface electroencephalogram (EEG), electrooculogram, and chin electromyography (EMG). Airflow, rib cage movement, abdominal movement, and oxyhemoglobin saturations are monitored to detect respiratory abnormalities. A continuous electrocardiogram detects arrhythmic events. Anterior tibialis EMG detects limb movements. The patient's position is noted. Additional monitoring may include expired or transcutaneous carbon dioxide sensing, esophageal pressure monitoring, or inductance plethysmography. EEG, electrooculogram, and chin EMG are used to determine wakefulness, sleep onset, sleep stage, and arousals. The limb EMG helps to detect arousals and sleep related movement disorders.[30]

Understanding a PSG interpretation requires knowledge of certain terminology. An obstructive apnea is defined as cessation of airflow for at least 10 seconds. The definition of a hypopnea is controversial and varies among sleep physicians. This incongruity can generate significant interinterpreter variability regarding the severity of the sleep disordered breathing.[31] The American Association of Sleep Medicine and the Centers for Medicare and Medicaid Services define a hypopnea as a reduction of thoracoabdominal movement or airflow of at least 30% from baseline lasting ≥10 seconds and associated with a ≥4% oxyhemoglobin desaturation.[29] An arousal is a change in the EEG to an awake frequency lasting ≥3 seconds. An arousal must be preceded by 10 seconds of normal sleep. Arousals caused by respiratory events that are not classifiable as hypopneas but appear related to increasing respiratory effort are called respiratory-effort related arousals. The AHI is the sum of apneas and hypopneas seen in an hour. An AHI of ≥5 is abnormal. OSAHS requires an abnormal AHI with daytime symptoms.[32] The arousal index refers to the number of arousals per hour and is an indicator of the level of sleep fragmentation. The arousal index may be a greater contributor to daytime symptoms than

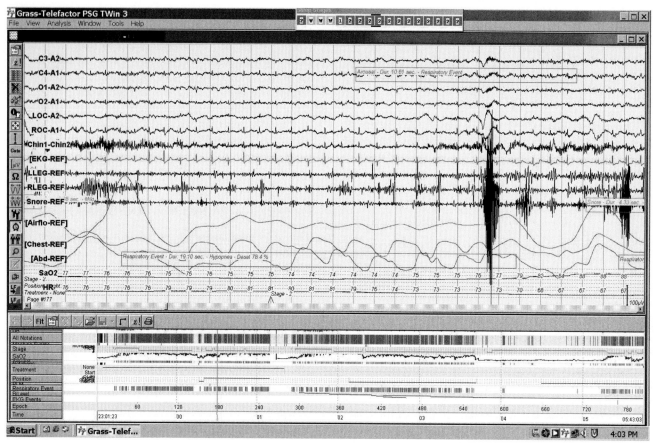

Figure 23-1. Typical polysomnogram 30-second epoch representing an obstructive hypopnea with a histogram at the bottom of the screen. The epoch represents airflow limitation with paradoxical abdominal and chest excursion followed by a snort, arousal and desaturation. The desaturation seen in this epoch is from the prior event.

the AHI.[3] Sleep efficiency is percent of the total time of the study that the patient is scored asleep. Upper airway resistance syndrome is defined as ≥5 respiratory events per hour with daytime symptoms but a normal AHI.[33] Lastly, an adequate sleep study should include all sleep stages and positions. Decreased amounts of supine sleep or rapid eye movement sleep seen during a study may reduce the sensitivity of a PSG in detecting sleep disordered breathing.

SPLIT-NIGHT STUDY

Traditionally, a second therapeutic PSG is conducted to obtain a best positive airway pressure level. As a result of prolonged wait times and increased costs associated with two separate studies, many laboratories incorporate the diagnosis and treatment of OSAHS into a single overnight session. If respiratory events are detected within the first 2 hours of the session, a therapeutic positive airway pressure titration is attempted. Split-night studies are less sensitive in diagnosing sleep disordered breathing. The sensitivity depends upon the amount of

time devoted to the diagnostic portion of the study. Conversely, lengthened diagnostic portions often lead to inadequate positive airway pressure titrations. A full-night positive pressure titration allows more time for changes in masks or positive pressure modalities.[24] Current recommendations suggest limiting split-night studies to patients with a high pretest probability of OSAHS.[29]

PORTABLE HOME MONITORING DEVICES

Timely access of obtaining a PSG is increasingly problematic. In response, various portable home monitoring devices have been developed as a substitute for the laboratory-based PSG. The sophistication of these devices varies greatly from recording only a single signal to performing a full PSG with EEG and respiratory channels.[34] Historically, the Centers for Medicare and Medicaid Services have not reimbursed studies utilizing devices without EEG. Recently, however, this agency proposed expanded coverage of CPAP devices for the diagnosis of OSAHS made by clinic evaluation and unattended home sleep monitoring without EEG. Current practice guidelines recommend unattended portable monitoring be reserved for patients with a high pre-test probability for moderate or severe OSAHS.[35]

TREATMENT

Treatment goals for OSAHS include significant improvement or resolution of the sleep disordered breathing, improvement in excessive daytime hypersomnolence and neurocognitive deficits, and improvement of clinical morbidities. Treatment options include weight loss, positional therapy, oral appliances, positive airway pressure, and surgical modification of the upper airway.[1]

LIFESTYLE MODIFICATIONS

Obesity is significantly and independently associated with OSAHS. A longitudinal study suggests that obesity increases the incidence and severity of OSAHS.[36] Conversely, weight loss leads to reduction in AHI, snoring, oxygen desaturations, blood pressure, and CPAP requirements. Large weight reductions from bariatric surgeries are associated with significant improvement and often cure OSAHS.[37] In many patients, the benefits seen after surgery persist at long-term follow-up. Extreme weight loss is not necessary to impact the severity of disease. In one small series, a loss of either 10 kilograms or 10% of total body weight is associated with a 50% improvement in AHI.[1]

Some patients have a significantly increased number of respiratory events in the supine position when compared to their nonsupine sleep. These patients can be prescribed positional therapy to limit the amount of their supine sleep. Avoidance of alcohol and sedative medications should also be stressed in patients with OSAHS.

ORAL APPLIANCES

An oral appliance is a viable treatment for OSAHS. Oral appliances include mandibular advancement devices and anterior tongue retainers. Both are constructed by dentistry. The mandibular advancement devices are produced with molds of the patient's bite and reposition the mandible anteriorly to increase the posterior oropharyngeal volume. The tongue retainers displace the tongue forward to achieve similar changes. These devices can also increase pharyngeal muscle tone. In a review of the literature, 50% of patients improve to a normal breathing level as defined by an AHI <10 per hour. Others improve but continue to have a significantly elevated AHI >20 per hour. Some worsen with treatment. Levels of oxyhemoglobin desaturations show modest improvement. Long-term cardiovascular mor-

bidity data is lacking. Long-term compliance ranges between 25% and 100%. Early side effects of excessive salivation and discomfort are usually transient. Rare late complications are not well defined but include temporal mandibular joint pain and dental occlusive alignment changes. Oral devices uniformly and significantly improve snoring. Cost of measuring, manufacturing, and fitting are significant and often not reimbursed by insurance.[38] Current practice parameters for oral appliances include:

- Snoring without OSAHS
- Mild OSAHS patients unresponsive to behavioral weight loss and positional therapies
- Moderate-to-severe OSAHS patients with intolerance of positive airway pressure
- Moderate-to-severe OSAHS patients unwilling or unable to undergo surgery for correctable craniofacial abnormalities, tonsillectomy and adenoidectomy, or tracheostomy.

Repeat PSG with the appliance is recommended for mild OSAHS if symptoms are not improved and for all moderate-to-severe OSAHS patients to confirm efficacy of treatment. Caution should be used in prescribing these devices to patients with temporal mandibular joint syndrome. Device fitting and manufacturing should be performed by trained professionals with extensive experience in this arena.[39]

POSITIVE AIRWAY PRESSURE

Standard of treatment for moderate-to-severe OSAHS is CPAP. The positive pressure serves as a pneumatic splint maintaining the patency of the oropharynx. An adequate CPAP titration eliminates all sleep disordered breathing and snoring during all sleep stages in all positions.[1] Substantial data, including a randomized control trial utilizing sham CPAP, supports its use to improve neurocognitive function, quality of life, perceived health status and daytime hypersomnolence.[40,41] Treatment with CPAP eliminates the increased risk for motor vehicle accidents.[20,42] Emerging evidence suggests improvement in blood pressure and left ventricular function with CPAP use.[43–46]

Unfortunately, compliance with CPAP therapy remains suboptimal. Satisfactory compliance is defined as an average CPAP use of ≥4 hours per night on ≥70% of nights. Using this definition, 25% to 50% of patients will discontinue or refuse CPAP therapy. Reasons for noncompliance include mask discomfort, nasal dryness and congestion, and difficulty adapting to the pressure setting.[47] Use of bi-level positive airway pressure does not objectively improve compliance.[48] The effect of an autotitrating CPAP device is unclear. One study suggests increased compliance with an autotitrating device begun at home versus CPAP introduced in the laboratory.[49] Early intervention to address compliance is important given long-term compliance equals rates achieved at 1 month.[1] An established program of early and frequent contact with the patient can improve 6-month compliance to approximately 85%.[50]

SURGERY

Because of this significant degree of positive airway pressure intolerance, surgical treatments for moderate-to-severe OSAHS continue to remain viable options. Current available surgeries include uvulopalatopharyngoplasty (UPPP), laser midline glossectomy and lingualplasty, inferior sagittal mandibular osteotomy and genioglossal advancement with hyoid myotomy and suspension (GAHM), maxillomandibular osteotomy and advancement, and tracheostomy. Of these, only tracheostomy achieves consistent resolution of nocturnal obstructive respiratory events, improvement in daytime symptoms, and improvement in cardiovascular measurements. The remaining surgical treatments are hindered by low success rates or by limited literature support. Of note, surgical success for these procedures is defined by a 50% reduction in AHI with an absolute value <20 events per hour. Subsequently, a patient with successful surgery may continue to have a moderate degree of OSAHS.

UPPP is the most commonly offered surgery. Overall success rate is approximately 40%. Similarly, glossectomy has a response rate of approximately 42%. These two treatments combined show higher response rates of 75% to 79% in small studies. GAHM carries variable success rates between 37.5% and 80% in preselected patients. Maxillomandibular osteotomy and advancement, alone or in conjunction with other surgeries, for example, UPPP or GAHM yields success rates from 40% to 100%.[51,52] Current practice recommendations include:

- Determination of presence and severity of OSAHS prior to surgery
- Initial treatment for moderate-to-severe OSAHS with positive airway pressure
- Surgery only for treatable craniofacial abnormalities and possibly for patients who reject positive airway pressure.

The candidates for surgery should be counseled on the effectiveness and rates of success of these procedures.[53]

PHARMACOTHERAPY

In general, CPAP, oral appliances, and surgery are superior to pharmacotherapy in maintaining airway patency for the treatment of OSAHS. Common sedative hypnotics for the treatment of chronic insomnia, for example, benzodiazepines, nonbenzodiazepine agents affecting the γ-aminobutyric acid/benzodiazepine complex, and melatonin-receptor agonists, have no role for the treatment of OSAHS. Limited data suggest that in patients with nasal obstruction from allergic rhinitis, treatment with intranasal corticosteroids may improve OSAHS symptoms.[54] Small, uncontrolled trials evaluating protriptyline and fluoxetine show that these agents may improve overall oxygen saturation by decreasing REM sleep, which is associated with more oxygen desaturations.[55] A systematic review of drug therapy for OSAHS in adults concludes, however, that there is insufficient evidence for the use of pharmacologic agents in the treatment of OSAHS.[56] Adjunctive therapy in patients with OSAHS who are tolerating CPAP but still have daytime sleepiness exists. Modafinil, a wake-promoting agent pharmacologically distinct from CNS stimulants, is approved in the United States for the treatment of excessive sleepiness in patients with OSAHS who are receiving nasal CPAP therapy. This agent has a low abuse potential and is well tolerated.[57]

CONCLUSION

In summary, OSAHS is a common disorder, frequently occurring with significant comorbid illness including hypertension, CAD, cerebral vascular disease, and diabetes mellitus (see Evidence-Based Summary below). Its detrimental effects on neurocognitive function are well established. The daytime hypersomnolence leads to increased motor vehicle accidents. Emerging evidence suggests a causative link to cardiovascular diseases. Treatment can alleviate much of the cognitive effects of OSAHS and positively impact morbidity from the cardiovascular complications. Diagnosis can be suggested by history and physical examination but requires objective testing for confirmation. The overnight laboratory-based PSG remains the gold standard and recommended diagnostic study. Treatment options include oral dental devices, positive airway pressure, and surgery. Adjunctive behavioral modifications such as weight reduction and exercise are important and are often under emphasized. Avoidance of alcohol and sedative medications should be stressed. Positive airway pressure is a proven treatment modality, but compliance is suboptimal. Overall success rates with surgery are not promising but are better with combined procedures. Surgery remains an option for patients who decline positive airway pressure treatment.

EVIDENCE-BASED SUMMARY

- Symptoms[1,24,25]
  - Hypersomnolence
  - Snoring
  - Witnessed apneas
  - Restlessness/diaphoresis
  - Morning headaches
- Physical exam[1,27]
  - BMI $\geq$ 30 mg/kg^2
  - Neck circumference > 40 cm
- Diagnosis[29]
  - Polysomnogram
- Treatment[1,37,39,41–47,53,56,57]
  - CPAP (standard therapy)
  - Oral appliances (selected patients)
  - Surgery (selected patients)
  - Insufficient evidence for drug therapy
  - Modafinil (for excessive sleepiness in patients on CPAP)
  - Weight loss, limit supine sleep, avoidance of alcohol and sedative medicines (all patients)

REFERENCES

1. Fogel RB, White DP. Obstructive sleep apnea. *Adv Intern Med.* 2000;45:351–389.
2. Strollo PJ Jr., Rogers RM. Obstructive sleep apnea. *N Engl J Med.* 1996;334(2):99–104.
3. Caples SM, Gami AS, Somers VK. Obstructive sleep apnea. *Ann Intern Med.* 2005;142(3):187–197.
4. Shamsuzzaman ASM, Gersh BJ, Somers VK. Obstructive sleep apnea: Implications for cardiac and vascular disease. *JAMA.* 2003;290(14):1906–1914.
5. Young T, Palta M, Dempsey J, Skatrud J, Weber S, Badr S: The occurrence of sleep-disordered breathing among middle-aged adults. *N Engl J Med.* 1993;328(17):1230–1235.
6. Ancoli-Israel S, Kripke DF, Klauber MR, Mason WJ, Fell R, Kaplan O. Sleep-disordered breathing in community-dwelling elderly. *Sleep.* 1991;14(6):486–495.
7. Punjabi NM, Sorkin JD, Katzel LI, Goldberg AP, Schwartz AR, Smith PL. Sleep-disordered breathing and insulin resistance in middle-aged and overweight men. *Am J Respir Crit Care Med.* 2002;165(5):677–682.
8. Kapur V, Strohl KP, Redline S, Iber C, O'Connor G, Nieto J. Underdiagnosis of sleep apnea syndrome in U.S. communities. *Sleep Breath.* 2002;6(2):49–54.
9. Young T, Evans L, Finn L, Palta M. Estimation of the clinically diagnosed proportion of sleep apnea syndrome in middle-aged men and women. *Sleep* 1997;20(9):705–706.
10. Shahar E, Whitney CW, Redline S, et al. Sleep-disordered breathing and cardiovascular disease. Cross-sectional results of the sleep heart health study. *Am J Respir Crit Care Med.* 2001;163(1):19–25.
11. Stoohs R, Guilleminault C. Cardiovascular changes associated with obstructive sleep apnea syndrome. *J Appl Physiol.* 1992;72(2):583–589.
12. Narkiewicz K, Montano N, Cogliati C, van de Borne PJ, Dyken ME, Somers VK. Altered cardiovascular variability in obstructive sleep apnea. *Circulation.* 1998;98(11):1071–1077.
13. Nieto FJ, Young TB, Lind BK, et al. Association of sleep-disordered breathing, sleep apnea, and hypertension in a large community-based study. Sleep Heart Health Study. *JAMA.* 2000;283(14):1829–1836.
14. Gami AS, Pressman G, Caples SM, et al. Association of atrial fibrillation and obstructive sleep apnea. *Circulation.* 2004;110(4):364–367.
15. Kanagala R, Murali NS, Friedman PA, et al. Obstructive sleep apnea and the recurrence of atrial fibrillation. *Circulation.* 2003;107(20):2589–2594.
16. Gami AS, Howard DE, Olson EJ, Somers VK. Day-night pattern of sudden death in obstructive sleep apnea. *N Engl J Med.* 2005;352(12):1206–1214.
17. Ip MSM, Lam B, Ng MMT, Lam WK, Tsang KWT, Lam KSL. Obstructive sleep apnea is independently associated with insulin resistance. *Am J Respir Crit Care Med.* 2002;165(5):670–676.
18. Greenberg GD, Watson RK, Deptula D. Neuropsychological dysfunction in sleep apnea. *Sleep.* 1987;10(3):254–262.
19. Findley LJ, Suratt PM. Automobile crashes and sleep. *Va Med Q.* 1996;123(4):258–259.
20. Findley L, Smith C, Hooper J, Dineen M, Suratt PM. Treatment with Nasal CPAP decreases automobile accidents in patients with sleep apnea. *Am J Respir Crit Care Med.* 2000;161(3):857–859.
21. Sassani A, Findley LJ, Kryger M, Goldlust E, George C, Davidson TM. Reducing motor-vehicle collisions, costs, and fatalities by treating obstructive sleep apnea syndrome. Comment. *Sleep.* 2004;27(3):453–458.
22. Howard ME, Desai AV, Grunstein RR, et al. Sleepiness, sleep-disordered breathing, and accident risk factors in commercial vehicle drivers. *Am J Respir Crit Care Med.* 2004;170(9):1014–1021.
23. Young T, Shahar E, Nieto FJ, et al. Predictors of sleep-disordered breathing in community-dwelling adults: The sleep heart health study. *Arch Intern Med.* 2002;162(8):893–900.
24. Chesson AL Jr., Ferber RA, Fry JM, et al. The indications for polysomnography and related procedures. *Sleep.* 1997;20(6):423–487.
25. Johns MW. Daytime sleepiness, snoring, and obstructive sleep apnea. The epworth sleepiness scale. *Chest.* 1993;103(1):30–36.
26. Silber MH. Clinical practice. Chronic insomnia. *N Engl J Med.* 2005;353(8):803–810.
27. Dixon JB, Schachter LM, O'Brien PE. Predicting sleep apnea and excessive day sleepiness in the severely obese: Indicators for polysomnography. *Chest.* 2003;123(4):1134–1141.
28. Zonato AI, Martinho FL, Bittencourt LR, de Oliveira Campones Brasil O, Gregorio LC, Tufik S. Head and neck

physical examination: Comparison between nonapneic and obstructive sleep apnea patients. *Laryngoscope.* 2005; 115(6):1030–1034.

29. Kushida C. Practice Parameters for the Indications of Polysomnography and Related Procedures: An Update for 2005. *Sleep.* 2005;28(4):499–519.

30. Meir H, Kryger T, Roth William C. *Dement: Principles and Practice of Sleep Medicine.* Philadelphia, PA: WB Saunders; 2000.

31. Redline S, Kapur VK, Sanders MH, et al. Effects of varying approaches for identifying respiratory disturbances on sleep apnea assessment. *Am J Respir Crit Care Med.* 2000; 161(2):369–374.

32. American Academy of Sleep Medicine. *International Classification of Sleep Disorders, Revised.* Westchester, IL: American Academy of Sleep Medicine; 2001.

33. Hosselet J-J, Ayappa I, Norman RG, Krieger AC, Rapoport DM. Classification of sleep-disordered breathing. *Am J Respir Crit Care Med.* 2001;163(2):398–405.

34. Flemons WW, Littner MR, Rowley JA, et al. Home diagnosis of sleep apnea: A systematic review of the literature: An evidence review cosponsored by the American Academy of Sleep Medicine, the American College of Chest Physicians, and the American Thoracic Society. *Chest* 2003; 124(4):1543–1579.

35. Portable Monitoring Task Force of the American Academy of Sleep Medicine Task Force Members. Clinical guidelines for the use of unattended portable monitors in the diagnosis of obstructive sleep apnea in adults patients. *J Clin Sleep Med.* 2007;3(7):737–747.

36. Peppard PE, Young T, Palta M, Dempsey J, Skatrud J. Longitudinal study of moderate weight change and sleep-disordered breathing. *JAMA.* 2000;284(23):3015–3021.

37. Hudgel DW. Treatment of obstructive sleep apnea. A review. *Chest.* 1996;109(5):1346–1358.

38. Ferguson KA, Cartwright R, Rogers R, Schmidt-Nowara W. Oral appliances for snoring and obstructive sleep apnea: A review. *Sleep* 2006;29(2):244–262.

39. Kushida CA, Morgenthaler TI, Littner MR, et al. Practice parameters for the treatment of snoring and obstructive sleep apnea with oral appliances: An update for 2005. *Sleep.* 2006;29(2):240–243.

40. Jenkinson C, Davies RJO, Mullins R, Stradling JR. Comparison of therapeutic and subtherapeutic nasal continuous positive airway pressure for obstructive sleep apnoea: A randomised prospective parallel trial. *Lancet.* 1999;353 (9170):2100–2105.

41. Ballester E, Badia Joan R, Hernandez L, et al. Evidence of the effectiveness of continuous positive airway pressure in the treatment of sleep apnea/hypopnea syndrome. *Am J Respir Crit Care Med.* 1999;159(2):495–501.

42. George CFP. Reduction in motor vehicle collisions following treatment of sleep apnoea with nasal CPAP. *Thorax.* 2001;56(7):508–512.

43. Kaneko Y, Floras JS, Usui K, et al. Cardiovascular effects of continuous positive airway pressure in patients with heart failure and obstructive sleep apnea. *N Engl J Med.* 2003; 348(13):1233–1241.

44. Pepperell JCT, Ramdassingh-Dow S, Crosthwaite N, et al. Ambulatory blood pressure after therapeutic and subtherapeutic nasal continuous positive airway pressure for obstructive sleep apnoea: A randomised parallel trial. *Lancet.* 2002;359(9302):204–210.

45. Becker HFMD, Jerrentrup AMD, Ploch TDP, et al. Effect of nasal continuous positive airway pressure treatment on blood pressure in patients with obstructive sleep apnea. Report. *Circulation.* 2003;107(1):68–73.

46. Mansfield DR, Gollogly NC, Kaye DM, Richardson M, Bergin P, Naughton MT. Controlled trial of continuous positive airway pressure in obstructive sleep apnea and heart failure. *Am J Respir Crit Care Med.* 2004;169(3): 361–366.

47. Zozula R, Rosen R. Compliance with continuous positive airway pressure therapy: Assessing and improving treatment outcomes. *Curr Opin Pulm Med.* 2001;7(6):391–398.

48. Reeves-Hoche MK, Hudgel DW, Meck R, Witteman R, Ross A, Zwillich CW. Continuous versus bilevel positive airway pressure for obstructive sleep apnea. *Am J Respir Crit Care Med.* 1995;151(2 Pt 1):443–449.

49. Means MK, Edinger JD, Husain AM. CPAP compliance in sleep apnea patients with and without laboratory CPAP titration. *Sleep Breath.* 2004;8(1):7–14.

50. Sin DD, Mayers I, Man GCW, Pawluk L. Long-term compliance rates to continuous positive airway pressure in obstructive sleep apnea: A population-based study. *Chest* 2002;121(2):430–435.

51. Sher AE, Schechtman KB, Piccirillo JF. The efficacy of surgical modifications of the upper airway in adults with obstructive sleep apnea syndrome. *Sleep.* 1996;19(2): 156–177.

52. Sher AE. Upper airway surgery for obstructive sleep apnea. *Sleep Med Rev.* 2002;6(3):195–212.

53. Thorpy M, et al. Practice parameters for the treatment of obstructive sleep apnea in adults: The efficacy of surgical modifications of the upper airway. *Sleep.* 1996;19:152–155.

54. Kiely. Effect of inhaled nasal fluticasone on OSA. *Am J Resp Crit Care Med.* 1998;157(3):A283.

55. Hanzel DA, Proia NG, Hudgel DW. Response of obstructive sleep apnea to fluoxetine and protriptyline. *Chest* 1991;100(2):416–421.

56. Smith I, Lasserson TJ, Wright J. Drug therapy for obstructive sleep apnoea in adults. *Cochrane Database Syst Rev.* 2006;(2):CD003002. PMID: 12076464.

57. Keating GM, Raffin MJ. Modafinil: A review of its use in excessive sleepiness associated with obstructive sleep apnoea/hypopnoea syndrome and shift work sleep disorder. *CNS Drugs* 2005;19(9):785–803.

PART 6

Endocrinologic Disorders

CHAPTERS

Chapter 24

Obesity

Kendra Boell

SEARCH STRATEGY

A systematic search of the medical literature was performed on April 6, 2007. The search, limited to human subjects and English language journals included Ovid, UpToDate®, and the Cochrane database. Search terms included obesity, pharmacotherapy, diabetes, insulin resistance, hypertension, dyslipidemia, orlistat, sibutramine, and phentermine.

INTRODUCTION

Long-term weight loss maintenance is a challenge in the treatment of obesity, especially in the primary care setting where time constraints and reimbursement are major issues. The prevalence of obesity is on the rise world wide, and is a major public health concern. There is little doubt that this disease needs to be treated; however the traditional strategies of weight reduction by behavior modification and physical activity have poor long-term outcomes, primarily as a result of lack of compliance.[1] Considerable evidence suggests that even a modest weight reduction of 5% to 10% of initial body weight can significantly impact the morbidity and mortality of obese patients.[2] Obesity is a multifactorial disease requiring individually tailored treatment strategies. Pharmacotherapy plays an important role in the appropriate patient.

CLINICAL EVALUATION

BODY MASS INDEX

Body mass index (BMI) is the most practical way to evaluate weight. It is calculated (metric formula) as follows:

$$BMI = (body\ weight\ in\ kilograms) \div (height\ in\ meters)^2$$

When measurements are recorded in pounds and inches, the following equation may be used:

$$BMI = [(body\ weight\ in\ pounds) \times 705] \div (height\ in\ inches)^2$$

BMI is relatively unaffected by height, and is highly correlated with body fat. A BMI of 18 to 25 kg/m² is considered normal or ideal body weight. Patients with a BMI of 25 to 30 kg/m² are low risk, while those with a BMI of 30 to 35 kg/m² are moderate risk. Patients with a BMI of 35 to 40 kg/m² are at high risk, and those with a BMI above 40 kg/m² are at very high risk for morbidity and mortality from their obesity. Irrespective of BMI, health risk is increased by more abdominal fat distribution (increased waist to hip ratio) (Fig. 24-1).

COMORBIDITIES

The Swedish Obese Subjects Study followed untreated obese subjects with an average BMI of 38 kg/m² for 2 years.[3] The 2-year incidence of the following comorbidities were:

- Hypertension: 13.6%
- Diabetes mellitus: 6.3%
- Hyperinsulinemia: 6.3%
- Hypertriglyceridemia: 7.7%
- Low serum high-density lipoprotein (HDL) cholesterol: 8.6%
- Hypercholesterolemia: 12.1%

A comparison of one of the above comorbidities, in the general population, yielded a 29% incidence rate

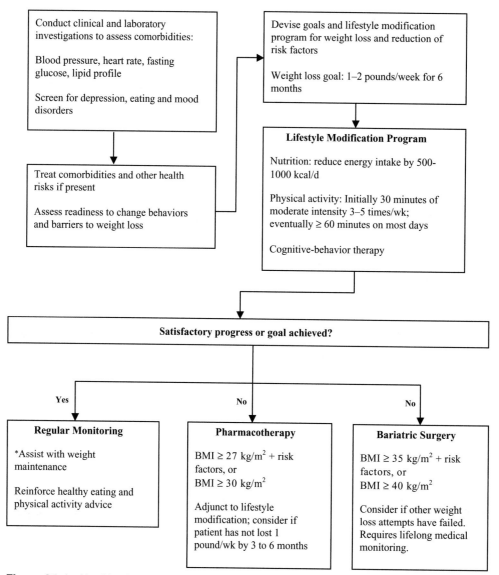

Figure 24-1. Algorithm for the assessment and stepwise management of the overweight or obese adult. *BMI and waist circumference cutoff points are different for some ethnic groups. LDL, low-density lipoprotein; HDL, low-density lipoprotein.

for hypertension[4] and an 8% incidence for diabetes.[5] The prevalence of insulin resistance is 5% in the nonobese population compared with 22% in those who are overweight, and 60% in persons who are obese.[6]

The Nurses' Health and the Health Professionals Studies also showed increased risk of developing a chronic disease including cholelithiasis, hypertension, heart disease, colon cancer, and stroke (in male subjects only), with increasing BMI.[7]

Diabetes Mellitus

Type 2 diabetes mellitus is strongly associated with obesity, regardless of ethnicity, with more than 80% of cases attributed to BMI greater than 30 kg/m^2.

Insulin Resistance

Insulin resistance probably results from a combination of genetic factors and obesity. Insulin resistance is defined as fasting serum insulin to serum glucose ratio less than five.

Hypertension

The risk for increased blood pressure is most prominent in patients whose fat distribution is primarily abdominal and upper body. The mechanism is not well understood. One theory suggests hyperinsulinemia may raise blood pressure by increasing sympathetic activity, renal sodium absorption, or vascular tone.[8]

Dyslipidemia

Obesity is associated with several changes in lipid metabolism, including low serum HDL cholesterol and elevated low-density lipoprotein and very-low-density lipoprotein cholesterol. Elevated triglycerides are also seen; however decreased HDL levels carry a greater relative risk of coronary heart disease.[9]

Stroke

BMI >27 kg/m^2 is associated with an increased risk of ischemic stroke. Elevated BMI is not correlated with hemorrhagic stroke, although the relationship is still present for total stroke risk, and is increased in men.[10]

Hepatobiliary Disease

The two prominent comorbidities seen in the hepatobiliary system of obese patients are symptomatic gallstones and steatosis. The increased risk of gallstones is likely because of the elevated production and excretion of cholesterol. When the rate of triglyceride synthesis exceeds the rate of clearance, the excess accumulates in the liver leading to steatosis.[11]

Degenerative Joint Disease

Osteoarthritis, seen predominantly in the knees and ankles of obese subjects, is most likely caused by repetitive trauma from excess body weight. It occurs more frequently in nonweight-bearing joints as well, suggesting that other components in the obese patient may alter cartilage and bone metabolism independent of weight bearing.[12]

Skin Changes

Several skin changes may be seen with increased weight, striae being the most common signaling strain on the skin from expanding fat deposits. Hirsutism in women is a result of increased testosterone production from visceral adiposity. Acanthosis nigricans may be seen around the neck, axilla, knuckles, and extensor surfaces, and is linked with insulin resistance.

Respiratory Disease

Obstructive sleep apnea and hypoventilation syndrome are the most serious respiratory problems associated with obesity. Increased abdominal pressure on the diaphragm can lead to decreased lung compliance, increased chest wall impedance, and higher residual lung volume which then decrease strength and endurance of respiratory muscles, and depress ventilatory drive. It is controversial as to whether or not obesity is a risk factor for asthma.[13]

Cancer

In both male and female subjects, increasing BMI has been associated with higher rates of death from cancer in the following areas: esophagus, colon, rectum, liver, gallbladder, pancreas, and kidney, in addition to increased rates of non-Hodgkin's lymphoma and multiple myeloma. Women were also at increased risk for breast, uterine, cervical, and ovarian cancer, while men were also at increased risk for stomach and prostate cancer.[14]

Polycystic Ovarian Syndrome

Anovulatory cycles, irregular menses, and decreased fertility are common in obese individuals.

Depression

The stigma associated with obese individuals is seen in schools, the workplace, and the health care arena, among other areas. This is evident in a study of more than 10 000 adolescents and women who had a BMI above the 95th percentile. This group completed fewer years of school, were less likely to be married, had lower household incomes, and higher rates of poverty than their normal weight counterparts, independent of their baseline socioeconomic status or aptitude test scores.[15]

COST OF OBESITY

In a 1998 study by Wolf and Colditz, the direct costs of obesity in the United States were estimated to be $51.6 billion dollars per year, with greater than 50% accounted for by type 2 diabetes. The indirect costs are calculated at approximately $95 billion per year.[16]

TREATMENT

OBESITY GUIDELINES

The goal of weight reduction must be realistic. It is unlikely that the obese patient will return to his or her ideal body weight. Rarely are patients happy with the weight loss they achieve. Accordingly the provider and patient must come to a mutual understanding of realistic weight loss goals.

Pharmacotherapy is a useful component of a weight management program in individuals with a BMI greater than 30 kg/m^2 or greater than 27 kg/m^2 with comorbid medical problems. (See Table 24-1) In order to be considered effective, weight loss should be in the range of 0.5 to 3 pounds per week, decrease more than 5% below baseline by 3 to 6 months, and have maintenance of the weight loss. Patients should be aware that drug therapy is not a cure for obesity, and only works in

Table 24-1. FDA Approved Drugs for the Treatment of Obesity.

Drug	Trade Names	Dosage (mg)	DEA Schedule
Orlistat	Xenical	120, three times daily before meals	N/A
Sibutramine	Meridia, Reductil	5–15, daily	IV
Diethylpropion	Tenuate	25, three times daily	IV
	Tenuate Dospan	75, daily	
Phentermine	Adipex	15–30, daily	IV
	Ionamin Slow Release		
Benzphetamine	Didrex	25–50, 3 times daily	III
Phendimetrazine	Bontril	17.5–70, 3 times daily	III
	Prelu-2	105, once daily	

conjunction with behavior modification and increased physical activity.

SYMPATHOMIMETIC DRUGS

The noradrenergic sympathomimetic drugs, including phentermine, diethylpropion, phendimetrazine, benzphetamine, and sibutramine mimic the neurotransmitter norepinephrine. They can increase blood pressure and heart rate. These drugs reduce food intake by causing early satiety. They are rapidly metabolized and reach peak concentrations in a few hours, although sibutramine has active metabolites. These drugs are metabolized to inactive products in the liver, and should not be used in patients with a history of heart disease or uncontrolled hypertension. Sibutramine should not be used in patients taking selective serotonin reuptake inhibitors, as the combination may precipitate serotonin syndrome.

Phentermine

Phentermine is approved by the U.S. Food and Drug Administration (FDA) for short-term use, loosely interpreted as up to 12 weeks. It is a Schedule IV drug, although the abuse potential is low. Both continuous and intermittent use of phentermine is associated with weight loss. However, weight loss decreased during the drug-free periods and accelerated once treatment resumed.

Diethylpropion

Diethylpropion is also only approved for short-term use and is a Schedule IV drug. It is available in a long acting form.

Benzphetamine

Benzphetamine is only approved for short-term use; however, it is a Schedule III drug.

Phendimetrazine

Phendimetrazine is also a Schedule III drug, and is only approved for short-term use.

Sibutramine

Sibutramine is a norepinephrine and serotonin reuptake inhibitor. It not only has anorectic properties, but has been shown to stimulate thermogenesis in experimental animals.[17] Sibutramine is the only sympathomimetic drug approved for both short-term and long-term use. It is a Schedule IV drug.

LIPASE INHIBITOR

Orlistat

Orlistat inhibits pancreatic lipases. As a result, 30% of ingested fat is not absorbed and is excreted in the GI tract. Less than 1% of the drug is absorbed. This drug is generally well tolerated, although patients may experience gastrointestinal side effects including cramps, flatus, fecal incontinence, oily spotting, urgency, and flatus with discharge. Additionally, orlistat may decrease the uptake of fat-soluble vitamins.[18] It is helpful to give a vitamin supplement to minimize this effect.

OTHER

Metformin

In patients who are diabetic or insulin resistant, metformin has been shown to increase insulin sensitivity, as well as decrease appetite and promote weight loss. The mechanism of appetite suppression is presumed to be related to the more efficient use of the anabolic hormone, insulin.

Fluoxetine

Fluoxetine is a selective serotonin reuptake inhibitor which has been shown to have anorectic side effects. The mechanism is not known.

Herbal Preparations

Caution should be used when recommending herbal preparations to patients as these are not regulated by the FDA. There is limited research to substantiate the claims made by some of the producers. Some of the herbs claiming weight loss properties include garcinia cambogia, caffeine, guar gum, chromium picolinate, and green tea.

UPCOMING THERAPEUTIC AGENTS[19]

Rimonabant[20] is currently in clinical trials. This agent acts on the endocannabinoid system by selectively blocking CB_1 receptors both centrally and peripherally. Increased activity of the endocannabinoid system is associated with disproportionate food intake.

Bariatric surgery may be indicated for patients who have class III obesity (BMI ($>$40) with comorbid medical problems who have failed conservative medical management.[21,23] The most common surgery performed in the United States today is the roux-en-Y gastric bypass procedure, which restricts the capacity of the stomach and limits absorption of calories by shortening the small intestine. However, adjustable gastric banding is gaining popularity because it is less invasive and is reversible. Bariatric surgery is a tool and must be used in conjunction with continued, monitored diet and exercise programs.

SUMMARY

Obesity needs to be recognized as a chronic disease, and not a failure of will power. Behavior modification and exercise are the foundation for maintaining a healthy weight, or reducing body mass. Medications are a useful adjunctive therapy in the appropriate patient to reduce and treat comorbidities associated with obesity.

RESOURCES

Additional materials and resources can be found at the following websites:

The American Obesity Association at www.obesity.org

The International Association for the Study of Obesity at www.iaso.org

EVIDENCE-BASED SUMMARY

- Use BMI to assess overweight and obesity, and to estimate relative risk of disease compared to normal weight. Body weight alone can be used to follow weight loss, and to determine efficacy of therapy (C).
- Waist circumference should be used to assess abdominal fat content (C).
- Initial goal of weight loss therapy should be to reduce body weight by 10% from baseline (A).
- Low Calorie Diets (LCDs) are recommended for weight loss in overweight and obese persons (A). Reducing fat is a practical way to help reduce calories.
- An individually planned diet with a deficit of 500–1000 kcal/d should achieve a weight loss of 1–2 pounds per week (A).
- Physical activity should be an integral part of weight loss therapy and weight maintenance (B).
- Weight loss is recommended in overweight and obese persons for the following:
- Lower elevated blood pressure in patients with hypertension
- Lower elevated levels of total cholesterol, low-density lipoprotein cholesterol, triglycerides, and to raise low levels of HDL cholesterol in patients with dyslipidemia
- Lower blood glucose levels in patients with diabetes (A)
- Weight loss drugs approved by the FDA may be used in the appropriate patient in addition to diet and exercise. Ongoing assessment of the drugs efficacy and safety is essential. (B)

Adapted from: NIH Clinical Guidelines on the Identification, Evaluation, and Treatment of Overweight and Obesity in Adults. The letters in parentheses indicate the evidence categories.

REFERENCES

1. Guy-Grand B. Pharmacological Approaches to Intervention. *Int J Obes Relat Metab Disord.* 1997 Mar; 21 Suppl 1:S22-24.
2. Hauptman. *Arch Fam Med.* 2000;9(2):160–167.
3. Sjostrom CD, Lissner L, Wedel H, Sjostrom L. Reduction in incidence of diabetes, hypertension and lipid disturbances after intention weight loss induced by bariatric surgery: The SOS Intervention Study. *Obes Res.* 1999;7:477.
4. Hajjar I, Kotchen TA. Trends in prevalence, awareness, treatment, and control of hypertension in the United States, 1988-2000. *JAMA.* 2003;290(2):199–206.
5. Mokdad AH, et al. Prevalence of obesity, diabetes, and obesity-related health risk factors, 2001. *JAMA.* 2003; 289(1):76–79.
6. Park YW, et al. The metabolic syndrome: prevalence and associated risk factor findings in the US population from the Third National Health and Nutrition Examination Survey, 1988-1994. *Arch Intern Med.* 2003;163(4): 427–436.
7. Field AE, Coakley EH, Must A, et al. Impact of overweight on the risk of developing common chronic diseases during a 10-year period. *Arch Intern Med.* 2001;161:1581.

8. Hall JE. Renal and cardiovascular mechanisms of obesity. *Hypertension.* 1994;23:381.

9. Willett EC, Manson JE, Stampfer JM, et al. Weight, weight change, and coronary heart disease in women. Risk within the 'normal' weight range. *JAMA.* 1995;273:461.

10. Kurth T, Gaziano JM, Berger K, et al. Body mass index and the risk of stroke in men. *Arch Intern Med.* 2002;162: 2557.

11. Stamfer MJ, Maclure KM, Colditz GA, et al. Risk of symptomatic gallstones in women with severe obesity. *Am J Clin Nutr.* 1992;55:652.

12. Cicuttini FM, Baker JR, Spector TD. The association of obesity with osteoarthritis of the hand and knee in women: A twin study. *J Rheumatol.* 1996;23:1221.

13. Ray CS, Sue DY, Bray JE, et al. Effects of obesity on respiratory function. *Am Rev Respir Dis.* 1983;128:501.

14. Calle EE, Rodriguez C, Walker-Thurmond K, Then MJ. Overweight, obesity, and mortality from cancer in a prospectively studied cohort of U.S. adults. *N Engl J Med.* 2003;348:1625.

15. Gortmaker SL, Must A, Perrin JM, et al. Social and economic consequences of overweight in adolescence and young adulthood. *N Engl J Med* 1993;329:1008.

16. Wolf AM, Colditz GA. Current estimates of the economic cost of obesity in the United States. *Obes Res.* 1998;6:97.

17. Hansen DL, Toubro S, Stock MJ, et al. Thermogenic effects of sibutramine in humans. *Am J Clin Nutr.* 1998;68:1180.

18. Hill JO, Hauptman J, Anderson JW, et al. Orlistat, a lipase, inhibitor for weight maintenance after conventional dieting: A 1-y study. *Am J Clin Nutr.* 1999;69:1108–1116.

19. Cota D Marsicano G, Tschop M, et al. The endogenous cannabinoid system affects energy balance via central orexigenic drive and peripheral lipogenesis. *J Clin Invest.* 2003;112:423–431.

20. Snow Vincenza, et al. Pharmacologic and surgical management of obesity in primary care: A clinical practice guideline from the American College of Physicians. *Ann Intern Med.* 2005;142(7):525–530.

21. *Clinical Guidelines on the Identification, Evaluation, and Treatment of Overweight and Obesity in Adults.* The Evidence Report. NIH Publication. *No. 98-4083 September 1998. National Institutes of Health.*

22. Padwal RS, Majumdar SR. Drug treatments for obesity: Orlistat, sibutramine, and rimonabant. *Lancet.* 2007;369: 71-77.23. DeMaria EJ. Bariatric surgery for morbid obesity. *N Engl J Med.* 2007;356:2176–2183.

Chapter 25

Diabetes Mellitus Management

Caryl Sumrall and Marshall J. Bouldin

SEARCH STRATEGY

A search for specific references and reviews was conducted in PubMed. Diabetes Care provides a use for search for position papers and clinical practice guidelines and can be accessed at http://care.diabetesjournals.org1

BACKGROUND

An epidemic of diabetes mellitus is sweeping the United States and the developing world. Since 1958, the prevalence of diabetes has increased more than 5-fold. Between 1991 and 2001, the prevalence of diabetes has increased by 49% overall, by 76% in the 30 to 39 age group, and as much as 10-fold in the pediatric population. As the population ages and becomes more overweight, the two major risk factors for type 2 diabetes, the epidemic of diabetes continues to accelerate. The cost of this disease for our society is shocking. Diabetes accounts for 15% of health care costs and 25% of Medicare costs in the United States. The total expenditure of our society on diabetes is greater than any other disease entity, including heart disease, cerebrovascular disease, cancer, and HIV. Most of this cost is from preventable complications of diabetes.[1]

Diabetes is a risk equivalent for cardiovascular disease (CVD) and is the leading cause of renal failure, adult blindness, and nontraumatic limb amputation in the United States. The Diabetes Control and Complications Trial showed significant risk reduction in the development of cardiovascular events, retinopathy, nephropathy, and neuropathy in patients with Type 1 diabetes mellitus with more tightly controlled diabetes than those with suboptimal control.[2] Glycemic control in addition to control of hypertension (HTN) and dys-

lipidemia are important in the management of diabetes. Clinical trials have shown that diabetes is highly preventable in those most at risk by moderate exercise and modest weight loss, and that this is more effective than drug therapy in preventing diabetes.[3,4] With these sobering facts in mind, it is important for primary care providers to be aware of the current standards of care for treating diabetes and preventing its complications as well as to understand effective therapies for diabetes in all its stages.[5]

CLASSIFICATION

There are two main clinical classifications of diabetes mellitus: type 1 diabetes and type 2 diabetes. Other specific types of diabetes (genetic defects in pancreatic β-cell function or insulin action, diseases of the exocrine pancreas, and drug or chemical induced diabetes) and gestational diabetes are less common and will be deferred to more detailed texts.[6]

TYPE 1 DIABETES

In type 1 diabetes there is little or no pancreatic secretion of insulin as a result of autoimmune β-cell destruction, requiring the patient to be treated with insulin replacement therapy in order to survive. While this type of diabetes most frequently appears in childhood or adolescence, it is possible to develop type 1 diabetes in adulthood. Patients with type 1 diabetes are classically thin or underweight, the result of chronic insulin deficiency and the resultant inability to utilize and store carbohydrate calories. Insulin resistance plays no part in pure type 1 diabetes. In the absence of exogenous insulin, type 1 diabetes patients develop ketosis, which can move quickly through ketoacidosis to death. While the prevalence of type 1 diabetes has been increasing, this disease still accounts for only a small percentage of patients with diabetes.[6]

TYPE 2 DIABETES

Type 2 diabetes mellitus (T2DM) accounts for 90% to 95% of all patients with diabetes, and occurs when there is significant resistance to the effects of insulin at tissue levels coupled with an insufficient insulin secretory response to overcome this resistance. This manifests as increased hepatic output and decreased muscle absorption of glucose, and long-term relative failure of β-cell function. The combination of these abnormalities leads to elevations in serum glucose levels and eventually to symptoms of overt diabetes, usually after many years of asymptomatic undiagnosed disease. Age, sedentary lifestyle, and adiposity are the major risk factors for T2DM. The typical type 2 diabetic patient is older and overweight; 85% to 90% of type 2 diabetic patients are overweight or obese.[6]

With the increase in obesity in the US population in all ages and the increasing prevalence of T2DM, T2DM is now quite common at younger ages. Indeed, some pediatric epidemiologic surveys have reported that T2DM is now the most common form of diabetes in children, some emergency department series are now reporting that diabetic ketoacidosis is now more often caused by T2DM (although it remains an uncommon complication of that disease), and it is no longer uncommon to find patients with type 1 diabetes who have become overweight and developed insulin resistance and T2DM as well. Children and adolescents diagnosed with T2DM are generally between 10- and 19-year-olds, obese, have a strong family history for T2DM, and have insulin resistance. Those affected with T2DM belong to all ethnic groups, but it is more commonly seen in non-white groups, particularly among American Indian youth.[1]

CLINICAL PRESENTATION

SYMPTOMS

Although type 1 patients are usually easily recognized early in the course of disease, T2DM likely presents no symptoms at all for many years. While not all patients exhibit symptoms of hyperglycemia, those patients with significant hyperglycemia may experience, either alone or in combination, the following symptoms: polyuria, polydipsia, unexplained weight loss, polyphagia, fatigue, and blurred vision. Women may have frequent vaginal candidiasis. Men may experience erectile dysfunction. In addition, susceptibility to certain infections

and impairment of growth may also be experienced. Those patients who have severe hyperglycemia for extended periods of time may develop nonketotic hyperosmolar syndrome or DKA. Presenting symptoms in these conditions may range from the insidious onset of dehydration and lethargy to nausea, vomiting, and severe electrolyte disturbances.[5]

DIAGNOSIS

A normal fasting glucose is considered to be less than 100 mg/dL. The diagnosis of diabetes is established by a fasting plasma glucose of ≥126 mg/dL on two separate occasions, symptoms of diabetes with a random plasma glucose of ≥200 mg/dL, or a 2-hour glucose tolerance test with a plasma glucose of ≥200 mg/dL. Although a glucose tolerance test is seldom used clinically it is useful for research purposes. Prediabetes is defined by impaired fasting glucose or by impaired glucose tolerance (IGT). Impaired fasting glucose is defined as a fasting plasma glucose between 100 mg/dL to 125 mg/dL. A random plasma glucose or glucose following a 2-hour glucose tolerance test of 140 mg/dL to 199 mg/dL is considered evidence of IGT. Those patients with prediabetes are at high risk for a future diagnosis of diabetes, and patients with prediabetes should be strongly encouraged to incorporate appropriate changes in their diet and exercise regimens to prevent development of diabetes.[6] Currently, no evidence exists to advocate screening for diabetes in all primary care patients (Table 25-1), although there is much evidence demonstrating improved risk for cardiovascular events and other complications with early detection and aggressive control.[8] Screening for diabetes is recommended in those patients who are at risk for T2DM which includes the following: being overweight or obesity; having first degree relatives with T2DM; being of African American, Asian, and Hispanic, or Native American ethnicity; having a history of gestational diabetes or polycystic ovarian syndrome; having CVD or risks including HTN, dyslipidemia, or metabolic syndrome.[9]

MANAGEMENT OF COMPLICATIONS

The major morbidity, mortality, and cost of diabetes is associated with its chronic complications. These complications of diabetes include macrovascular sequelae (CVD, stroke, peripheral vascular disease [PVD]) and microvascular complications (renal failure, retinopathy, neuropathy). It is now well known that tight control of blood glucose, blood pressure, and lipids can prevent or significantly delay the macrovascular and microvascular complications of diabetes. The management of multiple

Table 25-1. Criteria for Screening Adults for Diabetes

Date	Organization	Recommendations
2007	American Diabetes Association[6]	Diabetes screening for adults every 3 y starting at age 45 y
		Screen adults <45 y of age if they are overweight and other diabetes risk factors
2003	U.S. Preventative Services Task Force[7]	Insufficient evidence exists to recommend diabetes screening for asymptomatic adults
		Adults with HTN or hyperlipidemia should be screened for diabetes

risk factors and comorbidities in the diabetic patient requires a systematic evaluation and assessment with frequent visits to the primary care provider. Reminder systems such as flow sheets are useful in achieving recommended rates in patients with diabetes. Table 25-2 gives a list of recommended evaluations.

MACROVASCULAR DISEASE

Cardiovascular Disease

CVD is a major cause of death in patients with diabetes; it is also a major contributor to both direct and

Table 25-2. Recommended Evaluation for Diabetes Care

Evaluation	
Body weight/BMI	Each office visit
Blood pressure	Each office visit
Hemoglobin A1C	Every 10–12 weeks if not at goal; every 6 months if at goal
Lipids	Annually; more frequently to achieve treatment target
Foot examination	Physical examination each visit; monofilament annually
Urine microalbumin	Annually
Smoking cessation	Annually
Dilated eye examination	Annually
Treatment of CVD risks	
Antihypertensive	Optimal Blood Pressure Control. Include ACE-I or ARB if microalbuminuria is confirmed.
HMg CoA reductase (statin)	LDL reduction is primary target
Anti-platelet agent	Aspirin or clopidogrel
Pneumonia vaccine	At least one lifetime vaccine; revaccinate adults >64 if previous vaccine was >5 y ago
Flu vaccine	Annually unless contraindicated for all patients ≥6 months

indirect costs of diabetes and to morbidity associated with diabetes.[8] Of the 18.2 million Americans with diabetes, approximately 75% die of CVD. With the significant increase in the number of patients diagnosed with diabetes each year, complications of diabetes, in particular CVD, are a major health and economic problem.[8] The risk of myocardial infarction for a diabetic patient is equivalent to the risk of a patient who has known CVD, so that diabetes is now considered an independent CVD risk equivalent. A careful history and physical should be taken to evaluate patients for preexisting CVD.

Peripheral Vascular Disease

PVD caused by atherosclerosis is accelerated in patients with diabetes and increases morbidity caused by ischemia. Assessment of the carotid arteries, abdominal aorta, and femoral arteries should be included in the physical examination. Randomized controlled trials have demonstrated that CVD and PVD can be prevented or its progression slowed in diabetic patients by improving other cardiovascular risk factors (blood pressure, low-density lipoprotein (LDL), and smoking cessation) in addition to improving overall diabetes control.[10] Currently, the ADA guidelines recommend screening for CVD with thallium imaging in asymptomatic diabetic patients who have an abnormal testing electrocardiogram indicative of myocardial infarction or ischemia, peripheral arterial disease or two or more additional CVD risk factors.[11]

MICROVASCULAR DISEASE

Nephropathy

Diabetic nephropathy occurs in 20% to 40% of patients with diabetes and is the leading cause of end-stage renal disease. Annual screening for microalbuminuria is recommended in patients who have had type 1 diabetes for >5 years and in patients with T2DM, at initial diagnosis. Microalbuminuria in the range of 30–299 mg/24 h has been shown to be the earliest clinically discernable stage of diabetic nephropathy and is also independently associated with increased CVD risk. Measurement of the microalbumin to creatinine ratio in a random urine sample is recommended for screening. Less than 30 mg of albumin per gram of creatinine is normal. The role of annual microalbumin assessment after the onset of microalbuminuria is unclear.

In addition to annual screening for proteinuria, improved glucose and blood pressure control are necessary to reduce the risk for nephropathy. Treatment with angiotensin-converting enzyme inhibitors (ACE-I) or angiotensin receptor blockers (ARBs) with or without the presence of HTN can reduce the incidence of microalbuminuria and slow the development of overt nephropathy. Appropriate consultation with a nephrologist for those patients with diabetic nephropathy whose estimated GFR has fallen below 60 mL/min/1.73 m² has been found to delay progression of diabetic nephropathy and the initiation of dialysis, improve quality of care, and reduce costs.[5]

Retinopathy

Diabetic retinopathy is a vascular complication that is specific to diabetes and is the most frequent cause of blindness. Retinopathy can be prevented and its progression delayed by optimizing glycemic control. Optimal blood pressure control can independently reduce the risk and progression of diabetic retinopathy. For patients with type 1 diabetes, a dilated, comprehensive eye examination is recommended within 5 years after the onset of the disease and at least annually thereafter. Patients with T2DM should have a dilated, comprehensive eye examination soon after their diagnosis and at least annually thereafter. If retinopathy has developed or is progressing, more frequent eye examinations may be necessary. Treatment with laser therapy can reduce the risk of vision loss. Aspirin therapy does not increase the risk of hemorrhage in diabetic retinopathy or prevent diabetic retinopathy.[5]

Neuropathy

Lower extremity neuropathy leads to increased incidences of pain, foot ulceration, and amputation. Those patients at increased risk for developing foot ulcers are those who have poorly controlled diabetes, who have had diabetes for >10 years, or who have developed renal, retinal, or cardiovascular complications. In addition, patients with bony deformities of the foot, PVD, or a previous history of ulcers are also at risk. A foot examination should be performed at each office visit, with assessment of pedal pulses and a sensory examination performed annually using a Semmes–Weinstein 5.07 monofilament. Patients should be educated on appropriate foot care and advised on risk reduction for PVD, progressive neuropathy, and infection. Referral to a diabetic foot specialist or podiatrist is useful for treatment of calluses, ulcers, or other abnormalities that may be outside the scope of care provided by the primary diabetes provider.[5] The progression of painful diabetic neuropathy may be slowed with tight glycemic control. In the event that the patient does develop painful diabetic neuropathy, antidepressants and anticonvulsants are often used to decrease the intensity of pain experienced, often described as burning or stinging pain.[12]

Other forms of neuropathy, diabetic gastroparesis and autonomic dysfunction, result in major complications for patients. Such patients should be referred to a diabetic specialty center if available.

CONCOMITANT RISK FOR CVD IN DIABETES

Hypertension

The United Kingdom Prospective Diabetes Study demonstrated that intensive antihypertensive therapy had beneficial effects on macrovascular and microvascular diabetes-related outcomes. Furthermore, the benefit of blood pressure control was greater than that derived by glycemic control.[13] Blood pressure is an independent risk factor for both macrovascular and microvascular complications in patients with diabetes and most diabetics are hypertensive. Blood pressure should be measured at each office visit. The systolic blood pressure goal is <130 mm Hg, while diastolic blood pressure goal is <80 mm Hg. Patients who develop elevated blood pressure (systolic blood pressure >140 mm Hg or diastolic blood pressure >90 mm Hg) should be educated on diet and lifestyle recommendations to lower blood pressure and, depending on other cardiovascular risk factors, can be given a 3-month trial of diet and exercise modifications without medications to attempt to reduce their blood pressure readings. Medication treatment revolves around lowering overall blood pressure while providing cardiovascular protection (see Chapter 1). Initial drug therapy should be with a class shown in randomized controlled clinical trials to reduce CVD events in patients with diabetes: diuretics, ACE-I, ARBs, or calcium channel blockers. Multiple drug therapy (two or more agents) will usually be necessary to achieve blood pressure targets. Ideally, all patients with diabetes and HTN should be treated with a regimen containing an ACE-I or an ARB if possible, as both offer significant renal protection in patients with diabetes in addition to cardiovascular protection. ACE-I and ARBs are contraindicated in pregnancy.[5]

Dyslipidemia

Primary and secondary prevention of CVD in the diabetic patient requires the evaluation and management of dyslipidemia and is considered the standard of care.[5,14] Clinical trial evidence supports the use of lipid lowering agents to present primary and secondary CVD in diabetes treatment[14] (see Chapter 6). Patients with diabetes should be tested annually to screen for lipid abnormalities, and more frequently if necessary to evaluate treatment. Education on exercise, weight loss, and a diet of reduced saturated fat and cholesterol is essential and may be effective in improving lipid levels. For patients with diabetes and without overt CVD, an LDL goal of <100 mg/dL is advised. HMG CoA reductase inhibitor ("statin") therapy is recommended as initial drug therapy to achieve a LDL reduction of 30% to 40%. Patients with overt CVD and diabetes are at very high risk for further events, and should be treated with statin therapy if at all possible. A tighter LDL goal of <70 mg/dL is an option in this group. A pattern of high triglycerides and low HDL is characteristic of the insulin resistant state. Combination therapy with statins and fibrates or niacin may be required to achieve lipid goals but has not yet been evaluated in outcomes studies for CVD event reduction or safety. Statins are contraindicated in pregnancy.[5]

Anti-Platelet Agents

Aspirin in a dose of 75–162 mg/d is utilized in patients with diabetes to prevent CVD events. Daily aspirin is recommended as primary prevention in patients with T2DM who are >40 years or who have additional CVD risk factors, such as smoking, strong family history of CVD, HTN, dyslipidemia, or albuminuria. Daily aspirin is recommended for secondary prevention in all diabetic patients with known macrovascular disease. Aspirin is not recommended for patients with diabetes who are less than 21 years of age because of the increased risk of Reye's syndrome; in addition, it is contraindicated in pregnancy. For those patients who are intolerant of aspirin (history of aspirin allergy, history of GI bleeding, history of hepatic disease), other anti-platelet agents may be considered as an alternative (clopidogrel). The presence of retinopathy is not a contraindication to aspirin therapy.[5]

Smoking Cessation

Smoking is a known risk factor for CVD and is one of the most preventable causes of premature death. Smoking significantly multiplies the already significant CVD risk of diabetic patients and contributes to the progression of PVD. All patients with diabetes should be advised not to smoke. Smoking cessation counseling and other forms of treatment should be a routine component of diabetes care.[5]

PREVENTION

Individuals with "prediabetes" are at risk for diabetes.[6] Patient with prediabetes should be counseled on prevention strategies and be followed closely. Clinical trials have demonstrated that regular exercise and dietary changes may prevent or delay the onset of diabetes. In overweight subjects with IGT moderate exercise, personal dietary counseling to reduce fat intake and increase dietary fiber resulted in a significant reduction in new onset diabetes.[15] The Diabetes Prevention Project (DPP) showed that lifestyle modification in prediabetics reduced the incidence of diabetes.[4] In the DPP

trial metformin reduced the onset of diabetes but not as well as lifestyle intervention.[4] Other pharmacotherapeutics that have been shown to delay the onset of diabetes include rosiglitazone and acarbose.[5]

TREATMENT

LIFESTYLE RECOMMENDATIONS

Thorough, intensive education is essential to any diabetes treatment plan. Patients should be educated on the importance of weight loss (if necessary) and regular physical activity. The American Diabetes Association recommends 150 minutes of moderate-intensity exercise each week to improve glycemic control, promote weight loss, and to decrease CVD risk. In addition to aerobic exercise, resistance exercise is recommended three times a week.[16]

Referral to diabetes educators for diabetes self-management education and/or nutritionists for medical nutritional therapy can ensure appropriate dietary counseling and behavioral modifications specific to the individual patient's needs. Dietary recommendations are individually designed to reduce caloric intake if weight loss is needed and to improve glycemic control. It is recommended that saturated and trans fats be reduced. Carbohydrate intake should also be monitored to achieve glycemic control.[5,16]

Follow up and reinforcement are key to ensuring successful incorporation of these measures into the patient's diabetes care plan. A variety of strategies and techniques should be used to provide education and develop problem-solving skills in the various aspects of diabetes management. Crucial to the implementation of any management plan is that each aspect should be understood and agreed upon by the patient and the care providers, and that the treatment plan and goals are reasonable for that individual patient.

In addition, patients with diabetes should be counseled on the importance of self-monitored blood glucose (SMBG) testing. In addition to monitoring A1C levels, SMBG testing is critical in helping both providers and patients determine what their individual glucose patterns are and therefore where treatment should be adjusted. Table 25-3 is an example of a SMBG chart which patients are encouraged to keep. SMBG testing not only helps to identify hyperglycemia, but also episodes of hypoglycemia, when the patient may not experience symptoms. Clinical trials using insulin have shown that SMBG is an integral part of tight diabetes control. SMBG should be utilized three times a day or more in patients on multiple insulin injection therapy. SMBG has not been shown to improve glycemic control in noninsulin-treated diabetes.[17]

Table 25-3. Self Monitoring Blood Glucose (SMBG) and Diet Log

NAME: _____

DATE _____

DAY _____

COMMENTS

BG Readings	1	2	3	4	5	6	7	8	9	10	11	12	1	2	3	4	5	6	7	8	9	10	11	12
400																								
300																								
200																								
100																								

Carbohydrate		

Basal Rates		
Carb Bolus		
High BG Bolus		

BREAKFAST

Time	Food Description	Carbs	Time

MORNING SNACKS

LUNCH

Food Description	Carbs	Time

AFTERNOON SNACKS

DINNER

Food Description	Carbs

EVENING SNACKS

Hemoglobin AIC correlates with glycemic control and is used to monitor therapy. It is not recommended in the diagnosis of diabetes. Evaluation of the AIC should be a routine part of diabetes care and measured at least two times a year. More frequent measurements should be taken after 2 to 3 months to assess the therapeutic effects of pharmocotherapeutic agents. The American Diabetes Association currently recommends a target AIC of less than 7 % in most patients with diabetes.[5]

PHARMACOTHERAPY

There are numerous pharmacologic agents and delivery systems now available for the treatment of T2DM. In recent years new classes and combination therapies have been developed. An individualized approach to treatment is required and should take into consideration many variables including comorbid conditions, lifestyle, access to medications, patient adherence, and level of glycemic control. In general, oral therapy is initiated in patients to achieve glycemic control and is maximized by dose titration and use of combined oral therapy. Oral agents may also be used in combination with insulin. Insulin therapy should be used as initial therapy in those with weight loss, severe symptoms of hyperglycemia, or fasting glucoses of >250 mg/dL. Oral agents may be added to an insulin-based regimen.[5]

Lifestyle intervention combined with metformin is recommended for early treatment.[18] Fig. 25-1 illustrates an algorithm for pharmacotherapeutic choices in the treatment of T2DM. If the AIC is >7%, a second class (and third class) of therapy may be added (sulfonylureas, thiazolidinediones [TZDs], or insulin) in a stepwise fashion to achieve optimal glycemic control.[5] Other classes of antidiabetic agents and combination therapeutic agents are available as illustrated in Table 25-4.

SULFONYLUREAS

The oldest class of oral diabetes medications, the sulfonylureas, have been in use for approximately 50 years and are the most frequently prescribed oral agents. The sulfonylureas stimulate insulin secretion from β-cells of the pancreatic islets by binding to the sulfonylurea receptor on the β-cell surface. This class of oral diabetes agents is divided into first and second generation agents, with the first generation having a shorter duration of action (<12 hours) than the second generation (>24 hours) as a result of differences in metabolism rates, activity of metabolites, and rates of elimination. These medications are metabolized through the liver and reach their peak plasma concentrations within 2 to 4 hours. They are highly bound to plasma proteins and may interact with medications that have a similar binding effect, such as warfarin, salicylates, and sulfonamides. The response to this class of medications depends on the presence of β-cell function, and doses may have to be increased over time or additional agents added depending on the continued gradual loss of β-cell function that typically occurs with the progression of T2DM. On average, this class can lower A1C levels by 1% to 2%.[19]

The most common side effects of sulfonylureas are weight gain, with an average gain of 1 to 4 kilograms that stabilizes more than 6 months, and hypoglycemia, which may occur more frequently with the longer-acting second-generation sulfonylureas. This class should be used cautiously in patients with renal and hepatic disease, as decreased excretion can lead to more hypoglycemia. Rarely, sulfonylureas have been associated with fever, jaundice, blood dyscrasias, and erythema multiforme. Although some older data suggested that this class increases the risk for cardiovascular events in diabetic patients, more modern large randomized trials have not demonstrated this effect. The sulfonylureas may be used as monotherapy or with other oral diabetes agents and may be used safely with insulin.[20]

MEGLITINIDES

The nonsulfonylurea insulin secretagogues are also known as the meglitinides or rapid acting prandial insulin releasers. The agents in this class, repaglinide and vateglinide, stimulate rapid but short-lived insulin secretion to compensate for the defect in insulin response to meal consumption in diabetes. These medications are taken orally immediately before meals and can be useful in patients with irregular meal patterns or lifestyle needs. They reach peak plasma concentrations within 1 hour and are metabolized by the liver; their insulin releasing effect typically lasts for 3 hours. They carry a decreased risk of hypoglycemia and have a small amount of weight gain. They may be used as monotherapy for those patients who experience hyperglycemia strictly related to meals or in combination with other diabetes agents. They can typically lower A1C by 1% to 2%, and are most valuable when postprandial hyperglycemia is a significant problem.[19]

α-GLUCOSIDASE INHIBITORS

Acarbose and miglitol retard the rate of carbohydrate digestion resulting in a delay in glucose absorption. They can decrease postprandial hyperinsulinemia and triglyceride levels. They may be used as monotherapy or in combination with other diabetes medications. Patients do not experience weight gain and typically do

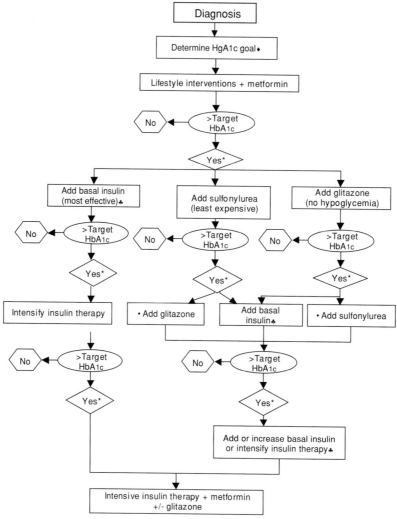

Figure 25-1. Management of hyperglycemia in T2DM.

(Copyright © 2006 American Diabetes Association. From Diabetes Care® ,Vol. 29, 2006; 1963–1972. Reprinted with permission from *The American Diabetes Association*.)

not have hypoglycemia unless used in conjuction with insulin or sulfonylureas. However, their use has been limited by an increased incidence of gastrointestinal (GI) disturbances, including flatulence, abdominal discomfort, and diarrhea. These drugs may therefore be difficult to use in patients with a history of chronic intestinal disease. These GI side effects may be minimized by gradually titrating dosages upward and by ensuring that patients eat meals containing complex carbohydrates instead of simple carbohydrates. Higher doses may result in increased liver enzyme concentrations. This class may lower A1C levels by 0.5% to 1%.[19]

BIGUANIDES

The biguanides improve diabetes control by decreasing hepatic output of glucose and increasing insulin-mediated glucose utilization in tissues. Metformin is currently the only biguanide available in the United States; phenformin was withdrawn in the 1970s, as a result of increased incidences of lactic acidosis. The biguanides are absorbed quickly, distributed widely, not metabolized, and eliminated unchanged in the urine. They decrease endogenous insulin requirements and basal plasma insulin concentrations. Metformin is now recommended in conjunction with lifestyle intervention

Table 25-4. Oral Antidiabetic Agents*

Drug Class (Generic Name)	Daily Dosage Range	Dose(s)/d	Duration of Action (h)	Main Adverse Effects
Insulin secretagogues sulfonylureas				
First generation				Weight gain, hypoglycemia
Tolbutamide	0.5–2.0 g	2–3	12	
Acetohexamide	0.25–1.5 g	1–2	12–24	
Tolazamide	0.1–0.5 g	1–2	12–24	
Chlorpropamide	1.25–20.0 mg	1	36–72	
Second generation				Weight gain, hypoglycemia
Glyburide	5–40 mg	1–2	16–24	
Glipizide	5–40 mg	1–2	12	
Glimepiride	1–8 mg	2–4	24	
Meglitinides				Hypoglycemia, weight gain
Netaglinide	60–360 mg	2–4	1–2	
Repaglinide	1–16 mg	2–4		
Biguanide				GI intolerance, lactic acidosis
Metformin	1.0–2.5 g	2–3	6–12	
α-Glucosidase inhibitors				GI intolerance
Acarbose	75–300 mg	3	NA	
Miglitol	75–300 mg	3	NA	
TZDs				Fluid retention, congestive heart failure, hepatoxicity, weight gain, hypoglycemia
Rosiglitazone	4–8 mg	1–2	12–24	
Pioglitazone	15–45 mg	1	24	
Incretin mimetics				GI intolerance
Pramlintide	0.6 mg	3	3	
Exanatide†	5–10 mg sq	2	2	
Dipeptidyl peptidase (DDP) IV inhibitors				Headache, upper respiratory infection
Sitagliptin	25–100 mg	1	1–4	
Combination medications	Dosage and interval are dependent upon specific combination			
Sulfonylurea/biguanide				Weight gain, hypoglycemia
Sulfonylurea/thiozolidinedione				Weight gain, hypoglycemia
Biguanide/ thiozolidinedione				GI intolerance, weight gain, hypoglycemia
DDP-IV inhibitor/biguanide				GI intolerance, headache

*Modified from multiple sources.
†Given subcutaneously.

as first line therapy in most type 2 diabetics. Metformin may also be used in combination with other diabetes agents and is now marketed in combination with several other oral antidiabetic drugs (Table 25-4).[19]

Biguanides carry no risk of serious hypoglycemia. They are contraindicated in patients with impaired renal function, in patients with liver disease, alcohol abuse, and a history of metabolic acidosis, and in patients with cardiac or respiratory insufficiency. Renal function should be assessed before initiating therapy and during the course of therapy, and metformin should be discontinued prior to procedures utilizing intravenous radiographic contrast media. They can be taken with meals or immediately after the meal to minimize GI side effects, which can include diarrhea, flatulence, and abdominal discomfort.[19] Metformin should be discontinued if serum creatinine exceeds 1.4 mg/dL in women and 1.5 mg/dL in men.

THIAZOLIDINEDIONES (TZDs)

TZDs, (pioglitazone and rosiglitazone) were introduced in the late 1990s. They contribute to improved insulin sensitivity, reduction in hyperinsulinemia, and increase peripheral glucose disposal rates while decreasing hepatic glucose production.[16] Their ability to improve glucose control relies on the presence of adequate insulin production by the pancreas. They are metabolized in the liver and bind to plasma proteins but have no known interference with other protein binding drugs. They have a slow onset of action, and overall improvement in glucose control may not be seen for 3 to 4 months. The TZDs have been shown to reduce A1C levels by 0.5% to 1.5% and may be used as monotherapy or in combination with other oral diabetes medications or insulin. They are contraindicated in patients with active liver disease and in patients with class III or IV congestive heart failure, as well as in pregnancy. Prior to starting this therapy, it is recommended that baseline liver enzymes be drawn to evaluate for pre-existing liver disease, and repeat liver enzymes periodically as determined by the clinician thereafter. Side effects include weight gain (an average of 1 to 4 kilograms that stabilizes more than 6–12 months), edema, hypoglycemia, and elevated liver enzymes.[21] Recent data have emerged regarding the potential risk with rosiglitazone and increased incidence of cardiovascular events and death in patients taking the medication; providers need to make an educated decision regarding its continued use as treatment for diabetes.[22]

GLUCAGON-LIKE PEPTIDE RECEPTOR AGONISTS—INCRETIN MIMETICS

Glucagon-like peptide 1 (GLP-1) is a gut-derived incretin hormone that stimulates insulin and suppresses glucagon secretion, inhibits gastric emptying, and reduces appetite and food intake. Currently available GLP-1 agonists include exenatide and pramlintide. Exenatide is administered by subcutaneous injection twice daily for patients with T2DM suboptimally controlled on oral antidiabetic agents (metformin, sulfonylureas, a combination of both, or TZDs). The starting dose of exenatide is 5 μg twice daily for 4 weeks, followed by an increase to 10 μg twice daily. Exenatide reduced A1C concentrations by 0·8% to 1·0 % more than 30 weeks, with prevention of weight gain or modest weight loss of 1·5 to 3 kilograms. The most frequent adverse events with exenatide were nausea, or more rarely vomiting or diarrhea. Exenatide has a circulating half-life of 60 to 90 minutes, with increases in plasma exenatide concentrations lasting 4 to 6 hours after a single subcutaneous injection.[23] Randomized controlled clinical trials with GLP-1 therapy result in improved fasting and postprandial blood sugars in nonpregnant patients with diabetes and have a favorable weight profile.[24] Further evaluation of long-term efficacy and safety with these agents are needed.

Preclinical studies indicate that the neuroendocrine actions of the peptide hormone amylin, produced in pancreatic α-cells, complement those of insulin in glucose homeostasis by targeting suppression of postprandial glucagon, delaying gastric emptying time, and enhancing satiety, which leads to decreased caloric intake and potential weight loss.[23] Amylin also replenishes hepatic glycogen stores and glucagon-like insulinotropic polypeptide, which increases insulin production in response to a meal.[23] Human amylin has a very short half-life and is too thick to inject as such not useful in diabetic patients.

Pramlintide, the first soluble, stable, nonaggregating, synthetic peptide analog of human amylin is now available. The time to achieve maximum concentration of pramlintide is 20 minutes, with the effect lasting up to 3 hours after drug administration. Its elimination half-life is approximately 20 to 45 minutes. Pramlintide is metabolized and eliminated predominantly by the kidneys. Since pramlintide possesses a wide therapeutic index, dosage adjustments are not required regardless of meal size or in the presence of mild-to-moderate renal insufficiency. Pramlintide has clearly been shown to reduce A1C by 0.1% to 0.4% in patients with type 1 diabetes and 0.3% to 0.7% in patients with T2DM. Trials also demonstrated that pramlintide therapy was associated with a weight reduction of 0.7 kg to 1.7 kg. Side effects include nausea, vomiting, and anorexia. Pramlintide is available in 30 mg and 60 mg doses bid subcutaneously Pramlintide is rated as pregnancy category C and is contraindicated in patients with gastroparesis.[25]

DIPEPTIDYL PEPTIDASE-4 ACTIVITY INHIBITORS (INCRETIN ENHANCERS)

Dipeptidyl peptidase-4 (DPP-4) inhibitors degrade the natural breakdown of incretins by DPP-4 and mimic many of the actions ascribed to GLP-1 agonists, including stimulation of insulin and inhibition of glucagon secretion, and preservation of β-cell mass through stimulation of cell proliferation and inhibition of apoptosis. By contrast, DPP-4 inhibitors are generally not associated with deceleration of gastric emptying or weight loss. Typically, these agents reduce serum DPP-4 activity by more than 80%, with some inhibition maintained for 24 hours after one dose or with once daily treatment. DPP-4 inhibition is accompanied by a rise in postprandial levels of intact GLP-1. Sitagliptin is well-tolerated at doses of 100 mg once daily, either as monotherapy, or in combination with metformin or pioglitazone, without significant hypoglycemia or weight gain. No characteristic pattern of adverse events has been associated with the use of DPP-4 inhibitors, despite the large number of potential substrates for DPP-4. In view of the widespread expression of DPP-4 on many cell types, including lymphocytes, there is considerable interest in the long-term safety profile of DPP-4 inhibitors.[23]

COMBINATION ORAL MEDICATIONS

With the natural progression of diabetes and decline of β-cell function, it may be necessary to add additional agents to maintain glycemic control. Combinations of different classes of oral agents are particularly effective, as each class targets a different mechanism contributing to elevated blood glucose. In fact, many oral medications are now available in combination form (Table 25-4). As with the use of these medications individually, appropriate laboratory values and side effects should be monitored, and therapy adjusted as necessary based on individual patient needs.

INSULIN

The introduction of insulin therapy in the 1920s was the most significant innovation in the treatment of diabetes.[26] Over time, new insulin types and methods of delivery have allowed patients who require insulin better control, more options, and more flexibility with regards to their diet, lifestyles, and insulin administration. For many patients with T2DM the gradual decline of β-cell function and increasing peripheral insulin resistance often renders insulin treatment necessary, either as monotherapy or in combination with oral agents. Figure 25-2 illustrates a method of initiation of insulin. Insulin therapy in patients with T2DM may be necessary at the time of diagnosis to reduce glucose toxicity, with the possibility of weaning insulin and converting to oral medications as hyperglycemia improves. Insulin is also indicated for severe or symptomatic hyperglycemia. Insulin may be temporarily required for a transient increase in insulin resistance such as in acute severe physical stress, injury, infection, or glucocorticoid therapy.[26]

Patient instructions for insulin therapy should emphasize the importance of timing of meals to insulin injections, of rotating insulin injection sites to minimize lipodystrophy, of regularity in the schedule of doses and meals, and of appropriate recognition and treatment of hypoglycemia. As with sulfonylureas, the most common side effects of insulin are hypoglycemia and weight gain. In patients with renal disease, insulin absorption and excretion will be affected, leading to decreasing insulin requirements as renal function declines and to more frequent episodes of hypoglycemia if not appropriately monitored. The importance of SMBG testing cannot be overemphasized in patients receiving insulin injections.[26]

Insulin can be classified into four different categories: rapid- (lispro aspart and glulisine), short- (regular), intermediate- (NPH, lente), and long-acting (ultralente, glargine, detemir) insulin.[27] Table 25-5 illustrates the currently available insulins. While each category has its own onset, peak, and duration, it is important to remember that individual patients respond individually to various insulin regimens, and

adjustment of predicted insulin dosages should be made with the aid of SMBG testing. These insulins may be used as monotherapy for treatment or in combination with oral medications, depending on the individual patient needs for optimal glucose control. In addition, combinations of intermediate and short or rapid acting insulins are available (70/30—NPH and R, Humalog 75/25—NPL and lispro, Novolog 70/30—NPA and aspart).[27] These mixed insulins may be useful in patients who have difficulty in mixing insulins but are limited in their flexibility. Titration increases or decreases mean that both components of the mixture are changed, so that there is no way to adjust only one component of their particular insulin regimen, which can lead to more frequent episodes of hypoglycemia.[28]

Insulin is stable at room temperature for approximately 1 month but will retain its stability longer if refrigerated. It should not be exposed to extreme cold or hot temperatures. With the exception of aspart, lispro, glulisine, detemir, and glargine, all other insulins are in suspension and require gentle mixing by rolling to ensure uniform suspension before the insulin is used. Regular insulin, aspart, lispro, glulisine, and detemir may be mixed with NPH without any variation in the stability in any of the types of insulin. Glargine may not be mixed with other insulins. Absorption occurs more quickly in the abdomen with slower absorption in the arms, buttocks, and thighs. Physical exercise increases blood flow to the active body part and therefore will increase insulin absorption from that region, which can lead to hypoglycemia. Patients should be counseled on the importance of SMBG when exercising to minimize the incidence of hypoglycemia.[27]

Methods of delivery of insulin have changed over time, and many modalities are now available. In addition to traditional syringes, many insulins are available for administration as insulin pens, which some patients find more convenient, safer, simpler, more accurate, or easier to see. Insulin pumps are becoming increasingly more common as therapy for type 1 diabetics and selected type 2 patients and offer considerable accuracy and flexibility at the cost of more complex maintenance, increased expense, and increased patient responsibility.[29]

Insulin and Surgery

In general, patients who are on insulin injections may continue those injections during the perioperative phase. Nighttime long-acting insulin doses may need to be decreased on the night prior to the procedure to prevent hypoglycemia, depending on when the patient will be allowed to eat following the procedure. For

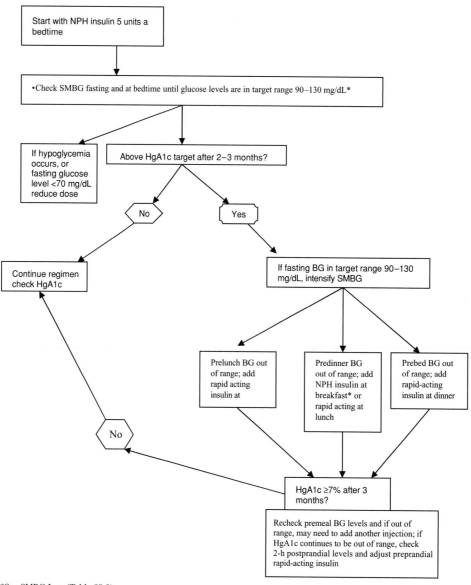

*See SMBG Log (Table 25-3).

Figure 25-2. Initiation and adjustment of insulin.
(Copyright © 2006 American Diabetes Association. From Diabetes Care® ,Vol. 29, 2006; 1963–1972.
Reprinted with permission from *The American Diabetes Association*.)

patients undergoing procedures that are long and/or complex, sliding scale or intravenous insulin is usually required in place of their injections.[30]

CONCLUSION

Diabetes is an extremely disease process that requires intensive management on the part of both the patient and the provider. For many, optimal control can only be achieved by a multidisciplinary approach involving the primary care provider, the diabetes educator, the nutritionist, and often other subspecialists. Particular attention must be given to comorbid conditions, in particular HTN and dyslipidemia, as modification of these risk factors contributes most directly to improvement in cardiovascular risk in diabetic patients. Macrovascular complications (CAD, cerebrovascular disease, and PVD) should be routinely screened for and preventive measures implemented (aspirin therapy and smoking cessation). Microvascular complications

Table 25-5. Insulins by Comparative Action*

Type	Onset(h)	Peak (h)	Effective Duration (h)	When to Take (min)
Rapid acting				
Lispro	0.25–0.5	05–2.51	≤5	0–15 prior to meal
Aspart	<0.20	1–3	3–5	0–15 prior to meal
Glulisine	<0.20	1–3	3–5	0–15 prior to meal
Short acting				
Regular	0.5–1	2–3	3–6	30 prior to meal
Intermediate				
NPH	2–4	4–10	10–16	45–60 prior to meal
Lente	3-	4–12	12–18	
Long acting				
Ultralente	6–10	10–16	18–20	N/A
Glargine	1–2	Peakless	Up to 24 h	N/A
Detemir	1–2	Peakless	Up to 24 h	N/A
Combinations				
50% NPH, 50% regular	0.5–1	Dual	10–16	
70% NPH, 30% regular	0.5–1	Dual	10–16	
70% NPH, 30% aspart	<0.25	Dual	10–16	
75% NPL, 25% lispro	<0.25	Dual	10–16	

*Modified from multiple sources.

(diabetic nephropathy, retinopathy, and neuropathy) should be routinely screened for and treated. Frequent follow-up with A1C levels and SMBG testing is essential to monitor control and adjust therapy according to individual patient needs.

EVIDENCE-BASED SUMMARY

- Risk factors for diabetes include obesity, sedentary lifestyle, and increasing age.
- Diabetes is a leading risk factor for macrovascular (CVD and PVD) and microvascular disease (retinopathy, neuropathy, nephropathy).
- Diabetes is usually associated with other risk factors for heart disease, including HTN and dyslipidemia.
- Management of the diabetic patient requires comprehensive medical management to prevent primary and secondary CVD which includes optimal control of HTN, lipids, as well as glycemic control.
- Treatment of diabetes requires comprehensive lifestyle intervention in addition to a multi-drug regimen to achieve glycemic control and optimization of other CVD risks.
- Diabetic patients often require combination antidiabetic agents to control their disease and often must utilize insulin for optimal glycemic control.

REFERENCES

1. Center for Disease Control and Prevention. Prevalence of diabetes. http://www.cdc.gov.diabetes/pubs. Accessed December 15 , 2007.
2. The DCCT Research Group. The effect of intensive treatment of diabetes on the development and progression of long-term complications in insulin-dependent diabetes mellitus. *N Engl J Med.* 1993;329:978–986.
3. Tuomilehto J, Lindstrom J, Eriksson JG, et al. Prevention of type 2 diabetes mellitus by changes in lifestyle among subjects with impaired glucose tolerance. *N Engl J Med.* 2001;344:1343–1350.
4. Knowler WC, Barrett-Conner E, Fowler SE, et al. Reduction in the incidence of type 2 diabetes with lifestyle intervention or metformin. *N Eng J Med* 2002;346:393–403.
5. American Diabetes Association, Inc. Standards of medical care in diabetes. *Diabetes Care.* 2007;30:S4–S41.
6. American Diabetes Association, Inc. Diagnosis and classification of diabetes mellitus. *Diabetes Care.* 2007;30:S42–S47.
7. U.S. Preventive Services Task Force. Screening for type 2 diabetes mellitus in adults: Recommendations and rationale. *Ann Intern Med.* 2003;138:212–214.
8. Grundy SM, Benjamin IJ, Burke GL, et al. Diabetes and cardiovascular disease: A statement for healthcare professionals from the American Heart Association. *Circulation.* 1999;100:1134–1146.
9. Laine C, Wilson JF. In the Clinic: Type 2 Diabetes. *Ann Intern Med.* 2007;146(1):ITC1–ITC16.
10. UK Prospective Diabetes Study Group. Tight blood glucose control and risk of macrovascular and microvascular complications so type 2 diabetes. *BMJ.* 1998;317:703–713.
11. Moore TD, Linn WD, Blodgett JL, O'Rourke RA. Hot topic: Should all asymptomatic diabetic patients undergo

noninvasive studies for stress induced myocardial ischemia? www.Accessmedicine.com. January, 2005.

12. Wong M, Chung JWY, Wong TKS. Effects of treatments for symptoms of painful diabetic neuropathy: Systematic review . *BMJ.* 2007;335:1–10.

13. UK Prospective Diabetes Study Group. Efficacy of atenolol and captopril in reducing risk of macrovascular and microvascular complications in type 2 diabetes. *BMJ.* 1998;317:713–720.

14. Snow V, Aronson MD, Hornbake ER, et al. Lipid control in the management of type 2 diabetes mellitus; a clinical practice guideline from the American College of Physicians. *Ann Intern Med.* 2004;140:644–649.

15. Tuomilehto J, Lindstrom J, Eriksson JG, et al. Prevention of type 2 diabetes mellitus by changes in lifestyle among subjects with impaired glucose tolerance. *N Engl J Med.* 2001;344:1343–1350.

16. Buse JB, Ginsberg HN, Bakris GL, et al. American Heart Association and the American Diabetes Association. Primary prevention of cardiovascular diseases in people with diabetes mellitus: A scientific statement from the American Heart Association and the American Diabetes Association. *Diabetes Care.* 2007;30(1):162–172.

17. Farmer A, Wade A, Goyder E, et al. Impact of self-monitoring of blood glucose in the management of patients with non-insulin treated diabetes: Open parallel group randomised trial. *BMJ.* 2007;335:105–106.

18. Nathan D, Buse J, Davidson M, et al. Management of hyperglycemia in type 2 diabetes: A consensus algorithm for the initiation and adjustment of therapy. *Diabetes care.* 2006;29:1963.

19. Krentz AJ, Bailey CJ. Oral antidiabetic agents: current role in type 2 diabetes mellitus. *Drugs.* 2005;65:385–411.

20. Korytkowski MT. Sulfonylurea treatment of type 2 diabetes mellitus: Focus on glimepiride. *Pharmacotherapy.* 2004;24: 606–620.

21. Day C. Thiazolidinediones: A new class of antidiabetic drugs. *Diabet Med.* 1999;16:179–192.

22. Nissen SE, Wolski K. Effect of Rosiglitazone on the Risk of Myocardial Infarction and Death from Cardiovascular Causes. *NEJM.* 2007;356:2457–2471.

23. Drucker DJ, Nauck MA. The incretin system: glucagon-like peptide-1 receptor agonists and dipeptidyl peptidase-4 inhibitors in type 2 diabetes. *Lancet.* 2006;368:1696–1705.

24. Amori RE, Lau J, Pittas AG. Efficacy and safety of incretin therapy in type 2 diabetes; systematic reivew and meta-analysis. *JAMA.* 2007;298:194–206.

25. Nogid A, Pham DQ. Adjunctive therapy with pramlintide in patients with type 1 or type 2 diabetes mellitus. *Pharmacotherapy.* 2006;26(11):1626–1640.

26. Kelley DB, et al. *Medical Management of Type 2 Diabetes*, 4th ed. Alexandria, VA: American Diabetes Association; 1998: 27–86.

27. Campbell RK, White JR. *Insulin Use in Type 2 Diabetes and in Gestational Diabetes. Medications for the Treatment of Diabetes.* American Diabetes Association, Alexandria, VA. 2000:113–126.

28. Klingensmith GJ. Multiple-component insulin regimens. *Intensive Diabetes Management*, 3rd ed. Alexandria, VA: American Diabetes Association; 2003:73–98.

29. Kelley DB, et al. *Routine Management: Tools. Medical Management of Type 1 Diabetes*, 3rd ed. Alexandria, VA: American Diabetes Association; 1998:49–116.

30. Hirsch IB, McGill JB. Role of insulin in management of surgical patients with diabetes mellitus. *Diabetes Care.*1990; 13:980–991.

Chapter 26

Metabolic Syndrome

Jimmy L. Stewart and Marion R. Wofford

SEARCH STRATEGY

A search of PubMed was conducted for specific references. Guidlelines for reference were obtained from www.guide-line.gov. UptoDate was queried for general content.

The term metabolic syndrome refers to a constellation of interrelated conditions that directly promote the development of atherosclerotic cardiovascular disease (CVD) and type 2 diabetes mellitus. The term metabolic syndrome has become widely accepted in the medical literature. The primary care provider is faced with the implications of the diagnosis of the metabolic syndrome for patients. Identification of one risk component of the metabolic syndrome should prompt evaluation of other components.[1] Early identification of the cluster of risks of CVD and diabetes may be important in educating patients on lifestyle interventions to avert or delay the development of CVD and type 2 diabetes. Pharmacologic treatment for metabolic syndrome does not differ from the treatment for the traditional risks for CVD including diabetes, hypertension, and hyperlipidemia, although more research on prevention and treatment of metabolic syndrome is clearly needed.

DEFINITION AND DIAGNOSIS

In 1988, Reaven first described a cluster of risk factors associated with CVD, which included hyperglycemia, low high-density lipoprotein, hypertriglyceridemia, and hypertension. He coined the phrase "syndrome X" and proposed that the pathophysiology leading to CVD is related to insulin resistance resulting in hyperinsulinemia. Reaven recognized an association with obesity and syndrome X but did not consider obesity a central component of syndrome X.[2]

Since Reaven's landmark presentation, other names have been applied to the syndrome including metabolic syndrome X, dysmetabolic syndrome, plurimetabolic syndrome, and the insulin resistance syndrome. Failure to reach consensus on a universally acceptable title stems from the fact that the exact causes of metabolic syndrome remain elusive. Strictly speaking, this is an association of conditions, not a syndrome[3], however, the term gained popularity during the last few years. Extensive research in the areas of epidemiology, pathophysiology, and clinical care related to metabolic syndrome has been done.

Multiple methods have been used during the last 10 years to define the metabolic syndrome criteria. The World Health Organization proposed diagnostic criteria of metabolic syndrome in 1998.[4] These guidelines were not widely accepted, as there is a requirement for evaluation of insulin resistance either by oral glucose tolerance test or euglycemic clamp. Both methods are difficult to conduct in the clinical setting. The National Cholesterol Education Program (NCEP) Adult Treatment Panel III (ATP III) proposed a set of criteria in 2001 based on common clinical measures including waist circumference, triglycerides (TG), HDL cholesterol, blood pressure (BP), and fasting glucose level. Abnormal findings in 3 of the 5 areas constitute a positive diagnosis.[1] Modifications to these criteria have been suggested by several organizations since 2001, including the American Heart Association (AHA), the National Heart, Lung, and Blood Institute,[5] and the International Diabetes Foundation (IDF).[6] Table 26-1 lists the diagnostic criteria for the modified ATP III guidelines as suggested by the AHA and National Heart, Lung, and Blood Institute.

Table 26-1. Diagnostic Criteria for Metabolic Syndrome

Any 3 of 5 Criteria Constitute the Diagnosis of Metabolic Syndrome	Cut Points
Elevated waist circumference	≥102 cm (≥40 inches) in men ≥88 cm (≥35 inches) in women
Elevated TG	≥150 mg/dL (1.7 mmol/L) or Drug treatment for elevated TG*
Reduced HDL cholesterol	<40 mg/dL (0.9 mmol/L) in men <50 mg/dL (1.1 mmol/L) in women or Drug treatment for reduced HDL cholesterol*
Elevated BP	≥130 mm Hg systolic BP or >85 mm Hg diastolic BP or Drug treatment for hypertension
Elevated fasting glucose	≥100 mg/dL or Drug treatment for elevated glucose

*Fibrates and nicotinic acid are the most commonly used drugs for elevated TG and reduced HDL cholesterol. Patients taking one of these drugs presumed to have high TG and low HDL.

Recently, modified guidelines of World Health Organization have been published, which are more consistent with NCEP guidelines.[6] These guidelines, like NCEP, include cut points for BP, HDL cholesterol, TG, and central obesity. The IDF guidelines differ in that they include adjusted waist circumference cut points for different ethnic groups. The IDF guidelines take into account the greater sensitivity of Asian Americans for insulin resistance with increasing waist circumferences.[6]

PREVALENCE

Metabolic syndrome is very common in the United States, particularly in individuals more than the age of 50. It is largely an entity of westernized societies and is highly associated with increasing weight, particularly abdominal obesity. An increasing prevalence of metabolic syndrome allows projection of increases in the prevalence of CVD and type 2 diabetes.[7] Approximately 35% of the population more than 50 years of age meet the original ATP III criteria.[8] Among the population as a whole, the age-adjusted prevalence from the Third National Health and Nutrition Examination Survey 1998–1994 (NHANES III) and NHANES 1999–2000 were 23.1% and 26.7% ($p = 0.043$), respectively, based on the original NCEP/ATP III criteria, which defined the glucose threshold of 110 mg/dL. When using the AHA and National Heart, Lung, and Blood Insitute

modified criteria (glucose threshold of 100 mg/dL), the age-adjusted prevalence is 29.2% with NHANES III.[9] Variability is seen with gender and ethnicity. Women have a greater increase in prevalence with Hispanic women having the highest prevalence (36%) and African American men having the lowest (16%).[8] Approximately 50 million US adults had metabolic syndrome in 1990 compared to the current estimates of nearly 64 million adults with metabolic syndrome and risk for diabetic and atherosclerotic disease in the future.[9]

Metabolic syndrome occurs in children and adolescents, but there is no consensus on the diagnostic criteria. The presence of metabolic syndrome is high is obese children and adolescents, and its prevalence increases with the degree of obesity.[10] In the period of adolescence there are physiologic alterations related to developmental changes making criteria development challenging.[11] A modified ATP III definition requires at least three of the following: TG levels >95th percentile, HDL in <5th percentile, systolic or diastolic pressure 95th percentile, and impaired glucose tolerance.[12] In another proposed criteria, the syndrome as it applies to children and adolescents was defined as serum TG ≥110 mg/dL, HDL cholesterol ≤40 mg/dL, waist circumference ≥90th percentile, fasting plasma glucose ≥110 mg/dL, and BP ≥90th percentile.[13] Without consensus on the definition of metabolic syndrome in children and adolescents, it is difficult to estimate the prevalence or risk in this age group. Furthermore, recommendations that apply to adults may not be generalizable to children and adolescents.[11]

PATHOPHYSIOLOGY

Although the exact mechanisms for the development of metabolic syndrome remain elusive, the major underlying risk factors include obesity and insulin resistance. Insulin resistance leads to worsening of each of the components of the metabolic syndrome, which together increase cardiovascular risk. Genetics appears to play an important role in predisposing certain individuals and populations to the development of metabolic syndrome. Multiple environmental factors modify this genetic predisposition and include physical inactivity, advancing age, cigarette smoking, and endocrine dysfunction.[1,5,14]

Although composite criteria are established to define the metabolic syndrome, it is the underlying constellation of individual conditions of metabolic origin that contribute to the increased risk for CVD. These include atherogenic dyslipidemia (small LDL particles, elevated TG and apolipoprotein B, low HDL cholesterol concentrations), elevated BP, elevated plasma glucose, a prothrombotic state identified by increases in fibrinogen and factor VIII, antifibrinolytics associated with plasminogen activator inhibitor-1, and a proinflammatory state associated by markers such as C-reactive protein.[14] Both obesity and insulin resistance are associated with inflammation.[15] A growing list of novel transcription factors, cytokines, and inflammatory mediators are associated with metabolic syndrome.[16] While these are not used in diagnosis and management, they are important in understanding the underlying pathophysiology of the metabolic syndrome. Interventions, including a Mediterranean diet, exercise, and the use of some medications used to modify traditional CVD risks such as statins, ACE inhibitors, and angiotensin receptor antagonists, have been shown to alter markers of inflammation in the metabolic syndrome.[16]

There is debate on whether the atherosclerotic risk imparted by the metabolic syndrome is more than the "sum of its parts."[14,17] Several longitudinal studies have established an increased multiplicative risk of developing both diabetes and CVD in subjects with metabolic syndrome.[14] Adults followed in the Framingham cohort without CVD or type 2 diabetes at baseline had a prevalence of metabolic syndrome of 26.8% in men and 16.6% in women. Over an 8-year period, the metabolic syndrome increased the relative risk for CVD in men and type 2 diabetes in men and women. The metabolic syndrome accounted for up to one-third of CVD in men and half of new type 2 DM diagnoses in this cohort.[7]

CLINICAL MANAGEMENT

The management of the metabolic syndrome depends on thorough identification of risk and appropriate stratification for intensive treatment of each individual CVD risk factor. Secondary goals include delaying or preventing the development of type 2 diabetes. In view of the complexities of multiple medications with possible side effects and interactions, multiple dosing regimens, adherence to therapy, access to medications prescribed, and challenging lifestyle modifications, a global approach to all risk factors is crucial in reaching all goals for treatment.

The ultimate choice and intensity of treatment depends on the calculated global risk of the patient. Diabetics and patients with established CVD should receive more intensive therapy based on established guidelines. Using Framingham Heart Study data, the 10-year risk for CHD for non-diabetics with the metabolic syndrome depends more on the individual risk factors. For these individuals, without type 2 diabetes and/or established CVD, the absolute 10-year Framingham risk score is a better predictor of cardiovascular endpoint risk.[14]

Lifestyle modifications targeted at improving the individual components of metabolic syndrome remain the first-line intervention to prevent metabolic syndrome and lower the risk for CVD and type 2 diabetes.[5] Weight loss, increased physical activity, an antiatherogenic diet, and smoking cessation are integral and powerful tools when closely followed by patients. Such lifestyle modifications are too often overlooked or ignored by medical personnel, but are essential for a long-term benefit by decreasing all risk factors simultaneously. Recently, the AHA guidelines have be modified so that they are applicable to patients with traditional risks for CVD (hypertension, hyperlipidemia, hyperglycemia) and metabolic syndrome with a focus on CVD prevention.[18] The AHA recommended lifestyle interventions are summarized in Table 26-2.

The AHA recommends maintaining a healthy body weight defined by a body mass index between 18.5 and 24.9 kg/m^2. This may be achieved with attention to caloric intake and expenditure. An overall healthy diet rich in fruits, vegetables, whole grains, low-fat dairy products, poultry, lean meats, and oily fish twice weekly applies to all groups including patients with metabolic syndrome, CVD or diabetes and in those aiming for primary prevention of CVD. Limited intake of saturated fats, trans-fats, and cholesterol is recommended. Low sodium intake and avoidance of alcohol are important.[18]

Regular physical activity improves all components of the metabolic syndrome.

Daily moderate-intensity activity such as brisk walking for at least 30 minutes is the standard recommendation but increased intensity increases the beneficial effects.[19]

Table 26-2. Lifestyle Goals for CVD Risk Reduction

Consume a healthy diet daily
High in fruits, vegetables, and whole grains
Low-fat dairy products
Low cholesterol, low saturated and trans-fats
Low sodium
Avoidance of alcohol
Aim for a healthy body weight
Body mass index of 18.5–24.9 kg/m^2
Aim for a desirable lipid profile
LDL <100 mg/dL
HDL >40 mg/dL in men and >50 mg/dL in women
TG <150 mg/dL
Aim of an optimal BP
BP <120/80 mm Hg
Aim for a normal glucose
Fasting glucose ≤100 mg/dL
Perform regular physical activity
Avoid exposure to tobacco products

Adapted from: American Heart Association Diet and Lifestyle Recommendations, Revision 2006.

Currently, no specific pharmacotherapeutic regimen is recommended to the treat the metabolic syndrome other by than medications approved for use in individual components. These include lipid lowering drugs, antidiabetic agents, antihypertensives, weight loss agents, and antiplatelet therapy. Therapeutic targets for each individual entity are not modified by the additional diagnosis of the metabolic syndrome. More detailed discussions are included in other chapters of this text.

Dyslipidemic targets should follow NCEP guidelines, targeting LDL as the primary goal based on Framingham risk, with non-HDL cholesterol and HDL cholesterol as secondary targets. Mainstays of therapy are currently the statins, bile acid sequestrants, and ezetimibe. Other medications targeting the secondary goals noted above and severe hypertriglyceridemia include nicotinic acid and the fibrates.[1]

Impaired glucose tolerance, resulting in elevated fasting glucose and overt type 2 diabetes, should be appropriately diagnosed according to the current American Diabetic Association guidelines.[20] Currently, no medications are recommended to treat elevated fasting glucose levels outside of type 2 diabetes. Once diabetes develops, multiple medications may be needed to modify endogenous insulin secretion and effectiveness, decrease gluconeogenesis, and increase insulin sensitivity in peripheral tissues.[20] Lifestyle modifications are again very important and are the foundation of appropriate care of the patient with impaired glucose tolerance or type 2 diabetes.

Elevated BP should be assessed with a reliable device according to the seventh Report of the Joint National Commission (JNC7).[21] Lifestyle modifications should be recommended for all individuals regardless of the level of BP. Medications should be considered for individuals whose BP is ≥140/90 mm Hg. For individuals with diabetes or chronic renal disease, the target BP should be <130/80 mm Hg, utilizing both lifestyle changes and medications. Drug choice should be driven by JNC7 recommendations and appropriate compelling indications for particular drug classes.[21]

For those individuals at higher risk for CVD (10-year risk for coronary heart disease ≥10%, type 2 diabetes, or current diagnosis of CVD), low-dose aspirin therapy should be initiated. Clopidogrel should be considered in situations precluding the use of aspirin.

CONCLUSION

The associated risk factors comprising the metabolic syndrome represent a challenging dilemma of comprehensive CVD risk assessment and treatment. As the prevalence of obesity and physical inactivity increase in developing societies, the metabolic syndrome will continue to present global healthcare challenges. Healthcare providers have a critical role in preventing the development of metabolic syndrome in patients. Attention to and aggressive management of all risk factors with lifestyle modifications and medication therapy will ensure primary and secondary prevention of atherogenic endpoints. Further understanding of the pathophysiologic changes leading to the disorder may help to identify various pharmacologic targets aimed at prevention and treatment of metabolic syndrome, CVD, and type 2 diabetes.

EVIDENCE-BASED SUMMARY

- Metabolic syndrome is a cluster of risk factors that are associated in increased risk for CVD and type 2 diabetes.
- The prevalence of metabolic syndrome is increasing worldwide as obesity and physical inactivity increase.
- Metabolic syndrome is associated with insulin resistance and proinflammatory, prothrombotic, and atherogenic markers.
- Lifestyle intervention with diet, exercise, and weight reduction are the fundamental to prevention and treatment of metabolic syndrome, CVD, and type 2 diabetes.
- Pharmacotherapy in metabolic syndrome is used to target individual components of the syndrome including dyslipidemia, hyperglycemia, and hypertension.

REFERENCES

1. Expert Panel on Detection, Evaluation, and Treatment of High Blood Cholesterol in Adults (Adult Treatment Panel III) final report. Executive Summary of the Third Report of the National Cholesterol Education Program (NCEP) *JAMA*. 2001;285:2486.
2. Reaven GM. Banting lecture 1988. Role of insulin resistance in human disease. *Diabetes*. 1988;37:1595.
3. Kahn R. Metabolic syndrome: Is it a syndrome? Does it matter? *Circulation*. 2007;115:1806.
4. Alberti KG, Zimmet PZ. Definition, diagnosis and classification of diabetes mellitus and its complications. Part 1: Diagnosis and classification of diabetes mellitus provision report of a WHO consultation. *Diabet Med*. 1998;15:539.
5. Grundy SM, Cleeman JI, Daniels SR, et al. Diagnosis and management of the metabolic syndrome. An American Heart Association/National Heart, Lung, and Blood Institute Scientific Statement. *Circulation*. 2005;112:2735.
6. Alberti KG, Simmet P, Shaw J. The metabolic syndrome-a new worldwide definition. *Lancet*. 2005;366:1059.

7. Wilson PW, D'Agostino RB, Parise H, et al. Metabolic syndrome as a precursor of cardiovascular disease and type 2 diabetes mellitus. *Circulation.* 2005;112:3006.

8. Ford ES, Giles WH, Dietz WH. Prevalence of the metabolic syndrome among US adults: Findings from the third National Health and Nutrition Examination Survey. *JAMA.* 2002;287:356.

9. Ford ES, Giles WH, Mokdad AH. Increasing prevalence of the metabolic syndrome among U.S. adults. *Diabetes Care.* 2004;27:2444.

10. Meigs JB. The metabolic syndrome (insulin resistance syndrome or syndrome X). www.uptodate.com. Accessed June 30, 2007.

11. Goodman E, Daniels SR, Meigs JB, et al. Instability in the diagnosis of metabolic syndrome in adolescents. *Circulation.* 2007;115:2316.

12. Weiss R, Dziura J, Burgert TS, et al. Obesity and the metabolic syndrome in children and adolescents. *N Eng J Med.* 2004;350:2362.

13. Cook S, Weitzman M, Auinger P, et al. Prevalence of a metabolic syndrome phenotype in adolescents: Findings form the third national health and nutrition examination survey, 1988–1994. *Arch Pediatr Adolesc Med.* 2003;157:821.

14. Grundy SM. Metabolic syndrome: Connecting and reconciling cardiovascular and diabetes worlds. *J Am Coll Cardiol.* 2006;47:1093.

15. Dandona P, Aljad A, Chaudhuri A, et al. Metabolic syndrome: A comprehensive perspective between obesity, diabetes, and inflammation. *Circulation.* 2005;111:1448.

16. Koh KK, Han SH, Quon MJ. Inflammatory markers and the metabolic syndrome; insights from therapeutic interventions. *J Am Coll Cardiol* 2005;46:1978.

17. Kahn R, Buse J, Ferrannini E, et al. The metabolic syndrome: Time for a critical appraisal joint statement from the American diabetes Association and the European Association for the study of diabetes. *Diabetes Care.* 2005;28:2289.

18. Lichtenstein AH, Appel LJ, Brands M, et al. Diet and lifestyle recommendations revision 2006: A scientific statement from the American Heart Association Nutrition Committee. *Circulation.* 2006;113:82.

19. Thompson PD, Buchner D, Pina IL, et al. Exercise and physical activity in the prevention and treatment of atherosclerotic cardiovascular disease: A Statement from the council on clinical cardiology (Subcommittee on Exercise, Rehabilitation, and Prevention and the Council on Nutrition, Physical Activity, and Metabolism (Subcommittee on Physical Activity). *Circulation.* 2003;107:3109.

20. Nathan DM, Buse JB, Davidson MB, et al. Management of hyperglycemia in type 2 diabetes: A consensus algorithm for the initiation and adjustment of therapy: A consensus from the American Diabetes Association and the European Association for the Study of Diabetes. *Diabetes Care.* 2006;29:1963.

21. Chobian AV, Bakris GL, Black HR, et al. The Seventh Report of the Joint National Committee on Prevention, Detection, Evaluation, and Treatment of High Blood Pressure. *JAMA.* 2003;289.2560.

Chapter 27

Thyroid Gland Disorders

Christina L. Barlow and Dana Dale

SEARCH STRATEGY

A comprehensive search of the medical literature was performed on Endocrinology texts, UpToDate®, and www.guidlelines.gov These resources were queried for general content. PubMed was accessed for specific references during January 2008.

THYROID GLAND DISORDERS

Disorders of the thyroid gland are a common problem encountered in a primary care setting. Normal thyroid function is essential to many cellular and metabolic processes which are important throughout the life cycle. Abnormalities of function may lead to a wide variety of nonspecific and subtle or overt signs and symptoms. Among the disorders that present to the primary care provider are hypothyroidism, hyperthyroidism, thyroid nodules, goiter, thyroid cancers, and even nonthyroidal illness. The routine screening for thyroid disease is not recommended by most consensus groups, thus the primary care provider must recognize the need for evaluation of thyroid function when appropriate.

PHYSIOLOGY

The thyroid is an endocrine gland controlled by a feedback loop involving the hypothalamus, pituitary gland, and the thyroid gland. The hypothalamus produces thyrotropin-releasing hormone (TRH) which stimulates the pituitary gland to produce thyroid-stimulating hormone (TSH). TSH controls the formation and release of the hormones serum thyroxine (T_4) and serum triiodothyronine (T_3). All of T_4 is made in the thyroid gland while only 20% of T_3 is formed in the thyroid. Eighty percent of T_3 is formed by the deiodination of T_4 to T_3 in the peripheral tissue (predominately in the liver and kidneys) in the presence of 5′ monodeiodinase. Serum T_3 and T_4 regulate the release or suppression of the TRH and TSH from hypothalamus and pituitary, respectively, in a feedback loop.[1]

Nearly all of T_3 and T_4 is protein-bound by thyroxine-binding protein or albumin. The unbound portion of thyroid hormone is referred to as free T_4 and free T_3 which are the physiologically active forms of hormone. Protein binding is important in regulation of uptake by tissues and for providing a reserve of hormone.[1]

Testing for thyroid abnormalities varies depending on the clinical situation but generally begins with the evaluation of the TSH and free T_4 levels. Other tests of thyroid function may be necessary. The measurement of Total T_4 and Total T_3 is seldom indicated. Free T_4 and free T_3 will be referred to as T_4 and T_3 throughout this text.

HYPOTHYROIDISM

Hypothyroidism is the manifestation of a deficiency of thyroid hormones. The symptoms may vary from severe as seen with myxedema coma to absent as with subclinical hypothyroidism.

CLASSIFICATION/CAUSES

There are many different causes of hypothyroidism including autoimmune disorders, iatrogenic causes, and secondary to other disease processes. Table 27-1 illustrates many of the conditions that may cause hypothyroidism.[1]

Table 27-1. Conditions Resulting in Hypothyroidism

Failure of the thyroid gland
Thyroidectomy
Radioactive iodine treatment
External beam radiation therapy
Immune-mediated hypothyroidism
Chronic autoimmune thyroiditis
Transient subacute lymphocytic thyroiditis
Postpartum thyroiditis
Drugs
Lithium
Amiodarone
Interferon alfa
Interleukin-2
Stavudine
Aminoglutethimide
Betaroxine
Infiltrative diseases
Fibrous thyroiditis
Hemochromatosis
Scleroderma
Leukemia
Cystinosis
Amyloid
Sarcoid
Infections
Hypothalamic or pituitary disease

Primary hypothyroidism accounts for approximately 99% of cases of hypothyroidism. In the United States, overt hypothyroidism occurs in 0.8% to 1% of the population.[2] Worldwide iodine deficiency is the most common cause; however, in regions that are iodine sufficient, chronic autoimmune (Hashimoto's) thyroiditis is the most common form of primary hypothyroidism. Infiltrative diseases such as amyloidosis, hemochromatosis, or fibrous thyroiditis are rare forms of primary thyroid failure. Hypothyroidism can be transient if caused by subacute lymphocytic thyroiditis or in postpartum thyroiditis.[2]

Iatrogenic causes of hypothyroidism include thyroidectomy, radioactive iodine treatment for Graves' disease, and external radiation therapy. The most common drugs that can cause hypothyroidism are lithium and amiodarone.[2]

Central hypothyroidism is caused by hypothalamic or pituitary disease. These patients generally have other hormonal deficiencies or a pituitary mass causing compressive symptoms such as visual field deficits or headaches.[1]

Congenital hypothyroidism occurs in newborns at a rate of one in 3000 to 4000 and is the leading cause of hypothyroidism in iodine-deficient regions of the world.[3] It can be transient, but it is usually permanent and may result in severe neurological consequences such as mental retardation, if untreated. Newborn screening programs are in place in developed countries. After the diagnosis is confirmed, immediate therapy with T_4 is essential to prevent impaired cognitive development.[3]

CLINICAL MANIFESTATIONS OF HYPOTHYROIDISM

Generally, the onset of hypothyroid symptoms is gradual. Some of the most common symptoms early on are fatigue, weakness, dry skin, menorrhagia, cold intolerance, or constipation. A careful review of systems may lead to early diagnosis of hypothyroidism.[4] Table 27-2 summarizes many of the symptoms related to hypothyroidism.

Skin/Hair
Patients may complain of dry, thickened, or scaly skin which may appear yellow in color. Hair loss and thinning of the outer-third of eyebrows are common. The extremities may be cool and peripheral edema (a condition referred to as myxedema) is common.

Cardiopulmonary
Hypothyroidism is considered in the evaluation of a patient with diastolic hypertension or resistant hypertension and is considered a form of secondary hypertension. Bradycardia may occur. In severe cases, pericardial effusions or pleural effusions may occur.

Table 27-2. Signs and Symptoms of Hypothyroidism

Weakness
Fatigue
Forgetfulness
Slow speech
Cold intolerance
Weight gain
Menstrual irregularities
Constipation
Decreased appetite
Hair loss
Cool skin
Dry or yellow skin
Periorbital puffiness
Bradycardia
Pericardial or pleural effusion
Ascites
Hoarseness
Diastolic hypertension
Sleep apnea
Paresthesias
Muscle cramps
Delayed tendon reflexes
Carpel tunnel syndrome
Dupuytren's contracture

Hypothyroidism should be considered in patients with hypercholesterolemia.

Patients may be hoarse because of vocal cord edema and may have enlargement of the tongue. Obstructive sleep apnea may result from sequelae of hypothyroidism.

Gastrointestinal

Hypothyroidism may contribute to weight gain although it does not cause morbid obesity. Constipation is a common complaint. In patients with unexplained ascites evaluation of thyroid function should take place.

Musculoskeletal and Neurologic

Patients may complain of muscle cramps, or muscle weakness. Carpal tunnel syndrome and Dupuytren's contracture may be found.[5] Severe cases may result in ataxia or there may be gradual development of paresthesias or hearing loss. On examination, there may be delayed relaxation phase of deep tendon reflexes.

Gynecologic

Menstrual irregularities such as menorrhagia or amenorrhea can occur. Thyroid function is one component of an infertility evaluation.

Psychiatric

Patients may suffer from depression, memory loss, or slow speech.

Laboratory Manifestations

Hypothyroidism should be considered when unexplained lab tests are found (Table 27-3).

A normochromic, normocytic anemia or pernicious anemia caused by vitamin B_{12} malabsorption may result from hypothyroid disease. Elevated creatinine phosphokinase levels can be seen on laboratory testing. Hyperlipidemia may occur with even mild hypothyroidism. Unexplained hyponatremia should prompt an evaluation for thyroid disease.

DIAGNOSIS

Serum TSH is the most sensitive test for thyroid dysfunction and the first indication of hypothyroidism. In

Table 27-3. Lab Abnormalities Associated with Hypothyroidism

Increased creatinine
Hyponatremia
Pernicious anemia
Normochromic normocytic anemia
Elevated transaminases
Elevated cholesterol
Elevated creatinine kinase

mild cases, there is only a slight elevation of serum TSH level. A repeat TSH in 2 to 3 months should be considered. Anti-TPO antibody is associated with autoimmune hypothyroidism. In patients with an elevated TSH but normal T_4; the titer of anti-TPO is predictive of progression to thyroid failure.[2] As the condition progresses serum T_4 declines, resulting in a compensatory rise in TSH. Clinical hypothyroidism is characterized by a very high TSH level with low T_4 and a low serum T_3. Diagnosis of hypothyroidism is made with an elevated TSH level and a low free T_4.[2]

Patients with central hypothyroidism, caused by hypothalamic or pituitary disease, have a low serum T_4 and low or normal serum TSH concentration. These patients should be referred to an endocrinologist for evaluation of other hormonal deficiencies and the presence of pituitary adenomas.[2]

TREATMENT

Treatment of hypothyroidism involves supplement with levothyroxine (T_4) at an average replacement dose of 1.6 mcg/kg per day.[2] Synthetic T_4 has a half-life of 7 days, so the serum TSH should be evaluated a minimum of 6 weeks after starting the replacement dose.[2] Thyroid supplement is best taken without food to increase bioavailability and avoid binding to other compounds that may be taken at the same time. If a dose is missed, it can be taken with the next day's dose. Patients should be advised to use the same brand or a specific generic formulation of levothyroxine, as different products may not be bioequivalent. Since T_4 has a narrow therapeutic range, the TSH should be measured at a minimum of 6 weeks after a change in thyroid products. Nonadherence to therapy should be considered when the TSH is mildly elevated and the free T_4 is normal.

TSH levels should be maintained within the normal range (~1.0 uM/L) in patients with primary hypothyroidism. Levels below the normal range indicate over replacement of T_4. Long term a supratherapeutic dose of T_4 can increase bone turnover and can also lead to cardiac arrhythmias. Patients on long-term therapy should have TSH level monitored annually.[2]

Patients with secondary hypothyroidism caused by thyroidectomy for thyroid carcinoma should be treated with T_4; the goal in these patients is to suppress the TSH below the normal range. For more detailed information on this topic, see the section on thyroid carcinoma. Patients with central hypothyroidism should be treated to a target serum free-T_4 in the upper-half of the normal range.[4]

In the elderly patients or those with coronary artery disease, therapy should be started with a low dose of levothyroxine (25 mcg) and increased slowly.[2,4] In pregnancy the levothyroxine requirement increases.[6] On confirmation of pregnancy, the levothyroxine dose should be increased by approximately 30%. This can be accomplished by taking two extra tablets per week. Follow-up measurement of the TSH should occur after 6 weeks on the increased dose.[6] By 16 to 20 weeks of gestation, increased levothyroxine doses are not required in most women.[6,7] Postpartum requirements return to the prepregnancy requirement.

Decreased requirements occur with aging. Malabsorption syndromes may also affect thyroid hormone requirements. If patients are allergic to the dye in a preparation of levothyroxine, a white tablet free from dye should be used.[4]

Levothyroxine is the usual hormone replacement although there are exceptions. Treatment with T_3 is recommended as temporary therapy in those with thyroid carcinoma who are to have radioiodine imaging and treatment. Dessicated thyroid can also be used for replacement but it might result in varying potency.[4]

Recent trials have not supported the use of levothyroxine plus T_3 for primary hypothyroidism. One trial did not show improvement in body weight, serum lipid levels, symptoms, or measures of cognitive performance when comparing levothyroxine alone to combination therapy.[8] Patients with depressive symptoms did not find any improvement on treatment with T_3.[9]

DRUG INTERACTIONS

Drugs may affect requirements of levothyroxine (see Table 27-4).[10] Calcium carbonate reduces T_4 absorption and increases serum thyrotropin levels when taken with the levothyroxine.[11] Cholestyramine, colestipol, ferrous sulfate, aluminum hydroxide, and sucralfate can decrease the absorption of levothyroxine, therefore, patients should be advised to take these medications several hours apart. Patients with impaired acid secretion caused by *Helicobacter pylori*-related gastritis, atrophic gastritis, or therapy with proton pump inhibitors may require an increased dose of thyroxine.[12] Other drugs such as phenobarbital, rifampin, phenytoin, and carbamazepine increase T_4 requirement by increasing hepatic metabolism.[10]

SUBCLINICAL HYPOTHYROIDISM

Subclinical hypothyroidism is diagnosed when the TSH is slightly elevated in the 5 to 10 mU/L range, the free thyroxine (T_4) is normal, and the patient is asymptomatic or may have vague complaints. The etiologies include early chronic autoimmune thyroiditis, history of ablative therapy for Graves' disease, history of radiation therapy, and inadequate T_4 replacement. Some of

Table 27-4. Drugs Causing Increased Levothyroxine Requirements

Aluminum containing antacids
Bile acid resins
Ferrous sulfate
Calcium supplements
Fiber supplements
Sucralfate (Carafate)
Rifampin
Carbamazepine (Tegretol)
Estrogens
Raloxifene (Evista)
Phenytoin (Dilantin)
Phenobarbital
Amiodarone (Cordarone, Pacerone)
Omeprazole
Propranolol (Inderal)
Glucocorticoids

these patients develop overt hypothyroidism. The risk of progression is higher in those with elevated antibodies to TPO and in those given radioiodine therapy or external radiation to the neck.[4]

Mortality and morbidity trials of patients treated for subclinical hypothyroidism have not been conducted but there may be benefit of treatment in these patients. A double-blind controlled trial in patients with subclinical hypothyroidism showed that physiological L-thyroxine replacement reduced total cholesterol and LDL by 3.8 % and improved clinical symptoms of hypothyroidism.[13] In another study, patients with increased baseline Lp(a) levels who were treated for subclinical hypothyroidism had a reduction in Lp(a) concentrations.[14] In women with subclinical hypothyroidism, replacement T_4 reduced LDL-C and Lp(a).[15] Treatment of subclinical hypothyroidism improves endothelial function.[16] The Tromso study concluded that there is an association between total cholesterol and LDL levels and the serum TSH levels. Treatment with thyroxine reduced those lipid levels.[17]

Guidelines have been issued regarding the evaluation and management of subclinical hypothyroidism.[18] Patients with TSH >10 mIU/L should be treated. The benefit of treating patients with serum TSH between 4.5 to 10 mIU/L is less clear. Treatment should be considered for symptoms of hypothyroidism or to those patients with positive anti-TPO titers, elevated cholesterol, or goiter. There are no recommendations regarding the routine screening for anti-TPO antibodies in patients with subclinical hypothyroidism. TSH levels should be evaluated every 6 to 12 months. TSH should be reduced to the normal range in those who are treated. The risk of treatment is the development of subclinical hyperthyroidism.[18]

MYXEDEMA COMA—SEVERE HYPOTHYROIDISM

Patients with this rare condition have a high mortality rate and should be treated aggressively. Myxedema coma may occur in patients with preexisting hypothyroidism or may even be the initial presentation. Myxedema coma may be associated with hypothermia, trauma, burns, surgery, sepsis, and severe infections.[19] Patients present with severe symptoms including decreased mental status, hypothermia, hypotension, hypoglycemia, bradycardia, hyponatremia, and decreased respirations. Patients suspected of having this should begin treatment immediately and not wait on confirmatory labs. Broad spectrum antibiotics are also recommended until infection has been ruled out.[20] Patients should also be evaluated for adrenal insufficiency which may coexist in patient with thyroid disease. Until adrenal insufficiency is ruled out, stress doses of hydrocortisone 100 mg IV every 8 hours should be given.[19]

There are no clinical trials regarding treatment of myxedema coma since it is so rare, although several treatment regimens have been recommended. One regimen is an initial loading dose of 200 to 500 mcg T_4 intravenously, followed by daily intravenous (IV) doses of 50 to 100 mcg until the patient is able to take T_4 orally.[19,20] Others prefer T_3 10 to 25 mcg IV every 8 hours.[18] A third option is combination therapy with T_3/T_4, with a T_4 loading dose of 4 mcg/kg IV daily and T_3 10 mcg IV every 8 hours.[18]

SCREENING FOR HYPOTHYROIDISM

Screening for thyroid disease with laboratory measures of various hormones in asymptomatic individuals is not recommended by the U.S. Preventive Services Task Force.[21] The American Thyroid Association recommends screening for hypothyroidism in the following populations: women more than 60 years of age, history of thyroid disease, autoimmune disease, unexplained depression, cognitive dysfunction, or hypercholesterolemia.[22] The U.S. Preventive Services Task Force recommends that patients with Down's syndrome be screened. These patients are at high risk for hypothyroidism and the symptoms of hypothyroidism may be difficult to appreciate.[21] Subclinical hypothyroidism is associated with poor obstetric outcomes and with poor cognitive development in the affected children. It is not, however, recommended to screen women of childbearing potential or who become pregnant. If pregnant patients are at risk for or have a prior history of thyroid disease, a TSH should be measured.[22]

HYPERTHYROIDISM

Thyrotoxicosis is the physiological and biochemical manifestations of excessive amounts of thyroid hormones, which may be secondary to hyperactivity of the thyroid gland or excessive exogenous hormone. Hyperthyroidism occurs when excessive amounts of thyroid hormones result from excessive production or release from the thyroid gland. The clinical manifestations of hyperthyroidism depend on the severity and duration of the abnormality, age of the patient, and susceptibility.[4]

CLASSIFICATION/CAUSES

Graves' disease is the most common cause of hyperthyroidism. Graves' disease is an autoimmune disease caused by the production of antibodies against the TSH receptor site which may cause stimulation of the gland. Graves' disease usually has one or more of the following: goiter, exophthalmos, dermopathy, or thyrotoxicosis.[4,22] Other causes of hyperthyroidism include toxic adenoma and toxic multinodular goiter which results from focal or diffuse hyperplasia of thyroid cells whose function is independent of regulation by TSH.[4]

Iodine-induced hyperthyroidism may occur after an iodine load is given in the forms of IV contrast used for CT or angiography or in the form of medications containing iodine such as amiodarone. This usually occurs in patients with a multinodular goiter and may be self-limiting after the iodine is stopped. Iatrogenic hyperthyroidism may result if a patient is taking excessive amounts of thyroid hormone which should be treated by decreasing the dose of the medication.[22]

The TSH receptor may be stimulated by high levels of hCG, thus hyperthyroidism may occur in patients with a hydatidiform mole or choriocarcinoma.[22]

Subacute thyroiditis is an acute inflammatory disorder of the thyroid gland which may be painful, and is usually secondary to a viral process. This initial hyperthyroid phase of subacute thyroiditis is usually followed by a hypothyroid phase before recovery occurs. Painless thyroiditis usually occurs in the postpartum period. As in subacute thyroiditis, there may be an initial hyperthyroid phase, followed by a hypothyroid phase and normal thyroid function. Other causes of hyperthyroidism may be secondary to a TSH-producing pituitary adenoma or struma ovarii in which functioning thyroid tissue is present in an ovarian neoplasm.[4,22]

CLINICAL MANIFESTATIONS

The classic symptoms of hyperthyroidism typically occur in younger patients. Patients more than 60 years of age may present with only weight loss or cardiac signs such as atrial fibrillation and congestive heart failure. The classic manifestations of hyperthyroidism are anxiety, weight loss despite increased appetite, palpitations, tachycardia, irritability, heat intolerance, tremor, and increased frequency of bowel movements. Symptoms that may be seen in Graves' disease, but not in the other causes of hyperthyroidism, include ophthalmopathy (proptosis, impaired eye muscle function, and periorbital edema), goiter, and dermopathy (thickening of the skin especially over the shins).[23]

Eyes

Eye findings related to hyperthyroidism include exophthalmos, as seen in Graves' disease. The increased sympathetic activity in patients with hyperthyroidism gives the appearance of a stare and lid lag.

Skin

Skin findings include warmth secondary to increased blood flow, increased sweating, and onycholysis (separation of the fingernails from the nail beds). The patient may also complain of itching. In Graves' disease only, thyroid dermopathy may be seen.

Cardiovascular

In hyperthyroidism, patients may have increased cardiac output, heart rate, and a widened pulse pressure. Atrial fibrillation occurs in up to 10% to 20% of patients with hyperthyroidism. In severe hyperthyroidism, congestive heart failure may occur.

Skeletal and Neuromuscular System

Since thyroid hormone increases bone resorption, long-term untreated hyperthyroidism is associated with osteoporosis and increased risk of fractures. Tremor is common in hyperthyroidism. One may also find muscle weakness that may be so profound that the patients are unable to stand from a seated position.

Gastrointestinal

Patients may have increased appetite with associated weight loss, although occasionally, a patient may have weight gain secondary to the increased appetite. Many patients will report diarrhea and hyperactive bowel sounds.

Geriatric

Geriatric patients may have relatively few signs and symptoms and may even appear depressed; this manifestation is called apathetic hyperthyroidism.[22]

DIAGNOSIS

The findings of an elevated T_4 with a suppressed TSH constitutes the diagnosis of hyperthyroidism. If the TSH is suppressed but the T_4 is normal, check a T_3 level to rule out T_3 thyrotoxicosis as the cause of the hyperthyroidism. Some asymptomatic patients have only a low TSH con-

centration with normal T_4 and T_3 levels, indicative of subclinical hyperthyroidism. If the T_4 and T_3 are high but the TSH is normal or high rather than the expected suppressed level, the diagnosis of a pituitary mass or a TSH-secreting adenoma should be considered.[22]

In cases where the diagnosis of hyperthyroidism is confirmed (low TSH, elevated T_4), a 24-hour radioiodine uptake and scan are performed to determine if the hyperthyroidism is secondary to Graves' disease or other causes (see Table 27-5). Since the treatment of hyperthyroidism differs depending on the cause of the hyperthyroidism, the etiology must be found prior to treatment. Increased radioiodine uptake is secondary to increased synthesis of thyroid hormone, but low uptake is secondary to damage of the thyroid with release of preformed hormone rather than increased synthesis of hormone.[4,22]

TREATMENT

Once the etiology of the hyperthyroidism is determined, the proper treatment must be decided. In patients with low radioiodine uptake determined to be subacute thyroiditis, treatment of symptoms is started with such medications as β-blockers for tachycardia and nonsteroidal antiinflamatory drugs if needed. Thionamides (methimazole and propylthiouracil [PTU]) are not used since the hyperthyroidism of thyroiditis is secondary to the release of preformed hormones rather than new hormone synthesis.[4]

In patients with Graves' disease, the goals of therapy include decreasing new thyroid hormone formation and resolution of the symptoms. Therapy to decrease new thyroid hormone formation includes radioactive iodine (treatment of choice in the United States), thionamides, and surgery (rarely used as first line).[4]

Table 27-5. Radioactive Iodine Uptake in Thyroid Disease

High uptake
  Graves' disease
  Toxic multinodular goiter
  Toxic adenoma
  Hashitoxicosis
  TSH-secreting adenoma
  Human chorionic gonadotropin mediated (hydatidiform mole, choriocarcinoma)
  Amiodarone-induced hyperthyroidism (nonthyroiditis)
Low uptake
  Subacute thyroiditis (painful thyroiditis)
  Painless thyroiditis (including postpartum thyroiditis)
  Amiodarone-induced thyroiditis
  Factitious ingestion of thyroid hormone
  Struma ovarii (functioning thyroid tissue in ovarian neoplasm)
  Metastatic thyroid cancer

β-Blockers

In hyperthyroidism, there is an increase in β-adrenergic tone causing such symptoms as anxiety, tachycardia, tremor, and palpitations. Therefore, if not contraindicated, a β-blocker should be initiated to help improve these symptoms. Examples of β-blockers that can be used include propranolol at higher doses, metoprolol, or the longer acting once-daily atenolol.[24]

Radioactive Iodine

Radioactive iodine ablation is the most common treatment for hyperthyroidism in the United States. Radioiodine is given orally at a dose which destroys thyroid tissue, and thus permanently cures hyperthroidism. Only approximately 5% of patients treated with radioactive iodine ablation require additional treatment with antithyroid medications after ablation. Most patients treated with radioiodine will develop hypothyroidism requiring replacement of thyroid hormone.

Radioactive iodine treatment is contraindicated in pregnancy. Hyperthyroid patients anticipating pregnancy should be encouraged to delay pregnancy for at least 6 months after ablation. There is a small chance of inducing radiation thyroiditis which is secondary to the release of stored hormone from the thyroid gland causing worsening of the hyperthyroid symptoms.[24] This can be dangerous in elderly patients and in patients with cardiac involvement. In these cases, consideration of pretreatment with antithyroid medications to render the patient euthyroid should be considered to decrease this risk. Pretreatment with methimazole is preferred over PTU since PTU may induce thyroid resistance to the effects of ^{131}I, which may last weeks to months. Methimazole may be stopped within 5 to 7 days of treatment with ^{131}I without affecting the radioiodine uptake.[24]

There continues to be controversy surrounding radioiodine therapy and worsening of Graves' ophthalmopathy. Some doctors will not use radioactive iodine in patients who already have moderate eye disease, but some physicians treat with radioactive iodine followed by 3 months of prednisone. In patients with moderate to severe eye disease, referral to an endocrinologist and ophthalmologist for specialized treatment should be considered.[4]

In patients with either a toxic adenoma or toxic multinodular goiter, the areas of autonomy cause suppression of the surrounding normal thyroid tissue. Radioactive iodine is taken up well within the autonomous areas while not affecting the surrounding areas leading to euthyroidism after ablation.[25]

Evaluation of patients who received radioactive iodine ablation initially requires a free T$_4$. The TSH may remain suppressed for months after the patient is euthyroid. A TSH should be ordered every 6 to 12 months to evaluate for the development of posttherapy hypothyroidism.

Thionamides

Antithyroid drugs (PTU and methimazole) are options for the treatment of hyperthyroidism. Treatment with these agents does not result in permanent hypothyroidism as with radioactive iodine ablation. Female patients more than 40 years of age with a small goiter, mild hyperthyroidism, and TSH-receptor antibody negative have high rates of hyperthyroid remission. In the United States, the frequency of remission is generally approximately 20% to 40%. Patients are usually given a 1 to 2 years' trial of antithyroid medication to determine if remission can be achieved. The side effects of the antithyroid medications include rash, GI upset, and arthralgias. The most dangerous side effect, agranulocytosis, occurs in 0.5% of patients.[24] Agranulocytosis with methimazole is dose-related and more likely when using doses greater than 40 mg/d. Rarely PTU causes hepatic necrosis and antineutrophil cytoplasmic antibody positive vasculitis. With methimazole, cholystatic jaundice is a possible side effect.[24]

Pretreatment with methimazole prior to radioactive iodine ablation is advised in the elderly patients or in patients with cardiovascular disease. Treatment is continued until the patient becomes euthyroid. Methimazole should be stopped 5 to 7 days before the radioactive iodine ablation is performed.[24]

In pregnancy, PTU and methimazole both cross the placenta. The patient should be given the smallest dose possible to control the hyperthyroidism. In pregnancy, PTU is preferred to methimazole because of the rare congenital side effect of aplasia cutis in the infant with methimazole.[2]

Surgery

Surgery for hyperthyroidism is seldom used in the United States. As one might expect, the disadvantages include permanent hypothyroidism, the risks of general anesthesia, hypoparathyroidism, and damage to the recurrent laryngeal nerve. Surgery should be considered in patients with very large goiters causing compressive symptoms, patients with a coexisting thyroid nodule, and pregnant women who have an allergy to antithyroid medication and are symptomatic of hyperthyroidism.[4]

THYROID STORM

When the effects of hyperthyroidism become life threatening, the term thyroid storm is used.[19] The crisis is usually found in patients with a previous history of Graves' disease that have not been completely treated, and is usually provoked by a severe illness or infection. The clinical signs include high fever which may reach 106°F, altered mental status, tachycardia, nausea/vomiting, and abdominal pain. If not diagnosed and treated properly, thyroid storm can be fatal. Treatment with antithyroid medication PTU is preferable to methimazole as PTU inhibits conversion of T_4 to T_3 when used in large doses. Iodine, in the form of SSKI (saturated solution of potassium iodide) or Lugol's solution, acutely blocks the release of hormone from the thyroid. PTU should be given 1 hour before the iodine to help in suppressing new thyroid hormone synthesis resulting from the dose of iodine. Steroids, dexamethasone or hydrocortisone, also help decrease the conversion of T_4 to T_3. If there are no contraindications, β-blockers should be used to help treat the cardiac manifestations. Propranolol is usually suggested as it also blocks T_4 to T_3 conversion. Initial improvement may be seen in 1 or 2 days with recovery taking a week. Steroids and iodine treatment are slowly stopped while long-term treatment plans are determined.[20]

SUBCLINICAL HYPERTHYROIDISM

Subclinical hyperthyroidism is defined as a suppressed TSH with a normal serum free T_4 and T_3.[4] Patients with subclinical hyperthyroidism may be asymptomatic, but there is an increased risk of developing atrial fibrillation and osteoporosis especially in elderly patients. Currently, there is an absence of complete evidence based guidelines recommending treatment. Strong consideration for treatment of subclinical hyperthyroidism should be made in elderly patients and patients with atrial fibrillation or osteopenia. Treatment should be considered in patients with goiters or high radioactive iodine uptake. Without the above mentioned risks, patients should have thyroid function tests every 6 months.[4]

EUTHYROID SICK SYNDROME

Euthyroid sick syndrome occurs when thyroid function is abnormal during nonthyroidal illness. There is usually a reduction in circulating T_3 with normal TSH and T_4 in mild illnesses with reduced T_4, T_3, and TSH in severe illnesses.

Drugs used during severe illness, such as dopamine, glucocorticoids, and dobutamine, can further cause TSH suppression which makes it more difficult to interpret the thyroid tests.[24] One should avoid checking thyroid function tests in ill patients unless the index of suspicion for myxedema or thyroid storm is high.

THYROID NODULES

Thyroid nodules are a common clinical problem evaluated in the primary care setting. In the United States, thyroid nodules have a prevalence of 4% to 7% and the incidence of cancer is 0.004%.[26] Nodules can be discovered by the patient, during a routine physical examination, or incidentally during radiologic procedures. The differential diagnosis of thyroid nodules includes thyroglossal duct cyst, pyramidal lobe of thyroid, delphian nodes, dermoid cyst, innominate artery, cervical lymphadenopathy, branchial cyst, carotid body tumor, thyroid lymphoma, subacute thyroiditis, and metastatic cancer.[27]

DIAGNOSTIC EVALUATION

Discovery of a thyroid nodule calls for a complete history and physical. A personal and family history may provide clues to the etiology of thyroid pathology. A history of head and neck irradiation, total body irradiation for bone marrow transplantation, or exposure to radiation increase the risk for thyroid carcinoma. A family history of thyroid carcinoma in a first degree relative is also predictive.[27] Findings that increase the suspicion of cancer include rapid growth, a very firm or hard nodule, fixation of the nodule, vocal cord paralysis, regional lymphadenopathy, and distant metastases.

The diagnostic approach begins by measurement of the serum TSH level. If TSH is low, then levels of free T_4 and free T_3 should be measured. Higher TSH levels with a higher serum anti-TPO antibody levels suggest Hashimoto's thyroiditis. However, a coexisting cancer can still be present. Radionuclide scanning is the next step in those with suppressed levels of TSH to evaluate functionality of the nodule. A functional nodule is nearly always benign. Nonfunctioning nodules have a 5% risk of being malignant.[26] Thyroid ultrasonography is recommended in patients with a solitary nodule discovered on physical examination, as additional nodules can be detected with ultrasound.[26] Diagnostic ultrasound should be done to evaluate the characteristics of the nodules. Sonographic appearance is better than nodule size for identifying nodules that are more likely to be malignant. Characteristics of malignant nodules include the presence of microcalcifications, hypoechogenicity of a solid nodule, and intranodular hypervascularity. If patients have more than two nodules larger than 1 to 1.5 cm, the nodules with suspicious sonographic appearance should be aspirated. CT scans are only recommended to evaluate substernal goiters.[26] Multi-slice CT is used when there is a suspicion of extracapsular extension.[28] In those with normal or high TSH levels, the next step is fine needle aspiration (FNA) biopsy with ultrasound guidance if needed. Ultrasound-guided FNA is recommended for thyroid nodules greater than 1.0 cm or those with suspicious ultrasound findings. Patients with multiple thyroid nodules are not at increased risk for malignancy compared to solitary nodules.[27]

The results of FNA can be categorized as benign, malignant, indeterminate, and nondiagnostic. For benign results, patients are followed clinically. For malignant cytologies, surgery is the next step. If the FNA results are nondiagnostic, repeat FNA with ultrasound guidance is recommended, if still nondiagnostic, surgery is recommended.[26] Indeterminate results can be managed with surgery or by performing radionuclide scanning if not performed previously. It is recommended to follow benign nodules clinically if palpable, and nonpalpabable nodules should be followed with serial ultrasound examinations 6 to 18 months after the initial FNA. If the nodule grows, it is recommended to repeat the FNA.[26]

THYROID CANCER

Thyroid cancer is uncommon. Radiation to the head and neck as a child increases the risk. There are familial forms of thyroid cancer. Also, metastases from other cancers can occur. There are four different types of thyroid cancer: papillary, follicular, anaplastic, and medullary. Papillary cancer is the most common and occurs more frequently in women. Recently there has been an increase in the number of cases with current estimates of 12 cases per 100,000.[1] Follicular cancer occurs more commonly in older patients and in women. Hurthle cell cancer is a variant of follicular and is more aggressive than other forms. Preoperative neck ultrasound should be performed to look for abnormal lymph nodes in the neck.[26]

The initial treatment of thyroid cancer is by near total or total thyroidectomy. Giving thyroxine after surgery for papillary and follicular cancer to suppress TSH and tumor growth, in addition to treating the hypothyroidism, is recommended. For high-risk patients, the TSH should be suppressed to below 0.1 mU/L. For low risk patients TSH can be maintained at lower limit of normal range. Radiation therapy is used for metastatic disease, adjunctive therapy, and recurrent disease. There should be regular follow-up of these patients after radiation.

Surveillance for metastatic disease requires additional testing. Serum thyroglobulin, a prohormone of T_4 and T_3, is made only by thyroid follicular cells. Thyroglobulin levels can be used to monitor for recurrences. There is a possibility of test interference by thyroglobulin antibodies which should be measured simultaneously by the lab.[26] TSH should be elevated to obtain the most reliable thyroglobulin assay which requires stopping levothyroxine therapy. Thyroglobulin, TSH levels, and thyroglobulin antibodies should be measured every 6 to 12 months after treatment of thyroid cancer. Thyroglobulin is the best tumor marker in those patients who have no thyroid tissue left. Thyroglobulin levels should be measured by the same lab as result of the variability of results.[26]

Recurrence of thyroid carcinoma may also be evaluated by administration of thyrogen, recombinant human TSH which stimulates any thyroid tissue, followed by thyroglobulin assay.[26] The American Thyroid Association recommends periodic chest X-rays in surveillance for metastatic disease.

Postoperative radioiodine remnant ablation is recommended for patients with stage III and stage IV disease, all patients younger than 45 and most patients older than 45 years with stage II, and in patients with high-risk features of nodal metastases. Ultrasound of the neck is recommended at 6 and 12 months then annually for 3 to 5 years depending on thyroglobulin status and the patient's risk for recurrence.[26]

Anaplastic carcinoma is highly malignant and can cause death from locally infiltrative disease. Medullary thyroid carcinoma can be sporadic or hereditary. Patients with medullary type should be evaluated for pheochromocytomas and hyperparathyroidism which may all coexist in the rare familial MEN (multiple endocrine neoplasia) syndrome. Lymphoma of the thyroid gland is uncommon and is managed with chemotherapy and radiotherapy.[1]

THYROIDITIS

Thyroiditis refers to inflammation of the thyroid gland. The classification of thyroiditis is based upon the presentation and etiology.[1] Painless thyroiditis can be caused by drugs such as interferon–alfa, interleukin-2, amiodarone, or lithium. It can occur in the postpartum period and can cause hyperthyroidism. It is similar to subacute painless lymphocytic thyroiditis which has a transient hyperthyroidism sometimes associated with subsequent hypothyroidism. The related hypothyroid state is also transient. Fibrous thyroiditis or Riedel's thyroiditis is a rare fibrosing disorder. It can be associated with fibrosclerosis in other organs.[29] Prednisone may be helpful or surgery may be needed to relieve compression. Chronic lymphocytic thyroiditis or Hashimoto's is very common in women and often leads to hypothyroidism. It is autoimmune in nature and high levels of thyroid antibodies can be found initially. Many present with a goiter and are euthyroid.[2] There is an increased incidence of lymphoma in Hashimoto's disease.

Painful thyroiditis can be caused by acute infections. Infectious thyroiditis is rare. More commonly, there is subacute painful thyroiditis. As compared with the other thyroid diseases, it is more common in women, and it tends to occur following viral infections. Erythrocyte sedimentation rates are increased, and T_4 levels can be elevated. The RAI uptake is markedly decreased.[2] This condition is generally a self-limiting disorder that requires only symptomatic treatment.

EVIDENCE-BASED SUMMARY

- Evaluation of thyroid hormones requires consideration of synthesis and release by the thyroid gland and peripheral conversion of T_4 to T_3
- The most sensitive test for thyroid function in serum TSH.
- Anti-TPO is predictive of autoimmune thyroid disease and progression to primary thyroid failure.
- Hashimoto's thyroiditis is the most common form of hypothyroidism in iodine sufficient regions
- Sufficient thyroid replacement with levothyroxine should achieve a goal TSH of 1 to 2 mU/L.
- Pregnant women with hypothyroidism require increased doses of levothyroxine during pregnancy.
- Radioactive iodine uptake is increased in Graves' disease but decrease in thyroiditis.
- Treatment for hyperthyroidism caused by Graves' disease, toxic adenoma, and toxic multinodular goiter includes radioiodine, antithyroid drugs, and rarely surgery.
- Thyroid nodule evaluation includes measures of TSH and T_4 and FNA.
- Myxedema coma and thyroid storm are life threatening conditions.

REFERENCES

1. Larsen PR, Kronenberg HM, Melmed S, Polonsky KS. *Williams Textbook of Endocrinology*. Philadelphia, PA: Saunders; 2003:457–490.
2. Roberts CG, Ladenson PW. Hypothyroidism. *Lancet*. 2004; 363:793.
3. Rose SR, American Academy of Pediatrics, Section on Endocrinology and Committee on Genetics, American Thyroid Association, Brown RS, Public Health Committee, Lawson Wilkins Pediatric Endocrine Society. Update of newborn screening and therapy for congenital hypothyroidism. *Pediatrics*. 2006;117:2290.
4. Baskin HJ, Cobin R, Duick D, et al. American Association of Clinical Endocrinologists Medical Guidelines for Clinical Practice for the evaluation and treatment of hyperthyroidism and hypothyroidism. *Endocr Pract*. 2002;8:457.
5. Cakir M, Samanci N, Balci N, Balci MK. Musculoskeletal manifestations in patients with thyroid disease. *Clin Endocrinol*. 2003;59:162.
6. Alexander E, Marqusee E, Lawrence J, et al. Timing and magnitude of increases in levothyroxine requirements during pregnancy in women with hypothyroidism. *N Engl J Med*. 2004;351:241.
7. Bach-Huynh TG, Jonklass J. Thyroid medications during pregnancy: *Ther Drug Monit*. 2006;28:431.
8. Clyde PW, Harrai AE, Getka EJ, et al. Combined levothyroxine plus liothyronine compared with levothyroxine alone in primary hypothyroidism: A randomized controlled trial. *JAMA*. 2003;290:2952.
9. Sawka AM, Gerstein HC, Marriott MJ, et al. Does a combination regimen of thyroxine (T4) and 3,5,3'-triiodothyronine improve depressive symptoms better than T4 alone in patients with hypothyroidism? Results of a double-blind, randomized, controlled trial. *J Clin Endocrinol Metab*. 2004;89:1486.
10. Surks M. Drug interactions with thyroid hormones. www.uptodate.com. Accessed January 15, 2006.
11. Singh N, Singh PN, Hershman JM. Effect of calcium carbonate on the absorption of levothyroxine. *JAMA*. 2000; 283:2822.
12. Centanni M, Gargano L, Canettieri G, et al. Thyroxine in goiter, Helicobacter pylori infection, and chronic gastritis. *N Engl J Med*. 2006;354:1787.
13. Meier C, Staub JJ, Roth CB, et al. TSH-controlled L-thyroxine therapy reduces cholesterol levels and clinical symptoms in subclinical hypothyroidism: A double blind, placebo-controlled trial (Basel Thyroid Study). *J Clin Endocrinol Metab*. 2001;86:4860.
14. Milionis HJ, Efstathiadou Z, Tselepis AD, et al. Lipoprotein (a) levels and apolipoprotein (a) isoform size in patients with subclinical hypothyroidism: Effect of treatment with levothyroxine. *Thyroid*. 2003;13:365.
15. Ganotakis ES, Mandalaki K, Tampakaki M, et al. Subclinical hypothyroidism and lipid abnormalities in older women attending a vascular disease prevention clinic: Effect of thyroid replacement therapy. *Angiology*. 2003; 54:569.
16. Taddei S, Caraccio N, Virdis A, et al. Impaired endothelium-dependent vasodilation in subclinical hypothyroidism: Beneficial effect of levothyroxine therapy. *J Clin Endocrinol Metab*. 2003;88:3731.
17. Iqbal A, Orde RJ, Figenschau Y. Serum lipid levels in relation to serum thyroid-stimulating hormone and the effect of thyroxin treatment on serum lipid levels in subjects with subclinical hypothyroidism: The Tromso Study. *J Intern Med*. 2006;260:53.
18. Subclinical thyroid disease. Scientific review and guidelines for diagnosis and management. Consensus Conference Panel on Subclinical Thyroid Disease—Independent

Expert Panel. January 14, 2004. www.guideline.gov. Accessed November 18, 2007.

19. Kearney T, Dang C. Review Diabetic and endocrine emergencies. *Postgrad Med J.* 2007;83:79.

20. Goldberg PA, Inzucchi SE. Critical issues in endocrinology. *Clin Chest Med.* 2003;24:583.

21. Screening for thyroid disease: Recommendation statement. *Ann Intern Med.* 2004;140:125.

22. Ladenson PW, Singer PA, Ain KB, et al. American Thyroid Association guidelines for detection of thyroid dysfunction. *Arch Intern Med.* 2000;160:1573.

23. Ross DS. Overview of the Clinical Manifestations of Hyperthyroidism in Adults. www.uptodate.com. Accessed March 16, 2007.

24. Singer PA. Treatment guidelines for patients with hyperthyroidism. *JAMA.* 1995;273.800.

25. Ross DS, Ridgway EC, Daniels GH. Successful treatment of solitary toxic thyroid nodules with relatively low-dose iodine-131, with low prevalence of hypothyroidism. *Ann Intern Med.* 1984;101:488.

26. Cooper DS, Doherty GM, Haugen BR, et al. The American Thyroid Association Guidelines Taskforce. Management guidelines for patients with thyroid nodules and differentiated thyroid cancer. *Thyroid.* 2006;16:109.

27. Hegedus L. The thyroid nodule. *N Engl J Med* 2004;351:1764.

28. Ishigaki S, Shimamoto K, Satake H, et al. Multi-slice CT of thyroid nodules: Comparison with ultrasonography. *Radiat Med.* 2004;22:346.

29. Tutuncu NB, Erbas T, Bayraktar M, Gedik O. Multifocal idiopathic fibrosclerosis manifesting with Riedel's thyroiditis. *Endocr Pract.* 2000;6:447.

Chapter 28

Contraception

C. Shannon Carroll, Sr. and Wendy S. Dean

SEARCH STRATEGY

A systematic search of medical literature pertaining to contraception was performed during November 2007. The search was limited to human subjects and journals in English language and included PubMed, UpToDate®, and the American College of Obstetricians and Gynecologists Practice Bulletin.

INTRODUCTION

Unintended pregnancy is a major public health problem worldwide. The overwhelming evidence that oral contraceptives are effective for reversible birth control has led to their widespread use in preventing pregnancy. Despite the availability of many contraceptive options, unplanned pregnancy rates remain high even in developed countries. The need for effective contraceptive methods with few side effects has led to a myriad of dose options and delivery systems.

Oral contraception pills (OCPs) were first introduced in the United States by the Food and Drug Administration (FDA) in the early 1960s for the control of irregular menses and infertility. Early preparations contained high estrogen and progestin concentrations, which were later found to result in adverse effects including weight gain, acne, and bloating and thus led to a high rate of discontinuation. The risk of cardiovascular events including stroke, myocardial infarction, and pulmonary embolism was not recognized until well after the approval of OCPs.[1] Safety concerns and the adverse side effects associated with high dose formulations have led to the development of OCP preparations with low doses of estrogen and progestin. Preparations containing more than 50 mcg of estrogen are no longer marketed in the United States as a result of the increased risk of thrombosis with higher doses. A variety of progestins, in a range of doses, have been developed in an effort to reduce side effects related to cardiovascular risks and also to reduce androgenic effects related to various progestins.[2] As a result of improved safety and efficacy, the age limit for OCP use, previously defined as less than 35 years for smokers and less than 40 years for nonsmokers, has recently been lifted by the FDA.[3] Currently, OCPs may be considered as an effective option for birth control until menopause in all healthy, nonsmoking women.

Primary care providers are often called upon to recommend contraceptive therapy for birth control. Appropriate use requires a basic knowledge of the pharmacology, indications, contraindications, efficacy, and the noncontraceptive benefits of OCPs. Making a choice of the many therapeutic options requires consideration of the specific progestins, dosing intervals, and delivery systems available for contraception.

PATIENT EVALUATION

A thorough medical, social, and family history of the patient is important prior to the recommendation of hormonal contraception. Absolute and relative contraindication to the use of OCPs should be identified. On review of systems, the physician may identify an opportunity to choose particular hormones that provide potential benefits in addition to contraception (Table 28-1).

A body mass index and accurate blood pressure measurement should be documented. Although pelvic and breast examinations are important, consensus groups agree that these procedures are not necessary prior to initiating therapy.[3]

Table 28-1. Potential Noncontraceptive Benefits with Oral Contraceptives

- Reduction in dysfunctional uterine bleeding
- Decrease in the amount of blood lost during menses
- Decrease in the incidence of anemia
- Alleviation of the symptomatology of benign cystic breast disease
- Decrease in the functional ovarian cysts
- Decrease in the incidence of pelvic inflammatory disease and ectopic pregnancies
- Reduction in acne
- Prevention of ovarian cancer
- Prevention of endometrial cancer

Table 28-2. Contraindications to Estrogen-containing Contraceptives

- History of thromboembolism or coagulation disorders
- History of vascular diseases including stroke, coronary heart disease, structural heart disease
- Diabetes associated with vascular disease
- Unexplained genital bleeding
- Smoker with age > 35 y
- Active liver disease or presence of benign or malignant liver tumor
- Known or suspected pregnancy
- History of breast cancer
- Classic migraine headaches
- Breast feeding

ADVERSE EFFECTS

Common side effects associated with OCPs include breakthrough bleeding, water retention, nausea, and breast tenderness. OCPs may cause an increase in blood pressure, mild insulin resistance, and lipid abnormalities.[3] Estrogens elevate serum triglycerides and high-density lipoprotein levels while decreasing low-density lipoprotein levels. On the other hand, progestins have an adverse effect on a patient's lipid panel by increasing low-density lipoprotein levels and decreasing high-density lipoprotein levels.[2]

CONTRAINDICATIONS

Patients with a history of thromboembolism or coagulation disorders should avoid OCPs. Patients with a history of vascular disease including stroke, coronary heart disease, and structural heart disease should avoid estrogen-containing OCPs. Oral contraceptive products may increase blood pressure, so these should be used with caution in patients with this cardiovascular risk factor. Patients with conditions increasing the risk for thrombosis, such as lupus, should avoid contraceptive hormonal therapy. Women older than 35 years of age who smoke should avoid combination OCPs as a result of the increased risk of cardiovascular disease.[2-4] Most estrogen and progestins are metabolized in the liver so should be avoided in patients with liver diseases. Patients with a history of breast cancer should also avoid estrogen-containing products because of the possibility of estrogen-dependent tumors. Pregnancy is a contraindication to OCP use.[3] Table 28-2 lists contraindications to the use of hormonal contraceptive.

DRUG INTERACTIONS

OCPs are metabolized by the liver so medications that interfere with hepatic enzyme activity may alter the effectiveness of OCPs.[2] Enzymatic inducers such as rifampin and phenytoin increase the metabolism of OCPs. Other medications that induce the metabolism of OCPs and potentially decrease their effectiveness include St. John's Wort and anticonvulsants including phenytoin, phenobarbital, carbamazepine, topiramate, and felbamate.[3,5] Fluconazole decreases the metabolism of estrogen, causing increased estrogen concentrations.[3] Any woman on a medication that interacts with the metabolism of OCPs should be instructed to use a backup contraceptive method.

Some women taking ethinyl estradiol along with certain antibiotics like tetracyclines or penicillin experience decreased concentrations of estrogen. As it is difficult to identify which patient may have a change in estrogen levels, it is currently recommended that all patients receiving an antibiotic use an alternative form of contraception.[3]

Women considering the use of hormonal contraception should be informed of the potential adverse effects, contraindications, and possible drug interactions in addition to the potential benefits.

MECHANISM OF ACTION/PHARMACOLOGY

Combination OCPs suppress pituitary gonadotropin secretion by interfering with the release of gonadotropin-releasing hormone from the hypothalamus thus preventing ovulation.[2,3] Estrogen suppresses follicle-stimulating hormone resulting in inhibition of the development of a dominant follicle. Estrogen also stabilizes the endometrium, thus controlling blood loss. Both estrogen and progestin together prevent a surge in the luteinizing hormone.[4] Progestins have several direct effects on the uterus that decrease the chances of pregnancy. First, progestins alter the endometrium by decreasing the production of glycogen and rendering the endometrium less suitable for implantation. Second, they thicken the cervical mucus making it more difficult for sperm penetration. Finally, they impair uterine and tubal motility preventing the transport of ova and sperm.[3]

All currently available OCPs contain either a synthetic estrogen and progestin or progestin alone. There are only two synthetic estrogens, ethinyl estradiol and mestranol, available in the United States.[4] Mestranol undergoes hepatic conversion to ethinyl estradiol. Mestranol may only be half as potent as ethinyl estradiol in some patients depending on the degree of conversion and is, therefore, not widely used.[4] Ethinyl estradiol is found in most available hormone contraceptives.[6,7]

Synthetic progestins derived from testosterone are combined to ethinyl estradiol to improve safety and efficacy, to reduce breakthrough bleeding that may occur with low-dose estrogen, and to improve tolerability. The various progestins differ in the estrogenic and androgen activity. The estrogenic activity results from metabolism of progestin to estrogenic substances. The androgenic activity is related to the structural similarity between progestins and testosterones. Progestin binds to the sex-hormone-binding globulin and affects free testosterone concentrations.[4] The degree of estrogenic and androgenic activity exhibited by a particular progestin is responsible for the associated side effects (Table 28-3).[8] Earlier forms of progestins include norethindrone, norethindrone acetate, levonorgestrel, and medroxyprogesterone. These have low progesterone-receptor selectivity and high-androgenic activity. While lower doses of these progestins may improve androgenic side effects, there may be poorer menstrual cycle control. The more selective, but less androgenic, progestins include norgestrel, ethynodiol diacetate, desogestrel, drospirenone, and norgestimate.

Table 28-3. Adverse Effects Associated with Hormonal Contraception Components

Component	Adverse Effects
High estrogen	Nausea, breast pain, increase in blood pressure, headache, bloating
Low estrogen	Early-cycle breakthrough bleeding, hypomenorrhea
High progestin	Fatigue, irritability, breast tenderness, headaches
Low progestin	Late-cycle breakthrough bleeding
High androgen	Weight gain, acne, oily skin, increased LDL cholesterol, decreased libido

LDL, low-density lipoprotein.

CLASSIFICATION OF ORAL HORMONE CONTRACEPTIVES

COMBINATION ESTROGEN/PROGESTIN

The most common combination, estrogen plus progestin, OCPs are available as the classic "21 days of active ingredient followed by a 7-day drug-free period." The last 7 tablets of the 28-day cycle are placebo tablets that are given to help improve patient compliance during the hormone-free interval. This cessation of hormone, specifically progesterone, causes the endometrium to slough in 1 to 3 days.[3] In patients taking OCPs, withdrawal bleeding usually lasts for 3 to 4 days and normal amount of blood loss is approximately 25 mL. This is approximately 10 mL less than the normal amount of blood loss that occurs in patients not taking OCPs.[2]

The dose of estrogen and progestin supplied throughout the dosing interval can be classified as follows: monophasic, biphasic, and triphasic formulations (Table 28-4). The monophasic formulations contain a consistent dose of estrogen and progestin for all 21 active tablets. The biphasic oral contraceptive tablets contain a fixed dose of estrogen and increasing amounts of progestin. The triphasic oral contraceptive tablets contain varying doses of either progestin or estrogen in combination with a fixed dose of the other agent.[2,3] Multiphasic oral contraceptive formulations were developed in the 1970s to lower the total hormone dose without increasing breakthrough bleeding.

A chewable combination formulation is now available. The Femcon Fe tablet contains ethinyl estradiol, 35 mcg, and norethindrone, 0.4 mg. The placebo tablet contains ferrous fumarate to help prevent iron deficiency, commonly found in menstruating women.[9]

LOW-DOSE FORMULATIONS

Several low-dose ethinyl estradiol, containing 20 to 25 mcg oral contraceptive formulations, are currently available. Perimenopausal women who desire contraception but prefer the lowest estrogen dose possible may benefit from low-dose formulations. These products may alleviate vasomotor symptoms and mood swings associated with menopause. Estrogen doses less than 35 mcg may be less effective in obese patients and should therefore be avoided.[3]

THIRD-GENERATION PROGESTIN FORMULATIONS

Reference to the classification by "generations" of progestins is widely used although there is no uniform agreement as to the meaning of this nomenclature. In general the term "first generation" refers to those

Table 28-4. Oral Contraceptive Pills by Estrogen/Progestin Content

Product	Estrogen	Dose (mcg)	Progestin	Dose (mg)
50-mcg Estrogen				
Necon 1/50 M, Norinyl 1/50, Ortho-Novum 1/50	Mestronol	50	Norethindrone	1
Ovcon 50	Ethinyl estradiol	50	Norethindrone	1
Ogestrel	E. estradiol	50	Norgestrel	0.5
Demulen 1/50, Zovia 1/50	E. estradiol	50	Ethynodiol diacetate	1
Monophasic (<50-mcg Estrogen)				
Alesse, Aviane, Lessina, Levlite, Lutera	E. estradiol	20	Levonorgestrel	0.1
Levlen, Levora 0.15/30, Nordette, Portia	E. estradiol	30	Levonorgestrel	0.15
Brevicon, Modicon, Necon 0.5/35, Notrel 0.5/35	E. estradiol	35	Norethindrone	0.5
Necon 1/35, Norinyl 1/35, Norethin 1/35, Notrel 1/35, Ortho-Novum 1/35	E. estradiol	35	Norethindrone	1
Demulen 1/35, Kelnor 1/35, Zovia 1/35	E. estradiol	35	Ethy. diacetate	1
Apri, Desogen, Ortho-Cept, Reclipsen, Solia	E. estradiol	30	Desogestrel	0.15
Junel 21 1/20, Junel Fe 1/20	E. estradiol	20	Northindrone acetate	1
Loestrin 1/20, Loestrin Fe 1/20, Microgestin 1/20	E. estradiol	20	Nor. acetate	1
Junel 21 1.5/20, Junel Fe 1.5/20	E. estradiol	20	Nor. acetate	1.5
Loestrin 1.5/30, Loestrin Fe 1.5/30, Microgestin 1.5/30,	E. estradiol	30	Nor. acetate	1.5
Cryselle, Lo-Ovral, Low-Ogestrel	E. estradiol	30	Norgestrel	0.3
Ortho-Cyclen, Mononessa, Previfem, Sprintec	E. estradiol	35	Norgestimate	0.25
Ovcon-35, Femcon Fe (chewable)	E. estradiol	35	Norethindrone	0.4
Yasmin	E. estradiol	30	Drospirenone	3

Biphasic	Estrogen	Dose in mcg (days)	Progestin	Dose in mg (days)
Mircette, Kariva	E. estradiol	20 (21), 10 (5)	Desogestrel	0.15 (21)
Necon 10/11, Gencept 10/11, Ortho-Novum 10/11	E. estradiol	35	Norethindrone	0.5 (10), 1 (11)
Triphasic				
Cyclessa, Cesia, Velivet	E. estradiol	25 (21)	Desogestrel	0.1 (7), 0.125 (7), 0.150 (7)
Estrostep Fe	E. estradiol	20 (5), 30 (7), 35 (9)	Norethindrone	1 (21)
Ortho-Novum 7/7/7, Notrel 7/7/7, Necon 7/7/7	E. estradiol	35 (21)	Norethindrone	0.5 (7), 0.175 (7), 1 (7)
Ortho Tri-Cyclen, Tinessa, Tri-Previfem, Tri-Sprintec	E. estradiol	35 (21)	Norgestimate	0.18 (7), 0.215 (7), 0.25 (7)
Tri-Levlen, Triphasil, Trivora	E. estradiol	30 (6), 40 (5), 30 (10)	Levonorgestrel	0.05 (6), 0.075 (5), 0.125 (10)
Tri-Norinyl, Leena, Aranell	E. estradiol	35 (21)	Norethindrone	0.5 (7), 1 (9), 0.5 (5)
Progestin Only				
Micronor/Nor-Q.D.			Norethindrone	0.35
Ovrette			Norgestrel	0.075
Extended Cycle				
Seasonale (84 d hormone + 7 d placebo)	E. estradiol	30	Levonorgestrel	0.15
Seasonique (84 d hormone + 7 d estrogen 10 mcg)	E. estradiol	30	Levonorgestrel	0.15
Loestrin 24 FE (24/4 d cycle)	E. estradiol	20	Norethindrone	1
YAZ (24/4 d cycle)	E. estradiol	20	Drospirenone	3
Lybrel (Continuous)	E. estradiol	20	Levonorgestrel	90 mcg

Adapted from: Several sources.

formulations developed before 1973 and "second generation" refers to those developed between 1973 and 1989.

The combination oral contraceptive formulations containing estrogen and the newer progestins (norgestimate and desogestrel) are referred to as third-generation OCPs.[1] These progestins have no estrogenic effects and less androgenic effects when compared to older progestins, and their contraceptive efficacy is similar to the older formulations.[4] When compared to levonorgestrel, these progestins have lesser effect on carbohydrate and lipid metabolism.[3]

The use of the newer progestins is controversial. European studies have demonstrated an association between the newer progestins and an increased risk of nonfatal venous thromboembolism; however, these epidemiologic studies did not establish a direct cause-and-effect relationship. Currently, there is insufficient evidence to support a labeling change in the package insert or to withdraw these progestins from the market. The use of these agents remains widespread.[4]

SPIRONOLACTONE ANALOG FORMULATION

Drospirenone is a new progestin derived from spironolactone that has an antimineralocorticoid, antiandrogenic activity. It is available in monophasic oral contraceptive product, containing 30 mcg ethinyl estradiol combined with 3 mg drospirenone, under the trade name Yasmin and as YAZ 24/4, containing 20 mcg ethinyl estradiol combined with 3 mg drospirenone. As a result of its antimineralocorticoid activity, drospirenone may be useful to prevent water retention and weight gain associated with the menstrual cycle. Women with androgen effects such as hirsutism or acne may derive additional benefits.[9] Drospirenone has potassium-sparing effects like spironolactone so should be used with caution in women at risk for hyperkalemia, including those with renal or hepatic disease, or in patients taking medications that increase potassium levels.[3]

EXTENDED-CYCLE FORMULATIONS

The purpose of the extended-cycle oral contraceptive product is to reduce the frequency of menses to once every 3 months and to reduce the withdrawal symptoms of headache and dysmenorrhea.[6] Seasonique, approved in 2006, and Seasonale, approved in 2003, both provide 30 mcg of ethinyl estradiol combined with levonorgestrel 0.15 mg daily for 12 weeks. During the 13th week, the Seasonale packets contain placebo tablets whereas the Seasonique tablets contain 10 mcg of ethinyl estradiol. The low-dose estrogen taken during the 13th week may prevent the hormonal withdrawal symptoms of headache, dysmenorrhea, and heavy menstrual bleeding.[9]

Lybrel, approved in 2007, is the first extended-interval OCP approved for continuous use. Each tablet contains 90 mcg levonorgestrel and 20 mcg ethinyl estradiol. With extended use, the incidence of breakthrough bleeding and spotting decreases although it still occurs in approximately 40% of users.[9]

Extended-cycle OCPs are an attractive option for some women who desire minimal bleeding. The long-term risks and benefits of these agents are unknown.

PROGESTIN-ONLY FORMULATIONS

Progestin-only tablets are a contraceptive option for women unable to use estrogen-containing products, such as lactating women. Progestin-only OCPs do not consistently inhibit ovulation, so the effectiveness is less than the combination estrogen and progestin products. It is very important that these progestin-only products be taken at the same time every day to help maintain consistent blood levels that do not fall below the minimal effective level. Progestin-only OCPs are taken daily without a hormone-free interval.[2] Table 28-4 provides a summary of currently available oral contraceptives.

OTHER HORMONAL CONTRACEPTION

VAGINAL RING FORMULATION

The hormone vaginal ring (NuvaRing) has a similar mechanism of action as oral contraceptive tablets, but does not require daily administration. The ring is inserted into the vagina for 3 weeks; during this time, the vaginal ring releases 15 mcg of ethinyl estradiol and 120 mcg of etonogestrel daily. After 3 weeks, the ring is removed for 1 week during which withdrawal bleeding occurs. If the vaginal ring needs to be removed for a period of 3 hours or longer, an alternative method of contraception should be used for 7 days.[10]

TRANSDERMAL PATCH FORMULATION

The contraceptive patch (Ortho Evra) delivers 20 mcg of ethinyl estradiol and 150 mcg of norelgestromin daily. Its mechanism of action is similar to OCPs. The patch is worn for 3 weeks and then discarded for 1 week during which time withdrawal bleeding occurs. The patch should be applied to the upper arm, lower abdomen, buttocks, or upper torso (excluding the breasts).

It has similar efficacy as oral contraceptive tablets; however, it may be less effective for women weighing more than 90 kg.[10] An additional concern is the increased risk for thrombosis. With the use of the oral agents, there is a peak estradiol level after ingestion followed by a decrease throughout the day. The transdermal patch results in hormone levels that are 25% lower than those caused by oral contraceptives; however, the levels remain consistent throughout the day. Women on the patch containing 20 mcg estradiol have 60% more serum estrogen than women on a 35-mcg estradiol oral agent.[9] In 2005, the FDA changed the labeling of the transdermal patch to warn physicians of the increase in estrogen levels with this delivery system.[6] The implications of this increase are unclear but may lead to an increased risk for thrombosis.[9]

INJECTABLE PROGESTIN

Depomedroxyprogesterone acetate (DMPA) is currently the only injectable contraceptive available in the United States. It is formulated as an aqueous suspension of microcrystals with a low solubility at the injection site which allows the progestin activity to last for 3 to 4 months after a single dose.[11] It is given as a 150-mg intramuscular injection within 5 days after the onset of menses to ensure that the patient is not pregnant.[4] Administering DMPA at this time prevents ovulation during the first month of use.[11] The injection should be repeated every 3 months to ensure continuous efficacy. If a patient presents to clinic more than 1 week late for her DMPA injection, she should be administered a pregnancy test before the next dose is given.

Breakthrough bleeding and spotting are common during the first months of use. With increased duration of use, amenorrhea is common, and at 1 year, nearly half of all patients using DMPA are amenorrheic. Return of fertility may be delayed several months with DMPA use. DMPA does not appear to affect blood pressure or increase the risk of venous thromboembolism but is associated with weight gain.[4] One serious adverse effect with the use of DMPA is bone demineralization, which may not be entirely reversible after discontinuation. Women using DMPA should take vitamin D and calcium supplements and be monitored by bone densitometry.[6]

INTRAUTERINE DEVICES

The use of intrauterine devices (IUDs) declined in the 1970s when the Dalkon Shield was linked to the pelvic inflammatory disease. Recent studies on newer devices have shown that IUDs provide a safe and effective method of contraception in women at low risk for pelvic inflammatory disease. IUDs are the most widely used nonpermanent contraceptive used worldwide.[12]

There are two IUDs currently available in the United States: the copper T380A IUD and the levonorgestrel-releasing IUD (Mirena IUS). Both IUDs are approved for long-term use; the copper-releasing IUD is implanted in the uterus for a 10-year duration and the levonorgestrel-releasing IUD for a 5-year duration.[9] The mechanism of action contributing to the effectiveness of IUDs is unclear. The copper T380A IUD appears to have an adverse effect on sperm. The levonorgestrel-releasing IUD releases approximately 20 mcg of hormone daily.[12]

With proper insertion, the expulsion of an IUD is unlikely. Once inserted, these T-shaped devices may result in menstrual abnormalities and increased spotting although this usually resolves by 6 months. If pregnancy should occur while the IUD is in place, removal is recommended (if this can be accomplished noninvasively).[12]

ROD IMPLANTS

A single rod implant for subdermal placement was approved in July 2006. The Implanon rod releases 40 mcg of etonogestrel (a metabolite of desogestrel) daily for 3 years. This highly effective contraceptive is easily reversible, and can be reversed by the removal of the rod. Ovulation resumes within 1 month of removal. Although there are no long-term studies to evaluate the side effects with Implanon, the absence of estrogen seems to pose a low risk for venous thromboembolism. The risk of bone demineralization seen in long-term DMPA is not known with Implanon.[9]

NONHORMONAL CONTRACEPTION

BARRIER METHODS

Male condoms are the most effective barrier for prevention of sexually transmitted diseases. Pregnancy rates with this form of contraception have been shown to be around 3% to 9%. The pregnancy rate for patients older than 30 years is half the pregnancy rate of those younger than 30 years.[2]

The female condom is also an effective form of barrier birth control and appears to provide external coverage to the labia and base of the penis. The female condom can be inserted prior to sexual activity and can be left in place after ejaculation has occurred. Pregnancy rates are comparable to its male counterpart with rates ranging from 3% to 5%. To date, no direct comparison of barrier methods has been undertaken.

Two other female barrier contraception methods include the cervical cap and the diaphragm. Both of these methods require fitting by a physician. Failure rates for both methods are comparable at 16% to 17%. Both barriers have to be removed after use. The cap has the advantage of being able to be left in for up to

48 hours. The diaphragm is recommended to be removed every 24 hours. The diaphragm method requires that spermicide be applied with each act of intercourse for the most effective contraception.[2]

NATURAL FAMILY PLANNING

Natural family planning has been reported to have varying degrees of effectiveness. It is usually instituted by having the patient record a strict menstrual calendar for 3 months. Abstinence is then instituted by subtracting 18 days from shortest cycle and 11 days from longest cycle. This form of contraception can mean that abstinence is required for greater than half of the menstrual cycle. It has been shown that the majority of couples fail to abstain for these lengths of time. Other forms of family planning have used evaluation of cervical secretions and basal body temperature measurements.[2]

CONCLUSION

The choice of oral contraceptive should be based on careful consideration of the patient. The healthcare provider must determine if there are any contraindications to a combination oral contraceptive product and encourage patients to discuss concerns or side effects. All combination oral contraceptive products have similar efficacy; however, products with the lowest dose of estrogen and progestin may have fewer side effects. Patients with a history of or concern for nonadherence may benefit from products such as the contraceptive patch, vaginal ring, injectable forms, or IUDs. These products do not require daily administration for efficacy.

Table 28-5. Patient Education Regarding Oral Contraceptive Use

- Oral contraceptive tablets should be started on the first day of menses or the first Sunday after menstruation.
- Patients who incorporate pill taking with a daily ritual have improved compliance.
- Patients should be advised that neither oral contraceptive tablets nor DMPA protects against STDs or HIV.
- If a patient misses one or two combination oral contraceptive tablets, she should take one tablet as soon as possible and followed by one tablet twice daily until all the missed tablets have been taken.
- Patients who miss more than two tablets should be advised to use a backup form of contraception.
- Progestin-only oral contraceptive products should be taken at the same time every day. If the patient is late in taking this product by 3 h or more, she should use a backup form of contraception.
- Patients should inform their healthcare provider if they are or plan to become pregnant.

DMPA, depomedroxyprogesterone acetate; STD, sexually transmitted disease; HIV, human immunodeficiency virus.

The healthcare provider should explain the advantages and disadvantages of agents and choose the agent that fits the patient's lifestyle and likelihood for adherence.[4,11] The prescription for a contraceptive agent should be accompanied by careful instructions given to the patient (Table 28-5).

EVIDENCE-BASED SUMMARY

- Low-dose estrogen/progestin combinations are effective in the prevention of pregnancy.
- The risk and benefits of hormonal contraception should be considered in all patients.
- The risk of thromboembolic disease is decreased with lower doses of estrogen.
- The side effects of a given hormonal contraceptive agent are related to its estrogen, progestin, and antiandrogen properties.
- In addition to oral contraceptives, other hormone delivery systems are available including hormone injections, patches, transdermal systems, and intrauterine devices.

REFERENCES

1. Pettiti DB. Combination estrogen–progestin oral contraceptives. *N Engl J Med.* 2003;349:1443–1450.
2. Mishell DR, Jr. Family planning: Contraception, sterilization, and pregnancy termination. In: Stencheuer MA, Droegemueller W, Herbst A, Mishell D, eds. *Comprehensive Gynecology*, 4th ed. St Louis, MO: Mosby; 2001:295–358.
3. Martin KA, Barbieri RL. Overview of the use of estrogen–progestin contraceptives. www.uptodate.com. Accessed November 13, 2007.
4. Dickerson LM, Bucci KK. Contraception. In: Dipiro JT, Talbert RL, YeeGC, Matzke GR, Wells BG, Posey LM, eds. *Pharmacotherapy: A Pathophysiologic Approach*, 5th ed. New York, NY: McGraw-Hill; 2002:1445–1460.
5. The use of hormonal contraception in women with coexisting medical conditions. *ACOG Pract Bull.* 2000;18:674–687.
6. David PS, Boatwrisht EA, Tozer BS, et al. Hormonal contraception update. *Mayo Clinic Proc.* 2006;81(7):949–955.
7. AHFS DI© Essentials™. http://online.statref.com. Accessed November 13, 2007.
8. Allen J. Cupp M. Hormonal contraception. *Pharmacist's Letter/Prescriber's Letter.* 2007;231207.
9. Masimasi N, Sivanandy MS, Thacker H. Update on hormonal contraception. *Cleve Clin J Med.* 2007;74:186–198.
10. Herndon EJ, Zieman M. New contraceptive options. *Am Fam Physician.* 2004;69:853–860.
11. Hormonal contraception. *ACOG Tech Bull.* 1994;198:506–513.
12. Peterson HB, Curtis KM. Long-acting methods of contraception. *N Engl J Med.* 2005;353:2169–2175.

Chapter 29

Menopausal Hormone Therapy

T. Kristopher Harrell and Annette K. Low

SEARCH STRATEGY

A systematic Medline search using "menopause" and "hormone replacement therapy" was performed in March 2007, which was limited to human subjects and articles from journals in English language. The American College of Obstetricians and Gynecologists Women's Health Care Physicians have published guidelines on their website at http://www.greenjournal.org

BACKGROUND

Menopause is defined by 12 consecutive months without menstrual periods; it naturally occurs between 45 and 55 years of age. Women experience variable symptoms during the perimenopausal period and frequently seek advice from their health care provider regarding the short- and long-term management of the changes related to menopause. For many years, the mainstay of menopausal treatment has been estrogen alone or in combination with progesterone. Hormone replacement therapy was thought to be beneficial in women in preventing heart disease. In the last decade, the approach to treatment of menopause has changed as findings from randomized, controlled clinical trials have shown detrimental effects of estrogen on breast cancer and no improvement in cardiovascular outcomes. Recently, a National Institutes of Health State of the Science Panel has recommended only short-term use of hormone therapy (HT) for menopausal symptom relief and, as such, used the term menopausal hormone therapy (MHT) rather than hormone replacement therapy.[1] Primary care providers should be familiar with the available evidence regarding MHT to be able to counsel patients in the short- and long-term

use of MHT. Given the potential risk related to HT, many patients and providers consider the use of alternative therapy to treat menopausal symptoms.

RESEARCH IN MENOPAUSAL HORMONE THERAPY

Observational studies reported positive effects with HT in postmenopausal women in the prevention of chronic diseases, which resulted in the widespread use of estrogen and progesterone.[2] The largest of these observational studies was the Nurses' Health Study that began in 1976 and was renewed in 1993 and 2002.[3] It enrolled over 121 000 nurses initially and remains the largest and longest-running study of women's health. A 10-year follow-up of postmenopausal participants, who were taking estrogen and did not have coronary heart disease or cancer at baseline, showed a reduction in incident coronary heart disease.[3] In 1997, the Postmenopausal Estrogen/Progestin Interventions Trial was one of the first randomized trials to demonstrate potential benefits of HT on surrogate markers for heart disease and osteoporosis.[4] This trial also led to the recommendation of combined estrogen and progesterone in women with an intact uterus. Until 2001, HT was widely recommended to prevent cardiovascular disease (CVD).

In 1998, the Heart and Estrogen/Progestin Replacement Study (HERS) showed an increase in coronary heart disease during the first year of HT; among women with established heart disease, there was no overall CVD benefit compared to placebo.[5] Another surprising result was an increase in the risk of venous thrombosis in the HERS study.[6]

The Women's Health Initiative (WHI) randomized control study consisted of a series of randomized clinical trials designed to compare estrogen alone[7] or combined estrogen–progesterone[8] with placebo in primary prevention of CVD. Over 16000 women, aged 50 to 79 years, were randomized to the combined estrogen plus progestin arm of the study. Compared to placebo, there was an increased risk for coronary heart disease, stroke, and venous thromboembolus in the first 5 years. For these reasons, the study was discontinued early in 2002.[8]

The WHI estrogen plus progestin study also showed a low but modest increased risk for breast cancer in women on the combined hormone regimen[8]; however, there was no increased risk for breast cancer in the unopposed estrogen arm of the study.[7]

The WHI estrogen-alone trial enrolled over 11000 women who had undergone hysterectomy. This trial also failed to show cardiovascular benefit and because of an increase in incident stroke was terminated early.[7]

The WHI study showed a reduction of risk for hip fracture in women on estrogen/progestin, and a significant reduction in risk for colon cancer for those women on combined HT, supporting previous findings in observational studies investigating the effects of MHT.[9] In the WHI study, there was a 2-fold increase in dementia among women older than 65 years on treatment with estrogen/progestin.[10]

Critics of these studies have pointed out that the age of the participants in the HERS and WHI trials was much more than women who routinely taking MHT given that the mean age in the HERS trial was 67 years at baseline and, in the WHI, it was 63 years at baseline. The findings may not be generalizable to younger women.[11] The age of menopause and initiation of HT may influence coronary heart disease, stroke, and other outcomes. Nevertheless, the HERS and WHI studies have had a remarkable impact on the use of HT for prevention of CVD and treatment of menopausal symptoms.[12] MHT should no longer be recommended for primary or secondary prevention of CVD.[13] Further research is needed to address this issue.[14]

STAGES OF MENOPAUSE

The normal ovarian cycle involves complex hormonal regulation from the hypothalamus, pituitary, and ovaries. During the menopause transition, there is a physiologic decline in ovarian function and the number of ovarian follicles. This results in a decreasing number of mature eggs, irregular ovulation, and menstrual irregularity. The pituitary gonadotropin, follicle-stimulating hormone (FSH), increases to promote continued estradiol secretion by the remaining ovarian follicles. Because of the fluctuations in FSH levels, measurement of FSH while a woman is still menstruating is not helpful. When the ovarian follicles are depleted, estradiol

levels decline. The ovary continues to produce androgens as a result of continued production of the pituitary gonadotropin, luteinizing hormone. Once menstruation ceases, an FSH of more than 30 mU/mL is considered diagnostic of menopause, although it is not usually needed for the diagnosis of menopause.[15]

The stages of menopause have recently been revised to clarify the nomenclature and to relate staging to the biochemical and clinical changes related to menopause.[16] The Stages of Reproductive Aging Workshop guidelines describe the stages of menopause as menopausal transition, perimenopause, menopause, and postmenopause. Progression to menopause reflects gradual ovarian follicular failure with a decline in estrogen levels. The effects of declining ovarian function begin several years before actual menopause occurs. Menopausal transition begins with variation in menstrual cycles. FSH levels may be normal to high and women are likely to have vasomotor symptoms during this stage. Perimenopause overlaps with the menopausal transition and begins when the menstrual cycles are more than 7 days different from the normal period. The perimenopausal period is greater than 60 days of amenorrhea or 2 skipped menstrual periods and in many women results in symptoms related to the genitourinary, neuroendocrine, and integumentary systems. Menopause is defined retrospectively after 12 months of anovulation; the mean age at menopause is 51 years.[16]

ASSESSMENT OF MENOPAUSE

CLINICAL PRESENTATION

Women in menopausal transition may experience changes in menstruation including the shortening of the follicular phase with heavier, lighter, or even absent menses. Hot flashes ("flushes") occur in up to 75% of women. Young women who have undergone surgical menopause have greater frequency and severity of hot flashes. The hot flash is a sensation of heat that typically begins in the face and chest and quickly spreads. The hot flash may be accompanied by palpitations and anxiety. These vasomotor symptoms may occur 1 to 2 times daily or as often as hourly and are most common at night (night sweats). The flash lasts for 2 to 4 minutes, is associated with perspiration, and followed by chills. The prevalence of hot flashes varies with ethnicity and may be related to obesity, sedentary lifestyle, smoking, and higher socioeconomic status.[1]

Vaginal dryness and dyspareunia (painful intercourse) are common in perimenopausal and postmenopausal women. These changes are related to decreased estrogen secretion and relieved by topical or systemic estrogen replacement.

Table 29-1. Common Symptoms Associated with Menopause

Vasomotor symptoms
   Hot flashes
   Night sweats
Urogenital symptoms
   Vaginal dryness, itching
   Dysuria, urgency, incontinence
   Recurrent urinary tract infections
Psychologic symptoms
   Anxiety, difficulty in concentration
   Depression, loss of interest, irritability
   Memory loss
Neurologic symptoms
   Headaches
   Dizziness
   Numbness and tingling

Table 29-3. Components of an Initial Menopause Assessment

Past medical history
   Reproductive history
   Sexual and social history
   Family history
   Psychiatric history
   Dietary habits
   Medication use
Physical examination
   Height and weight
   Thyroid palpation
   Cardiovascular examination
   Breast examination
   Pelvic examination
Diagnostic evaluation
   Chemistries
   Lipid panel
   Hormone levels
   Pap smear
   Mammogram
   Bone density
   Colonoscopy (if age-appropriate)

Sleep disturbance is a common complaint in menopause transition and may be caused by nocturnal hot flashes. There is evidence that menopausal transition causes sleep disturbance independent of vasomotor symptoms.[1]

Other symptoms described by women in menopausal transition include bladder dysfunction, body aches, sexual dysfunction, cognitive dysfunction, mood swings, and fatigue.[1] Table 29-1 lists the most common symptoms associated with menopause.

DIAGNOSTIC EVALUATION OF THE WOMEN IN MENOPAUSE

A recommendation for treatment of menopausal symptoms should be individualized and with consideration of the patient's past medical history, family history, lifestyle habits, and risk factors for CVD, malignancy, and other chronic diseases. A thorough medical history should be taken to determine the stage of menopause and to evaluate both absolute and relative contraindications for MHT (see Table 29-2). Absolute contraindi-

Table 29-2. Contraindications to Hormone Replacement Therapy

Absolute contraindications
   Vaginal bleeding
   History or evidence of breast or endometrial cancer
   Active venous thrombosis
Relative contraindications
   Uterine fibroids
   Endometriosis
   History of cholelithiasis
   History of migraine
   Hypertriglyceridemia
   Liver disease

cations for HT include vaginal bleeding, suspected or history of breast or endometrial cancer, or active venous thrombosis. Relative contraindications include uterine fibroids, endometriosis, history of cholelithiasis or migraine, hypertriglyceridemia, or liver disease. The determination of menopause is based upon a careful review of systems as the differential includes thyroid dysfunction, depression, and a variety of other conditions depending upon the chief complaints.

The physical assessment of the perimenopausal woman should include an examination of the thyroid gland, breasts, cardiovascular system, and the pelvis. A mammogram and Papanicolaou smear should be performed. A bone mineral density evaluation should be considered if it is age-appropriate and also if risk factors for osteoporosis exist.

Laboratory studies should include thyroid function tests, a complete blood count, lipid profile, and liver enzymes. Laboratory tests to determine ovarian hormone status can be performed although they are not required for the evaluation of menopausal transition. A circulating FSH with level greater than 30 mU/mL is consistent with menopause. Table 29-3 outlines the recommended evaluation for the perimenopausal patient.

MANAGEMENT OF MENOPAUSAL SYMPTOMS

The treatment of perimenopausal symptoms and the long-term treatment of the woman in menopause must be individualized. The decision to recommend MHT is made after evaluation of risks and benefits of MHT. The type and duration of therapy remains controversial and should be carefully weighed and discussed with each individual woman. Some symptoms related to perimenopause may be managed by lifestyle changes including exercise, avoidance of alcohol, smoking cessation, and relaxation techniques. For women with more severe symptoms, the use of HT is an option that may be considered. Many women consider alternative therapies and herbal compounds.

MENOPAUSAL HORMONE THERAPY

The choice and dosage regimen of MHT should be based on patient preference and previous medical history. MHT relieves women of menopausal symptoms such as vasomotor symptoms, vaginal dryness, and sleep disturbances.[1] Estrogen alone or in combination with progesterone is highly effective in the treatment of vasomotor symptoms but should be used at a low dose and only as a short-term treatment.[17,18] Specific estrogen and progesterone products are listed in Table 29-4. Since most MHTs will cause almost immediate breast tenderness, it is recommended to start at a low dose and increase the dose after 2 to 4 weeks. For women who have had a hysterectomy, estrogen alone is the preferred option. When initiating cyclic MHT in women with an intact uterus, it is recommended to give estrogen first for 1 to 2 months on a daily basis. This can then be followed by the addition of progesterone after 1 to 2 months of successful treatment with the estrogen. The cyclic regimen will avoid erratic bleeding or spotting in menopausal women, which is one of the most common reasons why women discontinue taking HT. All patients starting MHT should return to clinic in 2 months for further evaluation and discussion of relief of menopausal symptoms. Adherence to MHT can be maximized by allowing discussion, explaining the risks and benefits of MHT on an individualized basis, including patient preferences into the recommendations, and planning for frequent follow-up.[19]

Table 29-4. Estrogen and Progesterone Products

Estrogen products
Conjugated equine estrogens
Esterified estrogens
Estropiate sulfate
Estrone sulfate
Micronized estradiol
Ethinyl estradiol
Transdermal estradiol
Vaginal estrogen preparations
Progesterone products
Medroxyprogesterone
Levonorgestrel
Norethindrone
Micronized progesterone
Transvaginal progesterone

Estrogen and progesterone creams may also be beneficial but sporadic absorption rates may only offer local effects; thus, vaginal application of the creams offers the most relief of vaginal symptoms.[1]

ALTERNATIVES TO MENOPAUSAL HORMONE THERAPY

In those women with menopausal symptoms who do not wish to use any form of MHT or have contraindications to MHT, the primary care provider may discuss alternative therapies. Table 29-5 includes alternative therapies suggested to be effective in reducing menopausal symptoms although little data is available for most of the given therapies.

The selective serotonin reuptake inhibitors (fluoxetine, paroxetine, sertraline) and the serotonin—norepinephrine reuptake inhibitors (venlafaxine) have been shown to decrease menopausal hot flashes and improve quality of life. In clinical trials, gabapentin has shown benefit in comparison to clonidine, which is of little benefit, in the treatment of hot flashes.[20]

The use of complementary and alternative (CAM) therapy is frequently considered, yet, there are few well-designed studies for the use of CAM therapy for menopausal symptoms. Herbal products including the phytoestrogens found in foods containing soy or red clover may also be beneficial in reducing symptoms. These agents are not regulated by the Food and Drug Administration and therefore should be used with caution, as little information is available regarding their efficacy and adverse effects.[21]

Table 29-5. Alternative Therapies Used in the Treatment of Menopausal Symptoms

Medications
Selective serotonin reuptake inhibitors (fluoxetine, paroxetine, sertraline)
Venlafaxine
Gabapentin
Clonidine
Herbal supplements
Black cohosh
Phytoestrogens (isoflavones)
Soy products (tofu, soy milk, soy nuts)
Red clover
Ginseng
Kava
Primrose oil
Nonpharmacologic options
Exercise therapy (aerobic exercise several times weekly)
Relaxation techniques (meditation, stress management)
Environmental measures (avoiding warm places, air conditioning)
Acupuncture
Massage therapy

Other botanical agents reported to reduce menopausal hot flashes include black cohosh, ginseng, and kava although clinical trials evidence is scant.[1,20] Black cohosh, a widely used botanical agent for hot flashes, failed to show a reduction in vasomotor symptoms when used alone or in combination with multibotanical regimen in women treated for 12 months.[22] Women should be cautioned regarding the long-term use of alternative botanical therapies until there is clinical trial evidence of safety and efficacy.

Acupuncture, massage therapy, aerobic exercise, appropriate nutrition, and improved sleep hygiene have also been recommended, yet, there are few data confirming the benefits of reduction in menopausal symptoms.[23] Beneficial alternatives for the treatment of menopausal symptoms are important. Research in the use of CAM therapy with well-designed, randomized, controlled trials is imperative.

EVIDENCE-BASED SUMMARY

- The use of MHT in postmenopausal women remains controversial.
- Decisions about the use of MHT require the careful examination of the risks and benefits in each individual woman.
- MHT should no longer be used for the primary or secondary prevention of CVD.
- If MHT is used, it should only be used at the lowest dose for the shortest duration possible.
- If progesterone is used, it should only be used in females who have a uterus to provide protection of the endometrium.
- For those females already taking MHT, discontinuation should be considered.
- Alternative therapies for treatment of menopausal symptoms are based on little clinic trial evidence.
- Further research in the use of HT and alternative therapies is needed.

REFERENCES

1. National Institutes of Health State-of-the Science Conferences Statement: Management of menopause-related symptoms. *Ann Intern Med.* 2005;142:1003.
2. Barrett-Conners E, Grady D. Hormone replacement therapy, heart disease, and other considerations. *Ann Rev Public Health.* 1998;19:55.
3. Stampfer MJ, Colditz GA, Willett WC, et al. Postmenopausal estrogen therapy and cardiovascular disease. Ten-year follow-up from the nurses' health study. *N Engl J Med.* 1991;11:756.
4. Writing Group for the PEPI Trial. Effects of estrogen or estrogen/progestin regimens on heart disease risk factors in postmenopausal women. *JAMA.* 1995;273:199.
5. Hulley S, Grady D, Bush T, et al. Heart and Estrogen/Progestin Replacement Study (HERS). Randomized trial of estrogen plus progestin for secondary prevention of coronary heart disease in postmenopausal women. *JAMA.* 1998;280:605.
6. Grady D, Herrington D, Bittner V, et al. HERS Research Group. Cardiovascular disease outcomes during 6.8 years of hormone therapy: Heart and Estrogen/Progestin Replacement Study follow-up (HERS II). *JAMA.* 2002; 288:49.
7. Anderson GL, Limacher M, Assaf AR, et al. Effects of conjugated equine estrogen in postmenopausal women with hysterectomy: The women's health initiative randomized controlled trial. *JAMA.* 2004;291:1701.
8. Manson JE, Hsia J, Johnson KC, et al. Estrogen plus progestin and the risk of coronary heart disease. *N Engl J Med.* 2003;349:523.
9. Writing Group for the Women's Health Initiative Investigators. Risks and benefits of estrogen plus progestin in healthy postmenopausal women: Principal results from the women's health initiative randomized controlled trial. *JAMA.* 2002;288:321.
10. Shumaker SA, Legault C, Thal L, et al. Estrogen plus progestin and the incidence of dementia and mild cognitive impairment in postmenopausal women; the women's health initiative randomized controlled trial. *JAMA.* 2003; 289:2651.
11. Aubuchon M, Santoro N. Lessons learned from the WHI: MHT requires a cautious and individualized approach. *Geriatrics.* 2004;59:22.
12. Hing E, Brett MK. Changes in US prescribing patterns of menopausal therapy, 2001–2003. *Obstet Gynecol.* 2006; 108:33.
13. Mosca L, Collins P, Herrington DM, et al. Hormone replacement therapy and cardiovascular disease: A statement of healthcare professionals from the American Heart Association. *Circulation.* 2001;104:499.
14. Hulley SB, Grady D. The WHI estrogen-alone trial—Do things look any better? *JAMA.* 2004;291:1769.
15. Hall JE. Neuroendocrine physiology of the early and late menopause. *Endocrinol Metab Clin North Am.* 2004; 33:637.
16. Soule MR, Sherman S, Parrott E, Rebar R. Executive summary: Stages of Reproductive Aging Workshop (STRAW). *Fertil Steril.* 2001;76:874.
17. Stephenson J. FDA orders estrogen safety warnings: Agency offers guidance for HRT use. *JAMA.* 2004;289: 537.
18. North American Menopause Society. Treatment of menopause-associate vasomotor symptoms. Position statement of The North American Menopause Society. *Menopause.* 2004;11:11.

19. Nelson HD. Commonly used types of postmenopausal estrogen for treatment of hot flashes: Scientific review. *JAMA.* 2004;291:1610.
20. Grady D. Management of menopausal symptoms. *N Engl J Med.* 2007;355:2338.
21. National Center for Complementary and Alternative Medicine. *Do CAM Therapies Help Menopausal Symptoms?* http://nccam.nih.gov/. Accessed March 15, 2007.
22. Newton MN, Reed SD, LaCroix AZ, et al. Treatment of vasomotor symptoms of menopause with black cohosh, multibotanicals, soy, hormone therapy, or placebo. *Ann Intern Med.* 2006;145:869.
23. Nedrow A, Miller J, Walker M, et al. Complementary and alternative therapies for the management of menopause-related symptoms. *Arch Intern Med.* 2006; 166:1453.

PART 7

Urologic Disorders

CHAPTERS

Chapter 30

Erectile Dysfunction

Sunny A. Linnebur and Jeffrey I. Wallace

SEARCH STRATEGY

A systematic search of the medical literature was performed on March 14, 2007. The search, limited to human subjects and journals in English language, included the National Guideline Clearinghouse, the Cochrane database, MEDLINE, and International Pharmaceutical Abstracts.

Erectile dysfunction (ED) is defined as the inability to achieve an erection sufficient for satisfactory sexual intercourse.[1] It is estimated that approximately 52% of men in the United States who are 40 years and older suffer from some degree of ED.[2] The etiology can be due to psychological, vascular, endocrine, neurologic, urologic, or pharmacologic causes, and may often be multifactorial. The development of effective oral therapies has revolutionized the treatment of ED. More men are seeking treatment and most are seeking it through primary care providers.

CLINICAL PRESENTATION

ED typically occurs in men older than 40 years and the risk increases with age and comorbidities. Men may present to their primary care provider with a complaint of ED, but a full workup may reveal more serious underlying causes such as depression or cardiovascular disease. In fact, many patients with ED may have subclinical atherosclerosis and those without a clear etiology should be evaluated for vascular disease, as ED appears to be an independent predictor of cardiovascular disease.[3,4] Severity of ED varies from patient to patient but usually increases with age. Men suffering from ED may also complain of problems with libido and/or ejaculation, depending on the cause of their ED.

PHYSICAL FINDINGS

All patients with ED should be evaluated for abnormalities in the size and consistency of the prostate, testicles, and penis. The physical examination should also include blood pressure measurement and femoral and pedal pulse evaluations to further identify cardiovascular-related ED. Endocrine evaluation should include inspection for thyroid gland abnormalities, breasts for gynecomastia, and hair distribution or general masculine development. Perineal sensation and bulbocavernous reflex are part of an appropriate neurologic evaluation. Patients with abnormalities in the systems above should be further evaluated and may require referral to an appropriate specialist (e.g., urologist, endocrinologist).

DIAGNOSTIC EVALUATION

To aid successful treatment, an accurate diagnosis of ED must be made through a thorough history and physical findings including ED screening; sexual, medical, social, and medication histories; a physical examination; laboratory tests; and possibly additional cardiovascular testing. Screening patients for ED can be easily accomplished by using a patient-focused questionnaire. The Sexual Health Inventory for Men is a standard clinical tool that aids in diagnosing ED (Fig. 30-1).[5] It includes five questions from the ED portion of the International Index of Erectile Function related to confidence, penetration, maintenance, and satisfaction; a score of 21 or less indicates the patient is likely to have ED. In addition to screening male patients for ED, primary care providers should discuss sexual history as a means to improve and clarify diagnoses. Some sexual changes may be related to aging rather than to ED. As

Over the past 6 months:

1) How do you rate your confidence that you could get and keep an erection? (Very low =1, Low =2, Moderate = 3, High = 4, Very high = 5)

2) When you had erections with sexual stimulation, how often were your erections hard enough for penetration (entering your partner)? (No sexual activity = 0, Almost never or never = 1, A few times [much less than half the time] = 2, Sometimes [about half the time] = 3, Most times [much more than half the time] = 4, Almost always or always = 5)

3) During sexual intercourse, how often were you able to maintain your erection after you had penetrated (entered) your partner? (Did not attempt intercourse = 0, Almost never or never = 1, A few times [much less than half the time] = 2, Sometimes [about half the time] = 3, Most times [much more than half the time] = 4, Almost always or always = 5)

4) During sexual intercourse, how difficult was it to maintain your erection to completion of intercourse? (Did not attempt intercourse = 0, Extremely difficult = 1, Very difficult = 2, Difficult = 3, Slightly difficult = 4, Not difficult = 5)

5) When you attempted sexual intercourse, how often was it satisfactory for you? (Did not attempt intercourse = 0, Almost never or never = 1, A few times [much less than half the time] = 2, Sometimes [about half the time] = 3, Most times [much more than half the time] = 4, Almost always or always = 5)

Add the numbers corresponding to the questions 1–5. If your score is 21 or less, you may want to give this form to your health care professional who can determine if you have erectile dysfunction.

Figure 30-1. Sexual health inventory for men.
(Adapted with permission from Rosen RC, Cappelleri JC, Smith MD, Lipsky J, Pena BM. Development and evaluation of an abridged, 5-item version of the International Index of Erectile Function (IIEF-5) as a diagnostic tool for erectile dysfunction. *Int J Impot Res* 1999;11: 319–326.)

men age they sometimes require increased sexual stimulation, time, and concentration to obtain and maintain an erection compared to their younger selves. Men with these symptoms may benefit from reassurance that they do not have ED, and pharmacologic treatment is usually not indicated. Moreover, a sexual history is necessary to fully identify if the patient is suffering from erectile, libido, and/or ejaculatory dysfunction.

A full medical history, including history of diabetes, hypertension, dyslipidemia, cardiovascular disease, peripheral vascular disease, and hypogonadism is essential to identifying precipitating factors for ED.[6] Patients with these conditions should be evaluated for disease control, and those with poor control should have appropriate interventions to optimize disease management. A social history should be taken in patients complaining of ED to evaluate for tobacco, alcohol, and illicit drug use, all of which can contribute to ED. Psychological causes such as stresses, interpersonal relationship problems, and depression should be explored. Rapid-onset ED may be more psychogenic or medication-related in origin, whereas complete loss of nocturnal and stimulated erections is usually vascular or neurologic in origin. Finally, a complete medication history is important to identify medications used to treat concomitant illnesses that may be causing or contributing to ED. Common medical conditions, social factors, and medications that increase ED risk are listed in Table 30-1.

As discussed above, a physical examination in patients with suspected ED should focus on identifying abnormalities in systems that can increase ED risk (cardiovascular, urologic, endocrine, and neurologic). Laboratory tests should also be performed to help identify causes of ED. All patients should be screened with a fasting blood glucose to assess diabetes risk or control, fasting lipid profile to assess cardiovascular risk, blood chemistry to evaluate electrolytes and serum creatinine, hemogram to assess for anemia, and serum testosterone. Although hypogonadism is rarely the single cause of ED in men, low testosterone levels are associated with decreased libido and are an important part of the ED evaluation. Evaluating free testosterone and/or bioavailable testosterone is the preferred method of detecting hypogonadism.

Table 30-1. Common Medical, Social, and Medication-Related Causes of ED

Medical	Social	Medications
Diabetes	Smoking	Hydrochlorothiazide
Hypertension	Alcohol	Metoprolol, atenolol,
Dyslipidemia	Cocaine	propranolol
Peripheral vascular disease	Marijuana	Spironolactone
Cardiovascular disease		Methyldopa, clonidine, reserpine
Obesity		Digoxin
Sleep apnea		Fluoxetine, paroxetine,
Thyroid disease		sertraline, citalopram, escitalopram
Stroke		Amitriptyline, nortriptyline, imipramine, desipramine, doxepin
Parkinson disease		Lithium
Urologic surgery		Thioridazine, fluphenazine, thiothixene
Benign prostatic hypertrophy		Metoclopramide
		Finasteride, dutasteride
Hypogonadism		Cimetidine
Depression		Phenytoin, carbamazepine,
Psychologic		primidone, phenobarbital

Morning measurements are optimal since testosterone is secreted in a diurnal pattern, and at least two morning concentrations should be obtained. Total testosterone is not recommended as a measure of hypogonadism, as levels are affected by the increase in sex-hormone-binding globulin that occurs with aging. If free or bioavailable testosterone concentrations are found to be low, serum luteinizing hormone and prolactin concentrations should be drawn to aid in discriminating primary from secondary hypogonadism.

Additional cardiovascular testing is based on risk stratification. Consensus guidelines suggest that cardiologic evaluation be performed before sexual activity in those patients with intermediate and high cardiovascular risk (Table 30-2) to determine if sexual activity and ED treatment are safe.[7] An exercise treadmill test and/or echocardiogram are recommended. Patients with high cardiovascular risk should also be referred to a cardiologist for evaluation before ED treatment is initiated. Updated guidelines corroborate the above recommendations, provide some clarification on certain cardiac conditions, and emphasize that ED may be an early or sole symptom of atherosclerotic vascular disease.[8] As such, it appears prudent to perform an evaluation of cardiac risk factors in almost all patients presenting with ED.

RISK STRATIFICATION

Risk stratification for ED is necessary to determine appropriate management. Once a diagnosis of ED is made and a cause determined, patients should be separated into those with modifiable risks and those with unmodifiable risks. Modifiable risks include poor glycemic, hypertensive, and dyslipidemic control; smoking, alcohol, and illicit drug use; hypogonadism; depression; endocrine disorders; and use of medications that can cause ED. Unmodifiable risks for ED include urologic surgery, vascular disease, and neurologic disease. An evaluation and management algorithm designed for men with diabetes can also be utilized for most other men presenting with ED, and is shown in Figure 30-2.[7]

MANAGEMENT

NONPHARMACOLOGIC TREATMENT

Risk-Factor Modification

All patients with ED and modifiable risk factors should be initially managed by modifying their ED risk.[6] Improving glycemic control, dyslipidemia, and hypertension can potentially improve erectile function. Tobacco, alcohol, and illicit drug cessation should be encouraged. Increased exercise, weight loss, and a balanced diet have also been shown to improve erectile function, especially in obese men. Additionally, underlying medical conditions such as depression, hypogonadism, and thyroid dysfunction should be treated and effect on ED assessed. Risk-factor modification can help to improve erectile function and overall health, but many patients may still need pharmacologic therapy for ED. Pharmacologic therapy can be prescribed concomitantly with risk-factor modification, but patients may be less motivated to modify risk factors if their ED is quickly improved by pharmacologic treatment. Finally, medications causing ED can be stopped or replaced with similar medications that are associated with a lower ED risk (Table 30-3).[6,9,10]

Table 30-2. Cardiovascular Assessment in ED Patients

Grade of Risk	Categories of CVD	Management Recommendations
Low risk	Asymptomatic, <3 major risk factors for CAD; controlled HTN; mild, stable angina; post-successful coronary revascularization; uncomplicated past MI (>6–8 wk); mild valvular disease; LVD/CHF (NYHA Class I)	Primary-care management Consider all first-line therapies Reassess at 6–12 mo intervals
Intermediate risk	≥3 major risk factors for CAD, excluding gender; moderate, stable angina; recent MI (>2, <6 wk); LVD/CHF (NYHA Class II); noncardiac sequelae of atherosclerotic disease (e.g., CVA, peripheral vascular disease)	Specialized CV testing (e.g., ETT, Echo) Restratification into high risk or low risk based on the results of CV assessment
High risk	Unstable or refractory angina; uncontrolled HTN; LVD/CHF (NYHA class III/IV); recent MI (<2 wk), CVA; high-risk arrhythmias; hypertrophic obstructive and other cardiomyopathies; moderate/severe valvular disease	Priority referral for specialized CV management Treatment for sexual dysfunction to be deferred until cardiac condition stabilized and dependent on specialist recommendations

CAD, coronary artery disease; HTN, hypertension; CHF, congestive heart failure; CVA, cerebrovascular accident (stroke); CVD, cardiovascular disease; Echo, echocardiogram; ETT, exercise tolerance test; LVD, left ventricular dysfunction; NYHA, New York Heart Association; MI, myocardial infarction; CV, cardiovascular.
Adapted with permission from: DeBusk R, Drory Y, Goldstein I, Jackson G, Kaul S, Kimmel SE, et al. Management of sexual dysfunction in patients with cardiovascular disease: Recommendations of the Princeton Consensus Panel. *Am J Cardiol.* 2000;86:175–181.

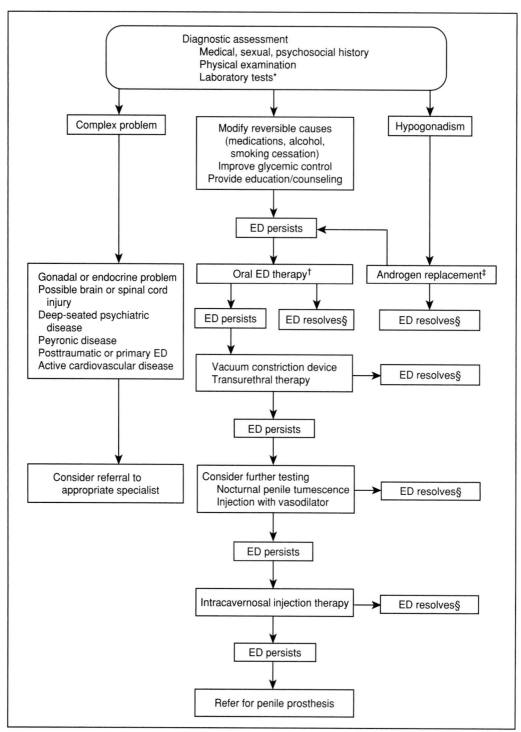

Figure 30-2. Primary management of ED: Treatment algorithm.

*Hemoglobin A$_{1C}$, thyrotropin, and AM total testosterone levels. Testosterone deficiency should be further evaluated by measuring luteinizing hormone, follicle-stimulating hormone, and prolactin levels to elucidate a specific etiology. (Bioavailable testosterone should be considered in men >50 years or body mass index >30 kg/m^3.)

†Phosphodiesterase inhibitors or others.

‡Androgen replacement and oral ED therapy are often initiated simultaneously in men with hypogonadism.

§Perform follow-up and reassessment.

(Reprinted with permission from: Dey J, Shepherd MD. Evaluation and treatment of erectile dysfunction in men with diabetes mellitus. *Mayo Clin Proc*. 2002;77:276–282.)

Table 30-3. Common Medications That Induce ED and Alternative Agents

Medication/ Class Associated with ED	Alternative Agent(s)
Thiazide diuretics, spironolactone	Loop diuretics (furosemide, bumetanide)
Beta-blockers, methyldopa, clonidine, reserpine	Angiotensin-converting-enzyme inhibitors (captopril, enalapril, lisinopril)
	Angiotensin-receptor blockers (losartan, valsartan, candesartan, irbesartan)
	Nebivolol
Finasteride, dutasteride	Alpha-blockers (terazosin, doxazosin, tamsulosin, alfuzosin)
Cimetidine	Other histamine-2 blockers (ranitidine, nizatidine) or proton pump inhibitors (omeprazole, lansoprazole, rabeprazole)
Serotonin reuptake inhibitors, tricyclic antidepressants	Bupropion, mirtazapine, trazodone
Lithium	Valproic acid
Metoclopramide	Erythromycin, proton pump inhibitors
Phenothiazine antipsychotics agents	Atypical antipsychotics (e.g., risperidone, olanzapine, quetiapine, aripiprazole)
Phenytoin, carbamazepine, primidone, phenobarbital	Valproic acid, gabapentin
Digoxin	Diltiazem

Psychological Counseling

Psychological counseling for patients with ED and their partners should play an integral role for any patient demonstrating a psychological component to their ED.[6] Proper psychosexual therapy can improve ED and eliminate need for pharmacologic therapy. Primary care providers can provide reassurance of the normal sexual changes with aging, such as decreased spontaneous erections in men and vaginal dryness in women, and can also encourage couples to seek counseling for relationship problems in general.

Pelvic Floor Muscle Exercises

Men suffering from ED may have weakness in their pelvic floor muscles. Recent reports have suggested that pelvic floor muscle exercises focusing on the bulbocavernosus and ischiocavernosus muscles, which are important for penile rigidity, can improve erectile function. Men can easily implement pelvic floor muscle exercises into their daily routine. For example, in one study, men were instructed to tighten their pelvic floor muscles as strongly as possible twice daily along with additional exercises while walking and after voiding.[11]

Vacuum Devices

The vacuum pump is an effective, noninvasive method of treating ED that is approved by the US Food and Drug Administration (FDA) for over-the-counter distribution. Typically, vacuum pumps are best accepted by men in stable relationships, but they are effective for essentially all types of ED. One report indicates that up to 84% of men are satisfied with results from a vacuum pump device.[12] Electric or battery-powered vacuum devices are the easiest to use, but all require reasonable dexterity. The device draws venous blood into the penis by negative pressure, and the patient must place a tension ring on the base of the penis to maintain the erection. Vacuum devices reduce spontaneity as they take several minutes to create an erection, and the tension ring must be removed after 30 minutes. Typical adverse effects include numbness, bruising, penile pain, delayed ejaculation, and a cyanotic color in the penis, most of which may decrease with improved technique.

Although vacuum pumps are effective and can be considered as first-line therapy, they remain second-line treatments for most patients with ED because of difficulties in use, adverse effects, and cost. However, patients with ED and concomitant severe cardiovascular disease or those taking nitrates are good candidates for vacuum pump therapy.

Other nonpharmacologic interventions include intraurethral inserts and surgical insertion of a penile prosthesis.

PHARMACOLOGIC TREATMENT

Phosphodiesterase Type-5 Inhibitors

Phosphodiesterase type-5 (PDE-5) inhibitors (sildenafil, vardenafil, and tadalafil) are first-line treatment for most men with ED. They increase nitric oxide availability in the penis, allowing men to obtain and maintain an erection with sexual stimulation. Each medication varies slightly in its dosing, onset, and duration (Table 30-4). Sildenafil is the most extensively studied of the three agents and has been found to be about 57% effective overall.[13] Clinically, all three agents are thought to be similarly effective, but some patients may respond to one PDE-5 inhibitor better than another.[14,15] Tadalafil has a longer duration of effect, which can increase spontaneity but also increase duration of side effects. Vardenafil should be avoided in patients with preexisting QT prolongation and in those taking medications such as quinidine, procainamide, sotalol, and amiodarone, which can cause QT prolongation. Choice of PDE-5 inhibitor should be based on effectiveness, safety, cost, and insurance coverage.

Each PDE-5 inhibitor is metabolized by the cytochrome P450 system, and serum concentrations can be

Table 30-4. Phosphodiesterase Type-5 Inhibitors for ED Treatment

	Sildenafil	Vardenafil	Tadalafil
Tablet availability	25, 50, 100 mg	5, 10, 20 mg	5, 10, 20 mg
Starting dose	50 mg daily	10 mg daily	10 mg daily
Onset	30–60 min	30–60 min	30 min–6 h
Duration	4 h	4 h	24–36 h
Best absorption	Empty stomach	Empty stomach	No preference

increased by drugs that inhibit this metabolic system. Thus, the lowest doses of PDE-5 inhibitors are recommended in patients taking cytochrome P450 inhibitors such as erythromycin, clarithromycin, ritonavir, saquinavir, indinavir, ketoconazole, and itraconazole, and dosing intervals may also need to be increased. Maximum concentrations of ritonavir and indinavir can also be decreased significantly by vardenafil, making low-dose sildenafil a better choice for patients taking protease inhibitors. Lower doses of PDE-5 inhibitors are also recommended for the elderly, those with hepatic impairment, and those with severe kidney dysfunction. In patients taking cytochrome P450 enzyme inducers, such as phenytoin, rifampin, phenobarbital, and carbamazepine, concentrations of PDE-5 inhibitors may be decreased. Hence, PDE-5 inhibitor doses may need to be increased if efficacy is not achieved.

Blood pressure should be monitored in patients taking alpha-blockers concomitantly with PDE-5 inhibitors, as hypotension can occur from this drug combination. PDE-5 inhibitors should be initiated at the lowest possible dose in patients already stable on alpha-blockers. If patients are stable on PDE-5 inhibitors, the addition of alpha-blockers should be slow and at the lowest starting dose. Moreover, in patients with benign prostatic hypertrophy requiring combination alpha-blocker and PDE-5 inhibitor therapy, uroselective alpha-blockers such as tamsulosin and alfuzosin are preferred to lessen the risk of hypotension. Patients taking sildenafil, 50 to 100 mg, should separate these doses from those of alpha-blockers by 4 hours, and similar precautions should be taken with the other two PDE-5 inhibitors to reduce the likelihood of hypotensive adverse effects.

Adverse effects that occur in patients taking PDE-5 inhibitors are usually dose related and due to vasodilation or low-affinity inhibition of other PDE enzymes. The most common adverse effects reported in patients taking PDE-5 inhibitors are headache (10–30%), rhinitis (1–11%), flushing (10–20%), dyspepsia (3–16%), myalgia and back pain (0–10%), and dizziness (up to 5%).[16] Rare ocular changes can also occur in patients taking PDE-5 inhibitors, most commonly with sildenafil. Up to 10% of patients may experience reversible problems with color discrimination and sensitivity to light, both related

to PDE-6 inhibition in the rods and cones of the retina. Reports of irreversible vision loss associated with nonarteritic anterior ischemic optic neuropathy (NAION) are rare. The reports of vision loss have mostly been in men older than 50 years with low cup-to-disc ratios or other characteristics commonly associated with arteriosclerosis (and ED): smoking, diabetes, hypertension, coronary artery disease, and hyperlipidemia.[17] A causal relationship between vision loss and use of PDE-5 inhibitors has not been established, but patients should be educated about the potential risk. Moreover, product labeling now discusses NAION and includes instructions for patients with sudden vision loss to stop use of all PDE-5 inhibitors and seek immediate medical attention. It is also recommended that PDE-5 inhibitors be avoided in patients with a previous history of NAION.

Most importantly, use of PDE-5 inhibitors is contraindicated in patients taking any form of nitrates (including as needed sublingual nitroglycerin). The combination of nitrates and PDE-5 inhibitors can cause fatal hypotension-related cardiac or cerebrovascular damage. In patients with cardiac disease, who are not taking nitrates regularly, sexual activity can also precipitate angina and the need to use nitrate therapy. Hence, cardiovascular examination is prudent to help identify patients who might experience an adverse cardiovascular outcome due to sexual activity and taking a PDE-5 inhibitor. Moreover, clinical experience regarding use of PDE-5 inhibitors is lacking in patients with recent myocardial infarction, stroke, arrhythmias, unstable angina, hypotension (less than 90/50 mm Hg), and uncontrolled hypertension (greater than 170/110 mm Hg). If a patient taking a PDE-5 inhibitor experiences chest pain or signs and symptoms of a cardiovascular or cerebrovascular event, they should be instructed to seek care immediately at an emergency department, making sure to let the emergency staff know they took a PDE-5 inhibitor. In general, nitrates should be withheld for 24 hours after a dose of sildenafil or vardenafil and for 48 hours after a dose of tadalafil.

Testosterone Replacement

Testosterone replacement may improve erectile function and libido, but should be recommended only for men with hypogonadism. Testosterone therapy is contraindicated in patients with prostate or breast cancer and should be used cautiously in patients with benign prostatic hypertrophy, sleep apnea, peripheral edema, congestive heart failure, polycythemia, and hepatic disease. Before exogenous testosterone is initiated, patients should be screened with a prostate specific antigen, aspartate amino transferase, alanine amino transferase, fasting lipid panel, hematocrit, and hemoglobin. Once patients are treated with testosterone, the above laboratory monitoring should be repeated within a few months and then every 6 to 12 months to assess for adverse effects. Free and/or bioavailable testosterone concentrations should also be monitored after treatment to assess efficacy.

Three different routes of testosterone replacement exist: intramuscular, transdermal, and buccal. Intramuscular testosterone enanthate, 200 mg, or testosterone cypionate, 300 mg, is administered approximately every 2 to 3 weeks; the dosing and frequency are based on testosterone concentrations just before the next injection. Initial dosing should be lower in elderly men. If concentrations are too high, the dose should be decreased or the interval between doses increased. Alternatively, if testosterone concentrations are too low, the dose should be increased or the interval shortened. Intramuscular injection of testosterone often results in more erratic concentrations than other routes, so its use has declined as other options have become available.

Transdermal testosterone is available as scrotal and nonscrotal patches and gel. Scrotal patches are rarely used because of the need to shave the scrotum before application. Nonscrotal testosterone patches are available in 2.5 mg and 5 mg patches, but dosing can be increased to 7.5 mg (using one of each patch), if necessary. Nonscrotal patches are placed on the back, abdomen, upper arms, or thighs every evening. Patch placement should be rotated to prevent site reactions, and sites should not be reused for 7 days. Morning testosterone concentrations in patients using patches can be measured after 1 day of therapy to assess efficacy. Testosterone patches typically provide more stable concentrations of testosterone than intramuscular injections. However, testosterone gel has now become the preferred method of testosterone replacement for most patients, due to increased testosterone concentration stability and low incidence of site reactions. Testosterone 1% gel is initiated at 2.5 to 5 g daily, applied to the shoulders, upper arms, or abdomen. Morning testosterone concentrations should be measured after 2 weeks of therapy and the dose increased to 7.5 g or 10 g, if necessary. Site reactions are reduced if application sites are rotated, and patients should be counseled to avoid showering, washing, or skin contact with partners for 4 to 6 hours after application to prevent testosterone loss and/or transfer.

Buccal testosterone has been available since 2003, and it offers an additional mechanism for testosterone delivery. The system is inserted above an incisor tooth twice daily, and patients should remove the old system and rotate sides of the mouth with each dose. Patients should also verify that the system is still in place after eating, drinking, brushing teeth, and rinsing the mouth. Typical adverse effects include gum irritation, pain, tenderness, edema, bitter taste, and headache. Morning testosterone concentrations should be monitored after 4 to 12 weeks to assess for efficacy.

The type of testosterone replacement should be guided by patient preference for route and risk of adverse reactions. In general, adverse reactions are usually route and dose related. Application site reactions are the most common adverse effect, occurring in at least one-half of patients using patches and in approximately 5% of men using transdermal gel. Site reactions due to patches can be decreased if triamcinolone cream, 0.1%, is applied under the central drug reservoir of the patch. All patients prescribed testosterone therapy should also be monitored for acne, prostate/urinary problems, peripheral edema, increased cholesterol, decreased high-density lipoprotein cholesterol, increased liver function tests, increased level of prostate specific antigen, and increased hematocrit or hemoglobin.

If responsive to testosterone replacement, erectile function and libido should increase slowly over a few months of testosterone treatment. If results are not satisfactory, other treatments for ED should be initiated. Concomitant treatment with PDE-5 inhibitors and testosterone are appropriate for patients with moderate to severe ED. Patients with more complicated ED, difficult-to-regulate testosterone concentrations, or laboratory abnormalities should be referred to an endocrinologist and/or urologist.

Vasodilatory Treatments

Intraurethral alprostadil and intracavernosal alprostadil, papaverine, and phentolamine are available vasodilatory treatments for ED. Each drug relaxes smooth muscles and induces vasodilation. Although the intracavernosal route is slightly more effective than the intraurethral route (approximately 70–90%, compared with up to 60%), intraurethral suppositories can be prescribed by primary care providers and are usually recommended as second-line therapy because they are easy to use. The initial dose of intraurethral alprostadil is 125 mcg, onset of action is within 5 to 10 minutes, and duration of activity is approximately 30 to 60 minutes. Doses may be doubled over time up to 1000 mcg to establish efficacy, but no more than 2 doses per day should be used. The first dose should also be observed by a health care provider due to risk of syncope. Typical adverse effects include penile pain (32%) and urethral burning (12%). Patients receiving unsatisfactory results from intraurethral suppositories can use it in combination with an adjustable penile constriction band, but adverse effects may increase.

Intracavernosal routes require physician-established dosing and monitoring and are thus recommended as third-line treatments for more difficult-to-treat patients. Intracavernosal alprostadil is the only agent administered via this route that is approved by the FDA for ED. Patients wishing to attempt this treatment should be referred to a urologist or endocrinologist. This route should be avoided in anticoagulated patients. After instruction by a medical provider and verification of efficacy, patients can administer their doses at home. The onset of action is within 10 minutes and the erection may last for 30 to 60 minutes. However, adverse effects can be extensive and include penile pain (37%), cavernosal fibrosis/scarring (3–8%), hematoma (3%), ecchymosis (2%), and, rarely, priapism (0.4%). Oral decongestants, such as pseudoephedrine, can be recommended for patients experiencing prolonged erections secondary to alprostadil. However, emergency department treatment should be recommended for any patient with priapism (painful erection lasting longer than 4 hours), as permanent damage to the corpora cavernosa may occur.

Alternative Agents

Sublingual apomorphine, oral phentolamine, and oral yohimbine are unapproved alternative agents used by some practitioners for ED treatment. Although approved for use in Europe, Mexico, and South America, sublingual apomorphine was denied approval by the FDA in 2003 and will not be marketed in the United States. Apomorphine is a centrally acting dopamine agonist that can be used to treat ED in patients taking nitrates. It is less effective than PDE-5 inhibitors and can cause nausea, dizziness, drowsiness, yawning, and headache.

Oral phentolamine is a vasodilator approved for use in Mexico and Brazil, but approval is not being pursued in the United States because of a perceived lack of market for an additional oral agent. Typical adverse effects include nasal congestion, headache, tachycardia, dizziness, and nausea, and it should not be used in combination with PDE-5 inhibitors.

Yohimbine, marketed in the United States as a dietary supplement, is an alpha-2 antagonist that has uncertain efficacy for ED. Typical adverse effects include headache, dizziness, hypertension, insomnia, and anxiety. Because yohimbine is not regulated as a drug by the FDA, recommending it could present additional unknown risks to the patient. In addition, yohimbine was named one of "12 supplements you should avoid," by the May 2004 issue of *Consumer Reports*, as it is

"likely hazardous" with reports of deaths and cardiovascular adverse effects and events associated with its use.[18]

TREATMENT FAILURE

Patients failing treatment with PDE-5 inhibitors may receive some benefit from combination therapy with alprostadil, a vacuum device, psychotherapy, or pelvic floor muscle exercises. However, prolonged erections and priapism have developed in some patients using combination sildenafil and alprostadil. Vacuum devices can also be used in combination with psychotherapy in patients with psychosexual problems. If a patient fails one of the above combination therapies, they likely have a more complex form of ED and should be referred to a urologist for further evaluation. Penile prostheses are also available for refractory cases or those who have contraindications to other treatments.

FUTURE TREATMENTS

New agents are being investigated for the treatment of ED. One new drug class being investigated is the melanocortin-agonist class. This class affects the central nervous system rather than directly affecting the vascular system like some other available agents.

EVIDENCE-BASED SUMMARY

- Risk factors for ED include conditions such as hypertension, dyslipidemia, diabetes, and depression; social factors such as smoking, alcohol, and drug use; and drugs such as antidepressants, diuretics, beta-blockers, cimetidine, and 5-alpha reductase inhibitors.
- Cardiovascular risk factors should be assessed in most patients presenting with ED, and patients with intermediate to high cardiovascular risk should receive cardiologic testing prior to ED treatment.
- Nonpharmacologic therapy such as risk-factor modification, counseling, pelvic floor muscle exercises, and vacuum devices are effective for ED and can be attempted first-line in many patients.
- Sildenafil, vardenafil, and tadalafil are effective pharmacologic therapy for most patients, and dosing should be based on age, concomitant medications, and kidney and liver function.
- Sildenafil, vardenafil, and tadalafil should not be utilized in patients with severe cardiovascular diseases or those taking nitrates.
- Testosterone replacement is recommended for patients with hypogonadism.

REFERENCES

1. NIH Consensus Development Panel on Impotence. Impotence. *JAMA.* 1993;270:83–90.
2. Feldman HA, Goldstein I, Hatzichristou DG, Krane RJ, McKinlay JB. Impotence and its medical and psychosocial correlates: Results of the Massachusetts Male Aging Study. *J Urol.* 1994;151:54–61.
3. Thompson IM, Tangen CM, Goodman PJ, Probstfield JI, Moinpour CM, Coltman CA. Erectile dysfunction and subsequent cardiovascular disease. *JAMA.* 2005;294:2996–3002.
4. Billups KL. Erectile dysfunction as an early sign of cardiovascular disease. *Int J Impot Res.* 2005;17:S19–S24.
5. Rosen RC, Cappelleri JC, Smith MD, Lipsky J, Pena BM. Development and evaluation of an abridged, 5-item version of the International Index of Erectile Function (IIEF-5) as a diagnostic tool for erectile dysfunction. *Int J Impot Res.* 1999;11:319–326.
6. American Association of Clinical Endocrinologists. Medical guidelines for clinical practice for the evaluation and treatment of male sexual dysfunction: A couple's problem—2003 update. *Endocr Pract.* 2003;9:78–95.
7. DeBusk R, Drory Y, Goldstein I, et al. Management of sexual dysfunction in patients with cardiovascular disease: Recommendations of the Princeton Consensus Panel. *Am J Cardiol.* 2000;86:175–181.
8. Kostis JB, Jackson G, Rosen R, et al. Sexual dysfunction and cardiac risk (the Second Princeton Consensus Conference). *Am J Cardiol.* 2005;96:313–321.
9. Keene LC, Davies PH. Drug-related erectile dysfunction. *Adverse Drug React Toxicol Rev.* 1999;18:5–24.
10. Hafez ESE, Hafez SD. Erectile dysfunction: Anatomical parameters, etiology, diagnosis and therapy. *Arch Androl.* 2005;51:15–31.
11. Dorey G, Speakman MJ, Feneley RCL, Swinkels A, Dunn CDR. Pelvic floor exercises for erectile dysfunction. *BJU Int.* 2005;96:595–597.
12. Cookson MS, Nadig PW. Long-term results with vacuum constriction device. *J Urol.* 1993;290–294.
13. Fink HA, MacDonald R, Rutks IR, Nelson DB, Wilt TJ. Sildenafil for male erectile dysfunction. A systematic review and meta-analysis. *Arch Intern Med.* 2002;162:1349–1360.
14. Moore RA, Derry S, McQuay HJ. Indirect comparison of interventions using published randomised trials: Systematic review of PDE-5 inhibitors for erectile dysfunction. *BMC Urol.* 2005;5:18.
15. Stroberg P, Hedelin H, Ljunggren C. Prescribing all phosphodiesterase 5 inhibitors to a patient with erectile dysfunction—A realistic and feasible option in everyday clinical practice—Outcomes of a simple treatment regime. *Eur Urol.* 2006;49:900–907.
16. Mikhail N. Management of erectile dysfunction by the primary care physician. *Cleve Clin J Med.* 2005;72:293–310.
17. Anonymous. Viagra and loss of vision. *Med Lett Drugs Ther.* 2005;47:49.
18. Anonymous. Twelve supplements you should avoid. *Consumer Rep* 2004(May). Available at www.consumerreports.org/cro/health-fitness/drugs-supplements/dangerous-supplements-504/12-supplements-to-avoid/index.htm. Accessed March 3, 2007.

Chapter 31

Benign Prostatic Hyperplasia

Nicole Murdock, Ronald Solbing, and Cara Liday

SEARCH STRATEGY

A systematic search of medical literature was performed on July 21, 2005, and again on August 8, 2007, for relevant clinical trials and reviews using the terms *benign prostatic hyperplasia, BPH, lower urinary tract symptoms, LUTS, alpha-receptor antagonists, alpha-blockers, and 5-alpha-reductase inhibitors.* The search, limited to human subjects and journals in English language, included the Cochrane database, PubMed, and UpToDate®.

Benign prostatic hyperplasia (BPH) is a very common condition in aging men. Lower urinary tract symptoms (LUTS) are the clinical hallmark of BPH. Diagnosis of BPH is a process of exclusion of other potential causes of LUTS through history, physical examination, and selected laboratory tests. Once BPH is diagnosed, treatment may be safely undertaken using pharmacologic and/or surgical interventions.

The prostate is a chestnut-shaped gland responsible for the production of the milky fluid discharged during male ejaculation. It is also structured similar to a doughnut, with the male urethra passing through the doughnut hole, and it is highly innervated with alpha-1 adrenergic receptors (Fig. 31-1). BPH is common in men due to age and testosterone-related enlargement of the prostate. Smoking, ethnic origin, chronic diseases, and other factors may relate to enlargement of the prostate, but these have not been well defined. At autopsy, pathologically demonstrated BPH is frequently found in men, including about 8% of men, aged 30 to 40 years, 50% of men, aged 50 to 60 years, and more than 80% of men older than 70 years.[1,2] One study found a 45% chance that a 45-year-old asymptomatic man who lives to the age of 75 will develop symptomatic BPH.[3]

CLINICAL PRESENTATION

LUTS are the hallmark of symptomatic BPH. LUTS include weak stream, frequency, nocturia, intermittent stream, incomplete emptying, straining, and urgency. The American Urological Association (AUA) has developed a tool called the "Symptom Index for BPH" used to quantify the subjective symptom severity,[4] which asks the patient to grade the severity of these seven symptoms on a scale from 0 to 5. The score can help guide the need for intervention as well as evaluate efficacy of treatment.

Complications of BPH include acute urinary retention, urinary tract infection, chronic renal failure, overflow urinary incontinence, bladder stones, and the need for prostate surgery (including subsequent adverse effects discussed in the section on "Surgery").

PHYSICAL FINDINGS AND DIAGNOSTIC EVALUATION

The goal of the initial evaluation—history, physical examination, and laboratory tests—is to identify other medical conditions that might be the cause of LUTS so that an appropriate treatment can be instituted. Table 31-1 presents a summary of the diagnostic evaluation.[4,6]

To help identify underlying conditions, a thorough history should be taken. This includes detailed questions about prior urinary infections or surgeries, age at onset of symptoms, and known anatomic abnormalities. Diabetes, neurologic disorders, back injuries, stroke, and central nervous system trauma may suggest a neurogenic bladder (one that cannot contract normally due to inadequate innervation). Prior urologic instrumentation, urologic surgery, or urethritis raises the possibility of urethral stricture as a source of LUTS.

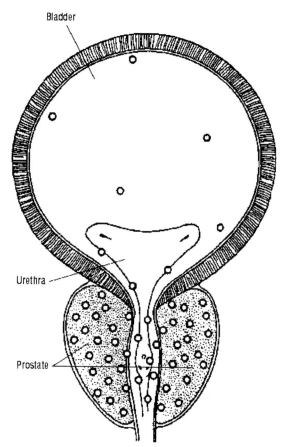

Bladder

Urethra

Prostate

Figure 31-1. Representation of the anatomy of and alpha-adrenergic receptor distribution in the prostate, urethra, and bladder. (From Narayan P, Indudhara R. *West J Med*. 1994;161:501. Reproduced with permission from the BMJ Publishing Group.)

Several medications can worsen LUTS, including some nonprescription drugs, dietary supplements, and drugs of abuse (Table 31-2). Drugs with sympathetic or anticholinergic properties are particularly likely to interfere with normal urinary functioning. Modification of medications that compromise urinary functioning may improve or resolve the LUTS regardless of other etiologies.

Physical examination should include a digital rectal examination to assess the prostate size and consistency as well as rectal sphincter tone. In BPH, the prostate gland is enlarged and has a smooth consistency. If nodules, asymmetry, or induration are found on examination, other diagnoses must be investigated, including cancer and infection.

A neurologic examination of the lower extremities should be performed, evaluating for neuromuscular diseases that may interfere with urinary function.

A urinalysis should be performed and evaluated to check for the presence of blood or infection.[4] Hematuria

Table 31-1. Diagnostic Evaluation of Men With Lower Urinary Tract Symptoms (LUTS)[4,5]

History
- Rule out other etiologies for LUTS
  - Prior urinary infections or surgeries
  - Age at onset of symptoms
  - Known anatomic abnormalities
  - Other diseases known to cause LUTS (e.g., diabetes mellitus, neurologic disorders, back injuries, stroke)
  - Use of medications known to cause or worsen LUTS (see Table 31-2)

Physical Examination
- Digital rectal examination (DRE)
  - Prostate size and consistency
  - Rectal sphincter tone
- Neurologic examination of lower extremities
  - Assess any neurologic deficiencies that may affect urinary function

Laboratory Tests
- Urinalysis
  - Hematuria
  - Proteinuria
  - Infection
- Prostate specific antigen assay
  - Determine risk for prostate cancer, may be elevated in benign prostatic hyperplasia as well

Other Studies
- Urine cytology: Cystoscopy
- Urinary flow studies: Prostate ultrasound
- Postvoid residual

Table 31-2. Medications That May Produce or Worsen Lower Urinary Tract Symptoms

Anticholinergic products	Mechanism: Decrease bladder detrusor muscle contractibility, causing a weakened ability to contract bladder to force urine out
	Agents: Tricyclic antidepressants
	Antispasmodic agents (e.g., dicyclomine, oxybutynin)
	First-generation antihistamines (e.g., diphenhydramine)
	Antiparkinson drugs (e.g., benztropine)
	Some muscle relaxants
	Some antipsychotic agents (e.g., clozapine, thioridazine)
Sympathomimetic products	Mechanism: Stimulates alpha-adrenergic receptors causing constriction of the prostate and urethra
	Agents: Pseudoephedrine, oxymetazoline (Afrin), ephedrine
Opioid analgesics	Mechanism: Urinary retention
	Agents: Narcotic analgesics (e.g., oxycodone, morphine)
Diuretics	Mechanism: Increased urinary frequency
	Agents: All types of diuretics (e.g., furosemide, torsemide)

and proteinuria require evaluation for urinary pathology that may not be related to BPH.

Further evaluation, if indicated by history and physical examination, may include prostate specific antigen (PSA), postvoid residual (PVR) measurement, urine cytology, urinary flow studies, cystoscopy, and prostate ultrasound. PSA and PVR are easily done in a primary care office. The remaining tests usually require urologic consultation. PVR volume is the urine volume remaining in the bladder after complete spontaneous emptying has been attempted by the patient. PSA is used to screen for prostate cancer, although BPH may elevate this to some extent. The age of the patient and the absolute level of PSA elevation have been shown to be related to the risk of prostate enlargement and adverse events from BPH.[6] This information may allow selection of individuals who need closer surveillance and earlier treatment for prostate enlargement; however, clinical application of this data is still uncertain. If moderate-to-severe symptoms are reported by the patient, urinary flow studies may indicate the degree of bladder outlet obstruction or detrusor dysfunctions.

RISK STRATIFICATION

Treatment of BPH is guided by the degree to which symptoms are bothersome to the patient. Validated tools have been designed to stratify the severity of these symptoms. The AUA Symptom Score defines 0 to 7 as mild, 8 to 19 as moderate, and 20 or greater as severe (Table 31-3). This tool consists of seven questions about LUTS the patient may be experiencing. The survey asks the patient to rank the severity of the symptoms on a scale of 0 to 5 (5 being most severe). The International Prostate Symptom Score[7] is identical to the AUA Index but also includes the question: "If you were to spend the rest of your life with your urinary condition just the way it is now, how would you feel about that?" This additional question is important as it serves to clarify the patient's perception of the impact of the LUTS on his life. If the patient is not bothered by symptoms, no treatment may be needed. Routine use of one of these measurement instruments is recommended for all patients with symptomatic BPH to assist in diagnosis and to measure the efficacy of therapeutic interventions.

MANAGEMENT

When considering treatment for LUTS, patients are stratified into three groups using the AUA symptom index (Table 31-3). Recommendations for BPH treatment can be found in the AUA Guideline on Management of BPH.[4] Treatment of BPH consists of lifestyle modification (any symptoms), watchful waiting (mild symptoms), pharmacotherapy (mild and moderate symptoms), and/or surgery (severe symptoms). Treatment decisions may be based on criteria set by the AUA and are summarized in Fig. 31-2. These criteria have been set somewhat arbitrarily, and the decision to treat should include patient preference and individualized benefit and risk, including comorbidities that may exclude some types of treatment (i.e., alpha blockers in ventricular systolic dysfunction). Therapeutic goals include relieving symptoms, delaying disease progression, preventing complications of BPH, minimizing adverse effects, and ultimately improving the patient's quality of life.

Lifestyle modifications should be suggested to all patients with LUTS. These include limiting fluid intake in the evening, especially those containing alcohol or caffeine (both of which can trigger urination urge). Educate patients to take the time to empty their bladder completely and often. As discussed in the initial evaluation, educate patients about the medications to avoid (Table 31-2).

Watchful waiting is recommended for patients with mild LUTS. In some patients, symptoms may improve or stabilize without treatment while in others it may progress over time. Watchful waiting comprises reassessment of

Table 31-3. Categories of BPH Disease Severity Based on Symptoms and Signs

Disease Severity	AUA Symptom Score	Typical Symptoms and Signs
Mild	#7	Asymptomatic Peak urinary flow rate, 10 mL/s Postvoid residual urine volume >25–50 mL Increased BUN and serum creatinine
Moderate	8–19	All the above signs plus obstructive voiding symptoms and irritative voiding symptoms (signs of detrusor instability)
Severe	≥20	All the above plus one or more complications of BPH

AUA, American Urological Association; BUN, blood urea nitrogen.
Reprinted with permission from: Lee M. *Management of benign prostatic hyperplasia*. In: DiPiro JT, Talbert RL, Yee GC, et al. eds. *Pharmacotherapy: A Pathophysiologic Approach*. 7th ed. New York, NY: McGraw-Hill; 2008.

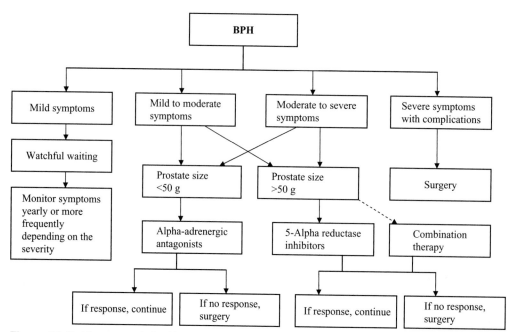

Figure 31-2. Management algorithm for benign prostatic hyperplasia.
(Adapted with permission from Lee M. *Management of benign prostatic hyperplasia*. In: DiPiro JT, Talbert RL, Yee GC, et al., eds. *Pharmacotherapy: A Pathophysiologic Approach*, 7th ed. New York, NY: McGraw-Hill; 2008.)

symptoms on an annual basis or more frequently, depending on symptom severity and rate of progression. Reassessment should include completion of a survey tool (i.e., AUA Symptom Index for BPH) to help determine changes in symptom severity. This is particularly useful if symptoms have worsened or are more bothersome to the patient. A subsequent workup, as previously described in initial evaluation, should follow as necessary. For patients who are symptomatic, watchful waiting may lead to worsening PVR urine volumes, infection, and many other BPH complications. For these reasons, watchful waiting should not be recommended for patients with moderate-to-severe LUTS.

PHARMACOTHERAPY

Pharmacotherapy is first-line treatment for men with moderate LUTS. Medications are reversible, safe, and noninvasive and provide significant symptomatic improvement. However, pharmacotherapy is considered an interim therapy in most patients, as medications at best either manage symptoms without affecting disease progression or only slow the progression of BPH complications and thereby delay the inevitable need for surgical intervention.

The two drug classes approved by the Food and Drug Administration (FDA) for the treatment of BPH symptoms are alpha-adrenergic antagonists and 5-alpha

reductase inhibitors. Other therapies include antiandrogenic compounds, gonadotropin-releasing hormone agonists, and herbal products. These therapies are less desirable as they have not been well studied and may have objectionable adverse effects.

ALPHA-1 ADRENERGIC ANTAGONISTS

The prostate gland is highly innervated, predominantly by alpha-1 adrenergic receptors (Fig. 31-1).[8] Stimulation of these receptors by catecholamines, such as norepinephrine, causes contraction of the tissue, leading to compression of the urethra resulting in LUTS as discussed above. Alpha-adrenergic antagonists, which promote smooth-muscle relaxation in both the prostate and bladder neck and thereby decrease obstruction and allow urination to proceed, are approved by the FDA for the treatment of BPH (Table 31-4).[4,6,9–16] These include the second-generation agents doxazosin (Cardura®), terazosin (Hytrin®), and alfuzosin (Uroxatral®), and the third-generation agent tamsulosin (Flomax®). Prazosin (Minipress®), a second-generation alpha-1 antagonist, requires multiple daily doses and has considerable cardiovascular effects; it is therefore not recommended or FDA approved for use in BPH.

The alpha-1 adrenergic antagonists that are approved for treatment of BPH seem to have comparable efficacy, although few direct comparisons have been performed.

Table 31-4. Comparison of Treatments for BPH[4,6,9–16]

Class	Alpha-antagonists				5-Alpha reductase inhibitors	
Generation		Second		Third		
Descriptor	Alfuzosin (Uroxatral®)	Doxazosin (Cardura®)	Terazosin (Hytrin®)	Tamsulosin (Flomax®)	Finasteride (Proscar®)	Dutasteride (Avodart®)
Available strengths	10 mg extended release	1, 2, 4, 8 mg	1, 2, 5, 10 mg	0.4 mg	5 mg	0.5 mg
Initial dosage in healthy adults	10 mg daily	1 mg at bedtime; titrate up depending on efficacy over several weeks	1 mg at bedtime; titrate up depending on efficacy over several weeks	0.4 mg; may titrate up to 0.8 mg after 2–4 wk, if symptoms are not controlled	5 mg	0.5 mg
Dosing range for healthy adults	10 mg	1–8 mg	1–10 mg	0.4–0.8 mg	5 mg	0.5 mg
Use in renal impairment	Caution in severe renal dysfunction	Actions may be prolonged	Yes	Yes	Yes	Yes
Use in hepatic impairment	Contraindicated in Child–Pugh B and C classification	Close monitoring, if used at all	Precaution in severe cases	Yes	Caution in severe disease	Caution; dosage adjustment may be necessary in severe disease
Time to effect of BPH symptoms	1–2 d	2–4 wk	2–4 wk	1–2 d		~6 mo
Average increase in urinary flow rates (mL/s)			2–3			1.6–2.0
Decreases prostate size?		No	No			Yes, by 25%
Decreases PSA?		No	No		Yes, by ~40%–50%*	
Adverse effects (major)	• Least amount of ejaculatory problems	• Orthostatic hypotension • Cardiovascular effects • Ejaculatory dysfunction • Fatigue		• Highest rate of ejaculatory problems (with alpha-antagonists) • Preferred alpha-antagonist in patients with underlying coronary disease, decreased circulatory volume, orthostasis, or cardiac arrhythmias	• Erectile dysfunction (higher than with alpha-antagonists) • Ejaculatory problems	

(continued)

341

Table 31-4. Comparison of Treatments for BPH[4,6,9–16] (Continued)

	Alfuzosin (Uroxatral®)	Doxazosin (Cardura®)	Terazosin (Hytrin®)	Tamsulosin (Flomax®)	Finasteride (Proscar®)	Dutasteride (Avodart®)
Class	Alpha-antagonists				5-Alpha reductase inhibitors	
Generation		Second		Third		
Descriptor	Alfuzosin (Uroxatral®)	Doxazosin (Cardura®)	Terazosin (Hytrin®)	Tamsulosin (Flomax®)	Finasteride (Proscar®)	Dutasteride (Avodart®)
Duration of efficacy	Medications will lose effect, if discontinued by patient in 1–2 d				Unknown how long effects may last; will eventually wear off by 3–12 mo	
Elimination half-life (h)	10	19–22	12	14–15	6–8	5 wk
Metabolism	Hepatic	Hepatic	Hepatic	Hepatic	Hepatic	Hepatic
Take with food	Yes	With or without	With or without	No	With or without	With or without
Clinically relevant drug interactions	• CYP 3A4 inhibitors (e.g., ketoconazole) • Phosphodiesterase inhibitors • With other medications that prolong the QT interval (sotalol, amiodarone, erythromycin)	• Phosphodiesterase inhibitors • Antihypertensive agents		• May be taken safely with phosphodiesterase inhibitors (specifically tadalafil) at lowest doses possible	• None	• CYP 3A4 inhibitors (e.g., ketoconazole)
Patient instructions	• Take with same meal each day • Do not crush or chew tablets	• Rise slowly from sitting/lying position as this drug may cause dizziness • May experience syncope or dizziness with first dose • Take at bedtime to minimize side effects of dizziness		• Patient should take drug 30 min after the same meal each day • Do not crush, chew, or open capsules	• Women of childbearing age (including health professionals) should not handle tablets due to potential teratogenicity • May cause impotence • (Dutasteride) Do not donate blood for at least 6 months after last dose (to avoid pregnant female receiving blood containing drug) • No cardiovascular adverse effects are associated with these agents	
Cost†	Brand $81	Generic $20–24 Brand $45–50	Generic $14–36 Brand $67	Brand $80–160	Generic $70 Brand $93	Brand $92

*For valid interpretation of laboratory results, consider doubling the PSA in patients taking these medications.
†30-day supply ranging from lowest to highest dose possible. (Cited from http://www.drugstore.com. Accessed August 19, 2007.)

Studies show that they increase urinary flow rates and reduce PVR volume, but have little effect on prostate size.

The second-generation agents in this class are administered once or twice daily. With the exception of alfuzosin, the second-generation agents are nonselective alpha-1-antagonists. They block prostatic alpha-1 receptors, as well as alpha-receptors found on the peripheral vasculature, which results in vasodilatation. Because of this nonselectivity, orthostatic hypotension may occur, particularly first-dose syncope. Patients should be started on low doses initially, with slow titration over 4 to 8 weeks. Patients should take these agents at bedtime to minimize orthostatic effects.

The effects of these agents on blood pressure can be either beneficial or excessive, depending on the particular patient situation. In patients with hypertension who are already on hypotensive agents, second-generation alpha-1 adrenergic antagonists should generally be avoided or used with caution, as blood pressures may be lowered too much. However, in those whose hypertension is inadequately treated, the agents may be preferred for their additional hypotensive effects.

As seen in the Antihypertensive and Lipid-Lowering Treatment to Prevent Heart Attack Trial, more patients treated with the alpha-antagonist doxazosin as monotherapy for hypertension developed congestive heart failure than did patients on other antihypertensive therapies.[12] These agents are thus not recommended for lone treatment for high blood pressure in patients with BPH and hypertension.[12,13] Alfuzosin is the exception among the second-generation agents. Compared with the other agents in this category, it is more uroselective and therefore unlikely to result in hypotensive or congestive heart failure adverse effects.[13]

Tamsulosin, the only third-generation agent, is selective for urologic alpha-1A adrenergic receptors. These account for 70% of the alpha-1 receptors in the prostate.[14,15] Antagonism of these receptors allows for the prostatic effects without peripheral vascular dilation. Tamsulosin, unlike the other alpha-antagonists, has very little blood pressure lowering effect and as a result, dose titration is unnecessary. However, two doses are recommended, and therapy should be initiated with the lower dose, 0.4 mg once daily. This may be increased to 0.8 mg daily after 2 to 4 weeks if symptoms are not controlled with the lower dose.

When selecting an alpha-blocking agent for a patient with BPH, therapy should be individualized. Doxazosin and terazosin, which may be beneficial in patients who need additional blood-pressure-lowering effects, are less expensive than alfuzosin and tamsulosin. On the other hand, tamsulosin or alfuzosin may be used in patients who are on other antihypertensive agents without having an additive hypotensive effect. Severe life-threatening hypotension has been reported when terazosin or doxazosin are used concomitantly with phosphodiesterase inhibitors such as sildenafil or vardenafil. Tamsulosin may be used cautiously in men with erectile dysfunction being treated with these agents because its selectivity reduces the likelihood of severe hypotension.

The benefits seen with the alpha-antagonists are seen only during current therapy; symptoms are likely to recur if the patient discontinues the medication. If LUTS worsen while on pharmacologic treatments, the patient should be reassessed for dosage increase or the need for surgical intervention.

5-ALPHA REDUCTASE INHIBITORS

Two 5-alpha reductase inhibitors are approved by the FDA for treatment of BPH, finasteride (Proscar®) and dutasteride (Avodart®). These drugs reduce prostate size by inhibiting enzymes that convert testosterone to an active metabolite dihydrotestosterone (DHT). These agents are most useful for patients with a prostate of 50 g or more in size.[16–18] As a result of reduction in prostate size, symptoms—including urinary flow, urgency, and frequency—improve in many patients. Unfortunately, the therapy generally takes 6 to 12 months before prostate size is adequately reduced to improve symptoms. Serum PSA concentrations decrease by about 50% during therapy with these agents. This should be considered when using this marker to determine the risk of prostate cancer, as values may appear falsely normal or even low.

Dutasteride is an inhibitor of both types of 5-alpha reductase enzymes, whereas finasteride inhibits only type II. As a result, dutasteride may be more potent although no direct comparisons have been performed. The major adverse effects of these agents include decreased libido and ejaculatory dysfunction; some studies indicate that these may worsen during the first year of therapy.

These agents appear most useful in men with moderate-to-severe symptoms and an enlarged prostate. Unlike alpha-antagonists, 5-alpha reductase inhibitors have been shown to delay the progression of BPH complications and the need for surgery.[18] They may also be preferred in patients with BPH who have uncontrolled arrhythmias or unstable angina, are on antihypertensive agents, or are unable to tolerate the hypotensive adverse effects of the second-generation alpha-antagonists. The overall percentage of patients who report improvement in BPH symptoms is lower and sexual dysfunction more prevalent with 5-alpha reductase inhibitors than with alpha-blockers. In addition, the delayed onset of action of 5-alpha reductase inhibitors is not ideal for patients with bothersome symptoms. In men with less severe disease and smaller prostate volumes, alpha-blockers may be more beneficial.

COMBINATION THERAPY

For patients with severe symptoms and an enlarged prostate (40–50 g), combination therapy may be beneficial. When beginning concomitant therapy with agents in both classes, the alpha-blocker improves symptoms within days and the 5-alpha reductase inhibitor after 6 months. Some studies have shown no difference in improvement with combination therapy as compared to alpha-antagonist therapy alone, although the short duration of trials limited their sensitivity to an effect of 5-alpha reductase inhibitors.[18–20] The Medical Therapy of Prostatic Symptoms Study showed that combination therapy reduces the risk of symptom progression and development of BPH complications.[5] This area needs further evaluation, but if a patient has a large prostate and moderate-to-severe symptoms, combination therapy is a logical treatment approach, despite the increased cost and risk of adverse effects. Ejaculatory dysfunction in particular may be more likely when initiating or continuing combination therapy.

ALTERNATIVE THERAPIES

Several herbal therapies are marketed in the United States for prostate health. These include saw palmetto, stinging nettle, and African plum. Saw palmetto has been studied more extensively than other herbal remedies for BPH. It is believed to act through both inhibition of 5-alpha reductase and blockade of adrenergic receptors. Symptom reduction occurs approximately 1 month after the initiation of the therapy.

Herbal agents are not FDA regulated and therefore not recommended for use in men with BPH. Clinical trials of saw palmetto have yielded mixed results, with the most recently published study of 225 men showing no improvement in symptoms or objective measures of BPH during a 1-year comparison with placebo.[21,22]

MONITORING

Monitoring for pharmacotherapy efficacy includes reassessment of the patient's symptoms using the AUA Symptom Index or other validated tools. Other workups may include repetition of initial evaluation as discussed previously. If alpha-blockers are used, blood pressure and heart rate as well as orthostatic changes should be assessed at each visit. Frequency of follow-up is contingent upon the severity of symptoms and may range from every 3 months, for those patients with severe symptoms, to once a year, for patients with mild symptoms. A change in therapy, including increased dosage or surgical intervention, is warranted if the LUTS do not improve or worsen. PSA levels may be falsely normal or even low when the patient is on a 5-alpha reductase inhibitor. Some physicians believe that PSA levels should be doubled if the patient is on this class of medications.

SURGERY

Surgery is indicated for patients with moderate to severe symptoms or those unresponsive or nonadherent with pharmacotherapy. It may be required in patients whose symptoms worsen or complications arise while on pharmacotherapy. Such cases include recurrent urinary tract infections, recurrent or persistent gross hematuria, bladder stones, renal insufficiency, or refractory urinary retention. When considering surgery for a patient, referral to a urologist is appropriate to discuss all options. The Agency for Health Care Policy and Research (AHCPR) Clinical Practice Guidelines provides information for invasive procedures that have undergone prolonged use and evaluation before 1994.[23] There are currently several minimally invasive surgeries/therapies for treating the associated symptoms of BPH. Surgical options include transurethral resection of the prostate (TURP), transurethral incision of the prostate (TUIP), and transurethral vaporization (TUVP). An excellent review of minimally invasive therapies has also been published.[24] These include urethral stent, balloon dilation, hypothermia, transurethral microwave therapy (TUMT), laser therapy, transurethral needle ablation (TUNA), and high-intensity focus ultrasound (HIFU). Open prostatectomy is the oldest and most invasive procedure done for BPH. It has a higher rate of strictures and retrograde ejaculations compared with TURP and TUIP, but has an excellent cure rate of 98%.

TURP is the gold standard surgical treatment as it is less invasive than an open prostatectomy but has similar cure rates (ranging from 85% to 100%). Side effects include incontinence (3%), bladder neck contracture (3%–5%), erectile dysfunction (5–10%), and retrograde ejaculation (60%–80%).[5,25] This procedure should not be performed in men who wish to remain fertile.

If a man has a prostate gland mass of less than 50 grams, a TUIP may be appropriate. Symptom improvement is only slightly less effective than TURP, ranging from 85% to 95%. Adverse effects include incontinence (~1%), erectile dysfunction (0%–4%), bladder neck contracture (1%), and retrograde ejaculation (15%–20%).[23,26]

EVIDENCE-BASED SUMMARY

- Lifestyle changes are recommended for anyone with BPH and LUTS.
- Watchful waiting may be considered for patients with mild symptoms of BPH.
- Pharmacotherapy is considered first-line treatment for BPH in patients with mild-to-moderate symptoms.
- Therapy should be individualized, depending on patient preference, comorbidities, size of the prostate, and adverse effects of therapeutic interventions.
- In patients with severe symptoms or those who prefer surgery, less-invasive options are now available, including the gold standard TURP.
- No therapy is without risks, but ultimately all have beneficial effects on patient's quality of life.

REFERENCES

1. Berry SJ, Coffey DS, Walsh PC. The development of human benign prostatic hyperplasia with age. *J Urol.* 1976; 132(3):474.
2. Noltenius H, Haake A, Giersch H, et al. Pathological–anatomical findings in 70–102 year old Caucasians. *Med Klin.* 1976;71(49):2163.
3. Verhamme KMC, Dieleman JP, Bleumink GS, et al. Incidence and prevalence of lower urinary tract symptoms suggestive of BPH in primary care. *Eur Urol.* 2002;42:323.
4. American Urological Association Practice Guidelines Committee. AUA guidelines on management of benign prostatic hyperplasia (2003). *J Urol.* 2003;170:530–547.
5. McConnell JD for the MTOPS Steering Committee. The long-term effects of medical therapy on the progression of BPH: results from the MTOPS trial. *J Urol.* 2002;167:1042.
6. Madsen FA, Bruskewitz RC. Clinical manifestations of benign prostatic hyperplasia. *Urol Clin North Am.* 1995;22: 291–298.
7. Uzzo RG, Herzlinger D, Vaughan. Prostate development: Hormonal and cellular considerations. American Urological Association Update Series, Lesson 1, Vol. XV,1996;15:1.
8. Chapple CR, Burt RP, Anderson PO, et al. Alpha-1-adrenoreceptor subtypes in the human prostate. *Br J Urol.* 1994;74:585–589.
9. Steers WD. 5 alpha reductase activity in the prostate. *Urology.* 2001;58(1):17–24.
10. Wright EJ, Fang J, Metter E, et al. Prostate specific antigen predicts the long-term risk of prostate enlargement. *J Urol.* 2002;176(6):2484.
11. Dutkiewics S. Efficacy and tolerability of drugs for the treatment of benign prostatic hyperplasia. *Int Urol Nephrol.* 2001:32:423–432.
12. ALLHAT officers and Coordinators for the ALLHAT Collaborative Research Group. Major cardiovascular events in hypertensive patients randomized to doxazosin vs. chlorthalidone: The Antihypertensive and Lipid-Lowering Treatment to Prevent Heart Attack Trial (ALLHAT). *JAMA.* 2000;288:2981–2997.
13. Djavan B, Marberger M. A meta-analysis on the efficacy and tolerability of alpha-1 adrenoceptor antagonists in patients with lower urinary tract symptoms suggestive of benign prostatic obstruction. *Eur Urol.* 1999;36:1–13.
14. Chapple CR, Wyndaele JJ, Nordling J, et al. Tamsulosin, the first prostate-selective alpha 1A-adrenoceptor antagonist. A meta-analysis of two randomized, placebo-controlled, multicentre studies in patients with benign prostatic obstruction (symptomatic BPH). European Tamsulosin Study Group. *Eur Urol.* 1996;29:155–167.
15. Anonymous. Tamsulosin for benign prostatic hyperplasia. *Med Lett Drugs Ther.* 1997;39:96.
16. Anonymous. Dutasteride (Avodart) for benign prostatic hyperplasia. *Med Lett Drugs Ther.* 2002;44:109–110.
17. Boyle P, Gould AL, Roehrborn CG. Prostate volume predicts outcome of treatment of benign prostatic hyperplasia with finasteride: Meta-analysis of randomized clinical trials. *Urology.* 1996;48:398–405.
18. Logan YT, Belgeri MT. Monotherapy versus combination drug therapy for the treatment of benign prostatic hyperplasia. *Am J Geriatr Pharmacother.* 2005;3(2):103–114.
19. Kirby RS, Roehrborn C, Boyle P, et al. Efficacy and tolerability of doxazosin and finasteride, alone or in combination, in treatment of symptomatic benign prostatic hyperplasia: The Prospective European Doxazosin and Combination Therapy (PREDICT) trial. *Urology.* 2003;61(1):119–126.
20. McConnell JD, Bruskewitz R, Walsh P, et al., for the Finasteride Long-Term Efficacy and Safety Study Group. The effect of finasteride on the risk of acute urinary retention and the need for surgical treatment among men with benign prostatic hyperplasia. *N Engl J Med.* 1998;338:557–563.
21. Bent S, Kane C, Shinohara K, et al. Saw palmetto for benign prostatic hyperplasia. *N Engl J Med.* 2006;354:557–566.
22. DiPaola RS, Morton RA. Proven and unproven therapy for benign prostatic hyperplasia (editorial). *N Engl J Med.* 2006;354:632–634.
23. McConnell JD, Barry MH, Bruskewitz RC, et al. *Benign Prostatic Hyperplasia: Diagnosis and Treatment.* Clinical Practice Guidelines, No. 8. AHCPR publication No. 94-0582. Rockville, MD: Agency for Health Care Policy and Research, Public Health Service, US Department of Health and Human Services; 1994.
24. Jepsen JV, Bruskewitz RC. Recent developments in the surgical management of benign prostatic hyperplasia. *Urology.* 1998;51(4A):23–31.
25. Griffiths DA. Pressure flow studies of micturition. *Urol Clin North Am.* 1996;23:279–297.
26. Osterling JE. Benign prostatic hyperplasia: Medical and minimally invasive treatment options. *N Engl J Med.* 1995; 332:99.

Chapter 32

Urinary Incontinence

Ann E. Canales and Beverly D. Nixon-Lewis

SEARCH STRATEGY

A systematic search of the medical literature was performed in May 2007. The search, limited to human subjects and journals in English language, included the National Guideline Clearinghouse, the Cochrane database, PubMed, and UpToDate®. The most recent national guidelines for urinary incontinence were created in 1996 and are considered to be outdated. No revised national guidelines were available at the time of publication.

INTRODUCTION

Urinary incontinence (UI) is the involuntary loss of urine[1] and results from several different etiologies that may or may not present in combination with one another. Prevalence data for UI vary significantly across the literature; however, evidence shows that UI increases with age and is generally more prevalent in women.[2]

Many individuals suffering from UI attempt to cope with the condition without seeking medical intervention. This may be a result of the social stigma associated with UI or the misconception that UI is a normal part of aging.[3] UI is a medical condition that warrants evaluation and individualized management. Quality of life in individuals suffering from UI is diminished when compared with those without incontinence[4]; successful treatment of UI is the ultimate goal of therapy whenever feasible.

CLASSIFICATION

UI is classified on the basis of the duration and onset of symptoms. Accurate diagnosis is essential to ensure that the most appropriate treatment strategies are initiated. There are two general types of UI: acute and persistent

(or chronic). Acute UI is associated with a new or recent medical condition that can be treated independently from the resultant UI. Persistent UI is either not caused by a new treatable medical condition or persists over a long period of time. As described in the following sections, persistent UI is divided into subtypes on the basis of etiology: urge urinary incontinence (UUI), stress urinary incontinence (SUI), mixed UI, chronic retention of urine (formerly overflow UI), and functional UI.

ACUTE UI

Acute UI (or reversible UI) may present independently or in conjunction with long-standing UI. There are numerous causes or contributing factors for UI. A couple of useful mnemonics for identifying possible reversible causes are listed in Table 32-1[5].

URGE URINARY INCONTINENCE

UUI results from an overactive bladder (OAB), a syndrome in which the detrusor involuntarily contracts, either provoked or spontaneously, causing a sudden "urge" to urinate. The etiology is presumed to be uninhibited bladder contractions, but compensatory mechanisms and the functional requirements for continence can contribute. In UUI, the OAB syndrome progresses to undesirable urine leakage.

STRESS URINARY INCONTINENCE

SUI is a condition in which the patient is unable to postpone urination following an increase in intra-abdominal pressure. In SUI, involuntary loss of urine occurs as a result of activities or actions such as exercise, coughing, sneezing, or lifting. Urethral sphincter insufficiency is often noted as the underlying abnormality.[3]

Table 32-1. Acronyms for Potentially Reversible Causes of Urinary Incontinence

D	Delirium	D	Delirium
I	Infection (UTI), inflammation	R	Restricted mobility, retention
A	Atrophic urethritis/ vaginitis	I	Infection (UTI), inflammation, impaction
P	Pharmaceuticals	P	Polyuria, pharmaceuticals, psychologic
P	Psychologic		
E	Excessive urine output		
R	Restricted mobility, retention		
S	Stool impaction		

Source: Adapted from Kane RL, Ouslander JG, Abrass IB. *Essentials of Clinical Geriatrics*. 5th ed. New York, NY: McGraw-Hill; 2004.

MIXED INCONTINENCE

Mixed incontinence results when individuals experience urine leakage as a result of urgency combined with increases in intra-abdominal pressure from exertion, sneezing, or coughing; it is essentially a combination of UUI and SUI.

CHRONIC RETENTION OF URINE

Chronic retention of urine, in which a nonpainful bladder remains palpable or percussible following the passage of urine, has replaced the term overflow urinary incontinence as defined by the International Continence Society.[1,6] This condition results from the inability of the bladder to completely empty on urination so that the bladder expands to and beyond capacity with the potential for resultant urine leakage. The inability to completely empty the bladder may be a result of loss of detrusor tone or bladder outlet obstruction (as is often seen in benign prostatic hyperplasia—described in Chapter 31). This is the second most common cause of UI in older men, second to UUI, but is uncommon in women.[6]

FUNCTIONAL UI

Functional incontinence results from external factors hindering timely transfer to the toilet and diseases or medications that may prevent an individual from recognizing the need to urinate. Thus, its etiology is not related to lower urinary tract pathophysiology. Functional incontinence is more prevalent among older individuals who have concomitant conditions such as dementia, Parkinson's disease, limited mobility, and cognitive or musculoskeletal deficits.

CLINICAL EVALUATION

A complete evaluation of UI begins with taking a detailed history.[3] Screening questions directed at specific charac-

teristics and precipitating events that lead to incontinent episodes are important. Review of the patient's medical and surgical history, current medications, and social history help to identify risk factors. Bladder records or voiding diaries can be useful in characterizing symptoms and are particularly helpful in monitoring treatment response.

PHYSICAL FINDINGS

The physical examination is essential in the evaluation of all patients with UI. It should focus on the neurologic, abdominal, rectal, and pelvic examinations. Special attention should be given to the patient's mobility and mental status to qualify the patient's functional ability with regard to independent toileting. Knowing the functional status of the patient is paramount to developing a successful treatment plan. Table 32-2[5] describes the key aspects to the physical examination.

The neurologic examination should focus on the perineum and lower extremities to identify any motor or sensory deficits that may point to neurologic conditions

Table 32-2. Key Aspects of an Incontinent Patient's Physical Examination

Mobility and Dexterity
    Functional status compatible with ability to self-toilet
    Gait disturbance (parkinsonism, normal-pressure hydrocephalus)
Mental Status
    Cognitive function compatible with ability to self-toilet
    Motivation
    Mood and effect
Neurologic
    Focal signs (especially lower extremities)
    Signs of parkinsonism
    Sacral arc reflexes
Abdominal
    Bladder distention
    Suprapubic tenderness
    Lower abdominal mass
Rectal
    Perianal sensation
    Sphincter tone (resting and active)
    Impaction
    Masses
    Size and contour of prostate
Pelvic
    Perineal skin condition
    Perineal sensation
    Atrophic vaginitis (friability, inflammation, bleeding)
    Pelvic prolapse (i.e., cystocele, rectocele)
    Pelvic mass
    Other anatomic abnormality
Other
    Lower extremity edema or signs of heart failure (if nocturia is a prominent complaint)

Source: Adapted from Kane RL, Ouslander JG, Abrass IB. *Essentials of Clinical Geriatrics*. 5th ed. New York, NY: McGraw-Hill; 2004.

believed to cause or worsen UI. Cognitive assessment, perhaps conducted with a mini-mental status examination, is important to exclude cognitive disorders that can complicate participation in a patient-dependent treatment plan.

The abdominal examination focuses on identifying bladder distention or tenderness as well as looking for lower abdominal masses.

The pelvic examination in women should assess for perineal skin condition and irritation, vaginal atrophy, prolapse of the bladder or rectum, as well as pelvic mass. The pelvic floor muscle function should assess tone at rest and the strength of a reflex contraction.

The rectal examination should assess for sphincter tone, impaction, and rectal mass. In men, prostate size and contour is also evaluated.

DIAGNOSTIC EVALUATION

In the initial evaluation, several objective studies are routinely recommended. A urinalysis should be performed on all patients. A culture should be done only if infection is suspected. In the older or institutionalized patient, there is a high incidence of asymptomatic bacteriuria, which is not a cause of either incontinence or morbidity.[6] Cytology and cystoscopy are indicated only if hematuria or pelvic pain is present.[6]

An observed clinical stress test is a very sensitive means of evaluating the presence of UI and specifically SUI. It can be misleading if the patient is inhibited or uncooperative, or if the bladder volume is low.[6] This test is conducted with the patient standing in a comfortable and relaxed position. The patient's bladder must be comfortably full for the test to be optimal. The patient should give a single vigorous cough. Instantaneous leakage is diagnostic of SUI.[6]

The postvoid residual (PVR) test has been recommended based on expert opinion using catheterization or ultrasound on all patients with UI. PVR volumes of less than 50 mL are considered normal, whereas volumes of greater than 200 mL are considered abnormal and suggestive of an obstructive uropathy or poor bladder contractility.

PVR volumes between 50 and 200 mL should be assessed on an individual basis after evaluating the patient's history, bladder diary, and any other associated physical findings in helping to establish a treatment plan. An example bladder diary is shown in Fig. 32-1.[5]

Referral for complex urodynamic testing should be reserved for patients who have PVR volumes greater

Bladder Record

Day:_____   Date:_____

INSTRUCTIONS
1. In the first column make a mark every time during the 2-hour period you urinate in the toilet.
2. Use the second column to record the amount you urinate (if you are measuring amounts).
3. In the third or fourth column, make a mark every time you accidentally leak urine.

Time Interval	Urinated in Toilet	Amount	Leaking Accident	*or*	Large Accident	Reason for Accident*
6–8 AM						
8–10 AM						
10–Noon						
Noon–2 PM						
2–4 PM						
4–6 PM						
6–8 PM						
8–10 PM						
10–Midnight						
Overnight						

Number of pads used today:_____

*For example, if you coughed and had a leaking accident, write "cough."
If you had a large accident after a strong urge to urinate, write "urge."

Figure 32-1. Example of a bladder diary for ambulatory care settings. (Source: Adapted from Kane RL, Ouslander JG, Abrass IB. *Essentials of Clinical Geriatrics.* 5th ed. New York, NY: McGraw-Hill; 2004.)

than 200 mL, patients with inconclusive results, those not responding to treatment, and those being evaluated for possible surgical intervention.

Finally, some evidence supports laboratory evaluation of the patient, including tests of renal function, serum glucose, serum calcium, and in the older patients, serum vitamin B_{12} levels.

THERAPEUTIC GOALS

The main goal for treating UI is improvement of the patient's quality of life, and a patient's treatment plan must be individualized for optimal effect.[3] The goal for individuals with acute incontinence is effective treatment of the underlying cause with full resolution of the UI. For most patients with persistent incontinence, the ideal primary goal is the restoration of continence, but improvement of symptoms, health, and activity level as well as self-image and physical appearance are strong secondary goals.

A patient-centered approach is important to successfully meet individualized goals. In developing the treatment plan, the patient's goals should be considered. In the elderly population or in the institutionalized environment, goals are not static and may change over time. Patient dryness may be an initial goal of treatment; however, that goal may change over time to prevention of skin breakdown and maintenance of a clean environment.

MANAGEMENT

Because of the differing etiologies of UI, management strategies will depend upon the type of UI. The treatment of acute UI is aimed at correcting the underlying condition. The treatment for persistent UI includes first-line treatment with nonpharmacologic interventions in conjunction with appropriate pharmacotherapy when indicated.[2,7] With medications, the choice is patient-specific and should be guided by the following considerations: evidence-based efficacy for the type of UI being treated, patient tolerability (age, underlying medical conditions, concurrent medication use, and anticipated adverse drug reactions), and cost to the patient and society. Figure 32-2[5,8] outlines the management of acute and persistent UI.

NONPHARMACOLOGIC MANAGEMENT OF UI

Often, individuals initiate nonpharmacologic management techniques before seeking formal medical care. Numerous methods may be used; some are effective, while others are only coping strategies without any therapeutic benefit for the condition.[4] Effective nonpharmacologic management depends not only on the type

of UI being treated, but also multiple factors about the patient and their support system. Some methods are patient-dependent, meaning that their purpose is to restore some level of control over the condition.

Other interventions are caregiver-dependent, meaning that they are focused on keeping the patient dry and the environment clean to prevent secondary problems associated with UI. Included within this category of management options are lifestyle modifications, behavioral interventions, environmental modifications, and nonprescription products. The use of these management techniques may serve as the initial presenting sign(s) of UI.

Some common maladaptive techniques include reliance on absorbent pads, restroom mapping, toileting frequently, avoidance of social situations, and altering or avoiding activity that may precipitate an incontinence event. This is an appropriate time for health professional intervention.

Lifestyle Modifications

Obesity and smoking have both been positively correlated with UI, while weight loss and smoking cessation have proven to reduce the burden of UI in affected individuals.[3] Because caffeine acts as a diuretic and spicy foods and carbonated beverages act as bladder irritants, moderation of these types of foods may help with UI symptoms as well.[3,7] Scheduling fluid intake to minimize situational incontinence (i.e., avoiding evening fluids to manage night-time wetness) and maintaining adequate fluid intake to prevent constipation and the production of concentrated urine, which can be irritating to the bladder, are also important interventions.[3]

Behavioral Interventions

Numerous behavioral interventions for the management of UI have been identified and categorized as either patient-dependent or caregiver-dependent. Table 32-3[5] summarizes these interventions.

Environmental Modifications

Rearrangement of the environment to improve the likelihood of timely transfer to a toilet may be a useful measure in the treatment of functional UI and UUI. Placement of a bedside commode and providing access to alternate urine receptacles may be appropriate in some situations.

NONPRESCRIPTION DEVICES

A large variety of absorbent products are readily available. They differ in many ways including size, ease of use, intended method of use (e.g., undergarment vs

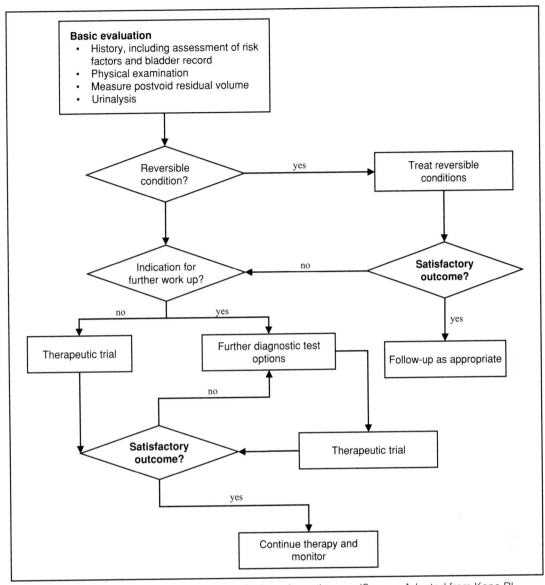

Figure 32-2. Algorithm for the management of urinary incontinence. (Source: Adapted from Kane RL, Ouslander JG, Abrass IB. *Essentials of Clinical Geriatrics.* 5th ed. New York, NY: McGraw-Hill; 2004; Fantl JA. *Urinary Incontinence In Adults: Acute and Chronic Management.* Rockville, MD: United States Department of Health and Human Services, Public Health Service, Agency for Health Care Policy and Research; 1996. Accessed October 11, 2005.)

bed pad), absorbency, odor protection, bacterial growth inhibition, disposability, and cost-effectiveness. The ready availability of such wide assortment of absorbent products is a large part of the reason that patients often attempt to self-manage UI before seeking professional help. Additionally, tampons and vaginal pessaries[3] may be useful for management of SUI in women during certain activities, such as exercise. A variety of other devices are available for the management of UI.

MANAGEMENT OF ACUTE UI

The treatment of acute UI is aimed at correcting the underlying condition whenever possible. Common reversible causes of UI may be found in Table 32-4.[8] If the management strategies listed there effectively reverse the UI, then no additional therapy for persistent UI should be necessary. If, however, these approaches fail to reverse the condition, additional testing should be undertaken to determine whether the UI has a

Table 32-3. Behavioral Interventions for Urinary Incontinence

Procedure	Definition	Comments
Types of Incontinence **Patient-dependent**		
Pelvic muscle (Kegel) exercises *Stress and urge*	Repetitive contraction and relaxation of pelvic floor muscles.	Requires adequate function and motivation. Biofeedback may be helpful in teaching the exercise.
Bladder training *Stress and urge*	Use of education, bladder records, pelvic muscle, and other behavioral techniques.	Requires trained therapist, adequate cognitive and physical functioning, and motivation.
Bladder retraining *Acute (e.g., postcatheterization with urge or overflow, poststroke)*	Progressive lengthening or shortening of inter-voiding interval, with intermittent catheterization used in patients recovering from overdistention injuries with persistent retention.	Goal is to restore normal pattern of voiding and continence. Requires adequate cognitive and physical function and motivation.
Urge-suppression training *Urge*	Purposeful postponement of urination following urge for a predetermined period of time. May use modified Kegel exercises, and distraction to aid in this method.	Requires adequate function and motivation.
Caregiver-dependent		
Scheduled toileting *Urge and functional*	Routine toileting at regular intervals.	Goal is to prevent wetting episodes. Can be used in patients with impaired cognitive or physical functioning.
Habit training *Urge and functional*	Variable toileting schedule based on patient's voiding patterns.	Requires staff or caregiver availability and motivation. Same as above.
Prompted voiding *Urge, stress, mixed, functional*	Offer opportunity to toilet every 2 h during the day; toilet only on request; social reinforcement; routine offering of fluids.	25–40% of nursing home residents respond well during the day and can be identified during a 3-d trial.

Source: Adapted from Kane RL, Ouslander JG, Abrass IB. *Essentials of Clinical Geriatrics.* 5th ed. New York, NY: McGraw-Hill; 2004.

persistent etiology. Inappropriate acute management may lead to persistent UI (e.g., indwelling-catheter use beyond an appropriate duration). In an older patient with new-onset or worsening UI, urinary tract infection should be suspected and appropriate antimicrobial therapy should be initiated.

PHARMACOLOGIC MANAGEMENT OF UUI

In patients with UUI, pharmacotherapy should be considered for anyone not achieving adequate relief of symptoms with nondrug measures. Medications should be used in conjunction with continued nonpharmacologic interventions.

Antimuscarinic Agents

This class of medications is the mainstay for the treatment of OAB and UUI.[9] Five muscarinic receptors, M1–M5, have been identified. Detrusor contraction has been associated with activation of the M3 receptor, while activation of the M1 receptors in the central nervous system (CNS) has been associated with disruption of cognitive function.[10] Common, and often dose-limiting, adverse effects (AEs) demonstrated by this class include dry mouth, blurred vision, and constipation.[11]

Inhibition of M3 receptors in the bladder is the primary focus of antimuscarinic agents for OAB and UUI. The chemical differences in the antimuscarinic medications include molecular size, polarity, and specificity for the M3 receptor. Multiple studies have demonstrated relative equivalence in efficacy as compared with placebo for oxybutynin and tolterodine, but these agents differ in tolerability, formulation availability, and to a limited extent cost (discussed later).[9] Some of the newer agents, such as solifenacin, trospium, and darifenacin, have not undergone as many comparative trials, but have received approval of the Food and Drug Administration for the treatment of UI (Table 32-5).

Oxybutynin chloride, one of the older and more thoroughly studied agents is a small, lipophilic molecule specific for the M1 and M3 receptors. It readily crosses the blood–brain barrier (BBB) and produces centrally mediated AEs such as somnolence, drowsiness, and fatigue. Dry mouth and blurred vision, particularly in older patients, result from the drug's peripheral effects on muscarinic receptors. It is available as an immediate-release tablet, an extended-release tablet, and a transdermal patch. The efficacy is relatively equivalent for all formulations, but the tolerability and cost are increased with the extended-release and transdermal

Table 32-4. Management of Reversible Conditions That Contribute to Urinary Incontinence

Condition	Management
Conditions affecting the lower urinary tract	
Urinary tract infection (symptomatic)	Antimicrobial therapy
Atrophic urethritis/vaginitis	Estrogen (topical)
Pregnancy/vaginal delivery/episiotomy	Behavioral intervention
	Avoid surgical therapy postpartum as condition may be self-limiting
Postprostatectomy	Behavioral intervention
	Avoid further surgery until certain that the condition will not resolve
Stool impaction	Disimpaction
	Appropriate use of stool softeners and laxatives
	High-fiber dietary intake
	Greater mobility
	Adequate fluid intake
Adverse drug effects	Discontinuation or change of therapy if clinically appropriate
	Dosage reduction or modification (i.e., flexible diuretic scheduling)
Increased urine production	
Metabolic (hyperglycemia, hypercalcemia)	Improved control of diabetes mellitus
	Therapy for hypercalcemia depends on underlying cause
Excess fluid intake	Reduction in intake of diuretic fluids (caffeinated beverages)
Volume overload	
Venous insufficiency with edema	Support stockings
	Leg elevation
	Sodium restriction
	Diuretic therapy
Heart failure	Medical management
Impaired ability or willingness to reach a toilet	
Delirium	Diagnosis and treatment of underlying causes of acute confusional state
Chronic illness, injury, or restraint that interferes with mobility	Regular toileting
	Use of toilet substitutes
	Avoiding restraints when possible
Psychologic	Pharmacologic and/or nonpharmacologic treatment

Source: Adapted from Fantl JA. *Urinary Incontinence in Adults: Acute and Chronic Management.* Rockville, MD: United States Department of Health and Human Services, Public Health Service, Agency for Health Care Policy and Research; 1996. Accessed October 11, 2005.

Table 32-5. Pharmacologic Options for Urge Urinary Incontinence

Drug	Dose	Comments
Oxybutynin hydrochloride	Generic available	Similar efficacy noted for all formulations.
Ditropan®	2.5–5 mg, 2–3 times daily (IR)	Tolerability improved with ER and transdermal formulations.
Ditropan XL®	5–30 mg daily (ER)	Transdermal may cause local skin irritation.
Oxytrol™	3.9 mg daily (transdermal) changed every 3–4 d	
Tolterodine	Generic available	Similar efficacy noted for both formulations.
Detrol®	1–2 mg, 2 times daily (IR)	Tolerability improved with ER formulation.
Detrol® LA	2–4 mg daily (ER)	Adjust dose for renal and hepatic impairment.
		Possible drug interactions with potent CYP3A4 inhibitors.
Trospium chloride	20 mg daily	Take on empty stomach
Sanctura™		Cognitive impairment not noted in clinical studies.
Solifenacin succinate	5–10 mg daily	Adjust dose for renal and hepatic impairment.
VESIcare®		Minimized CNS adverse effects likely due to M3 receptor selectivity.
Darifenacin hydrobromide	7.5–15 mg daily	Minimized CNS adverse effects likely due to M3 receptor selectivity.
Enablex®		Possible drug interactions with potent CYP3A4 inhibitors.
		Adjust dose for hepatic impairment
		No cognitive impairment noted in clinical studies.

ER, extended release; CNS, central nervous system.

formulations. No significant drug interactions have been identified.

Tolterodine tartrate is a large polar molecule that is unlikely to cross an intact BBB, but it is a nonselective muscarinic receptor antagonist and may cause significant AEs in a compromised BBB, such as may be found in the very elderly population.[10] Additionally, tolterodine is a CYP450 2D6 and 3A4 substrate, which creates several potentially significant drug interactions with strong inhibitors or inducers of these isoenzymes. For example, ketoconazole, a strong inhibitor, may warrant a dose decrease for tolterodine.

Trospium chloride, the least lipophilic antimuscarinic agent available, would be the least likely to cross the BBB under normal conditions. It is, however, a nonselective muscarinic receptor antagonist and may lead to significant AEs in the event of a breach of CNS permeability barriers[10] as has been described for tolterodine. Current studies have demonstrated no cognitive impairment with this agent compared with placebo,[10] but trospium produces anticholinergic AEs similar to those of other agents in this class.[12] Additionally, because trospium is renally eliminated, it poses less risk for drug interactions. However, dose adjustment is recommended in case of renal impairment and also in patients older than 75 years.

Solifenacin succinate and darifenacin hydrobromide are newer M3-specific antimuscarinic agents with the least potential of causing CNS AEs. Solifenacin requires dosage adjustments for renal and hepatic impairment and as a CYP450 3A4 substrate, drug interactions are possible. Darifenacin is a large polar molecule that is not only a specific M3 receptor antagonist, but is also a substrate for the P-glycoprotein active transport efflux pumps in the CNS, thereby minimizing CNS AEs. Darifenacin is a CYP450 3A4 substrate and a moderate 2D6 inhibitor, which may lead to drug interactions. Drugs that could cause accumulation of darifenacin, such as ketoconazole, should be coadministered cautiously.

Because the newer agents are somewhat less likely to induce CNS toxicity in older individuals, they may be preferred over oxybutynin and tolterodine. For individuals in whom the anticholinergic AEs are not bothersome or potentially dangerous, using the less-expensive agents (immediate-release oxybutynin or tolterodine) may be preferred; however, multiple daily doses are required and compliance must be considered. If compliance is likely to be a problem, the transdermal-patch formulation or any once-daily formulation may be more appropriate.

Several older agents with antimuscarinic effects have been used for the treatment of UI; however, flavoxate, propantheline, dicyclomine, hyoscyamine, and imipramine have essentially been replaced by the newer, more-specific agents with sufficient clinical trial efficacy and tolerability data.[3] Additionally, gabapentin and botulinum toxin A have been studied recently for the treatment of OAB, particularly OAB resistant to anticholinergic medications, but sufficient clinical evidence is still lacking. Although these agents are not currently considered first-line treatment options for UUI, they may be preferable in individuals with concomitant medical conditions for which they are useful (i.e., imipramine for UUI in an individual with depression who can tolerate the CNS AEs of the medication).

PHARMACOLOGIC MANAGEMENT OF SUI

Since SUI results from the inability of the sphincter mechanisms to remain closed during bladder filling, the medications used in the treatment of SUI act at the bladder neck and urethra or on the pelvic floor musculature to promote closure of the urethral sphincter. Table 32-6 provides a summary of individual agents that are used

Table 32-6. Pharmacologic Options for Stress Urinary Incontinence

Drug	Dose	Comments
Estrogen (topical) Women only	0.5 mg cream applied vaginally every night for 2 wks, then extended to 2–3 times weekly Estrogen-containing ring inserted every 3 mo	Oral formulation also studied, but efficacy and safety questionable. Topical formulation efficacy not validated in clinical trials. Avoid cream in women with absolute contraindication to estrogen.
Pseudoephedrine	15–60 mg, 3 times daily	Efficacy questionable. Use caution in hypertensive patients.
Ephedrine	25–50 mg, 3 times daily	Use caution in hypertensive patients. May cause agitation, insomnia, tremor, or cardiac arrhythmias.
Imipramine Tofranil®	10–50 mg, 1–3 times daily	Potential use in concomitant depression. May be useful for mixed incontinence (stress + urge). Avoid use in older patients due to possibility of CNS depression.
Duloxetine Cymbalta®	40 mg, 2 times daily	Unlabeled use and dose in the United States, investigational drug for SUI

for SUI. In addition to pharmacotherapy and surgery, some minimally invasive techniques have been studied for the treatment of SUI; these include injectable therapies and radiofrequency micro-remodeling.[13]

Estrogen

The urinary tract support systems decline following menopause in women. This is probably due to a thinning of the periurethral mucosa. Both local and systemic estrogen have been studied for the treatment of SUI; however, conflicting efficacy data and possible AEs with the use of systemic estrogen have essentially removed this option from current clinical use.[3] Local estrogen is still recommended as a safe and potentially effective treatment option for SUI in women without an absolute contraindication to the use of estrogen, but published efficacy data are lacking.

α-Adrenergic Agonists

α-Adrenergic agonists work at the bladder neck and urethra to enhance closing pressure via stimulation of α-1 adrenergic receptors. Potentially useful agents include pseudoephedrine, ephedrine, and imipramine. These agents must be used cautiously in individuals with pre-existing hypertension and avoided in individuals suffering from chronic retention of urine.

Duloxetine, an antidepressant that inhibits neuronal norepinephrine and serotonin reuptake and is also approved for diabetic peripheral neuropathic pain and generalized anxiety disorder, is being studied for the treatment of SUI in the United States. It is approved for SUI use in other countries. Other agents, such as Ro 115–1240, a selective α-1A/1I-adrenergic agonist, are also in the investigational pipeline.

Imipramine, a tricyclic antidepressant, has been used in SUI as well, with a proposed mechanism of action related to its α-adrenergic agonist activity.

PHARMACOLOGIC MANAGEMENT OF MIXED UI

Pharmacologic treatment for mixed UI should be aimed at the more bothersome and/or more treatable condition first while minimizing drug toxicity. For example, a patient with UUI and SUI may benefit from treatment with imipramine since it has a dual mechanism of action that is potentially effective for both types of UI; however, sufficient studies are lacking and potential toxicity should be considered, especially in older individuals.

PHARMACOLOGIC MANAGEMENT OF CHRONIC RETENTION OF URINE

Chronic retention of urine, formerly identified as overflow urinary incontinence, may be due to an atonic detrusor or bladder outlet or urethral obstruction. Atonic detrusor is treated with catheterization while the treatment of obstruction may be managed with α-1 adrenergic antagonists. A common cause of this condition is benign prostatic hyperplasia. This condition may be successfully treated with α-1 adrenergic antagonists and/or 5-α-reductase inhibitors. Table 32-7 provides a summary of individual agents that are used for chronic retention of urine.

α-1 Adrenergic Antagonists

These agents work by relieving the resistance of the bladder neck and urinary sphincter. Prazosin, doxazosin, terazosin, tamsulosin, and alfuzosin are all available on the market. Tamsulosin and alfuzosin are both

Table 32-7. Pharmacologic Options for Chronic Retention of Urine

Drug	Dose	Comments
α-1-Adrenergic agonists		
Prazosin	1–10 mg, 2 times/daily	Nonselective
Minipress™		Orthostatic hypotension is a common adverse effect
Doxazosin	1–8 mg daily (HS)	Useful for BPH
Cardura®		
Terazosin	1–10 mg daily (HS)	Useful in concomitant hypertension
Hytrin®		
Tamsulosin	0.4–0.8 mg daily	Selective for urinary tract
Flomax®		Useful for BPH
Alfuzosin	10 mg daily (ER)	Tamsulosin is a CYP3A4 and 2D6 substrate
Uroxatral™		Alfuzosin is a CYP3A4 substrate
5-α-Reductase inhibitors		
Finasteride	5 mg daily	Useful for BPH
Proscar®		Benefit not immediately observable
Dutasteride	0.5 mg daily	Sexual dysfunction adverse effect
Avodart™		Minor CYP3A4 substrates

HS, bedtime; ER, extended release; BPH, benign prostatic hyperplasia.

more selective for the α receptors in the urinary tract, they are associated with less orthostatic hypotension—a common AE of the nonselective drugs.

5-α-REDUCTASE INHIBITORS

Finasteride and dutasteride work by inhibiting the conversion of testosterone to dihydrotestosterone, thereby causing shrinkage of the prostate gland with long-term therapy.

SURGICAL OPTIONS

Surgery is an option for treatment of SUI, UUI, and chronic retention of urine. It is usually reserved for individuals who fail or cannot tolerate less-invasive therapeutic options, including pharmacotherapy. Referral to a surgeon should be considered for patients in whom the quality of life can be improved with successful intervention, regardless of age, but risks of the surgery should always be considered as well.

EVIDENCE-BASED SUMMARY

- UI is classified as acute or chronic and is best treated according to the etiology: urge, stress, mixed, chronic retention of urine, or functional.
- Acute UI is best treated by correcting the underlying cause, when possible.
- Voiding diaries can be helpful in characterizing symptoms of chronic UI and monitoring treatment response.
- The primary goal of treatment is to improve the patient's quality of life and should be individualized with reasonable expectations.
- Numerous environmental modifications, nonpharmacological devices, and medications are available for the management of UI.
- Antimuscarinic agents are the primary pharmacologic treatment options for UUI while various medications, including topical estrogen, alpha-adrenergic agonists, and selected antidepressants are available treatment options for SUI. Treatment of mixed UI is best aimed at the more bothersome subtype of UI—stress or urge.1
- Alpha-adrenergic antagonists and 5-α-reductase inhibitors are the primary pharmacological treatment options for chronic retention of urine.
- Surgery is a treatment option for SUI, UUI, and chronic retention of urine; however, it is best reserved for those not tolerating other options.

REFERENCES

1. Abrams P, Cardozo L, Fall M, et al. The standardisation of terminology of lower urinary tract function: Report from the standardisation sub-committee of the International Continence Society. *Neurourol Urodyn*. 2002;21:167–178.
2. Epstein BJ, Gums JG, Molina E. Newer agents for the management of overactive bladder. *Am Fam Physician*. 2006;74:2061–2068.
3. Davila GW, Guerette N. Current treatment options for female urinary incontinence—A review. *Int J Fertil Women Med*. 2004;49:102–112.
4. Serels S. The wet patient: Understanding patients with overactive bladder and incontinence. *Curr Med Res Opin*. 2004;20:791–801.
5. Kane RL, Ouslander JG, Abrass IB. *Essentials of Clinical Geriatrics*. 5th ed. New York, NY: McGraw-Hill; 2004.
6. DeBeau CE. *Clinical Presentation and Diagnosis of Urinary Incontinence*. Available at www.uptodate.com. Accessed May 4, 2007.
7. DeBeau CE. *Treatment of Urinary Incontinence*. Available at www.uptodate.com. Accessed May 4, 2007.
8. Fantl JA. *Urinary Incontinence In Adults: Acute and Chronic Management*. Rockville, MD: United States Department of Health and Human Services, Public Health Service, Agency for Health Care Policy and Research; 1996. Accessed October 11, 2005.
9. Herbison P, Hay-Smith J, Ellis G, Moore K. Effectiveness of anticholinergic drugs compared with placebo in the treatment of overactive bladder: Systematic review. *BMJ*. 2003;326:841–844.
10. Kay GG, Granville LJ. Antimuscarinic agents: Implications and concerns in the management of overactive bladder in the elderly. *Clin Ther*. 2005;27:127–138; Quiz 139–140.
11. Gray M. Assessment and management of urinary incontinence. *Nurse Pract*. 2005;30:32–33, 36–43; Quiz 43–45.
12. Singh-Franco D, Machado C, Tuteja S, Zapantis A. Trospium chloride for the treatment of overactive bladder with urge incontinence. *Clin Ther*. 2005;27:511–530.
13. Gilleran JP, Zimmern P. An evidence-based approach to the evaluation and management of stress incontinence in women. *Curr Opin Urol*. 2005;15:236–243.

PART 8

Rheumatologic Disorders

CHAPTERS

Chapter 33

Osteoporosis

Candis M. Morello, Renu F. Singh, and Leonard J. Deftos

SEARCH STRATEGY

A systematic search of the medical literature was conducted between March 7, 2007, and March 20, 2007. A search update was conducted between February 13, 2008, and March 11, 2008. The search, limited to human subjects and English language journals, included the National Guideline Clearinghouse, PubMed, and the Cochrane database. The National Osteoporosis Foundation can be found at www.nof.org and the *Clinician's Guide to Prevention and Treatment of Osteoporosis* can be found at http://www.nof.org/professionals/clinicians_ Guide.htm.

Osteoporosis is the most common human bone disease that is often recognized only after a patient experiences a fracture. Characterized by low bone mass and increased bone porosity, osteoporosis leads to reduced bone strength and an increased risk of bone fracture. Although the disease can affect any bone, most typical fracture sites include the hip, spine, wrist, and ribs. Osteoporosis is prevalent in the United States and considered a major public health threat, particularly as our population ages. U.S. Census data estimated that in 2002, more than 10 million women and men aged 50 and older had osteoporosis, and this number is projected to rise by 30% in 2020.[1] Approximately 44 million Americans have osteoporosis and osteopenia (low bone mass) and by 2020, more than 61 million are expected to be affected by these disorders. Osteoporosis most commonly occurs in Caucasian and Asian postmenopausal women, and 50% will experience an osteoporosis-related fracture during their lifetime. Table 33-1 describes other risk factors for developing osteoporosis and fractures. Osteoporotic fractures result in significant financial and individual costs. The United States spends approximately $18 billion annually treating fractures secondary to osteoporosis.[2] Adults who incur one fracture are 50% to 100% likely to sustain another. Moreover, the one year posthip fracture mortality rate for patients 50 years and older is approximately 24%.

Living bone undergoes a dynamic constant remodeling process of new bone formation (by osteoblasts) and bone resorption (by osteoclasts). Bone loss results when bone resorption occurs more rapidly than bone formation or vice versa. The skeleton consists of two types of bone: (1) cortical and (2) trabecular. Cortical bone is dense and forms the outer skeletal shell, trabecular bone is more porous and forms the interior honeycomb structure. Optimal peak bone mass is achieved by 20 to 35 years of age. Increasing bone mass during childhood, adolescence, and early adulthood years is imperative to preventing osteoporosis in the later years of life.

Osteoporosis can be classified as a primary or secondary disorder. Primary osteoporosis refers to bone loss associated with both menopause and osteoporosis of aging, also referred to as senile osteoporosis. Postmenopausal osteoporosis is mainly caused by trabecular bone loss as a result of declining estrogen production, while age-related osteoporosis is characterized by loss of trabecular and cortical bone, affecting women and men in a 2:1 ratio, after 75 years of age. Secondary osteoporosis results from bone loss associated with medical disorders such as hyperthyroidism or Cushing's syndrome or because of chronic medication use such as systemic glucocorticoid or anticonvulsant therapy. Through preventive care and treatment, primary care providers can play a significant role in reducing the prevalence of osteoporosis.

CLINICAL PRESENTATION AND PHYSICAL FINDINGS

Bone loss and resulting osteoporosis are often silent, occurring with few or no clinical indicators. Patients experiencing symptoms may present with lower thoracic or lumbar bone pain. Signs resulting from multiple vertebral fractures include kyphosis (excessive outward curvature of the spine, particularly near the shoulders), lordosis (also referred to as dowager's or widow's hump), or loss of height. Since the development of osteoporosis is commonly a silent process, the first signs of the disease are often minimal or nontraumatic fractures in the vertebra, hip, or wrist bones, sometimes symptomatic but frequently diagnosed by radiographs. Acute fracture pain may occur initially but typically resolves in a few months. Some patients, however, may experience a chronic dull pain near the fracture site. Patients may also suffer from psychological symptoms, such as depression and loss of self-esteem from the pain, physical limitations, and lifestyle and cosmetic changes associated with their condition.

DIAGNOSTIC EVALUATION

HISTORY AND PHYSICAL EXAMINATION

A complete history and physical examination are vital in evaluating a patient for osteoporosis, particularly assessing for nonmodifiable and potential modifiable risk factors such as those listed in Table 33-1.

LABORATORY EVALUATION

Although patients with osteoporosis usually have normal routine laboratory tests, certain tests may help rule out other metabolic bone diseases (e.g., hyperparathyroidism, osteomalacia, Paget's disease) or secondary causes of osteoporosis (e.g., glucocorticoid use, other immunosuppressants, hyperthyroidism, malabsorption disorders). Initial blood and urine tests include: serum calcium (corrected for serum albumin level), phosphorus, alkaline phosphatase, parathyroid hormone, thyroid stimulating hormone, 25-hydroxyvitamin D, testosterone (in men), creatinine, complete blood count, protein electrophoresis, and a 24-hour urine for creatinine and calcium.

BONE MINERAL DENSITY MEASUREMENT

Bone mineral density (BMD) measurement by central dual energy x-ray absorptiometry (DXA) is the gold standard for diagnosing osteoporosis. A continuous, inverse relationship exists between measured BMD and fracture risk; the lower the BMD, the greater the risk of fracture. With every one standard deviation decrease in BMD, fracture risk approximately doubles. The World Heath Organization classifies bone mass in terms of T-scores, or BMD scores (see Table 33-2). T-scores reflect the BMD mean standard deviation from a young normal adult female population. Osteoporosis is defined as a T-score of -2.5 or below, and these patients have an increased risk of bone fracture. Patients with osteopenia have low bone mass and are at risk of developing osteoporosis in the future. Z-scores are similar to T-scores but reflect mean BMD scores of age-matched, sex-matched, and ethnic-matched patients. Thus, Z-scores may be more useful in assessing premenopausal women, men <50 years of age, and children. A Z score of ≤ -2.0 is defined as the BMD being below the expected range for age, while a score of > -2.0 is defined as being within the expected range for age.

Diagnosis of osteoporosis can be made by directly quantifying bone mass or a fragility fracture history. The National Osteoporosis Foundation suggests several BMD tests that are good predictors of future fractures (see Table 33-3)[3]:

RISK STRATIFICATION

Risk factors for developing osteoporosis and the World Heath Organization definition of osteoporosis are in Tables 33-1 and 33-2, respectively. Using BMD in conjunction with risk factor assessment improves the accuracy of fracture predictions.[4] Since pharmacologic treatment can substantially reduce fracture risk, identifying and screening patients at high risk is indicated. The National Osteoporosis Foundation recommends BMD testing for the following patients:[3]

- Women 65 years and older, regardless of risk factors.
- Men 70 years and older, regardless of risk factors
- Younger postmenopausal women with one or more risk factors (other than being white, postmenopausal, and female).
- Men 50–70 years based on their risk factor profile
- Women in the perimenopausal period with a specific risk factor associated with increased fracture risk (e.g. low body weight, prior low-trauma fracture, taking a high-risk medication)
- Adults who fracture after age 50 (to confirm diagnosis and determine disease severity).
- Adults with a medical condition (e.g. rheumatoid arthritis) or taking a medication (e.g. prednisone $\geq$5mg/day for $\geq$3 months) associated with low bone mass or bone loss
- Anyone being considered for pharmacologic therapy for osteoporosis
- Anyone being treated for osteoporosis, to monitor treatment effect

Table 33-1. Risk Factors for Developing Osteoporosis and Fractures

Nonmodifiable Risk Factors	Potentially Modifiable Risk Factors
• Advanced age • Gender: Women >> Men (approximately 4:1 ratio, especially postmenopausal women) • Race: Caucasian or Asian > Hispanic or African American • Genetics: First-degree family history of osteoporosis or nontraumatic fracture, or personal history of low body weight or small body frame, cystic fibrosis, homocystinuria, osteogenesis imperfecta, Ehlers-Danlos, glycogen storage diseases, Gaucher's disease, hemochromatosis, hypophosphatasia, idiopathic hypercalciuria, Marfan syndrome, Riley-Day syndrome, Menkes steely hair syndrome, porphyria • Gonadal steroids: late menarche, early menopause or oophorectomy without hormone replacement (especially premenopausal), amenorrhea, nulliparity, gonadal failure or loss (androgen insensitivity, anorexia nervosa or bulimia, Turner's & Klinefelter's syndromes, hyperprolactinemia, panhypopituitarism, athletic amenorrhea) • Gastrointestinal disorders: GI surgery, inflammatory bowel disease, gastric bypass, celiac disease, primary biliary cirrhosis, pancreatic disease • Hematologic disorders: hemophilia, leukemia and lymphomas, rheumatic and auto-immune diseases, ankylosing spondylitis, multiple myeloma, sickle cell disease, systemic mastocytosis, thalassemia, lupus, rheumatoid arthritis) • History of a fracture as an adult, especially after age 50 and other contributing factors (poor balance, reduced proprioception, poor vision, orthostatic hypotension)	• Low BMD • Falling • Decreased gonadal steroid levels (estrogen in women and testosterone in men) • Lifestyle choices: sedentary (inadequate physical activity or immobilization), smoking (active or passive), low dietary intake of calcium and vitamin D (or inadequate sunlight exposure), excessive alcohol consumption (>2 drinks per day), excessive vitamin A, salt, and caffeine intake • Medications: excessive use of aluminum-containing antacids, chronic glucocorticoid use (≥ 5mg prednisone or equiv for ≥ 3 months) • adrenocorticotropin • immunosuppressants • tamoxifen (premenopausal use) • cytotoxic drugs • anticonvulsant therapy (enzyme inducers such as phenobarbital or phenytoin), • lithium • proton pump inhibitors (e.g. omeprazole, lansoprazole, esomeprazole, rabeprazole) • excessive levothyroxine • cholestyramine • long-term heparin use • parenteral medroxyprogesterone acetate • Selective serotonin reuptake inhibitors (SSRIs) • thiazolidines (rosiglitazone, pioglitazone) • long term total parenteral nutrition • Chronic treatable medical conditions (e.g., bulimia, anorexia nervosa, hyperthyroidism, primary hyperparathyroidism, Cushing's syndrome, or malabsorption syndromes)

BMD, bone mineral density

• Anyone not receiving therapy in whom evidence of bone loss would lead to treatment
• Postmenopausal women discontinuing estrogen therapy

Height loss and secondary causes of osteoporosis are also risk factors strongly associated with fracture risk and would also be logical indications for BMD measurement.[5] Figure 33-1 outlines a flow chart for screening patients. Additional guidelines for testing men, children, and premenopausal women as well as indications for specific densitometric tests are provided by the International Society for Clinical Densitometry and the American Association of Clinical Endocrinologists.[6,7]

Additional risk assessment tools include measuring biochemical markers of bone turnover, using vertebral fracture assessment (VFA), and the World Health Organization (WHO) absolute fracture risk algorithm (FRAX). VFA refers to densitometric spine imaging to detect vertebral fractures, as radiographically confirmed vertebral fractures are a strong predictor of vertebral fractures, independent of BMD, age and other clinical risk factors.[3,6] FRAX may be used to calculate the 10-year probability of a hip fracture and the 10-year probability of any major osteoporotic fracture (defined

Table 33-2. Definition of Osteoporosis

Bone Classification*	T-Score† (BMD Measurement)
Normal	At −1.0 and above
Osteopenia (low bone mass)	Between −1.0 to −2.5
Osteoporosis	At −2.5 or below

* Based on 1994 World Health Organization classification of BMD.
† Mean standard deviation from a young normal adult female population.
BMD, bone mineral density.

Table 33-3. BMD Testing Techniques

Method	Site of BMD Testing	Comment
DXA	Spine, hip, wrist, total body	Highly precise and accurate, quick, low radiation exposure, not portable; gold standard. Central DXA of hip and/or spine is the preferred measure for definitive diagnosis.
Peripheral dual-energy X-ray absorptiometry	Forearm, finger, heel	Trivial amounts of radiation exposure. Not applicable to axial skeleton. Used more for screening purposes to assess if DXA is indicated. Lack of evidence for fracture prediction in men.
Quantitative computed tomography	Spine, hip, wrist	Most radiation exposure and more expensive; measures trabecular and cortical bone density. Peripheral quantitative computed tomography can measure bone density in periphery (forearm, tibia).
Quantitative ultrasound densitometry	Fingers, heel, tibia, patella	No radiation; portable. Not as precise as DXA or single-energy X-ray absorptiometry, but good predictor of future fracture risk.

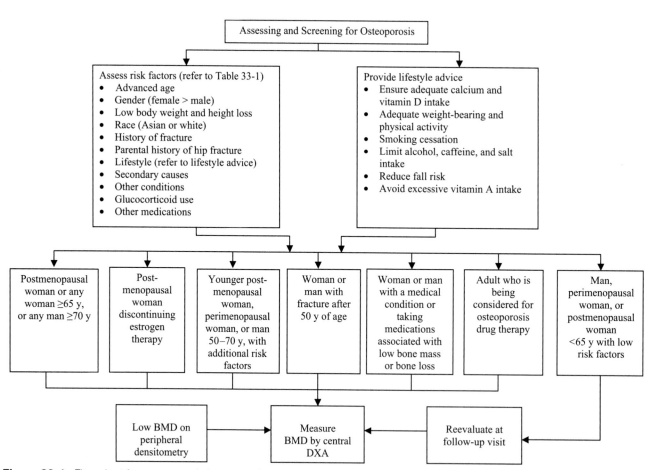

Figure 33-1. Flow chart for recommendations regarding selection of patients for dual-energy X-ray absorptiometry (DXA). For peripheral densitometry, each system will have different levels of T-score cutoff. In most cases, DXA will be recommended for patients with T-scores of −1.0 or lower. It is important to identify diseases or drugs that are likely to cause skeletal fragility or to increase the risk of falls. (Adapted from Raisz LG. Screening for osteoporosis. *N Engl J Med.* 2005;353:164–171 and National Osteoporosis Foundation: *Clinician's Guide to Prevention and Treatment of Osteoporosis*, 2008.)

as vertebral, hip, forearm, or humerous fracture).[3,8] The FRAX considers femoral neck BMD as well as several clinical risk factors. This algorithm may be most useful in identifying which patients with low bone mass (T score −1.0 to −2.5), or osteopenia, are most likely to benefit from treatment.[8]

MANAGEMENT[9]

PREVENTIVE STRATEGIES

Prevention of osteoporosis begins early in life. A well-balanced diet provides a variety of nutrients required for optimal bone health. Calcium is an essential mineral for healthy bones, and most Americans do not consume sufficient amounts. The recommended daily calcium requirements for ages 9–18 years are 1300 mg/day, for 18–50 yrs; 1000 mg/day, and over 50 yrs; 1200 mg/day.[3,10] Although dairy products are the major source of calcium for most people, Table 33-4 lists other food sources that provide calcium. Absorption of calcium is reduced when consumed from foods with oxalic or phytic acids, such as spinach, wheatbran, and other forms of unrefined flour.

Oral calcium supplements can be used when dietary sources do not meet the maximum daily calcium requirements. Calcium carbonate provides the highest amount of elemental calcium per tablet (40%), compared with calcium acetate (25%), calcium citrate (21%), calcium lactate (13%), and calcium gluconate (9%).

Calcium carbonate should be taken after meals to enhance absorption, whereas calcium citrate can be taken anytime. Doses of more than 500 mg per day of elemental calcium should be taken in 2 to 3 divided doses because overall intestinal absorption of calcium is reduced at higher doses. Achlorhydria, which frequently occurs with aging, reduces the absorption of calcium carbonate, whereas calcium citrate absorption is not impaired in achlorhydria. As such, calcium citrate may be a preferred calcium salt in older persons.

A major adverse effect of calcium supplementation is constipation, which may be managed by increasing dietary fiber and fluid intake, reducing the total daily calcium intake, or changing the calcium salt. Other side effects of calcium supplements include bloating, and gas. Doses should not exceed 2500 mg per day to avoid kidney stones.

Calcium salts also interact with a number of drugs. Calcium adsorbs or chelates antibiotics such as tetracyclines, azithromycin, fluoroquinolones in the gut. Also, by increasing intragastric pH, calcium salts reduce absorption of itraconazole, ketoconazole, and iron. These agents should be spaced at least 2 hours apart from calcium dosing. Long-term (>1 y) proton pump inhibitor (PPI) use has been shown to increase the risk of hip fractures in patients >50 years of age by impairing calcium absorption and/or inhibiting osteoclast activity. It is recommended that PPIs be given in the lowest dose for the shortest time period possible, and to use calcium salts other than calcium carbonate (which requires gastric acidity for absorption) when taking a PPI. Calcium supplements may also interfere with the absorption of other drugs such as thyroid hormone (levothyroxine) and should be spaced 6–12 hours apart.

Sufficient daily amounts of vitamin D are made by the body after 5 to 15 minutes of the skin exposure to sunlight, but the process can be attenuated by skin pigmentation and topical sunscreens. However, if regular sunlight exposure is not practical or feasible, vitamin D may be obtained from oral supplements. In addition, patients >70 years do not effectively convert provitamin D in their skin to vitamin D from sunlight. Recommended adequate daily intakes of vitamin D have been published for all life stages[10]. Vitamin D dosed at 800–1000 IU per day is required to prevent hip and nonvertebral fractures in patients ≥50 years of age. Newer guidelines recommend ages 19–50 years receive vitamin D at 400–800 IU/day, and over 50 years consume 800–1000 IU/day.[3]

Weight-bearing aerobic exercise and resistance training of at least 30 minutes a day for adults (60 min for children) should be encouraged to increase BMD in the spine, hips, and wrists. Regular exercise also has been linked to improvements in balance, stronger muscles, improved muscle tone, and reduced falls.

Patients at high risk for falls should be evaluated for fall prevention strategies aimed at minimizing fall risk. Strategies should include optimizing living conditions such as removing rugs, using night lights, installing shower seats and/or holding bars, and avoiding medications that are known to increase the risk of falls, such as sedating medications, anticholinergics, and narcotics.

Table 33-4. Selected Food Sources Containing High Amounts of Calcium[22,23]

Food	Calcium (mg)
Yogurt, plain, nonfat, 8 oz.	452
Soy beverage, calcium fortified, 8 fl. oz.	368
Fruit, yogurt, low fat, 8 oz.	345
Sardines, Atlantic, in oil, drained, 3 oz.	325
Mozzarella, part skim 1.5 oz.	311
Cheddar cheese, 1.5 oz.	307
Milk, (skim) nonfat, 8 fl. oz.	306
Milk, low fat (2%), 8 fl. oz.	285
Milk, whole, 8 fl. oz.	276
Salmon, pink, canned, 3 oz.	181
Spinach, cooked from frozen, ½ cup	146

The use of hip protectors should be considered for frail older people and patients at high risk for falling, although patient adherence is low because these devices are bulky and uncomfortable to wear.

Smokers should be strongly encouraged to quit, since smoking has been associated with an increase in risk of overall fractures, while cessation of smoking seems to reduce the fracture risk.[11] Consumption of more than 2 alcoholic beverages per day increases patient risk of low BMD. Both women and men should avoid excessive weight loss. Consumption of excessive doses of vitamin A may be associated with decreases in BMD and an increased risk of fracture.[12] Although current data are limited, patients should be advised not to exceed the dietary reference intake (DRI) of 700 to 900 mcg/d (2310 IU to 3000 IU) of vitamin A for women and men, respectively. Patients on chronic glucocorticoid therapy (doses of ≥ 5 mg/day of prednisone or equivalent for ≥ 3 months) are at risk for glucocorticoid-induced osteoporosis and should be advised to take calcium supplementation of 1200–1500 mg/day and vitamin D of 800 IU/day.

There are conflicting studies whether phytoestrogens, such as soy, are beneficial in improving BMD and reducing bone turnover in postmenopausal women. These may be as a result of varying content of isoflavones (the active agent) in different soy foods or products, increased sensitivity to the effects of soy isoflavones in Asian women, or whether soy is consumed in early or late postmenopause. As a result, phytoestrogens are not recommended for prevention or treatment in postmenopausal women with osteoporosis.

TREATMENT

Pharmacologic treatment should be initiated in women and men 50 years and older presenting with any of the following[3]:

- BMD T-scores ≤ -2.5 at the femoral neck, total hip, or spine after appropriate evaluation to exclude secondary causes
- Low bone mass (T score between -1.0 and -2.5 at the femoral neck, total hip, or spine) and secondary causes associated with high risk of fracture (e.g. glucocorticoid use or total immobilization)
- A hip or vertebral (clinical or morphometric) fracture
- Other prior fractures and low bone mass (T score between -1.0 and -2.5) at the femoral neck, total hip, or spine)
- Low bone mass (T score between -1.0 and -2.5 at the femoral neck, total hip, or spine) and 10-year probability of hip fracture $\geq 3\%$ or a 10-year probability of any major osteoporosis-related fracture $\geq 20\%$ based on the U.S. adapted WHO algorithm[8]

Adequate calcium and vitamin D intake have been associated with reduced bone loss, lower fall risk, and a lower risk of bone fractures. Calcium and vitamin D supplements may be needed to ensure adequate calcium intake (see Table 33-4). Both agents should be continued indefinitely for long-term efficacy. Cholecalciferol (vitamin D_3) is preferred over ergocalciferol (vitamin D_2) for vitamin D supplementation as cholecalciferol is more effective at raising serum 25(OH)D concentrations and is active for a longer period of time than ergocalciferol, especially in older patients. Adequate calcium (at least 1200 mg/day) and vitamin D_3 (800–1000 IU/day) intake must continue indefinitely with any pharmacologic therapy to obtain maximum benefit.

Table 33-5 summarizes the medications used in the treatment and prevention of osteoporosis. Bisphosphonates are the first-line pharmacologic agents for the prevention and treatment of postmenopausal osteoporosis, treatment of osteoporosis in men, and the prevention and treatment of glucocorticoid-induced osteoporosis. Bisphosphonates act to decrease bone resorption by inhibiting osteoclast function. They have been shown to halt bone loss and increase BMD, but their ability to improve bone strength is more related to their ability to preserve trabecular architecture than their effect on BMD.

The currently available bisphosphonates for osteoporosis management are alendronate, risedronate, ibandronate, and zoledronate (also called zoledronic acid). The agents vary in their effect on increasing BMD at vertebral and nonvertebral sites, fracture risk reduction at different sites, dosing regimens, route of administration, and administration instruction. Although the effect on BMD varies between these agents, there is not a clear relationship between degree of BMD increase and fracture risk reduction. Alendronate (Fosamax), risedronate (Actonel), and zoledronate (Reclast) have been shown to reduce both spine and hip fractures in women with postmenopausal osteoporosis.[13,14,15] Ibandronate (Boniva) reduces vertebral fractures. Ease of adherence to therapy may be a more important selection criteria than the choice of bisphosphonate, as there is a high discontinuation rate of bisphosphonates, especially during the first year. Postmenopausal women who consistently take a bisphosphonate have fewer bone fractures than nonadherent women.[16] Simplifying dosing regimens to once weekly (oral alendronate, oral risedronate), once monthly (oral ibandronate or oral risedronate), once every three months (intravenous ibandronate), or once yearly (intravenous zoledronate) may offer a distinct advantage over traditional once daily dosing. Further, patients who are unable to tolerate oral forms of bisphosphonates due to a contraindication or

Table 33-5. Medications Used in Treatment and Prevention of Osteoporosis*

Drug Class	Drug Name (Brand Name)	Dosing Guidelines
Bisphosphonates	Alendronate (Fosamax tablets or oral solution)	Treatment of postmenopausal osteoporosis • 70 mg tablet orally once weekly, or • 1 bottle of 70 mg oral solution once weekly, or • 10 mg tablet orally once daily Prevention of postmenopausal osteoporosis • 35 mg tablet once weekly, or • 5 mg tablet orally once daily Treatment to increase bone mass in men with osteoporosis • 70 mg tablet orally once weekly, or • 1 bottle of 70 mg oral solution once weekly, or • 10 mg tablet orally once daily Treatment of glucocorticoid-induced osteoporosis • 5 mg tablet orally once daily, except for postmenopausal women not receiving estrogen, for whom dosing is: • 10 mg tablet orally once daily
	Alendronate plus cholecalciferol (Fosamax Plus D tablets)	Treatment of postmenopausal osteoporosis • 70 mg/5,600 IU tablet orally once weekly (provides 7 days worth of 800 IU vitamin D_3 in a single once weekly dose) • 70 mg/2800 IU tablet orally once weekly (provides 7 days worth of 400 IU vitamin D_3 in a single once weekly dose) Treatment to increase bone mass in men with osteoporosis • 70 mg/2800 IU tablet orally once weekly
	Risedronate (Actonel tablets)	Prevention and treatment of postmenopausal osteoporosis • 150 mg tablet orally once monthly • 75 mg tablet orally, taken on two consecutive days each month • 35 mg tablet orally once weekly, or • 5 mg tablet orally once daily Treatment to increase bone mass in men with osteoporosis • 35 mg tablet orally once weekly Prevention and treatment of glucocorticoid-induced osteoporosis • 5 mg tablet orally once daily
	Risedronate with calcium (Actonel with calcium tablets)	Prevention and treatment of postmenopausal osteoporosis • 35 mg tablet orally once weekly with 500 mg elemental calcium (1250 mg calcium carbonate) for remaining six days of the week
	Ibandronate (Boniva tablets or injection)	Prevention and treatment of postmenopausal osteoporosis • 2.5 mg orally once daily, or • 150 mg tablet orally once monthly (on the same date each month) Treatment of postmenopausal osteoporosis • 3 mg intravenously every three months (administered as a bolus over 15–30 seconds)
	Zoledronate acid (Reclast injection)	Treatment of postmenopausal osteoporosis • 5 mg intravenously once a year (administered as an infusion over no less than 15 minutes)
Calcitonin	Calcitonin- salmon (Miacalcin nasal spray or injection; Fortical nasal spray-rDNA origin)	Treatment of postmenopausal osteoporosis in women >5 years postmenopause • 200 IU (1 spray) per day intranasally, alternating nostrils daily • 100 IU subcutaneously or intramuscularly every other day
Estrogen therapy	Estrogen (Premarin tablets)	Prevention of postmenopausal osteoporosis • 0.3 mg orally daily. Subsequent dosing adjustment based on individual and BMD response. Oral progestin should be added if woman has an intact uterus.
Selective estrogen receptor modulator	Raloxifene (Evista tablets)	Prevention and treatment of postmenopausal osteoporosis • 60 mg orally daily
Parathyroid hormone	Teriparatide (Forteo pen injection-rDNA origin)	Treatment of postmenopausal osteoporosis • 20 mcg injected subcutaneously into the thigh or abdominal wall once daily Treatment to increase bone mass in men with osteoporosis • 20 mcg injected subcutaneously into the thigh or abdominal wall once daily

*Dosing per FDA-approved indication.

gastrointestinal tolerance may be candidates for an intravenous (IV) bisphosphonate.

To maximize oral absorption, alendronate and risedronate must be taken at least 30 minutes before the first food, beverage, or medication of the day with 6 to 8 oz of plain water only. Oral ibandronate (Boniva) must be taken 60 minutes before the first food or beverage of the day. Patients must not chew or suck the tablet because of a potential for oropharyngeal ulceration. To minimize the risk of esophageal stricture or perforation, the patient must be instructed not to lie down for at least 30 minutes after dosing and then to do so only after consuming the first food of the day. Patients with an abnormality of their esophagus, stricture, achalasia, or inability to sit upright for 30–60 minutes should not receive an oral bisphosphonate. Patients at high risk of aspiration should not receive oral alendronate solution. Oral bisphosphonates may cause dysphagia, esophagitis, or esophageal or gastric ulcers. Concomitant use of nonsteroidal anti-inflammatory agents or aspirin may increase the risk of gastrointestinal side effects. In addition, patients with aspirin sensitivity resulting in bronchospasm should avoid bisphosphonates.

The bisphosphonates have recently been associated with osteonecrosis of the jaw.[17] While uncommon, patients receiving bisphosphonate therapy should receive a routine oral examination prior to initiating therapy, biannual dental examinations, minimize periodontal inflammation and avoid invasive dental procedures. Patients should inform their dentists that they are taking a bisphosphonate.

Other side effects associated with bisphosphonate therapy include bone, joint, or muscle pain, a slightly higher risk of atrial fibrillation in some studies, and an acute phase reaction with IV formulations (pyrexia, influenza-like symptoms). The latter may be minimized post-treatment with analgesics such as acetaminophen. Bisphosphonates should not be given to patients with poor renal function (creatinine clearance <35 mL/min), and IV bisphosphonates should be avoided in patients receiving nephrotoxic medications (e.g., aminoglycosides, NSAIDs). Any existing hypocalcemia should be corrected before starting bisphosphonate therapy.

Calcitonin-salmon (Miacalcin nasal spray or injection, Fortical nasal spray) is administered as a nasal spray or an injection for the treatment of postmenopausal osteoporosis in women who are more than 5 years postmenopausal. Calcitonin has been demonstrated to significantly increase vertebral BMD in osteoporotic women and reduce lumbar spine fractures. Calcitonin also relieves pain associated with spinal compression fractures. Calcitonin increases hip BMD, but does not reduce hip fractures. The intranasal dose of calcitonin is one spray (200 IU) per day intranasally, alternating nostrils daily while the injectable form is administered as a 100 IU subcutaneous or intramuscular injection every other day. The main adverse effects of intranasal calcitonin are mild to moderate rhinitis, nasal irritation, erythema, and excoriation, which seem to be more common in patients >65 years than younger patients. The injectable formulation may cause a local inflammatory reaction at the injection site, nausea, and flushing of the hands and face.

Estrogen therapy, with or without a progestin, has been shown to prevent postmenopausal bone loss. The Women's Health Initiative demonstrated that estrogen with or without a progestin reduces hip, vertebral, and total fractures in women without known osteoporosis.[18,19] Unfortunately, an increased risk of invasive breast cancer, myocardial infarction, venous thromboembolism and stroke occurred with conjugated equine estrogen combined with medroxyprogesterone acetate in the Women's Health Initiative, while conjugated equine estrogen alone in women with a hysterectomy also showed an increased incidence of venous thromboembolism, stroke, and dementia (although breast cancer risk was not increased). As such, the use of these agents for osteoporosis is no longer generally recommended in otherwise healthy postmenopausal women and if used, should be started at the lowest possible dose for the shortest time period possible.

Raloxifene (Evista), a selective estrogen receptor modulator, has been approved for both osteoporosis treatment and prevention in postmenopausal women. It reduces the risk of spine fracture in women with and without prior spinal fracture. However, it remains second line after bisphosphonates because it has not yet been shown to reduce the risk of hip fractures. Raloxifene has been associated with a reduction in risk of invasive breast cancer in postmenopausal women, suggesting that women at high risk of invasive breast cancer may benefit from raloxifene's protective effects. Raloxifene has a black box warning on its product labeling that it should be avoided in patients at high risk of thromboembolic events as it can increase the risk of deep venous thromboembolism, pulmonary embolism, and stroke. Its use should be discontinued at least 72 hours prior to and during prolonged immobilization. In addition, raloxifene increases hot flushes; women in perimenopause should avoid its use. The dose of raloxifene is 60 mg orally once daily.

Teriparatide (Forteo) is a parathyroid hormone formulation that is injected subcutaneously into the thigh or abdominal wall once a day. Teriparatide stimulates new bone formation, resulting in increased BMD. Teriparatide has been shown to reduce the risk of both vertebral and nonvertebral fractures in clinical trials of postmenopausal women with osteoporosis. Teriparatide increases BMD more effectively than alendronate in glucocorticoid-induced osteoporosis.[20] It may also reduce back pain in patients with vertebral fractures. The teriparatide product labeling carries a black-box warning of increased incidence of osteosarcoma based on observations in rats; the incidence was dependent on the dose and treatment duration. Teriparatide should be reserved for patients who are intolerant to, or have failed therapy with bisphosphonates, and it should not be prescribed for patients at risk for developing osteosarcoma such as Paget's disease or adolescents, or patients with cancer that may spread to bone. Further, if teriparatide is prescribed, treatment is limited to 2 years because of the lack of longer-term efficacy and safety data. Adverse effects of teriparatide are generally mild and include nausea and dizziness. Patients should be monitored for hypercalcemia and hypercalciuria. At present, teriparatide should not be given in combination with a bisphosphonate as the latter (specifically, alendronate) has been shown to significantly blunt the effect of teriparatide. However, teriparatide therapy followed by a bisphosphonate can maintain the gains in BMD obtained by teriparatide.

The use of combination therapy is still controversial. Combinations of the above agents (such as a bisphosphonate with estrogen therapy or raloxifene; teriparatide with raloxifene) may provide a further increase in BMD, but it remains to be seen if this translates to fewer hip and spinal fractures than individual agents alone. While, combination therapy may be considered for patients with severe osteoporosis or who continue to fracture with single drug therapy, combination treatment is associated with higher drug costs for patients and has the potential for more adverse effects. Initiating and monitoring combination therapies may be best decided by an endocrinologist.

Patients who have a bone fracture also experience severe pain from the fracture itself. Calcitonin may have a role in reducing pain in patients with vertebral fractures. However, these patients will most likely require analgesics to control the pain in addition to osteoporosis therapy.

MONITORING

The safety and efficacy of alendronate has been confirmed for up to 10 years of use. Women who discontinue alendronate after 5 years have a moderate decline in BMD but do not have a higher risk of nonvertebral fractures after five years without therapy compared to women who continued alendronate.[21] However, women who continued alendronate for 10 years had significantly fewer vertebral fractures than women who discontinued therapy after five years.[21] This suggests that women who

are at high risk for vertebral fractures should continue bisphosphonate therapy beyond 5 years.

Bisphosphonates can prevent bone fractures independently of whether they increase BMD. Hence, the need and frequency of follow-up BMD testing post-therapy has been debated. Unless a fracture occurs, BMD can be repeated every 2 years once on therapy. Changing therapy can be considered after at least 1 year of medication therapy if fractures continue or if bone or back pain develops. Monitoring should also address any troublesome side effects encountered, and medication adherence. Since less than 50% of patients persist with bisphosphonate therapy after 2 years of use, medication regimens requiring less frequent administration, such as once every three months IV ibandronate or once yearly IV zoledronate should be considered for poorly adherent patients.

RECENT DEVELOPMENTS

Denosumab, an antibody preparation that inhibits osteoclastogenesis, may have similar application. Newer selective estrogen receptor modulators are under development as are other agents that inhibit osteoclast function, such as cathepsin inhibitors. Strontium ranelate, with bone anabolic actions, is approved in Europe and Canada for osteoporosis treatment and may become available in the United States.

EVIDENCE-BASED SUMMARY

- Osteoporosis is often a silent disease until a fracture occurs. Symptomatic patients may experience bone pain, loss of height, or kyphosis. Fractures in the vertebra, hip, and wrist are common.
- Nonmodifiable risk factors (see Table 33-1) for osteoporosis include advanced age, female gender, race (white or Asian), family history of fracture, low body weight or short stature, personal history of fracture, gonadal steroid issues.
- Modifiable risk factors (see Table 33-1) include low BMD, falling, reduced gonadal steroids, poor lifestyle choices, long-term use of some medications (e.g., prednisone), and chronic treatable medical conditions.
- Screening is recommended for all women ≥ 65 y, all men >70 y, postmenopausal women <65 y, and men 50–70 y with risk factors, men or perimenopausal women with specific risk factors, all adults who fracture after age 50, medical conditions or medications associated with low bone mass, anyone being considered for pharmacologic treatment, anyone being treated for osteoporosis

- BMD testing at diagnosis is the most important predictor of fracture risk.
- Bone mineral density testing with a central DXA is the preferred tool for establishing a diagnosis of osteoporosis.
- Strategies to prevent osteoporosis start in childhood and include a well-balanced diet, adequate calcium and vitamin D intake, regular aerobic and weight bearing exercise, quitting smoking, limiting alcohol intake, and avoiding excessive dieting.
- Preventive strategies should be implemented in older persons at risk for falls
- First-line pharmacologic treatment of osteoporosis includes calcium, and vitamin D3 supplementation and a bisphosphonate.
- Choice of bisphosphonates should consider the regimen most likely to be adhered to by the patient.
- Other therapies, such as calcitonin, raloxifene, estrogen replacement therapy with or without a progestin, or teriparatide may be considered if fractures continue to occur or new bone or back pain develops after 1 year of bisphosphonate therapy.
- Simultaneous treatment with more than one antiresorptive agent may be initiated by an endocrinologist
- With initiation of pharmacologic treatment, BMD testing should be performed every two years to monitor bone loss
- Once initiated for osteoporosis, bisphosphonates therapy may be continued for beneficial effect on BMD, especially in patients at high risk for vertebral compression fractures.

REFERENCES

1. National Osteoporosis Foundation, American's bone health: The state of osteoporosis and low bone mass. http://www.nof.org/advocacy/prevalence. Accessed March 20, 2007.

2. National Osteoporosis Foundation, Disease Facts. http://www.nof.org/osteoporosis/diseasefacts.htm Accessed March 20, 2007.

3. National Osteoporosis Foundation: *Clinician's Guide to Prevention and Treatment of Osteoporosis.* http://www.nof.org/professionals/clinicians_Guide.htm. Accessed March 11, 2008.

4. Kanis JA, Johnell O, De Laet C, et al. A meta-analysis of previous fracture and subsequent fracture risk. *Bone* 2004; 35:375–382.

5. Raisz LG. Screening for osteoporosis. *N Engl J Med.* 2005; 353:164–171.

6. The International Society for Clinical Densitometry. *2007 ISCD Official Positions:* http://www.iscd.org/Visitors/positions/OfficialPositionsText.cfm. Accessed Feb 27, 2008.

7. Hodgson SF, Watts NB, Bilezikian JP, et al. American Association of Clinical Endocrinologists medical guidelines for clinical practice for the prevention and treatment of postmenopausal osteoporosis: 2001 Edition, with selected updates for 2003. *Endocr Pract.* 2003;9(6):544–564; Erratum, *Endocr Pract.* 2004;10(1):90.

8. The World Health Organization Fracture Risk Assessment Tool: http://www.shef.ac.uk/FRAX/. Accessed February 27, 2008.

9. U.S. Department of Health and Human Services. Bone health and osteoporosis: A report of the Surgeon General. Rockville, MD: U.S. Department of Health and Human Services, Office of the Surgeon General, 2004. http://www.surgeongeneral.gov/library or http://www.hhs.gov/surgeongeneral/library/bonehealth. Accessed March 11, 2007. Executive summary available at http://www.hhs.gov/surgeongeneral/library/ bonehealth/docs/exec_summ.pdf

10. Dietary Reference Intakes: the essential guide to nutrient requirements. The National Academies Press, Washington, D.C., 2006.

11. P. Vestergaard, L. Mosekilde. Fracture risk associated with smoking: A meta-analysis. *J Intern Med.* 2003;254(6): 572–583.

12. Jackson HA, Sheehan AH. Effect of vitamin A on fracture risk. *Ann Pharmacother.* 2005;39:2086–2090.

13. Hochberg MC, Thompson DE, Black DM, et al, for the FIT Research Group. Effect of alendronate on the age-specific incidence of symptomatic fractures. *J Bone Min Res* 2005;20(6):971–976.

14. McClung MR, Geusens P, Miller PD, et al, for the Hip Intervention Program Study Group. Effect of risedronate on the risk of hip fracture in elderly women. *New Engl J Med* 2001;344(5):333–40.

15. Lyles KW, Colon-Emeric CC, Magaziner JS, et al, for the HORIZON Recurrent Fracture Trial. Zoledronic acid and clinical fractures and mortality after hip fracture. *New Engl J Med* 2007;357(18):1799–1809.

16. Siris ES, Harris ST, Rosen CJ, et al. Adherence to bisphosphonate therapy and fracture rates in osteoporotic women: Relationship to vertebral and nonvertebral fractures from 2 US claims databases. *Mayo Clin Proc.* 2006; 81(8):1013–1022.

17. Woo S-B, Hellstein JW, Kalmar JR. Systematic review : Bisphosphonates and osteonecrosis of the jaw. *Ann Intern Med.* 2006;144(10):753–761.

18. Writing Group for the Women's Health Initiative Investigators. Risks and benefits of estrogen plus progestin in healthy postmenopausal women. Principal results from the Women's Health Initiative randomized controlled trial. *JAMA.* 2002;288(3):321–333.

19. The Women's Health Initiative Steering Committee. Effects of conjugated equine estrogen in postmenopausal women with hysterectomy. The Women's Health Initiative randomized controlled trial. *JAMA.* 2004;291(14): 1701–1712.

20. Saag KG, Shane E, Boonen S, et al. Teriparatide or alendronate in glucocorticoid-induced osteoporosis. *New Engl J Med* 2007;357(20):2028–2039.

21. Black DM, Schwartz AV, Ensrud KE, et al. Effects of continuing of stopping alendronate after 5 years of treatment. The Fracture Intervention Trial Long-Term Extension (FLEX): A randomized trial. *JAMA.* 2006; 296(24): 2927–2938.

22. *USDA Dietary Guidelines for Americans 2005.* Appendix B-4. Non-Dairy Food Sources of Calcium. Available at http://health.gov/dietaryguidelines/dga2005/document/html/appendixB.htm. Accessed March 10, 2007.

23. *USDA Dietary Guidelines for Americans 2005.* Appendix B-5. Food Sources of Calcium. Available at http://health.gov/dietaryguidelines/dga2005/document/html/appendixB.htm. Accessed March 10, 2007.

Chapter 34

Rheumatoid Arthritis

Arthur A. Schuna

SEARCH STRATEGY

A systematic search of the medical literature was conducted on December 27, 2006. The search, limited to human subjects and journals in the English language, included the National Guideline Clearinghouse, PubMed, and the Cochrane database

Rheumatoid arthritis (RA) is a systemic disease with symmetric inflammation of joints as a hallmark feature. Many other organ systems may also be involved. Joint destruction with loss of ability to perform daily functional activities often results if adequate treatment is not used. Early treatment with therapies that slow disease progression is recommended together with physical modalities to assist the patient to maintain normal activities of daily living and prevent disability.

RA occurs in approximately 1% of the population. The factors responsible for RA are not known.

CLINICAL PRESESNTATION

Symptoms of RA often are insidious with nonspecific symptoms such as fatigue, weakness, low-grade fever, and loss of appetite in addition to joint symptoms. Stiffness and myalgia may precede the development of synovitis. Joint stiffness tends to be more of a problem early in the morning. Duration of morning stiffness is a useful clinical parameter to follow as patients with more active inflammation remain stiff for longer periods of time and successful suppression of disease activity should reduce the duration ideally to less than 30 minutes. Fatigue onset tends to be earlier in the day for patients with more active disease and lessens with effective treatment. Joint involvement tends to be symmetrical

although early in the disease, it may involve a few joints and be asymmetrical in pattern.[1] No single physical finding or laboratory test can be used to make the diagnosis. The American College of Rheumatology has developed criteria for RA classification that can be useful in making the diagnosis (Table 34-1). These criteria have been criticized as they are not very useful for patients with early disease. For example, radiographic changes and rheumatoid nodules are late-disease manifestations and symmetric involvement may not be seen early in the disease.[2]

PHYSICAL FINDINGS

The joints of the hands and feet are most frequently affected by RA. Other joints commonly affected include the elbows, shoulders, hips, and knees. Palpation may reveal tenderness and swelling as well as increased skin temperature over inflamed joints. In the hand, metacarpal and proximal interphalangeal joints and the wrist tend to be involved. The distal interphalangeal joints are seldom involved in RA but may be inflamed in other rheumatic diseases.

Deformities of hand joints including subluxation, ulnar deviation of the metacarpals, and boutonniere and swan-neck deformities tend to be late manifestations of the disease. Tendon rupture may also lead to deformity and loss of function. Swelling may occur just over joints or more diffusely if involvement includes the tendon sheath (tenosynovitis). Swelling occurs as a result of proliferation of inflamed synovial membrane as well as the accumulation of joint fluid that extends the joint capsule. Functional difficulties in clasping, grasping, and pinching may result from inflammation or chronic deformity.

Table 34-1. Criteria for the Classification of Rheumatoid Arthritis

Criterion*	Definition
1. Morning stiffness	Stiffness of joints lasting at least 1 h before improvement
2. Arthritis of 3 or more joints	Soft-tissue swelling or fluid in joint
3. Arthritis in hand joints	At least one swollen wrist, MCP, or PIP
4. Symmetric joint swelling	Simultaneous involvement of bilateral joint areas
5. Rheumatoid nodules	Subcutaneous nodules over extensor tendons, bony prominences, or near joints
6. Positive rheumatoid factor	Significantly elevated rheumatoid factor concentration
7. Radiographic changes	Characteristic changes for rheumatoid arthritis noted on hand radiographs including erosions and periarticular osteoporosis

*A patient shall be classified as having rheumatoid arthritis if at least four of these criteria are met. Criteria 1–4 must be present for at least 6 weeks.
MCP, metacarpophalangeal; PIP, proximal interphalangeal.
Adapted from: Arnett FC, Edworthy SM, Bloch DA, et al. The American Rheumatism Association 1987 revised criteria for the classification of rheumatoid arthritis. *Arthritis Rheum.* 1988;31:315–324.

Swelling of the elbow is best assessed by palpation of the radiohumeral joint. Swelling of the olecranon bursa may also be seen but may also occur in patients without inflammatory arthritis. Reduced range of motion in the elbow may occur with long-standing inflammation and disuse.

Pain in the shoulder may result from synovitis of the shoulder joint or inflammation of tendons or bursa around the shoulder. Painful motion may be noted early in the disease with loss of motion with disuse.

Spine involvement is uncommon with RA but may be seen in other inflammatory rheumatic diseases. Cervical (C1–C2) instability and subluxation is rarely seen in RA.

The knee may be involved with swelling of the joint as well as surrounding bursae. With chronic synovitis, cartilage degradation and instability of the joint may be a factor. Loss of range of motion may result in changes in gait. Chronic joint pain can result in muscle atrophy, which can lead to ligamentous laxity and joint instability.

In the foot, involvement of the ankle and metatarsal joints is common. Callus formation, bunion, and other foot deformities may also contribute to foot pain.

EXTRA-ARTICULAR FINDINGS

Rheumatoid nodules are found in 20% of the patients with RA. They are usually found on extensor tendons of the hand, elbows, and forearm but may also be found elsewhere, including the lung and sclera.

Vasculitis may be seen particularly in patients with long-standing RA. Small-vessel vasculitis can result in tiny infarcts near the ends of digits, particularly around the nail bed. Skin ulcers similar to stasis ulcers may develop particularly in the lower extremities.

Lung manifestations of RA include pleural effusions, pulmonary fibrosis, and lung nodules. In addition to auscultation, chest radiographs are useful in assessing the patient.

RA is associated with a higher risk of cardiovascular disease. This risk appears to lessen with treatment of inflammation. Pericarditis and myocarditis may occur but are relatively uncommon. Cardiac conduction abnormalities and aortic valve incompetence may also occur.

Ocular manifestations include keratoconjunctivitis sicca and inflammation of the sclera, episclera, and cornea. Inflammation of the lacrimal ducts can lead to decreased tear formation resulting in keratoconjunctivitis. Inflammation of the episclera tends to be self-limiting but involvement of the sclera or cornea may require intervention.

Lymphadenopathy may be seen in patients with very active inflammation. Amyloidosis is a rare complication sometimes seen in patients late in the course of their disease.

DIAGNOSTIC EVALUATION

A careful history and physical examination should be done to assess whether the patient meets diagnostic criteria for RA. Additionally, laboratory and radiographic studies are useful to help confirm the diagnosis. Care must be taken to rule out other causes of arthritis, which can sometimes be very challenging due to similarities between these entities. Discussion of these differences is beyond the scope of this chapter.

Laboratory evidence for inflammation can be assessed using the erythrocyte sedimentation rate (ESR) and C-reactive protein (CRP). The ESR measures the rate of settling of erythrocytes through plasma over a period of 1 hour. The rate of settling is influenced by surrounding plasma proteins and tends to increase with active inflammation. The ESR is a very nonspecific marker and can be increased with a number of diseases as well as with advanced age. Another drawback is that patients with very active synovitis may have normal ESR and an elevated ESR may be seen in patients without any apparent disease. CRP is a protein made by the liver, which increases production during inflammation. It tends to parallel ESR changes but the rise and fall of CRP tends to be more abrupt. The CRP has limitations similar to ESR in terms of lack of specificity and sensitivity. Nevertheless, the presence of elevated CRP and

ESR can be useful in conjunction with physical findings in evaluating the patient.

Rheumatoid factor is an IgG antibody that is found in increased concentrations in patients with RA. A positive rheumatoid factor may be seen in 50% of patients early in the disease course but increases to as many as 85% over time. Rheumatoid factor can be elevated in patients with other diseases including systemic lupus erythematosus, polymyositis, chronic infection, and malignancy. About 5% of young patients without obvious disease may have a positive rheumatoid factor and the prevalence increases to about 9% to 14% of people older than 70 years. The high rate of positive rheumatoid factor in patients without disease may lead to false positives, particularly when the clinical suspicion for RA is low. Conversely, RA may be present in patients with a negative rheumatoid factor.

Anticyclic citrullinated peptide antibody is another test with similar sensitivity (50–85%) but higher specificity (90–95%) than rheumatoid factor. For this reason, it has been found to be clinically useful in diagnosing patients with RA.[3,4]

Other laboratory findings that are commonly seen include normochromic, normocytic anemia. This anemia is often termed "anemia of chronic disease." It is caused by high levels of proinflammatory cytokines, such as interleukin-1 (IL-1), which reduce the bone marrow's response to erythropoietin. Additionally, thrombocytosis is frequently seen in patients with active inflammation.

Radiographs of affected joints are also useful. Although these may be normal in very early disease, it is still worthwhile obtaining X-rays at baseline to be able to assess for disease progression with treatment. Radiographs of small joints of the hands and feet are particularly worthwhile due to the relatively high rate of involvement of these joints. Early radiographic changes include periarticular osteoporosis and loss of joint space due to cartilage degradation. Erosions usually develop later and tend to be first seen on bone near the joint margin.

In addition to radiographs, magnetic resonance imaging and ultrasound may be useful in documenting changes in joints and soft-tissue structures consistent with RA. These modalities may be useful to document early inflammatory arthropathy before bone and cartilage degradation occur, which radiographs are able to detect.

MANAGEMENT

The management of RA includes a combination of both nondrug and drug therapy. Nondrug therapies include exercise to maintain range of motion and prevent muscle atrophy, which may occur from disuse. Additionally, patients may need to recognize that physical exertion may aggravate symptoms particularly when the disease is active. Learning physical limits are important for the patient. In some cases, assistive devices such as canes, crutches, walkers, or wheelchairs may be necessary. In addition, braces may be of benefit for joints with instability. Occupational therapy may be useful to evaluate patients for devices to assist with activities of daily living, which may be important to help a patient maintain independence.

Podiatry may be needed to assist patients with foot deformities and other rheumatoid foot disorders. Orthotic shoe inserts or custom shoes may be necessary for some patients. Surgery may also be necessary in some patients with more severe joint destruction.

DRUG THERAPY

Drug therapy includes nonsteroidal anti-inflammatory drugs (NSAIDs), corticosteroids, and disease-modifying antirheumatic drugs (DMARDs). DMARDs, as the acronym implies, are those drugs that are believed to alter disease progression. Current guidelines for treatment recommend that an agent in this category be started within 3 months of the onset of symptoms.[5,6] It has been demonstrated that early initiation of DMARDs results in better long-term outcomes.[7] Earlier initiation of DMARDs may prevent the erosions and deformities that tend to occur later in the course of the disease. For this reason, early and accurate diagnosis of the patient is essential. Expedited referral to a rheumatologist may be needed in some patients, particularly when a patient has atypical features of presentation.

The choice of DMARD for first-line therapy is not clearly defined, though for patients with more severe disease methotrexate is frequently chosen due to superior long-term outcome data compared to other oral DMARDs and lower cost than biologic DMARDs.[8–10] See Fig. 34-1 for a schematic algorithm for the treatment of RA. For a list of DMARDs, common doses, and monitoring parameters, see Tables 34-2 and 34-3.

Combination therapy with two or more DMARDs may sometimes be useful when single DMARD therapy fails to achieve adequate responses. The combinations of cyclosporine plus methotrexate, and methotrexate plus sulfasalazine and hydroxychloroquine have been shown to be particularly effective.[6,11–18] Combinations of methotrexate plus biologic DMARDs have also been shown to be effective compared to single-agent therapy.[19]

Nonsteroidal Anti-Inflammatory Drugs

A variety of NSAIDs are available for the treatment of RA (see Table 34-4). It is important to recognize

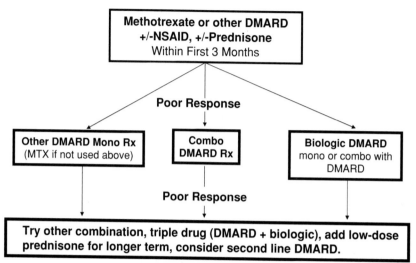

Figure 34-1. Treatment of rheumatoid arthritis.
Abbreviations: RA, rheumatoid arthritis; NSAID, nonsteroidal anti-inflammatory drug; Rx, therapy; DMARD, disease-modifying antirheumatic drug.

Table 34-2. Dosage and Laboratory Monitoring

Drug	Usual Dose	Initial	Maintenance
NSAIDs	See table	Scr or BUN, CBC q 2–4 wk p starting therapy × 1–2 mo Salicylates: Serum salicylate levels if therapeutic dose and no response	Same as initial plus stool guaiac q 6–12 mo
Methotrexate	Oral, SC, or IM: 7.5–15 mg q week	Baseline: AST, ALT, alk phos, t. bili, hep B and C studies, CBC w/plt, Scr	CBC w/plt, AST, alb q 1–2 mo
Leflunomide	Oral: 100 mg daily for 3 d then 10–20 mg daily	Baseline: ALT, CBC	ALT, CBC monthly initially and then periodically when stable
Hydroxychloroquine	Oral: 200 mg bid	Baseline: Color fundus photography and automated central perimetric analysis	Peripheral visual field testing q 9–12 mo or Amsler grid at home q 2 wk
Sulfasalazine	Oral: 500 mg bid, then 8 to 1 g bid max.	Baseline: CBC w/plt, then q week × 1 mo	Same as initial q 1–2 mo
Etanercept	50 mg SC weekly	None	None
Infliximab	3 mg/kg IV at 0, 2, 6 wk then q 8 wk	None	None
Adalimumab	40 mg SC q 2 wk	None	None
Anakinra	100 mg SC daily	None	None
Rituximab	1000 mg × 2 doses, 14 d apart	None	None
Abatacept	<60 kg = 500 mg 60–100 kg = 750 mg >100 kg = 1000 mg given at 0, 2, and 4 wk then every 4 wk by IV infusion	None	None
Azathioprine	Oral: 50–150 mg daily	CBC w/plt, AST q 2 wk × 1–2 mo	CBC w/plt, AST q 4–6 wk
d-Penicillamine	Oral: 125–250 mg daily, may 8 by 125–250 mg q 1–2 mo, max 750 mg daily	baseline: UA, CBC w/plt, then q week × 1 mo	CBC w/plt, UA q 4–6 wk
Cyclophosphamide	Oral: 1–2 mg/kg per day	UA, CBC w/plt q wk × 1 mo	UA, CBC w/plt q 4–6 wk
Cyclosporine	Oral: 2.5 mg/kg per day	Scr, blood pressure at 4 wk	Scr, blood pressure 4 wk
Corticosteroids	Oral, IV, IM, IA, and soft-tissue injections: variable	Glucose, blood pressure	Glucose, blood pressure q 3–6 mo, bone density annually

Alb, albumin; alk phos, alkaline phosphatase; ALT, alanine aminotransferase; AST, aspartate aminotransferase; BUN, blood urea nitrogen; CBC, complete blood count; hep, hepatitis; IA, intra-articular; IM, intramuscular; IV, intravenous; p, after; plt, platelet; q, every; Scr, serum creatinine; t. bili, total bilirubin; UA, urinalysis.

Table 34-3. Clinical Monitoring of Drug Therapy in Rheumatoid Arthritis

Drug	Toxicities Requiring Monitoring	Symptoms to Inquire About*
NSAIDs and salicylates	GI ulceration and bleeding, renal damage	Blood in stool, black stool, dyspepsia, nausea/vomiting, weakness, dizziness, abdominal pain, edema, weight gain, shortness of breath
Corticosteroids	Hypertension, hyperglycemia, osteoporosis[†]	Blood pressure if available, polyuria, polydipsia, edema, SOB, visual changes, weight gain, headaches, broken bones or pain in bones
Azathioprine	Myelosuppression, hepatotoxicity, lymphoproliferative disorders	Symptoms of myelosuppression (extreme fatigue, easy bleeding or bruising, infection), jaundice
Gold (intramuscular or oral)	Myelosuppression, proteinuria, rash, stomatitis	Symptoms of myelosuppression, edema, rash, oral ulcers, diarrhea
Hydroxychloroquine	Macular damage, rash, diarrhea	Visual changes including a decrease in night or peripheral vision, rash, diarrhea
Methotrexate	Myelosuppression, hepatic fibrosis, cirrhosis, pulmonary infiltrates or fibrosis, stomatitis, rash	Symptoms of myelosuppression, SOB, nausea/vomiting, lymph node swelling, coughing, mouth sores, diarrhea, jaundice
Leflunomide	Hepatitis, GI distress, alopecia	Nausea/vomiting, gastritis, diarrhea, hair loss, jaundice
Penicillamine	Myelosuppression, proteinuria, stomatitis, rash, dysgeusia	Symptoms of myelosuppression, edema, rash, diarrhea, altered taste perception, oral ulcers
Sulfasalazine	Myelosuppression, rash	Symptoms of myelosuppression, photosensitivity, rash, nausea/vomiting
Etanercept, adalimumab, anakinra	Local injection site reactions, infection	Symptoms of infection
Infliximab	Immune reactions, infection	Postinfusion reactions, symptoms of infection
Rituximab, abatacept	Infusion reactions, infection	Postinfusion reactions, symptoms of infection

*Altered immune function increases infection, which should be considered particularly in those patients taking azathioprine, methotrexate, and corticosteroids or other drugs as a symptom of myelosuppression.

[†]Osteoporosis is not likely to manifest itself early in treatment but all patients should be taking appropriate steps to prevent bone loss.

GI, gastrointestinal; SOB, shortness of breath.

Adapted from: American College of Rheumatology Ad Hoc Committee on Clinical Guidelines. Guidelines for monitoring drug therapy in rheumatoid arthritis. *Arthritis Rheum.* 1996;39:723–731.

Table 34-4. Dosage Regimens for Nonsteroidal Anti-inflammatory Drugs

Drug	Recommended Anti-inflammatory	Total Daily Dosage	Dosing Schedule
	Adult	Children	
Aspirin	2.6–5.2 g	60–100 mg/kg	qid
Celecoxib	200–400 mg		daily, bid
Diclofenac	150–200 mg		tid to qid / extended release-bid
Diflunisal	0.5–1.5 g	—	bid
Etodolac	0.2–1.2 g (max. 20 mg/kg)	—	tid to qid
Fenoprofen	0.9–3.0 g	—	qid
Flurbiprofen	200–300 mg	—	bid to qid
Ibuprofen	1.2–3.2 g	20–40 mg/kg	tid to qid
Indomethacin	50–200 mg	2–4 mg/kg (max. 200 mg)	bid to qid / extended-release, daily
Meclofenamate	200–400 mg	—	tid to qid
Meloxicam	7.5–15 mg		daily
Nabumetone	1–2 g	—	daily to bid
Naproxen	0.5–1.0 g	10 mg/kg	bid / extended release daily
Naproxen sodium	0.55–1.1 g	—	bid
Nonacetylated salicylates	1.2–4.8 g	—	bid to 6x/d
Oxaprozin	0.6–1.8 g (max. 26 mg/kg)	—	daily to tid
Piroxicam	10–20 mg	—	daily
Sulindac	300–400 mg	—	bid
Tolmetin	0.6–1.8 g	15–30 mg/kg	tid to qid

that these drugs do not alter the disease course, so they should be considered adjuncts to assist in pain and inflammation control but should not be considered definitive therapy. In many cases, if DMARDs are effective, patients may discontinue these drugs or use them on an as-needed basis only. NSAIDs can be particularly useful in early disease as they have a relatively prompt onset of action. They have similar adverse effects with gastrointestinal upset and ulceration, decreased renal function (particularly in patients with marginal renal function to begin with), and the potential to increase blood pressure as common adverse effects. With the exception of salsalate and celecoxib, they may also inhibit platelet function, which can prolong bleeding times. NSAIDs as a class have been implicated as increasing risk for coronary events though documentation is limited, and this risk appears to be small unless patients have preexisting coronary disease. Gastroprotection in patients with high risk of ulcers can be achieved by the use of proton-pump inhibitors or misoprostol. Celecoxib may also offer a decrease in gastrointestinal toxicity. The safety of NSAIDs in pregnancy has not been established but their use should be avoided in the third trimester of pregnancy as these drugs may prolong gestation and lead to bleeding and other complications during delivery. Misoprostol should be avoided in pregnancy as it may induce abortion.

Corticosteroids

Corticosteroids are useful for patients with RA. They may be given by the oral or intramuscular route for systemic effect or intra-articular or soft-tissue injection for management of inflammation in a single joint, tendon, or bursa. The advantages are that they are rapid acting and are effective in practically all patients given an adequate dose. The disadvantages are the wide variety of potentially serious toxicities associated with these drugs particularly if high doses or prolonged treatment is required.

Systemic corticosteroids may be used as "bridge" therapy to provide control of inflammation while waiting for DMARDs to work. They may also be given to manage acute flares of disease activity, which may be self-limiting. Finally, they may be used chronically as an adjunct to reduce disease activity when DMARDs alone are not enough. Oral prednisone is most commonly used in a once-daily or twice-daily divided dose. When given chronically, the lowest dose should be used, which provides adequate disease control. Consideration should be given to the use of calcium and vitamin D supplements, and periodic bone densitometry should be done to evaluate patients for osteoporosis. Close surveillance of other adverse effects should also be done including hypertension, diabetes, and cataracts.

Intra-articular and soft-tissue injections typically use long-acting depot dosage forms such as triamcinolone acetonide, which may have an effect for 4 to 6 weeks. In many cases, injection may induce prolonged remission in an actively inflamed joint, ligament, or bursa. The dosage used is dependent on joint size as smaller joints cannot accommodate large injection volumes. For example, in a finger joint 10 mg per 0.25 mL may be used while a knee joint can accommodate 60 to 80 mg. Repeated injections into a joint or tendon should be avoided as they may put the patient at risk for aseptic necrosis or tendon rupture, respectively. Patients should be instructed to avoid excessive usage for several weeks following injection as rest may help reduce inflammation of joint or soft tissue and reduce risk for complications. Local injections should not be repeated more than 2 to 3 times per year.

Disease-Modifying Antirheumatic Drugs

A number of drugs have been identified that appear to alter disease activity and are therefore considered "disease modifying" (Table 34-2). This includes older oral drugs and injectable gold, which suppress immune function in a general way, and injectable biologic agents, which target specific proinflammatory cytokines.

DMARDs include methotrexate, hydroxychloroquine, sulfasalazine, leflunomide, azathioprine, gold (both intramuscular and oral dosage forms), and penicillamine. Of these drugs, the best long-term outcome has been documented with methotrexate with fewer patients discontinuing it for lack of efficacy or toxicity. Leflunomide has been shown to have similar efficacy in long-term studies but there are no direct comparative trials with methotrexate. Cyclosporine and cyclophosphamide have been effective for RA but their toxicity risk is high and they are seldom used.

Methotrexate is given in a once-weekly dose of 7.5 to 25 mg. Doses greater than 15 mg should be given by subcutaneous injection as the bioavailability becomes less predictable for oral doses more than that. Patients need to be monitored with periodic complete blood counts for bone marrow toxicity and serum transaminases (alanine aminotransferase or aspartate aminotransferase) to assess for liver toxicity. Additionally, periodic serum albumin should be obtained to monitor the liver as patients may develop liver fibrosis without hepatitis. Patients taking methotrexate should be advised not to drink alcohol as there is some concern for additive hepatic toxicity and it is not known if there is a "safe" amount of alcohol that can be consumed with the drug. Periodic liver biopsy used to be recommended but the incidence of cirrhosis and fibrosis is so uncommon that the risk from biopsy exceeds the benefit for most patients. The only reason to do biopsy now may be as a baseline in patients with prior history of liver disease or significant alcohol intake or in those with persistent transaminase elevation or decrease in albumin on treatment. Pulmonary fibrosis may also occur rarely. Patients presenting with nonproductive cough and shortness of breath should have a chest X-ray to look for fibrosis. Fortunately, both liver and pulmonary toxicities are rare. Stomatitis and gastrointestinal adverse effects may occur with methotrexate use. These adverse effects can often be managed by reducing the dose or supplementing the patient with folic acid, 1 to 10 mg daily. Gastrointestinal toxicity may also be reduced by giving the drug in divided doses over 24 hours.

Hydroxychloroquine is an antimalarial drug that has been documented to be also useful for patients with RA. It is somewhat less effective when given long-term than methotrexate but does not need laboratory monitoring. Skin rash and gastrointestinal toxicity are the most common adverse effects. As there is a small risk for retinal toxicity, which may be manifest by scotomas and loss of vision, it is recommended that patients have annual ophthalmic examinations with visual field testing.

Sulfasalazine is somewhat less effective than methotrexate in long-term use but toxicity is relatively low for most patients and can be useful as monotherapy or in combination with other DMARDs. The most common adverse effect is gastrointestinal distress. This can be minimized by starting with low doses (e.g., 500 mg twice daily) and increasing gradually to 2 to 3 g in divided dose as maintenance. In addition, the use of an enteric-coated formulation may reduce gastrointestinal toxicity. Complete blood counts to monitor for myelosuppression, and transaminases to monitor for drug-induced hepatitis should be done periodically. History of sulfa allergy is a contraindication. Photosensitivity and other skin rashes may occur.

Although no direct comparisons with methotrexate have been done, long-term studies suggest that leflunomide has a similar long-term efficacy.[20] Liver and bone marrow toxicity have been reported with leflunomide, so alanine aminotransferase and complete blood counts should be done monthly for the first 6 months and then every 6 to 8 weeks. As combination therapy with other drugs with marrow toxicity increases risk for this toxicity, laboratory monitoring, done every 4 weeks, should continue long-term in patients on combinations. Other toxicities include alopecia and gastrointestinal toxicity and these effects seem to be dose related.

Lowering the dose may still prove to be effective without loss of efficacy. The drug has a prolonged half-life, so administration of a loading dose of 100 mg daily for 3 days followed by maintenance of 20 mg daily will result in much more rapid onset of action. Not using a loading dose reduces the frequency of toxicity in patients but failure to use a loading dose will increase the time to onset of effect from a few days to several months. As the drug undergoes enterohepatic circulation, the elimination half-life is 14 days. The drug should be avoided in pregnancy, and patients of childbearing potential should be advised to use adequate contraception. In patients who wish to become pregnant or those who have serious toxicity, the use of cholestyramine should be considered to rapidly remove drug from the body. Procedures to do this are outlined in the package insert.

Gold salts, azathioprine, penicillamine, cyclosporine, cyclophosphamide, and minocycline have all been used in RA. Although they may still have a place in select patients, it is seen that either their efficacy is low, toxicity is high, or both; hence, these drugs are not frequently used in RA.

Biologic DMARDs

Biologic DMARDs are drugs that target specific proinflammatory cytokines like IL-1 (anakinra) and tumor necrosis factor (TNF) (adalimumab, etanercept, and infliximab). Additionally, certain biologic DMARDs have been developed that cause peripheral B-cell depletion (rituximab) and block the costimulation necessary to activate T cells (abatacept). They are created using recombinant DNA technology. They may be effective when other therapies fail to achieve an adequate clinical response, but they are considerably more expensive than older drugs.[21]

Response rates with these agents in patients who fail to achieve adequate control with methotrexate alone are 50% to 75%. No laboratory monitoring is required. There appears to be a small increased risk for infections in patients treated with these drugs and they should be avoided in patients with active infection and used with caution in those with a history of recurrent infection. Patients who develop an infection while taking them should have a temporary interruption of therapy until the infection has been cured. Tuberculin skin testing should be done to screen for latent tuberculosis prior to initiation of these therapies.

Infliximab and etanercept have been noted to cause exacerbations of congestive heart failure. In patients with a history of decompensated heart failure or frequent admissions for this condition, alternative antirheumatic therapy should be considered. Inhibition of TNF has been theorized to carry some risk for cancer as this proinflammatory cytokine is important in ridding the body of tumor cells. Studies to date have failed to document an increase in incidence compared to patients with RA not treated with these drugs, but long-term surveillance studies are yet to be performed. Although biologic agents have been demonstrated to be effective in patients who fail to achieve adequate responses from methotrexate, when combined with methotrexate they appear to have increased efficacy than when used as monotherapy. Combinations of biologic agents should be avoided as they appear to increase infection risk.

Adalimumab

Adalimumab is a human IgG_1 antibody to TNF. It binds excess TNF to reduce the role of this cytokine in stimulating an inflammatory response. In addition to RA, the drug is approved by the Food and Drug Administration (FDA) for the treatment of psoriatic arthritis, and ankylosing spondylitis. The drug is given as a subcutaneous injection of 40 mg every 2 weeks. The most common adverse effect is injection site reactions. To date, congestive heart failure has not been reported with adalimumab.

Etanercept

Etanercept is a fusion protein combining the constant-region long chain of IgG_1 with two soluble TNF receptors. These receptors are naturally occurring anti-inflammatory cytokines. The binding of excess TNF molecules with etanercept prevents them from attaching to cell-surface TNF receptors, which would result in cell activation and stimulate the inflammatory response. The drug is given by subcutaneous injection and can be given either as 25 mg twice a week or 50 mg once a week. In addition to RA, the drug is FDA approved for the treatment of juvenile RA, psoriatic arthritis, and ankylosing spondylitis. In children, the dose is adjusted depending on their weight. In addition to the concerns regarding infection and congestive heart failure, the drug has been reported to worsen symptoms in patients with demyelinating disease such as multiple sclerosis. Also, there have been a few case reports of pancytopenia, but this complication does not appear to be common, and currently routine monitoring of patients for bone marrow toxicity is not recommended in the package insert.

Infliximab

Infliximab is a chimeric antibody consisting mostly of human IgG_1 with an attachment portion derived from mouse anti-TNF antibody. Infliximab is given by intravenous infusion at a dose of 3 mg/kg given at 0, 2, and 6 weeks and then every 8 weeks. Some patients need higher or more frequent doses to control inflammation throughout the time interval between injections. Doses of up to 10 mg/kg can be used, and shortening the dosing interval up to 4 weeks may be used if needed. To prevent the development of antibodies, methotrexate should be given in all patients receiving the infliximab. Infusion reactions may occur and sometimes can be prevented by slowing the rate of infusion. In more severe cases, these reactions may be managed by premedication with corticosteroids and antihistamines.

Anakinra

Anakinra is the only IL-1 receptor antagonist. It is the same as naturally occurring IL-1 receptor antagonist, which binds to receptors on the cell surface and prevents cell activation to promote inflammatory response by IL-1. The drug is available as prefilled syringes of 100 mg, which must be given by daily subcutaneous injection. Infection risk and other precautions are similar to TNF inhibitors.

Rituximab

Rituximab in combination with methotrexate is FDA-approved for use for the treatment of RA in patients who fail to achieve adequate control with TNF inhibitors. Combination therapy was shown to have better outcomes in clinical trials. This drug depletes B cells, which promote antibody response and play an important role in the humoral inflammatory response. It has been shown to reduce disease activity by 50% in 43% of patients treated with a combination of methotrexate and rituximab who received 1 g by intravenous infusion on day 1 and day 15, when patients were evaluated 24 and 48 weeks later.[22] Premedication with 100 mg methylprednisolone, given intravenously 30 minutes prior to infusion, reduces the likelihood and severity of infusion reactions. Unlike other biologic agents, it is not administered continuously but only given when RA flares. Experience with long-term repeated courses of the drug is limited at this time.[23]

Abatacept

Abatacept is a costimulation modulator that inhibits binding of antigen presenting cells to the CD28, cell-surface receptor of cytotoxic T lymphocytes, and decreases their activation. In a trial of patients who failed to achieve adequate response from anti-TNF therapy, 50% of patients responded to abatacept.[24] Dosing is based on patient weight (see Table 34-2). The drug is given every 4 weeks after the initial 3 doses given 2 weeks apart.

EVIDENCE-BASED SUMMARY

- Symmetrical inflammation of joints with pain, swelling, and morning stiffness are hallmarks of rheumatoid arthritis. Joint deformity and rheumatoid nodules are late manifestations. Pulmonary fibrosis, vasculitis, pericarditis, and scleritis are less common manifestations of the disease.
- Nondrug therapy includes therapeutic exercise to maintain muscle strength and joint range of motion, assistive devices to aid in activities of daily living, and surgery in some patients.
- Treatment with DMARDs should be initiated as soon as possible, preferably within 3 months of the onset of symptoms.
- Of the oral drugs for rheumatoid arthritis, methotrexate is more likely to be continued long-term with relatively low discontinuance rates for toxicity and loss of benefit. When combined with other drugs, it has the best documentation of added benefit.
- Hydroxychloroquine, leflunomide, and sulfasalazine are other frequently used oral DMARDs.
- Biologic agents such as etanercept, adalimumab, infliximab, rituximab, abatacept, and anakinra may prove effective when other DMARDs fail to achieve adequate responses
- NSAIDs should be considered adjuncts to DMARDs for most patients as they do not alter disease course. Corticosteroids are beneficial for many patients but toxicity limits their use as chronic therapy for most patients.

REFERENCES

1. Venables PJW, Mani RN. Clinical features of rheumatoid arthritis. http://www.utdol.com/utd/content/topic.do?topicKey=rheumart/3022&selectedTitle=6~150&source=search_result. Accessed February 27, 2008.
2. Visser H. Early diagnosis of rheumatoid arthritis. *Best Pract Res Clin Rheumatol.* 2005;19(1):55–72.
3. Shmerling RH. Diagnostic tests for rheumatic disease: Clinical utility revisited. *South Med J.* 2005;98(7):704–711.
4. Colglazier CL, Sutej PG. Laboratory testing in rheumatic diseases: A practical review. *South Med J.* 2005;98(2):185–191.
5. American College of Rheumatology Subcommittee on Rheumatoid Arthritis. Guidelines for the management of rheumatoid arthritis:2002 update. *Arthritis Rheum.* 2002; 46:328–346.
6. Goldbach-Mansky R, Lipsky PE. New Concepts in the treatment of rheumatoid arthritis. *Ann Rev Med.* 2003;54: 1797–1807.
7. Breedveld FC, Kalden JR. Appropriate and effective management of rheumatoid arthritis. *Ann Rheum Dis.* 2004; 63:627–633.
8. Sokka T, Hannonen P, Mottonen T. Conventional disease-modifying antirheumatic drugs in early arthritis. *Rheum Dis Clin North Am.* 2005;31(4):729–744.
9. Cronstein BN. Low-dose methotrexate: A mainstay in the treatment of rheumatoid arthritis. *Pharmacol Rev.* 2005; 57:163–172.
10. Emery P. Treatment of rheumatoid arthritis. *BMJ.* 2006; 332(7534):152–155.
11. Bingham S, Emery P. Combination therapy in rheumatoid arthritis. *Springer Semin Immunopathol.* 2001;23:165–183.
12. Calguneri M, Pay S, Claiskaner Z, et al. Combination therapy versus monotherapy for the treatment of patients with rheumatoid arthritis. *Clin Exp Rheumatol.* 1999;17:699–704.
13. Dougados M, Combe B, Cantagrel A, et al. Combination therapy in early rheumatoid arthritis: A randomised, controlled, double-blind 52-week clinical trial of sulphasalazine and methotrexate compared with single components. *Ann Rheum Dis.* 1999;58:220–225.
14. O'Dell JR. Combinations of conventional disease-modifying antirhuematic drugs. *Rheum Dis Clin North Am.* 2001; 27:415–426.
15. Pincus T, O'Dell JR, Kremer JM. Combination therapy with multiple disease-modifying antirheumatic drugs in rheumatoid arthritis: A preventive strategy. *Ann Intern Med.* 1999;131:768–774.
16. Verhoeven AC, Boers M, Tugwell P. Combination therapy in rheumatoid arthritis: Updated systemic review. *Br J Rheumatol.* 1998;37:612–619.
17. Kremer JM. Rational use of new and existing disease-modifying agents in rheumatoid arthritis. *Ann Intern Med.* 2001;134:695–706.
18. Nurmohamed MT, Dijkmans BA. Efficacy, tolerability and cost effectiveness of disease-modifying antirheumatic drugs and biologic agents in rheumatoid arthritis. *Drugs.* 2005;65(5):661–694.
19. Smolen JS, Aletaha D, Keystone E. Superior efficacy of combination therapy for rheumatoid arthritis: Fact or fiction? *Arthritis Rheum.* 2005;52(10):2975–2983.
20. Kalden JR, Schattenkirchner M, Sorension H, et al. The efficacy and safety of leflunomide in patients with active rheumatoid arthritis: A five year follow-up study. *Arthritis Rheum.* 2003;48:1513–1520.
21. Furst DE, Breedveld FC, Kalden JR, et al. Updated consensus statement on biological agents, specifically tumour necrosis factor α (TNF α) blocking agents and interleukin-1 receptor antagonist (IL-1ra), for the treatment of rheumatic diseases, 2005. *Ann Rheum Dis.* 2005;64(4):iv2–iv14.
22. Edwards JC, Szczepanski L, Szechinski J, et al. Efficacy of B-cell-targeted therapy with rituximab in patients with rheumatoid arthritis. *N Engl J Med.* 2004;350(25):2572–2581.
23. Smolen JS, Emery P, Keystone EC, et al. Consensus Statement on the Use of Rituximab in Patients With Rheumatoid Arthritis. *Ann Rheum Dis.* 2007;66:143–150.
24. Genovese MC, Becker JC, Schiff M, et al. Abatacept for rheumatoid arthritis refractory to tumor necrosis factor alpha inhibition. *N Engl J Med.* 2005;353(11):1114–1123.

Chapter 35

Osteoarthritis

Lucinda M. Buys and Mary Elizabeth Elliott

SEARCH STRATEGY

A systematic search of the medical literature was performed on August 20, 2007, using the terms osteoarthritis and arthritis. The search, limited to human subjects and English language journals, included the PubMed and Cochrane Collection databases.

Osteoarthritis (OA) is the most common of the rheumatic diseases, with a prevalence of approximately 200 per 100,000 person-years, and is responsible for enormous disability and loss of productivity.[1-3] The prevalence and severity of OA is higher in older age groups than in younger groups, affecting an estimated 46 million Americans.[4]

The most common risk factors for the development of OA, which is typically a multifactorial disease, include obesity, previous occupation, participation in certain sports, history of joint trauma, and a genetic predisposition to OA. Patients with osteoarthritis are less likely to have osteoporosis, probably because heavy individuals have higher bone density because of weight-bearing, but increased risk of OA as a result of excessive joint loading.[3]

CLINICAL PRESENTATION

The typical patient presenting with OA is older than 50 years of age and has had the presenting symptoms for months to years, often having treated them with nonprescription medications or dietary supplements. Pain in the affected joint is a nearly universal complaint, and hands, knees, or hips are the most commonly affected joints. Pain is most common with motion, unless the disease is advanced, in which case pain can be present at rest. Joint stiffness resolves with motion and recurs with rest.

Late-stage disease is associated with joint deformity (Fig. 35-1). Joint space narrowing and/or osteophytes may be evident in X-ray films (Fig. 35-2). Abnormal alignment of joints and joint effusion can occur in late disease (Fig. 35-3).

DIAGNOSTIC EVALUATION

The diagnosis of OA is made through history, physical examination, characteristic radiographic findings, and laboratory testing.[2,5] The major diagnostic goals are: (1) to discriminate between primary and secondary OA and (2) to clarify the joints involved, severity of joint involvement, and response to prior therapies, providing a basis for a treatment plan.

Physical examination reveals a patient in mild, moderate, or severe pain. Crepitus—a crackling or grating sound heard with joint movement that is caused by irregularity of joint surface—may be present. Limited range of motion may be accompanied by joint instability.

The American College of Rheumatology has published traditional diagnostic criteria and also "decision trees" for OA diagnosis.[5] As with all guidelines, these tools assist the clinician rather than replace clinical judgment.

RISK STRATIFICATION

The prognosis for patients with primary OA is variable and depends on the joint involved. If a weight-bearing joint or the spine is involved, considerable morbidity and disability are possible. In the case of secondary OA, the prognosis depends on the underlying cause. Treatment of OA may relieve pain or improve function, but it does not reverse preexisting damage to the articular cartilage.

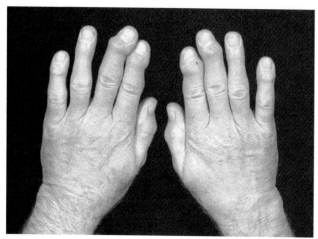

Figure 35-1. Typical appearance of the bony changes associated with Heberden's and Bouchard's nodes.

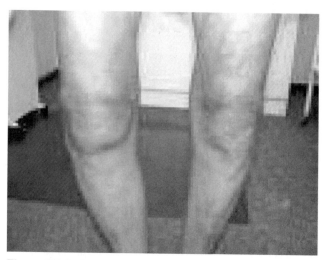

Figure 35-3. Physical findings of joint enlargement and genu varum of the knees.

MANAGEMENT

Management of the patient with OA should be tailored to each individual based on clinical findings and prognosis. Goals are to: (1) educate the patient, caregivers, and relatives, (2) relieve pain and stiffness, (3) maintain or improve joint mobility, (4) limit functional impairment, and (5) maintain or improve quality of life.[6–10]

Treatment for the patient with OA depends on the distribution and severity of joint involvement, comorbid disease states, concomitant medications, and allergies (Fig. 35-4). Management for all individuals with OA should begin with patient education, and physical and/or occupational therapy, and weight loss or assistive devices if appropriate.[6–12]

The primary objective of medication is to alleviate pain.[7–11] Scheduled acetaminophen, up to 4 g/d, should be tried initially. If this is ineffective, nonsteroidal anti-inflammatory drugs (NSAIDs) are prescribed, or possi-

bly a cyclooxygenase-2 (COX-2) selective inhibitor (celecoxib) if warranted. Application of capsaicin or methyl salicylate topical creams over specific joints can sometimes be helpful adjuncts for pain control. Glucosamine and chondroitin in combination can be helpful for those with moderate to severe arthritis. Joint aspiration followed by glucocorticoid or hyaluronate injection can relieve pain, and is offered concomitantly with oral analgesics or after an unsuccessful trial of these agents. Opioid analgesics are a last-resort medication to prescribe if other therapies are unsuccessful. When symptoms are intractable or there is significant loss of function, joint replacement may be appropriate if the patient is a surgical candidate.

Finally, for patients interested in clinical trials, investigational strategies with oral doxycycline, matrix metalloproteinase inhibitors, disease-modifying osteoarthritis drugs, or cartilage transplants may be considered.

For management of patients with OA, evidence-based recommendations have recently been summarized by the Third Canadian Consensus Conference Group (Table 35-1).[13] ACR recommends acetaminophen as the drug of first choice. In patients with risk factors for gastrointestinal (GI) complications, use of a nonselective NSAID plus a proton pump inhibitor (PPI), or a COX-2 selective inhibitor plus a PPI is supported by much recent evidence, as described below.

NONPHARMACOLOGIC THERAPY

The first step in OA treatment is patient education about the disease process, the extent of OA, the prognosis, and treatment options. Education is paramount, in that OA is often seen as a "wear and tear" disease, an inevitable consequence of aging for which nothing

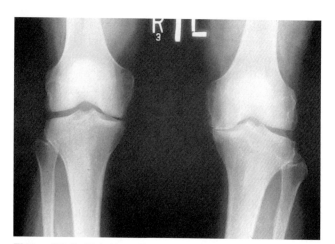

Figure 35-2. Plain X-ray films of the knee demonstrating joint space narrowing.

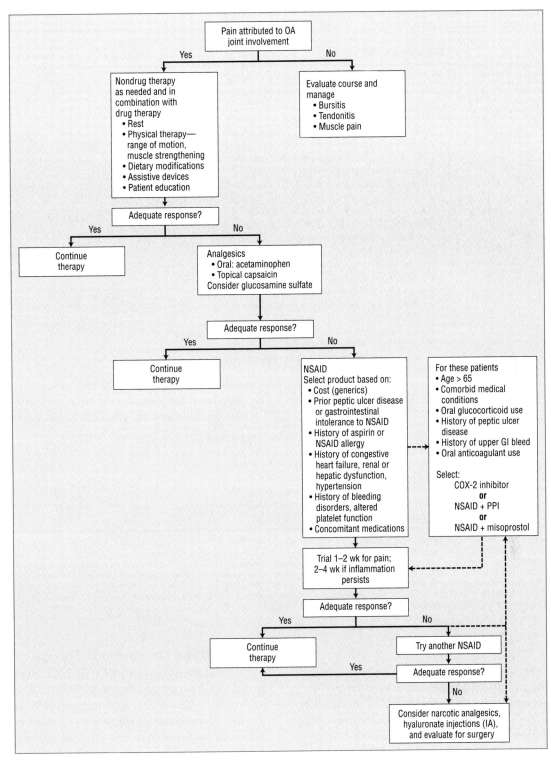

Figure 35-4. Treatment for osteoarthritis.

helps. Even worse, patients may resort to the use of alternative but unproven medications or quackery. Patients should be warned about these and encouraged to access information from local or national units of the Arthritis Foundation (www.arthritis.org). The Arthritis Foundation provides literature about OA and OA medications and information about local clinics and agencies offering physical and economic assistance. The Arthritis Foundation also sponsors support groups and public education programs.

Table 35-1. Summary of Recommendations for Osteoarthritis

	Recommendation	Level of Evidence	Grade of Recommendation
Patient–physician communication	Patients should be fully informed about evolving information regarding the benefits and risks of their treatment options.	3	C
Indications	NSAIDs and coxibs are generally more effective and preferred by patients over acetaminophen, although a trial of the latter is warranted for some patients. Topical NSAID formulations may confer benefit in knee OA	1	A
GI toxicity	In patients with risk factors for PUB, a coxib is still the anti-inflammatory drug of choice, depending on the patient's cardiovascular risks. High-risk patients who must use nonselective NSAIDs should have a PPI.	1	A
Renal	Before starting an NSAID or coxib, determine renal status and creatinine clearance in patients more than 65 years of age or in those with comorbid conditions that may affect renal function.	3	C
	Advise patients that if they cannot eat or drink on a given day, they should withhold that day's dose of NSAID/coxib.	4	D
Hypertension	In patients receiving antihypertensive drugs, measure blood pressure within a few weeks after initiating NSAID/coxib therapy and monitor appropriately; drug doses may need adjustment.	1	A
Cardiovascular	Patients taking rofecoxib have been shown to have an increased risk of CV events. Current data suggest that this increased CV risk may be an effect of the NSAID/coxib class. Physicians and patients should weigh the benefits and risks of NSAID/coxib therapy.	1	A
Geriatric consideration	NSAIDs/coxibs should be used with caution in elderly patients, who are at the greatest risk for serious GI, renal, and CV side effects.	3	C
Pharmacoeconomics	Although the data are ambiguous, coxibs may be more cost-effective than traditional NSAID + proprietary PPI among high-risk patients.	3	C

Categories of evidence: 1A, meta-analysis of RCT; 1, at least one RCT; 2A, at least one controlled study without randomization; 3, descriptive studies such as comparative, correlation, or case-control studies; 4, expert committee reports or opinions and/or clinical experience of respected authorities.
Grades of recommendations: A, category 1 evidence; B, category 2 evidence or extrapolated recommendation from category 1 evidence; C, category 3 evidence or extrapolated recommendation from category 1 or 2 evidence; D, category 4 evidence or extrapolated recommendation from category 2 or 3 evidence.
NSAID: nonsteroidal anti-inflammatory drug; GI: gastrointestinal; CV: cardiovascular; PUB: perforations, ulcers, and bleeds; PPI: proton pump inhibitor.
Adapted from: Tannenbaum H, Bombardier C, Davis P, Russell AS, Third Canadian Consensus Conference Group. An evidence-based approach to prescribing nonsteroidal antiinflammatory drugs. Third Canadian Consensus Conference. *J Rheumatol.* 2006;33:140–157.

DIET

Excess weight increases the biomechanical load on weight-bearing joints and is the single best predictor of need for eventual joint replacement.[3,12,14,15] Even a 5-kg weight loss can decrease the load on a weight-bearing joint. Weight loss is associated with decreased symptoms and disability, although results are variable.[15,16] At least one randomized, controlled trial has demonstrated improvement in pain and self-reported physical function using a combination of modest weight loss (5%) and exercise.[17] Although dietary intervention for overweight OA patients is reasonable, weight loss usually requires a motivated patient and a structured weight-loss program.

Physical and Occupational Therapy

Physical therapy—with heat or cold treatments and an exercise program—helps to maintain and restore joint range of motion and reduce pain and muscle spasms. Warm baths or warm water soaks may decrease pain and stiffness. Heating pads should be used with caution, especially in older people. Patients should be warned not to fall asleep on the heat source or to lie on it for more than brief periods in order to avoid burns.

Exercise programs and quadriceps strengthening can improve physical functioning and can decrease disability, pain, and analgesic use by OA patients.[1,17,18] Isometric exercise is preferred over isotonic exercise because the latter can aggravate affected joints. Exercises should be taught and then observed before the patient exercises at home, ideally three to four times daily. The patient should be instructed to decrease the number of repetitions if severe pain develops with exercise.

The decision about whether to encourage walking should be made on an individual basis. With weak or deconditioned muscles, the load is transmitted excessively to the joints, so weight-bearing activities can exacerbate symptoms. However, avoidance of activity by those with hip or knee OA leads to further deconditioning or weight gain. A program of patient education, muscle stretching and strengthening, and supervised walking can improve physical function and decrease pain in patients with knee OA.[1,17,18] Referral to the physical and/or occupational therapist is especially helpful for patients with functional disabilities. The therapist can assess muscle strength and joint stability, and recommend exercises and methods of protecting the affected joint from excessive forces. The therapist can also provide assistive and orthotic devices, such as canes, walkers, braces, heel cups, splints, or insoles for use during exercise or daily activities.

Surgery

Surgery can be recommended for OA patients with functional disability and/or severe pain unresponsive to conservative therapy. Criteria for total replacement (arthroplasty) of the knee were developed at an NIH consensus conference.[19] Likewise, criteria for total hip replacement, as well as a summary of clinical outcomes resulting from this procedure have been published.[20] These hip and joint replacement recommendations have been based on critical review of the literature as well as on expert opinion. For patients with advanced disease, a partial or total arthroplasty can relieve pain and improve motion, with the best outcomes after hip or knee arthroplasty.

PHARMACOLOGIC THERAPY

Drug therapy in OA is targeted at relief of pain. OA is commonly seen in older individuals who have other medical conditions, and OA treatment is often long-term. As such, a conservative approach to drug treatment, focusing on the needs of the individual patient, is warranted (Fig. 35-4). For mild or moderate pain, topical analgesics or acetaminophen can be used. If these measures fail, or if there is inflammation, NSAIDs may be useful. Even when drug therapy is initiated, appropriate nondrug therapies should be continued and reinforced. Nondrug modalities are the cornerstone of OA management and may provide as much relief as drug therapy.

The ACR recommends acetaminophen as first-line drug therapy for pain management in OA, as a result of its relative safety, efficacy, and lower cost compared with NSAIDs.[1,13,21] The ACR recommends consideration of NSAIDs for OA patients in whom acetaminophen is ineffective. NSAIDs all display comparable analgesic and anti-inflammatory efficacy and are similarly beneficial in OA (Table 35-2).[22,23]

For patients with elevated GI risk or cardiovascular risk who need treatment with an NSAID, a COX-2 selective inhibitor or a traditional NSAID taken with a PPI should be considered. For those taking regular low dose aspirin for cardiovascular risk (with or without increased GI risk), a traditional NSAID taken with a PPI, or a COX-2 selective inhibitor taken with a PPI can be considered. Given the current concerns regarding cardiovascular risk with COX-2 selective inhibitors or possibly any NSAIDs, and continuing concern about GI events, treatment with the lowest dose possible for the shortest duration possible is warranted.[13]

Topical products can be used alone or in combination with oral analgesics or NSAIDs. Capsaicin, isolated from hot peppers, releases and ultimately depletes substance P from afferent nociceptive nerve fibers. Data comparing topical capsaicin to other effective pharmacologic treatments for OA is lacking.

The exact role of glucosamine, chondroitin, or a combination of the two products is still unclear.[24–26] Because of the relative safety of these agents, a trial of glucosamine/chondroitin may be reasonable in patients considering alternatives to traditional OA treatments. Dosing should be at least 1500 mg/d of glucosamine and 1200 mg/d of chondroitin. The glucosamine component should be the sulfate salt rather than the hydrochloride salt as nearly all positive efficacy studies used the better absorbed sulfate salt. Glucosamine-related adverse events are generally mild and include gastrointestinal symptoms (gas, bloating, cramps). If made from shellfish, however, glucosamine should not be used in those with shellfish (shrimp, crab, lobster) allergies. The initial concerns regarding glucosamine-induced hyperglycemia had likely been overstated as later safety data in both healthy subjects and those with type 2 diabetes mellitus did not show significant elevations in blood glucose. Chondroitin is extremely well tolerated, with the most common adverse effect being nausea. Depending on the source of chondroitin (cattle, pig, or shark), this compound could also pose risk to persons who are allergic to shark, and some have expressed concern about the possibility of bovine spongiform encephalopathy (mad-cow disease) when the source of chondroitin is cow trachea.

Intraarticular glucocorticoid injections can provide excellent pain relief, particularly when a joint effusion is present.[1,27] Aspiration of the effusion and injection of

Table 35-2. Medications Commonly Used in the Treatment of Osteoarthritis

Medication	Dosage and Frequency	Maximum Dosage (mg/d)
Oral analgesics		
Acetaminophen	325–650 mg every 4–6 h or 1 g 3–4 times/d	4000
Tramadol	50–100 mg every 4–6 h	400
Acetaminophen/codeine	300 to 1000 mg/15 to 60 mg every 4 h as needed	4000 mg/360 mg[*]
Acetaminophen/oxycodone	325 to 650 mg/2.5 to 10 mg every 6 h as needed	4000 mg/40 mg[*]
Topical analgesics		
Capsaicin 0.025% or 0.075%	Apply to affected joint 3–4 times/d	—
Nutritional supplements		
Glucosamine hydrochloride/chondroitin sulfate	500 mg/400 mg 3 times/d	1500/1200
NSAIDs		
Carboxylic acids		
Acetylated salicylates		
Aspirin, plain, buffered, or enteric-coated	325–650 mg every 4–6 h for pain; anti-inflammatory doses start at 3600 mg/d in divided doses	3600[†]
Nonacetylated salicylates		
Salsalate	500–1000 mg 2–3 times a day	3000[†]
Diflunisal	500–1000 mg 2 times a day	1500
Choline salicylate[‡]	500–1000 mg 2–3 times a day	3000[‡]
Choline magnesium salicylate	500–1000 mg 2–3 times a day	3000[‡]
Acetic acids		
Etodolac	800–1200 mg/d in divided doses	1200
Diclofenac	100–150 mg/d in divided doses	200
Indomethacin	25 mg 2–3 times a d; 75 mg SR once daily	200; 150
Ketorolac[§]	10 mg every 4–6 h	40
Nabumetone[¶]	500–1000 mg 1–2 times a day	2000
Propionic acids		
Fenoprofen	300–600 mg 3–4 times a day	3200
Flurbiprofen	200–300 mg/d in 2–4 divided doses	300
Ibuprofen	1200–3200 mg/d in 3–4 divided doses	3200
Ketoprofen	150–300 mg/d in 3–4 divided doses	300
Naproxen	250–500 mg twice a day	1500
Naproxen sodium	275–550 mg twice a day	1375
Oxaprozin	600–1200 mg daily	1800
Fenamates		
Meclofenamate	200–400 mg/d in 3–4 divided doses	400
Mefenamic acid[f]	250 mg every 6 h	1000
Oxicams		
Piroxicam	10–20 mg daily	20
Meloxicam	7.5 mg daily	15
Coxibs		
Celecoxib	100 mg twice daily or 200 mg daily	200 (400 for RA)

[*]Maximum dosage in combination product limited by acetaminophen maximum of 4000 mg/d.
[†]Monitor serum salicylate levels over 3–3.6 g/day.
[‡]Only available as a liquid; 870 mg salicylate/5 mL.
[§]Not approved for treatment of OA for more than 5 days.
[¶]Nonorganic acid but metabolite is an acetic acid.
[f]Not approved for treatment of OA.
RA, rheumatoid arthritis; SR, sustained-release.

glucocorticoid are carried out aseptically, with examination of the aspirate recommended to exclude crystalline arthritis or infection. (This risk is low, however, approximately 1 in 50 000 procedures.) After injection, the patient should minimize activity and stress on the joint for several days. Initial pain relief may be seen within 24 to 72 hours after injection, with peak pain relief approximately 1 week after injection and lasting up to 4–8 weeks.

HA products are injected once weekly for either 3 or 5 weeks depending on the specific agent administered. Four preparations are commercially available: Hylagan® (20 mg sodium hyaluronate/2 mL), Supartz® (25 mg sodium hyaluronate/2.5 mL), Synvisc® (16 mg hylan polymers/2 mL) and Orthovisc® (30 mg hyaluronan/2 mL). Hylagan® and Supartz® are administered weekly for 5 injections, while Synvisc® and Orthovisc® are administered weekly for 3 injections. Injections are well tolerated, although acute joint swelling and local skin reactions, including rash, ecchymoses, and pruritus have been reported.

Low-dose opioid analgesics can be useful in patients who experience no relief with acetaminophen, NSAIDs, intraarticular injections, or topical therapy. These agents are particularly useful in patients who cannot take NSAIDs because of renal failure, or for patients in whom all other treatment options have failed and who are at high surgical risk, precluding joint arthroplasty. Low-dose opioids are the initial intervention, usually given in combination with acetaminophen. Sustained-release compounds usually offer better pain control throughout the day, and are used when simple opioids are ineffective. If pain is intolerable and limits activities of daily living, and the patient has sufficiently good cardiopulmonary health to undergo major surgery, joint replacement may be preferable to continued reliance on opioids.

EVIDENCE-BASED SUMMARY

- OA is a very common, slowly progressive disorder that affects diarthrodial joints and is characterized by progressive deterioration of articular cartilage, subchondral sclerosis, and osteophyte production.
- Clinical manifestations include gradual onset of joint pain, stiffness, and limitation of motion.
- The primary treatment goals are to reduce pain, maintain function, and prevent further destruction. An individualized approach based on education, rest, exercise, weight loss as needed, and analgesic medication can succeed in meeting these goals.
- Recommended drug treatment starts with acetaminophen ≤4 g/d and topical analgesics as needed. If acetaminophen is ineffective, NSAIDs may be used, often providing satisfactory relief of pain and stiffness. Individuals at increased risk for toxicity from NSAIDs, especially for GI, cardiovascular, or renal events, deserve special attention. Coxibs may have advantages in some OA patients, but their safety relative to other NSAIDS and their role in OA remains in a state of flux.
- Glucosamine/chondroitin may be useful in moderate to severe arthritis and is safe.
- Experimental therapy aimed at preventing the progression of OA requires further clinical investigation before entering widespread clinical use.

REFERENCES

1. ACR Subcommittee on Osteoarthritis Guidelines. Recommendations for the medical management of osteoarthritis of the hip and knee: 2000 Update. *Arthritis Rheum.* 2000; 43:1905–1915.
2. Solomon L. Clinical features of osteoarthritis. In: Kelly WN, Harris ED, Ruddy S, Sledge CB, eds. *Textbook of Rheumatology,* 6th ed. Philadelphia, PA: Saunders;2001: 1409–1418.
3. Felson DT, Lawrence RC, Dieppe PA, Hirsch R, et al. Osteoarthritis: New insights. Part 1: The disease and its risk factors. *Ann Intern Med.* 2000;133:635–646.
4. Hootman JM, Helmick CG. Projections of US prevalence of arthritis and associated activity limitations. *Arthritis Rheum.* 2006;54:226–229.
5. American College of Rheumatology Subcommittee on Osteoarthritis Guidelines. Recommendations for the medical management of osteoarthritis of the hip and knee. *Arthritis & Rheumatism* 2000;43:1905–1915.
6. Felson DT. Osteoarthritis of the Knee. *N Engl J Med.* 2006; 354:841–848.
7. Dieppe PA, Lohmander LS. Pathogenesis and management of pain in osteoarthritis. *Lancet.* 2005;365:965–973.
8. Chard J, Lohmander S, Smith C, Scott D. Osteoarthritis. *Clin Evid.* 2003;10:1402–30.
9. Roddy E, Zhang W, Doherty M, et al. Evidence-based recommendations for the role of exercise in the management of osteoarthritis of the hip or knee—the MOVE consensus. *Rheumatology (Oxford).* 2005;44:67–73.
10. Hunter DJ, Felson DT. Osteoarthritis. *BMJ.* 2006;332: 639–642.
11. Juni P, Reichenbach S, Dieppe P. Osteoarthritis: Rational approach to treating the individual. *Best Pract Res Clin Rheumatol.* 2006;20:721–740.
12. Lievense AM, Bierma-Zeinstra SM, Verhagen AP, et al. Influence of obesity on the development of osteoarthritis of the hip: A systematic review. *Rheumatology.* 2002;41:1155–1162.
13. Lievense AM, Bierma-Zeinstra SM, Verhagen AP, et al. Influence of obesity on the development of osteoarthritis of the hip: A systematic review. *Rheumatology.* 2002;41:1155–1162.
14. Gelber AC, Hochberg MC, Mead LA, et al. Body mass index in young men and the risk of subsequent knee and hip osteoarthritis. *Am J Med.* 1999;107:542–548.
15. Reijman M, Pols HA, Bergink AP, et al. Body mass index associated with onset and progression of osteoarthritis of the knee but not of the hip: The Rotterdam Study. *Ann Rheum Dis.* 2007;66:158–162.
16. Christensen R, Bartels EM, Astrup A, Bliddal H. Effect of weight reduction in obese patients diagnosed with knee osteoarthritis: A systematic review and meta-analysis. *Ann Rheum Dis.* 2007;66:433–439.
17. Messier SP, Loeser RF, Miller GD et al. Exercise and dietary weight loss in overweight and obese older adults with knee osteoarthritis: The Arthritis, Diet, and Activity Promotion Trial. *Arthritis Rheum.* 2004;50:1501–1510.
18. Fransen M, McConnell S, Bell M. Exercise for osteoarthritis of the hip or knee. *Cochrane Database Syst Rev.* 2003;3: CD004286.

19. National Institutes of Health (NIH) Consensus Development Panel on Total Knee Replacement. National Institutes of Health consensus statement on total knee replacement December 8–10, 2003. Final statement. Rockville (MD): U.S. Department of Health and Human Services (DHHS); 2004:18.

20. Learmonth ID, Young C, Rorabeck C. The Operation of the Century: Total Hip Replacement. *Lancet.* 2007;370:1508–19.

21. Towheed TE. Acetaminophen for osteoarthritis. *Cochrane Database Syst Rev.* 2006;(1):CD004257.

22. Eccles M, Freemantle N, Mason J, for the North of England Non-Steroidal Anti-Inflammatory Drug Guideline Development Group. North of England Evidence Based Guideline Development Project: Summary guideline for nonsteroidal anti-inflammatory drugs versus basic analgesia in treating the pain of degenerative arthritis. *Br Med J.* 1998;317:526–530.

23. Wolfe MM, Lichenstein DR, Singh G. Medical progress: Gastrointestinal toxicity of nonsteroidal anti-inflammatory drugs. *N Engl J Med.* 1999;340:1888–1899.

24. Clegg DO. Glucosamine, chondroitin sulfate, and the two in combination for painful knee osteoarthritis. *N Engl J Med.* 2006;354:795–808.

25. Richy F, Bruyere O, Ethgen O, et al. Structural and symptomatic efficacy of glucosamine and chondroitin in knee osteoarthritis: A comprehensive meta-analysis. *Arch Intern Med.* 2003;163:1514–1522.

26. Bruyere O, Compere S, Rovati LC, et al. Five-year follow up of patients from a previous 3-year randomized, controlled trial of glucosamine sulfate in knee osteoarthritis. *Arthritis Rheum.* 2003;48:S80.

27. Bellamy N, Intraarticular corticosteroid for treatment of osteoarthritis of the knee. *Cochrane Database Syst Rev.* 2006;(2):CD005328.

Chapter 36

Gout

Michael E. Ernst and Elizabeth C. Clark

SEARCH STRATEGY

A systematic search of the medical literature was performed on July 14, 2005, and again on February 16, 2007. The search, limited to human subjects and English language journals, included MEDLINER® (1999 to February 2007), the Cochrane Database of Systemic Reviews, ACP Journal Club, and Database of Abstracts of Reviews of Effectiveness. Search terms included gout and gouty arthritis. Selected review articles and clinical trials were examined. Pertinent references of the identified articles were also examined. Additionally, the American College of Rheumatology website, www.rheumatology.org was reviewed for information.

Gout is a disease characterized by deposition of monosodium urate crystals in the joints and tendons. It is the most common form of inflammatory arthritis in men more than 40 years of age.[1] Historically, gout was limited to affluent members of society; however, the incidence and prevalence of gout continue to increase in all social classes, probably because of growing waistlines, increased longevity, and changing dietary patterns.[2,3]

Men are affected with gout approximately 7 to 9 times more commonly than women, except in older age groups where approximately half of newly diagnosed cases will be in women.[3,4] The incidence of gout increases with age, with annual incidence ranging from one per 1000 for men aged 40 to 44 years to 1.8 per 1000 for those aged 55 to 64 years.[5] The lowest rates of gout are observed in younger women, in which there are approximately 0.8 cases per 10 000 patient-years.[6]

PATHOPHYSIOLOGY

Gout results from physiologic disturbances of urate metabolism which lead to hyperuricemia. Normal uric acid levels are near the limits of urate solubility because of a delicate balance that exists between the amount of urate produced and excreted.[7] Hyperuricemia is defined as a serum urate level of >7 mg/dL in men or >6 mg/dL in women.[4] In the hyperuricemic state, uric acid salts form crystals and are deposited in and around the joints and soft tissue. Hyperuricemia can result in four distinct clinical stages: asymptomatic hyperuricemia, acute gouty arthritis, intercritical gout (intervals between attacks), and chronic tophaceous gout.

Serum urate levels are the single most important risk factor for the development of gout; however, hyperuricemia and gout are not always concurrently present, and most patients with hyperuricemia remain asymptomatic.[4] The risk of gout increases in a parallel manner with serum urate levels. The 5-year cumulative risk of gout in patients with serum urate <7 mg/dL is 0.6%, compared to a risk of 30.5% with urate levels >10 mg/dL.[8]

Two distinct mechanisms can lead to hyperuricemia: decreased uric acid clearance or overproduction of uric acid. Several conditions (Table 36-1) are associated with either mechanism.[5,9,10] The vast majority (80–90%) of patients with gout have a relative deficit in the renal excretion of uric acid for an unknown reason (primary idiopathic hyperuricemia).[4]

COMPLICATIONS

Renal complications, including urolithiasis, acute renal failure, and chronic urate nephropathy can occur with gout. Nearly 10% of individuals who report the passage of a kidney stone on two or more occasions have a history of gout.[11] The frequency of urolithiasis depends on serum uric acid concentrations, acidity of the urine, and urinary uric acid concentration. Typically, patients

Table 36-1. Causes of Hyperuricemia

Underexcretion of Urate

Primary idiopathic hyperuricemia	
Renal	Renal insufficiency/renal failure, polycystic kidney disease
Metabolic/ endocrine	Diabetes insipidus, lactic acidosis, ketosis, hypothyroidism, hyperparathyroidism
Drugs	Diuretics, low-dose salicylates, cyclosporine, levodopa, niacin, ethambutol, pyrazinamide
Miscellaneous	Hypertension, Down syndrome, sarcoidosis, berylliosis, lead intoxication, toxemia of pregnancy

Overproduction of Urate

Primary idiopathic hyperuricemia	
Genetic	Hypoxanthine-guanine phosphoribosyl-transferase deficiency, phosphoribosyl-pyrophosphate synthetase overactivity, glucose-6-phosphate dehydrogenase deficiency, fructose-1-phosphate aldolase deficiency
Hematologic	Myeloproliferative and lymphoproliferative disorders, polycythemia vera, hemolytic anemias and anemias associated with ineffective erythropoiesis, cytotoxic drugs
Nutritional	Purine-rich diet, alcohol
Miscellaneous	Obesity, psoriasis, rhabdomyolysis, Paget's disease, exercise, hypertriglyceridemia

Table 36-2. American College of Rheumatology Criteria for the Classification of Acute Gouty Arthritis*

1. More than one attack of acute arthritis
2. Maximum inflammation developed within 1 d
3. Monoarthritis attack
4. Redness observed over joints
5. First metatarsophalangeal joint painful or swollen
6. Unilateral first metatarsophalangeal joint attack
7. Unilateral tarsal joint attack
8. Tophus (proven or suspected)
9. Hyperuricemia
10. Asymmetric swelling within a joint on x-ray films
11. Subcortical cysts without erosions on x-ray films
12. Monosodium urate monohydrate microcrystals in joint fluid during attack
13. Joint fluid culture negative for organisms during attack

*The combination of crystals, tophi, and/or six or more criteria is highly suggestive of gout.

with uric acid nephrolithiasis have a urinary pH of less than 6.0. Clinicians should be suspicious of hyperuricemic states in patients who present with kidney stones, and all patients with diagnosed gout should have renal function monitored regularly.

CLINICAL PRESENTATION OF ACUTE GOUTY ARTHRITIS

Approximately 90% of first attacks of gout present as an acute inflammatory monoarthritis of the first metatarsophalangeal joint, a condition known as "podagra." However, any joint of the lower extremity may be affected and occasionally gout will present as a monoarthritis of the wrist or finger.[12] The onset is rapid, and the joint is warm, erythematous, swollen, and tender. A low-grade fever may be present. The attack is usually self-limiting within 3 to 5 days, but may take up to a week to subside. Atypical presentations of gout can occur, such as in the older people or in women where it can present as a polyarticular arthritis easily mistaken for osteoarthritis.[2]

Acute gouty arthritis may occur without provocation. Fluctuations in serum uric acid brought about by binge amounts of alcohol or ingestion of large amounts of protein- or purine-rich foods can initiate an attack. Acute flares may occur infrequently, although with time the period between attacks may shorten if appropriate measures to correct hyperuricemia are not undertaken.[12] Later in the disease, tophaceous deposits of monosodium urate crystals in the skin or subcutaneous tissues may be found. These tophi can be anywhere but are often found on the hands, wrists, elbows, or knees. It is estimated to take 10 or more years for tophi to develop.[12]

DIAGNOSTIC EVALUATION

Table 36-2 shows the American College of Rheumatology classification criteria for an acute gouty arthritis attack. Although the diagnosis can be suspected clinically, gout is definitively diagnosed when monosodium urate crystals are observed in synovial fluid or a tophus.[4,13] Crystals are needle shaped and when examined under polarizing light microscopy they are strongly negatively birefringent (doubly refractive). Measuring 24-hour urinary uric acid excretion can help in determining whether hyperuricemia is caused by overproduction or underexcretion; however, because fewer than 10% of hyperuricemic patients are overproducers, this test is not often performed. Testing should be considered in patients with recurrent kidney stones, a strong family history of gout or kidney stones, or gout at a young age. Overproduction hyperuricemia is defined by excessive uric acid excretion of more than 1 g in 24 hours.[14]

In patients with long standing gout, radiographs may show punched-out marginal erosions and secondary osteoarthritis changes; however, in an acute first attack radiographs are unremarkable.[15] Alternatively, the presence of chondrocalcinosis on radiographs may

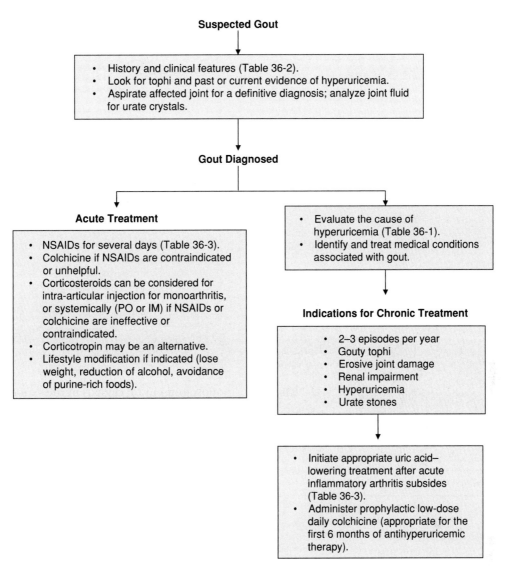

Suspected Gout

- History and clinical features (Table 36-2).
- Look for tophi and past or current evidence of hyperuricemia.
- Aspirate affected joint for a definitive diagnosis; analyze joint fluid for urate crystals.

Gout Diagnosed

Acute Treatment

- NSAIDs for several days (Table 36-3).
- Colchicine if NSAIDs are contraindicated or unhelpful.
- Corticosteroids can be considered for intra-articular injection for monoarthritis, or systemically (PO or IM) if NSAIDs or colchicine are ineffective or contraindicated.
- Corticotropin may be an alternative.
- Lifestyle modification if indicated (lose weight, reduction of alcohol, avoidance of purine-rich foods).

- Evaluate the cause of hyperuricemia (Table 36-1).
- Identify and treat medical conditions associated with gout.

Indications for Chronic Treatment

- 2–3 episodes per year
- Gouty tophi
- Erosive joint damage
- Renal impairment
- Hyperuricemia
- Urate stones

- Initiate appropriate uric acid–lowering treatment after acute inflammatory arthritis subsides (Table 36-3).
- Administer prophylactic low-dose daily colchicine (appropriate for the first 6 months of antihyperuricemic therapy).

Figure 36-1. Algorithm for evaluation and treatment of gout.

indicate pseudogout. The use of magnetic resonance or computed tomography imaging to diagnosis gout is not usually warranted.

TREATMENT

Figure 36-1 summarizes the clinical approach to the diagnosis and treatment of gout. The general goals of therapy are to terminate the acute painful attack, prevent recurrences by lowering excess uric acid stores, and prevent or reverse complications of urate deposition into joints, kidneys, or other sites. Because of the association between gout and conditions such as alcoholism, hypertension, obesity, metabolic syndrome, and myeloproliferative disorders, successful treatment of gout also involves addressing the underlying conditions

that may be contributing to it. In addition, because elevated uric acid levels have been associated with increased risk of coronary artery disease, a gout attack should be an incentive to assess the patient's overall cardiovascular risk profile.[16]

ACUTE GOUTY ARTHRITIS

Nonsteroidal Anti-Inflammatory Drugs

Table 36-3 summarizes the available pharmacotherapy for gout. In most patients without complications, nonsteroidal anti-inflammatory drugs (NSAIDs) are preferred for initial therapy. Indomethacin has been historically favored as the NSAID of choice for acute gout flares, but there is little evidence to support one NSAID as more efficacious than another.[4] The most

Table 36-3. Pharmacotherapy of Acute and Chronic Gout

Acute Gout (Treatment)

Drug NSAIDs* FDA-approved	Typical Regimen	Considerations
Indomethacin	25–50 mg four times daily initially for 3 d, then taper to twice daily for 4–7 d	Avoid use in patients with peptic ulcer disease, active bleeding. May cause nephropathy, gastritis, fluid overload in patients with congestive heart failure.
Sulindac	200 mg twice daily for 7–10 d	
Naproxen	500 mg twice daily initially for 3 d, then 250–500 mg once daily for 4–7 d	
Others studied		
Ketoprofen	75 mg four times daily	See above
Etodolac	300 mg twice daily	
Ibuprofen	800 mg four times daily	
Colchicine	0.5–0.6 mg every hour until adverse effects occur or maximum dosage of 6 mg is reached	Dose reduction necessary in patients with renal insufficiency. Dose-dependent gastrointestinal adverse effects (diarrhea, nausea, vomiting). Avoid using concurrently with macrolide antibiotics. Intravenous dosing not recommended.
Corticosteroids		
Oral	Prednisone 40–60 mg once daily × 3 d, then taper by 10–15 mg/d every 3 d until discontinuation	Use with caution in diabetics. Avoid long-term use. May cause fluid retention, impaired wound healing. Intra-articular administration is preferred for monarticular involvement; avoid use if joint sepsis is not excluded.
Intramuscular	Triamcinolone acetonide 60 mg IM once, or methylprednisolone 100–150 mg/d × 1–2 d	
Intra-articular	Triamcinolone acetonide 10–40 mg (large joints), 5–20 mg (small joints)	
Corticotropin	25 USP units subcutaneously for acute small joint monoarticular gout; 40 USP units IM or IV for larger joints or polyarticular involvement	Repeat injections may be needed. Requires intact pituitary–adrenal axis. Less effective in patients receiving long-term oral corticosteroid therapy.

Chronic Gout (Prevention)

Drug	Regimen	Comments
Allopurinol	50–300 mg once daily	Can be used in both urate overproduction and urate underexcretion. Adverse effects include rash, gastrointestinal symptoms, potential for fatal hypersensitivity syndrome. Dose reduction necessary in patients with renal insufficiency.
Colchicine	0.6 mg twice daily	Prophylaxis against acute gout during the initiation of antihyperuricemic therapy.
Uricosurics		
Probenecid	250 mg twice daily, titrated up to 500–2000 mg/d (target serum urate <6 mg/dL)	Useful in urate underexcretion. Avoid in patients with history of urolithiasis.
Sulfinpyrazone	50 mg twice daily, titrated to 100–400 mg/d (target serum urate <6 mg/dL)	

*Therapeutic benefit of NSAIDs in gout is considered to be a class effect.

important determinant of therapeutic success with NSAIDs appears not to be which one is chosen, but rather how soon it is initiated. Therapy should be initiated with maximum dosages at the onset of symptoms and continued for 24 hours after complete resolution of an acute attack, then tapered quickly over 2 to 3 days.[13]

Unfortunately, NSAIDs are associated with a number of adverse effects, including gastrointestinal (gastritis, bleeding, and perforation), renal (renal papillary necrosis, reduced creatinine clearance), cardiovascular (sodium and fluid retention, increased blood pressure), and central nervous system (impaired cognitive function). NSAIDs should be used with caution in the older people, and in patients with a history or increased risk of peptic ulcer disease, renal insufficiency, congestive heart failure, or receiving anticoagulants.

Colchicine

Colchicine has been used for the treatment of gout since ancient times. As a result of the high incidence of adverse effects, and low benefit-risk ratio, it is used less often than NSAIDs. When colchicine is begun within the first 24 hours of an acute attack, two-thirds of patients will respond within hours of administration.[17] Although it is a highly effective therapy, colchicine is limited by dose-dependent gastrointestinal adverse effects, including nausea, vomiting, and diarrhea. More than 80% of patients may experience these adverse effects at therapeutic dosages before complete relief of symptoms.[4,17]

Colchicine is usually administered orally. An initial dose of 1 to 1.2 mg is usually given, followed by 0.5 to 0.6 mg every hour until symptoms are relieved, gastrointestinal adverse effects develop, or a total of 5 to 7 mg have been given. It should be administered within 12 to 24 hours of symptom onset, and is less effective once an acute attack has persisted beyond a few days. It is rapidly absorbed and eliminated; however, in patients with renal insufficiency, the terminal half-life may be two to three times normal (up to 24 hours).[18] Because of fatalities associated with improper use of intravenous colchicine, it should be only be administered by experienced clinicians.[19]

Corticosteroids

Corticosteroids can be safely used in gout, particularly when NSAIDs or colchicine are contraindicated.[4] They can be used either systemically or by intra-articular injection. Monarticular gout attacks respond well to small intra-articular doses of triamcinolone.[20] Injection should be done under aseptic technique in a joint determined to be free of infection. Oral corticosteroids, such as prednisone 20 to 40 mg/d initially, can be used in patients experiencing polyarticular involvement.[4] Therapy should be tapered carefully over several days, as rebound flares can occur. A single intramuscular injection of a long-acting corticosteroid, such as methylprednisolone, can be used as an alternative to the oral route.[4] If not contraindicated, low-dose colchicine can be used as adjunctive therapy to injectable corticosteroids to prevent rebound flare-ups.[7]

Corticosteroids can have a number of adverse effects, and should be used with caution in patients with diabetes since they can increase blood glucose. In addition, patients with a history of gastrointestinal problems, bleeding disorders, cardiovascular disease, and psychiatric disorders should be monitored closely. Long-term corticosteroid use should be avoided because of the risk for osteoporosis, hypothalamus-pituitary axis suppression, and muscle deconditioning that can occur.

Corticotropin

Corticotropin, which stimulates the adrenal cortex to produce cortisol, corticosterone, and other androgens, can be administered in acute gout. It is typically given in a dose of 40 to 80 units as an intramuscular injection.[12] Studies with corticotropin are limited, but it appears to provide similar efficacy to systemic antiinflammatory doses of corticosteroids.[21] When administered alone or in combination with colchicine, corticotropin may provide earlier efficacy compared with indomethacin but with fewer adverse effects.[22] Several doses of corticotropin may be needed, and it cannot be used in patients with a recent prior use of systemic steroids. Since the studies have several limitations, the regimen should be considered only as an alternative, primarily in patients with comorbidities where other regimens are contraindicated.

PROPHYLACTIC TREATMENT OF CHRONIC (INTERCRITICAL) GOUT

Prevention of chronic gout attacks is aimed at lowering serum uric acid concentrations to less than 6 mg per dL, and preferably below 5 mg/dL.[23,24] Serum urate levels may return to normal with simple dietary and lifestyle modifications—including weight loss and purine-restricted diets—although these interventions may be only moderately effective in lowering serum uric acid levels.[25]

Evidence about when to start prophylactic therapy is controversial. Since gout attacks are generally infrequent and often self-limiting, initiation of long-term therapy after the first attack is often not indicated. Prophylactic therapy is cost-effective if patients have 2 or more attacks per year, or in patients with tophi or who have documented states of overproduction.[7,26] Urate-lowering therapy should not commence during an acute attack, but rather should be started 6 to 8 weeks after resolution.[18]

Urate-lowering therapies generally fall into two categories—those that reduce urate production (e.g., allopurinol), or those that increase urate excretion (uricosuric agents). Overproducers of urate can be identified using a 24-hour urinary urate excretion test, but it has a number of limitations, including patient inconvenience and possible misdiagnosis of patients who are not following strict low-purine diets. Also, the test cannot identify patients with combination urate overproduction and underexcretion.[7] Regardless of what type of urate-lowering therapy is selected, use of low-dose colchicine (0.6 mg twice daily) concurrently in first 6 months is recommended to help prevent acute flares if no contraindications exist.[27]

Allopurinol

Allopurinol, a xanthine oxidase inhibitor that prevents formation of uric acid, is the most widely used agent for prophylaxis because of its convenient once-daily dosing and its benefits to both underexcreters and overproducers.[7] Allopurinol lowers uric acid levels in a dose-dependent manner.[18] It is typically initiated at a dose of 100 mg/d and then gradually titrated to 300 mg/d to achieve a serum uric acid level of 6 mg/dL or less. The dose of allopurinol should be reduced in patients with renal insufficiency.[28] When prescribed, allopurinol should be used long-term, as intermittent administration is less effective in controlling gouty attacks.[29]

Although allopurinol is the most effective urate-lowering agent available, some patients are unable to tolerate the adverse effects such as rash, gastrointestinal upset, headache, and urticaria. More severe adverse reactions including severe rash (toxic epidermal necrolysis, erythema multiforme, or exfoliative dermatitis), hepatitis, interstitial nephritis, and eosinophilia reportedly occur in approximately 2% of patients, and is associated with a 20% mortality.[23,28] The greatest risk for this "allopurinol hypersensitivity syndrome" is with higher doses (200 to 400 mg/daily), especially in the presence of renal insufficiency.[28]

Uricosuric Agents

Probenecid and sulfinpyrazone are uricosurics that inhibit post-secretory renal proximal tubule reabsorption of uric acid. Of the two agents, probenecid is more commonly used. Both agents should be used only in patients with documented underexcretion of urate (less than 800 mg in 24 hours on a regular diet, or 600 mg on a purine-restricted diet). As a result of the increased risk for urolithiasis from the uricosuria that results after initiating probenecid or sulfinpyrazone, both agents are contraindiacated in patients with creatinine clearance of less than 50 mL/min or a history of renal calculi.[18] Probenecid can inhibit the tubular secretion of other organic acids; thus, increased plasma concentrations of penicillins, cephalosporins, sulfonamides, and indomethacin can occur. Sulfinpyrazone is less frequently used secondary to its adverse effect profile.[18]

MONITORING AND FOLLOW-UP

For a patient experiencing a first attack of gout, long-term therapy is generally not indicated. Many experts believe that long-term treatment should be started only after two or three attacks of gout. Patients having a first attack should be educated about the likelihood of recurrence and what to do if another attack occurs. Approximately 60% of patients have a second attack within the first year, and 78% have a second attack within 2 years. Only 7% of patients do not have a recurrence within a 10-year period.

When using medications chronically, renal function (serum creatinine, blood urea nitrogen), liver enzymes (aspartate aminotransferase, alanine aminotransferase), complete blood count, and electrolytes should be obtained at baseline and periodically thereafter. In patients without evident tophi, consideration can be given to discontinuing chronic therapy 6 to 12 months after normal serum urate levels are obtained.

ASYMPTOMATIC HYPERURICEMIA

Asymptomatic hyperuricemia does not usually require treatment or follow-up except for those individuals at high risk of complications, such as those with very high levels of uric acid, a personal or strong family history of gout, urolithiasis, or uric acid nephropathy. Some experts have recommended not treating asymptomatic hyperuricemia unless uric acid levels are at least 12 or 13 mg/dL in men or 10 mg/dL in women.[14] Although the treatment of asymptomatic hyperuricemia has not proven to reduce cardiovascular disease, evidence indicating a link between the two suggests patients with hyperuricemia should be evaluated for signs of cardiovascular disease and appropriate risk reduction measures undertaken. Correctable causes of hyperuricemia, such as medications, obesity, malignancy, and alcohol abuse should be treated.[9]

EVIDENCE-BASED SUMMARY

- Gout classically presents as an acute inflammatory monoarthritis and is definitively diagnosed when monosodium urate crystals are observed in synovial fluid or a tophus.
- NSAIDs are the first-line therapy for an acute gout attack. Colchicine and corticosteroids can also be used.
- Asymptomatic hyperuricemia is generally not treated.
- In patients who experience two or more gout attacks in a year, or who have tophi, long-term prophylactic treatment with allopurinol is recommended.
- Serum urate levels should be lowered below 6 mg/dL and preferably 5 mg/dL to reduce the risk of recurrent attacks.
- Lifestyle changes such as reduction of alcohol intake, weight loss, and avoidance of purine-rich foods are recommended to help reduce risk for gout attacks.

REFERENCES

1. Roubenoff R, Klag MJ, Mead LA, et al. Incidence and risk factors for gout in white men. *JAMA*. 1991;266:3004–3007.
2. Bieber JD, Terkeltaub RA. Gout: On the brink of novel therapeutic options for an ancient disease. *Arthritis Rheum*. 2004;50:2400–2414.
3. Wallace KL, Riedel AA, Joseph-Ridge N, et al. Increasing prevalence of gout and hyperuricemia over 10 years among older adults in a managed care population. *J Rheumatol*. 2004;31:1582–1587.
4. Rott KT, Agudelo CA. Gout. *JAMA*. 2003;289:2857–2860.
5. Choi HK, Atkinson K, Karlson EW, et al. Purine-rich foods, dairy and protein intake, and the risk of gout in men. *N Engl J Med*. 2004;350:1093–1103.
6. Mikuls TR, Farrar JT, Bilker WB, et al. Gout epidemiology: Results from the UK General Practice Research Database, 1990–1999. *Ann Rheum Dis*. 2005;64:267–272.
7. Terkeltaub RA. Gout. *N Engl J Med*. 2003;349:1647–1655.
8. Campion EW, Glynn RJ, DeLabry LO. Asymptomatic hyperuricemia. Risks and consequences in the Normative Aging Study. *Am J Med*. 1987;82:421–426.
9. Choi HK, Atkinson K, Karlson EW, et al. Obesity, weight change, hypertension, diuretic use, and risk of gout in men: The health professionals follow-up study. *Arch Intern Med*. 2005;165:742–748.
10. Lin KC, Lin HY, Chou P. The interaction between uric acid level and other risk factors on the development of gout among asymptomatic hyperuricemic men in a prospective study. *J Rheumatol*. 2000;27:1501–1505.
11. Kramer HM, Curhan G. The association between gout and nephrolithiasis: The National Health and Nutrition Examination Survey III, 1988-1994. *Am J Kidney Dis*. 2002;40:37–42.
12. Kim KY, Schumacher HR, Hunsche E, et al. A literature review of the epidemiology and treatment of acute gout. *Clin Ther*. 2003;25:1593–1617.
13. Schlesinger N, Baker DG, Schumacher HR Jr. How well have diagnostic tests and therapies for gout been evaluated? *Curr Opin Rheumatol*. 1999;11:441–445.
14. Dincer HE, Dincer AP, Levinson DJ. Asymptomatic hyperuricemia: To treat or not to treat. *Cleve Clin J Med*. 2002;69:594.
15. Pal B, Foxall M, Dysart T, et al. How is gout managed in primary care? A review of current practice and proposed guidelines. *Clin Rheumatol*. 2000;19:21–25.
16. Janssens HJ, van de Lisdonk EH, Bor H, et al. Gout, just a nasty event or a cardiovascular signal? A study from primary care. *Family Pract*. 2003;20:413–416.
17. Ahern MJ, Reid C, Gordon TP, et al. Does colchicine work? The results of the first controlled study in acute gout. *Aust N Z J Med*. 1987;17:301–304.
18. Schlesinger N. Management of acute and chronic gouty arthritis: Present state-of-the-art. *Drugs*. 2004;64:2399–2416.
19. Bonnel RA, Villalba ML, Karwoski CB, et al. Deaths associated with inappropriate intravenous colchicine administration. *J Emerg Med*. 2002;22:385–387.
20. Fernandez C, Noguera R, Gonzalez JA, et al. Treatment of acute attacks of gout with a small dose of intraarticular triamcinolone acetonide. *J Rheumatol*. 1999;26:2285–2286.
21. Siegel LB, Alloway JA, Nashel DJ. Comparison of adrenocorticotropic hormone and triamcinolone acetonide in the treatment of acute gouty arthritis. *J Rheumatol*. 1994;21:1325–1327.
22. Axelrod D, Preston S. Comparison of parenteral adrenocorticotropic hormone with oral indomethacin in the treatment of acute gout. *Arthritis Rheum*. 1988;31:803–805.
23. Wortmann RL. Gout and hyperuricemia. *Curr Opin Rheumatol*. 2002;14:281–286.
24. Shoji A, Yamanaka H, Kamatani N. A retrospective study of the relationship between serum urate level and recurrent attacks of gouty arthritis: Evidence for reduction of recurrent gouty arthritis with antihyperuricemic therapy. *Arthritis Rheum*. 2004;51:321–325.
25. Dessein PH, Shipton EA, Stanwix AE, et al. Beneficial effects of weight loss associated with moderate calorie/carbohydrate restriction, and increased proportional intake of protein and unsaturated fat on serum urate and lipoprotein levels in gout: A pilot study. *Ann Rheum Dis*. 2000;59:539–543.
26. Ferraz MB, O'Brien B. A cost effectiveness analysis of urate lowering drugs in nontophaceous recurrent gouty arthritis. *J Rheumatol*. 1995;22:908–914.
27. Borstad GC, Bryant LR, Abel MP, et al. Colchicine for prophylaxis of acute flares when initiating allopurinol for chronic gouty arthritis. *J Rheumatol*. 2004;31:2429–2432.
28. Hande KR, Noone RM, Stone WJ. Severe allopurinol toxicity. Description and guidelines for prevention in patients with renal insufficiency. *Am J Med*. 1984;76:47–56.
29. Bull PW, Scott JT. Intermittent control of hyperuricemia in the treatment of gout. *J Rheumatol*. 1989;16:1246–8.

PART 9

Disorders of the Eyes, Ears, Nose, and Throat

CHAPTERS

Chapter 37

Allergic and Nonallergic Rhinitis

S. Rubina Inamdar

SEARCH STRATEGY

Information in this chapter was obtained from published articles identified in a Medline search conducted in March 2008 using the search term allergic rhinitis.

INTRODUCTION

Rhinitis is a misunderstood and commonly trivialized problem despite its high prevalence. The defining symptoms of rhinitis are well known ("it's just a runny nose"), including nasal congestion, mucoid discharge, pruritus, and sneezing. What are less well known are the spectrum of secondary symptoms such as fatigue, sleep disturbance, cognitive and motor impairment, mood changes, and somnolence that often accompany nasal symptoms.[1] Cumulatively, these contribute to potentially serious and detrimental effects on quality of life, functionality, and productivity.

Approximately 40 million Americans have allergic rhinitis, another 17 million individuals are estimated to have nonallergic rhinitis, and 10 million suffer from mixed allergic and nonallergic conditions.[2] Global epidemiology studies have found similar proportions throughout the world. This makes rhinitis one of the most common of chronic human diseases and the most prevalent chronic disease of childhood.

Billions of dollars are spent each year on office visits and medications, while indirect costs such as decreased productivity in the workplace and at school and poor quality of life add untold dollars to the cost. Thus, what seems like a relatively innocuous disease has far-reaching impact.

CLASSIFICATION

More than a dozen forms of rhinitis are recognized in the "Global Resource in Allergy" consensus document, published by the World Allergy Organization. Rhinitis is classified by etiology and temporal criteria. The three most common types are allergic, nonallergic, and infectious. Infectious rhinitis, often manifested as the "common cold," and acute sinusitis typically occur together, as they share the same mucosal tissue. For this reason, infectious rhinitis and acute sinusitis have been retermed "acute rhinosinusitis,"[3] and these conditions are addressed in Chapter 38 of this textbook.

Allergic and nonallergic rhinitis are each further subdivided into "intermittent" and "persistent" conditions. Intermittent rhinitis is considered acute or occasional rhinitis with symptoms lasting fewer than 4 days per week or for fewer than 4 weeks. Patients with persistent rhinitis have symptoms for more than 4 days per week or for more than 4 weeks.[4] These conditions were formerly termed "seasonal" and "perennial," which were helpful terms for allergic rhinitis but nonsensical for nonallergic rhinitis.

Additionally, the newer classification scheme accounts for individuals who have symptoms intermittently from allergens that are traditionally perennial. For example, cats produce "perennial" allergens, but if a woman does not have a cat in her home and only gets symptoms when she visits friends or relatives who have cats, then she has intermittent allergic rhinitis secondary to cat allergens.

Severity classification of rhinitis is relatively straightforward from a qualitative standpoint:

- Patients with mild rhinitis have normal sleep, no impairment of daily activities, normal work and school, and no troublesome symptoms.

• Patients with moderate-to-severe rhinitis have one or more of the following symptoms: abnormal sleep, impairment of daily activities, interference with regular work and school attendance and performance, and troublesome symptoms.

Thus, most patients that present to a medical provider are likely to have more moderate-to-severe symptoms. In clinical testing of medications, more specific quantitative scales are used to measure symptoms of rhinitis.

CLINICAL PRESENTATION

For patients with symptoms indicative of rhinitis, taking a complete history will generally point the clinician toward a diagnosis. Determining the age of onset of symptoms, frequency of symptoms, triggers, and presence of comorbid conditions will lead to a correct differential diagnosis of one of the types of rhinitis in the majority of patients. Symptom presentation and differentiating features are listed in Table 37-1.

The most common presenting symptoms of rhinitis are nasal congestion and anterior or posterior drainage. This can be associated with sneezing, sinus pressure/pain, mouth breathing, and/or snoring. Patients may describe a chronic cough, hoarseness, or globus sensation as a result of postnasal drainage. Eustachian tube dysfunction with tinnitus, sensation of fluid in the ear, and "ear popping" can occur due to sinonasal inflammation.

Typically, allergic rhinitis is further characterized by pruritus of the nose, upper palate, inner ear, and conjunctiva. Serial sneezing, in which an individual has several sneezes in a row, is also associated with allergic rhinitis. Allergic rhinitis is differentiated from nonallergic rhinitis by a clinical history of allergen exposure and specific immunoglobulin E (IgE) testing demonstrating a response to a potentially causative allergen. IgE testing is performed using either skin prick testing or radioallergosorbent test (RAST) blood testing.[5] The most common allergens are dust mites, trees, grasses, weeds, cockroaches, pets, and molds. Repeated exposure to these allergens sensitizes the immune system prompting antigen specific B cells to activate and mature into IgE producing plasma cells. The antigen-specific IgE then circulates in the blood or binds to mast cells awaiting activation by allergens.

Nonallergic rhinitis presents very similarly to allergic rhinitis except for the absence of pruritic features. A collection of disorders associated with nasal symptoms but with a wide variety of etiologies and pathophysiologies, nonallergic rhinitis can be caused by medications such as β-blockers, endocrine abnormalities, irritants, and vasomotor instability. Recurrent nasal symptoms appear similar to allergic rhinitis but without specific IgE-mediated allergy (see Table 37-1). There is a strong female preponderance, and only 30% of patients present below 20 years of age.[3] Pathophysiology in this group of disorders is less well understood. Vasomotor rhinitis is not immune mediated, but can result in vascular engorgement and inflammation. Cerebrospinal fluid rhinorrhea, caused by leakage of cerebrospinal fluid into the nasal cavity, can be caused by craniofacial trauma or surgery. This can be mistaken for allergic or nonallergic rhinitis with disastrous consequences. Gustatory rhinitis, or nasal symptoms associated with eating, may be a result of an irritant response to spicy foods, vasomotor response to alcohol, or chemical sensitivity to certain preservatives.

Physical examination in these patients usually reveals some evidence of nasal pathology. Outer nares should be inspected for evidence of excoriation, swelling, and mucoid discharge. Anterior rhinoscopy will reveal swollen turbinates, some mucoid discharge, and occasionally nasal polyposis. Allergic patients may have pale bluish boggy nasal mucosa, while nonallergic patients may have a variety of findings ranging from normal mucosa to atrophic. Allergic patients have many classic findings including "allergic shiners," or under-eye pigmentation; Dennie–Morgan lines, which are creases below the eyes; and the "nasal crease" across the lower bridge of the nose. Children may rub their noses so often that they create the "allergic salute."

QUALITY OF LIFE AND SOCIOECONOMIC IMPACT

Allergic rhinitis is not simply a nuisance. Multiple studies confirmed what many patients with rhinitis have symptoms that can have a profound impact on quality of life.

An estimated 80% of rhinitis patients have sleep disturbances with resulting daytime fatigue.[3] This contributes to 2 million missed schooldays and 100 million missed workdays every year in the United States.[3] Employees with rhinitis have decreased productivity, are absent more frequently, and are at increased risk for work-related injury and motor vehicle accidents. Schoolchildren may have learning impairment, mood changes, shyness, fatigue, and depression.[1] Cognitive impairment, a well-known effect of rhinitis, is likely the result of the inflammatory cascade of rhinitis, sleep disturbance, and the nonprescription medications many patients take. In many states, driving while under the influence of sedating antihistamines can result in a traffic citation.

Table 37-1. Common Symptoms of Rhinitis and Potentially Differentiating Features

Type	Symptoms	Classic Triggers	Special Features	Testing
Allergic	Sneezing, pruritus, clear mucus drainage although may develop colored drainage with an increase in cellular byproducts. May be intermittent or persistent, possible seasonal worsening	Dust mites, animal dander, cockroaches, pollens, molds	Family history of atopic disease, other atopic illnesses such as asthma	Specific allergen testing through cutaneous allergy testing or RAST testing. Some specialty clinics may offer allergen challenges.
Infectious	Rhinitis symptoms without pruritus, transient. Purulent discharge, associated symptoms of systemic illness such as fever, sore throat, ear pain, malaise, fatigue	Virus, bacterial	Possible sick contact exposure	Generally none required
Nonallergic, drug-induced	Aspirin/NSAIDS, β-blockers, other medicines. May be intermittent or persistent depending on medication exposure	Acute onset symptoms within a 4 h of drug exposure. Alterations in vascular tone due to cardiovascular medications.	Aspirin allergy may have associated asthma and nasal polyps	May require subspecialty evaluation for formal challenge or aspirin desensitization
Occupational	Rhinitis symptoms that are present at work, but improve at home, over the weekend, or while on vacation	May be allergic or nonallergic. Fumes, aerosolized chemicals, animal dander,	May have associated asthma or conjunctivitis	May require subspecialty evaluation for specific IgE testing, direct challenge, and monitoring at work.
Hormonal	Symptoms of rhinitis associated with hormonal fluctuations	Menstruation, puberty, pregnancy, endocrine disorders		Pregnancy test or endocrine evaluation is indicated.
Gustatory	Rhinitis associated with food consumption	Spicy foods, alcohol	Can be socially debilitating	Usually none required.
Nonallergic with eosinophilia syndrome	Persistent rhinitis symptoms	None	Treated as if vasomotor rhinitis	Specific allergen testing is negative, but nasal cellular infiltrate is composed of eosinophils.
Atrophic	Atrophy of nasal mucosa resulting in crusting, malodorous discharge. Also known as ozena.	Dry environment, sino/nasal surgery	Discharge can be malodorous, but patient may not recognize it as they are anosmic	Culture for culprit bacteria, evaluate for nutritional deficiency
Vasomotor	Persistent rhinitis symptoms	Temperature, barometric or humidity changes, irritants such as cigarettes, perfume, paint, smoke, and emotional stress	90% of patients are women 40–60 y of age.	Specific allergen testing to determine possible mixed rhinitis.
Nasal polyps	Rhinitis symptoms but associated with anosmia, presence of nasal polyps seen on anterior rhinoscopy or CT scanning	Irritants, viral infections and NSAID ingestion can cause acute exacerbations	Can have high levels of localized staphylococcal enterotoxin sensitivity. Often associated with asthma	CT imaging. May require referral to allergy possible aspirin desensitization, or otolaryngology for surgery.
Mucociliary defects	Chronic nasal congestion, often from childhood, associated with chronic bronchitis, otitis, infertility	Recurrent infections	Can have a secondary form due to certain medications, infections, cystic fibrosis	Mucociliary transport testing. Sweat testing for cystic fibrosis
Cerebrospinal rhinorrhea	Clear nasal discharge days to months after sinus surgery or facial trauma. Symptoms worse with bending forward.	Sinus or facial manipulation		Subspecialty evaluation with otolaryngology is imperative

(continued)

Table 37-1. Common Symptoms of Rhinitis and Potentially Differentiating Features *(Continued)*

Type	Symptoms	Classic Triggers	Special Features	Testing
Tumors related	May have mild rhinitis symptoms, but congestion and nasal obstruction, or epistaxis may be the hallmark symptom.		Can have headache associated	Subspecialty evaluation is suggested. CT imaging may be required
Mechanical obstruction	Adenoidal hypertrophy, nasal septal deviation, foreign bodies, choanal atresia	May worsen with concomitant allergic disease	May become secondarily infected	Radiographic imaging, rhinoscopy
Granulomatous diseases	Symptoms of rhinitis, anosmia, purulent or bloody discharge, and other associated symptoms of systemic granulomatous diseases		Sarcoid, infectious granuloma, Wegener's granulomatosis, midline granuloma	Aggressive serologic and pathologic evaluation and referral is recommended

ANATOMY AND FUNCTION OF THE NOSE

As a passageway for oxygen and a channel to the brain for smells and taste, the nose and its complex structures (Figure 37-1) provide humidification and warming of air, filter particles, and protect the lungs and thereby assure optimal lung function. In patients with exercise-induced asthma, breathing through their nose resulted in less bronchospasm than taking breaths through the mouth.[6]

The nose has a normal cycle of congestion and decongestion with each side alternating being congested. This cycle can be exaggerated during inflammatory responses and result in airway obstruction. The lateral recumbent position is associated with congestion of the dependent side of the nose, which can be especially uncomfortable while trying to sleep while suffering from an upper respiratory tract infection. Interestingly, prolonged pressure on the axilla results in ipsilateral congestion in the nose ("crutch reflex").[7]

Mucus production in the nose begins from the anterior chamber, flows along the turbinates, and drains into the posterior pharynx. Normally, mucus is thin and not noticeable. As a result of inflammation, mucus thickens and with the release of inflammatory mediators, takes on any of several colors.[1]

COMORBID CONDITIONS

Rhinitis of all types can be associated with significant comorbid conditions. Chronic nasal congestion and mouth breathing can result in facial/cranial changes in children. Often an allergic rhinitis exacerbation or infectious rhinitis can result in asthma exacerbations, secondary infection with bacterial sinusitis, persistent cough, otitis media, otitis media with effusion, chronic snoring, or eustachian tube dysfunction.

The most important comorbid condition associated with rhinitis is asthma. The nose and the lungs are both lined with airway epithelium, and they are susceptible to the same types of insults. Well-conducted antigen challenge studies have demonstrated inflammation in the nose after challenge with ragweed in the left bronchus. In the same vein, patients challenged with antigen in the nose had decreased airflow consistent with exacerbations of asthma.[8] More than 95% of patients with asthma have concomitant rhinitis, and more than 50% of patients with rhinitis have some symptoms of asthma.[6] During allergy seasons, 30% of patients with allergic rhinitis but not asthma have bronchial hyperactivity. Allergic rhinitis is clearly a significant risk factor for asthma, and patients who present with rhinitis should also be screened for asthma by history or further

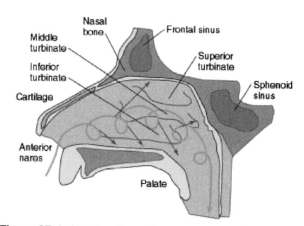

Figure 37-1. Nasal anatomy. The nose serves to filter inhaled air, removing dust, pollen, viruses, and bacteria, while also humidifying and warming the inhalant. The three turbinates provide a large surface area and generate a turbulent airflow that ensures maximal warming and humidification, while also forcing impact of particles onto the nasal mucosa. Mucus produced by the nose flows from the anterior chamber filtering and collecting debris and then drains down the back of the throat.

tests. Infectious rhinitis can also be a potent trigger of asthma exacerbations.

Another comorbid condition of rhinitis is rhinosinusitis. More than 50% of patients with chronic rhinosinusitis have specific IgE fractions associated with the condition. IgE-mediated rhinitis may prompt further inflammation in the sinuses, or the inflammation in the sinuses may lead to IgE differentiation and production.

TREATMENT

Therapies for rhinitis have not changed significantly over the past 20 years. As noted in Figure 37-2, patients generally present after nonprescription therapies fail to modulate symptoms of stuffiness, postnasal drip, scratchy throat, and difficulty breathing. Symptoms that likely have an infectious origin can be managed supportively, adding antibiotics only if the condition persists or worsens. Recently, deaths of infants and children from inadvertent overdoses and usual doses of antihistamines and decongestants have resulted in market withdrawals and controversy over the use of these medications in pediatric patients, especially those younger than 6 years. Use of nonpharmacologic approaches, other medications, and immunotherapy is thus increasing in this age group.

For allergic rhinitis, vasomotor rhinitis, and other conditions in which an identifiable external factor triggers symptoms, the first line of management—and the most poorly implemented—is avoidance. This is possible with uncommonly encountered irritants, such as cigarette smoke or spicy foods. However, other triggers

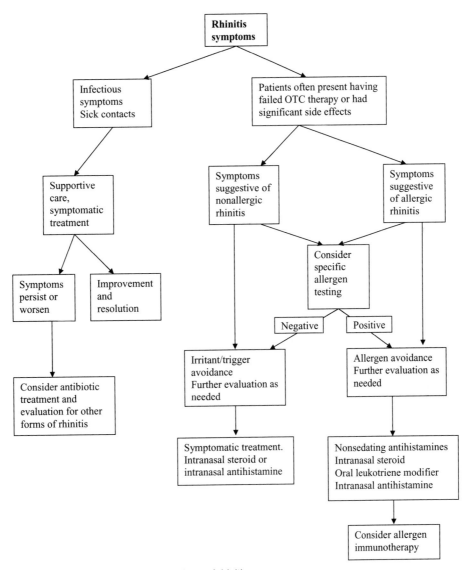

Figure 37-2. Diagnosis and treatment of rhinitis.

Table 37-2. Oral Dosages of Commonly Used Oral Antihistamines and Decongestants

Medication	Availability	Dosage and Interval* Adults	Children
Nonselective (first generation) antihistamines			
Chlorpheniramine maleate, plain†	OTC	4 mg every 6 h	6–12 y: 2 mg every 6 h 2–5 y: 1 mg every 6 h
Chlorpheniramine maleate, Sustained-release	OTC	8–12 mg daily at bedtime or 8–12 mg every 8 h	6–12 y: 8 mg at bedtime <6 y: not recommended
Clemastine fumarate†	OTC	1.34 mg every 8 h	6–12 y: 0.67 mg every 12 h
Diphenhydramine hydrochloride†	OTC	25–50 mg every 8 h	5 mg/kg per day divided every 8 h (up to 25 mg per dose)
Peripherally selective (second generation) antihistamines			
Loratadine†	OTC	10 mg once daily	6–12 y: 10 mg once daily 2–5 y: 5 mg once daily
Fexofenadine	R$_x$	60 mg twice daily or 180 mg once daily	6–11 y: 30 mg twice daily
Cetirizine†	OTC	5–10 mg once daily	>6 y: 5 mg once daily infants 6–11 Mo‡
Oral decongestants			
Pseudoephedrine, plain†	OTC¶	60 mg every 4–6 h	6–12 y: 30 mg every 4–6 h 2–5 y: 15 mg every 4–6 h
Pseudoephedrine, sustained-release§	OTC¶	120 mg every 12 h	Not recommended
Phenylephrine**	OTC	10–20 mg every 4 h	6–12 y: 10 mg every 4 h 2–6 y: 0.25% drops, 1 ml every 4 h

*Dosage adjustment may be needed in renal/hepatic dysfunction. Refer to manufacturers' prescribing information.
†Available in liquid form.
‡0.25 mg/kg orally demonstrated to be safe.[31]
§Controlled-release product available: 240 mg once daily (60 mg immediate release with 180 mg controlled release).
¶See text regarding OTC requirements.
**Phenylrine has replaced pseudoephrine in many OTC antihistamine–decongestant combination products. Read product labels carefully.
Source: Reprinted with permission from DiPiro JT, et al: *Pharmacotherapy: A Pathophysiologic Approach,* 7th ed., Chapter 98, published by McGraw-Hill, 2008.

such as barometric changes and aeroallergens are often impossible to avoid. A large body of allergens/irritants can be partially avoided, but the data for avoidance are mixed. For these reasons allergen avoidance is often coupled with medical therapy.

Nonpharmacologic means of treating symptoms of allergic rhinitis include maintaining an upright position to enhance nasal drainage, maintaining adequate fluid intake, increasing humidity of inspired air, irrigating the nose with saline drops, and clearing mucus from the nasal passageways with a bulb syringe.[9] These interventions can be used in patients of all ages.

Pharmaceutical therapy includes anticholinergic agents, oral antihistamines and decongestants (Table 37-2), topical decongestants (Table 37-3), intranasal corticosteroids (Table 37-4), intranasal antihistamines, and oral leukotriene modifiers (Table 37-5). The approach to therapy depends on the age of the patient, frequency and severity of the rhinitis, and the type of rhinitis. For allergic rhinitis, antihistamines and decongestants are convenient and effective, but they are often limited by adverse effects such as sedation (antihistamines) or

jitteriness and increased blood pressure (decongestants). Antihistamines have little effect in nonallergic rhinitis, but decongestants provide symptomatic relief. Nonsedating antihistamines—such as cetirizine, levocetirizine, fexofenadine, loratadine, and desloratadine—revolutionized the treatment of allergic rhinitis, allowing once-daily therapy for patients that does not

Table 37-3. Duration of Action of Topical Decongestants

Medication	Duration (H)
Short-acting	
Phenylephrine hydrochloride	Up to 4
Intermediate-acting	
Naphazoline hydrochloride	4–6
Tetrahydrozoline hydrochloride	
Long-acting	
Oxymetazoline hydrochloride	Up to 12
Xylometazoline hydrochloride	

Source: Reprinted with permission from DiPiro JT, et al: *Pharmacotherapy: A Pathophysiologic Approach,* 7th ed., Chapter 98, published by McGraw-Hill, 2008.

Table 37-4. Dosage of Nasal Steroids

Medication	Dosage and Interval
Beclomethasone dipropionate, monohydrate	>12 y: 1–2 inhalations (42–84 mcg) twice daily in each nostril
	6–12 y: 1 inhalation per nostril (42 mcg) twice daily to start
Budesonide	>6 y: 2 sprays (64 mcg) per nostril in AM and PM or 4 sprays per nostril in AM (maximum, 256 mcg)
Flunisolide	Adults: 2 sprays (50 mcg) per nostril twice daily (maximum, 400 mcg)
	Children: 1 spray per nostril 3 times a day
Fluticasone	Adults: 2 sprays (100 mcg) per nostril once daily; after a few days decrease to 1 spray per nostril
	Children >4 y and adolescents: 1 spray per nostril once daily (maximum, 200 mcg/d)
Mometasone furoate	>12 y: 2 sprays (100 mcg) per nostril once daily
Triamcinolone acetonide	>12 y: 2 sprays (110 mcg) per nostril once daily (maximum, 440 mcg/d)

Source: Reprinted with permission from DiPiro JT, et al: *Pharmacotherapy: A Pathophysiologic Approach,* 7th ed., Chapter 98, published by McGraw-Hill, 2008.

add to constitutional symptoms such as somnolence and cognitive impairment. These agents typically provide relief for pruritic symptoms but do not have a significant effect on congestion.[10–12]

Leukotriene modifiers are a popular treatment for allergic rhinitis, but have little role in nonallergic rhinitis. Zileuton, montelukast, and zafirlukast have efficacy in both allergic rhinitis and asthma. In studies comparing efficacy of leukotriene modification compared with nonsedating antihistamines as monotherapy, efficacy was equivalent.[13] These agents are advantageous in that they provide single agents that address the symptoms of individuals with mild asthma and mild rhinitis.

Intranasal antihistamines are approved for both allergic and nonallergic rhinitis, and unlike oral antihistamines, may have beneficial effects on nasal congestion and ocular pruritus. They are often used in combination with intranasal steroids. The strong unpleasant taste of intranasal antihistamines can hamper adherence.[10–12]

Intranasal steroids such as fluticasone propionate, mometasone, beclomethasone, ciclesonide, and triamcinolone are the mainstay of therapy currently for both allergic and nonallergic rhinitis. They improve all major rhinitis symptoms: nasal pruritus, congestion, rhinorrhea, and sneezing. Studies have demonstrated that intranasal steroids are more efficacious than antihistamines or leukotriene modifiers for all symptoms. Patients are sometimes reluctant to use products that they must spray into the nose, making adherence a concern. The most common adverse effect of intranasal steroids is epistaxis and nasal irritation, usually due to poor inhaler technique.[10–12]

Other agents such as intranasal cromolyn (mast cell stabilizer) and intranasal ipratropium (anticholinergic) are not used as frequently. Intranasal ipratropium can be very effective in treating intermittent nonallergic rhinitis such as gustatory rhinitis or exercise-associated vasomotor rhinitis. For patients who are bothered by these syndromes, treatment with intranasal ipratropium before exercise or eating can prevent symptoms.[10–12]

For patients with allergic symptoms caused by an identifiable allergen, immunotherapy is a possibility. The advent of subcutaneous immunotherapy, or SCIT, has increased interest in this approach, which is well established in adult patients with allergic rhinitis.[14] SCIT provides an emerging but not yet sufficiently studied option for children as young as 2 years of age.[15]

Table 37-5. Dosage Regimens for Montelukast in Treatment of Allergic Rhinitis

Age	Dosage*
Adults and adolescents >15 y	One 10-mg tablet daily
Children 6–14 y	One 5-mg chewable tablet daily
Children 2–5 y	One 4-mg chewable tablet or oral granule packet daily

*The timing of drug administration can be individualized. If the patient has combined asthma and seasonal allergic rhinitis, the dose should be given in the evening.
Source: Reprinted with permission from DiPiro JT, et al: *Pharmacotherapy: A Pathophysiologic Approach,* 7th ed. Chapter 98, published by McGraw-Hill, 2008.

EVIDENCE-BASED SUMMARY

- Allergic rhinitis is a common but also misunderstood disease that causes substantial and often unrecognized morbidity.
- Symptoms of nasal congestion, mucoid discharge, pruritus, and sneezing are categorized as allergic or nonallergic and as intermittent or perennial.
- Severity of allergic rhinitis is differentiated by the effect on sleep, with patients with mild conditions having normal sleep and daily activities and those with moderate-to-severe allergic rhinitis having compromised function in these areas.

- Allergic rhinitis is diagnosed through a complete history that focuses on the age of onset of symptoms, frequency of symptoms, triggers, and presence of comorbid conditions.
- Allergic rhinitis exacerbation or infectious rhinitis can result in asthma exacerbations, secondary infection with bacterial sinusitis, persistent cough, otitis media, otitis media with effusion, chronic snoring, or eustachian tube dysfunction.
- Avoidance of allergens is the first line of treatment, followed by use of nonprescription medications for symptoms present in a given patient.
- Antibiotics are indicated only if symptoms of allergic rhinitis appear to be infectious in origin and they persist or worsen.
- Immunotherapy is an emerging option, especially for adult patients and children older than 6 years but increasingly in younger patients as well.

REFERENCES

1. American College of Allergy. Asthma and immunology. Allergic diseases and cognitive impairment. www.acaai.org/public/advice/cogn.htm. Accessed November 9, 2007.

2. Howarth PH. Allergic and nonallergic rhinitis. In: Adkinson NF, Yuninger JW, Busse WW et al, eds. *Middleton's Allergy Principles and Practice,* 6th ed. Philadelphia, PA: Mosby; 2003:1391–1410.

3. Scarupa MD, Kaliner M. Allergic rhinitis www.worldallergy.org/professional/allergic_diseases_center/rhinitis.rhinitis_indepth.php. Accessed May 28, 2008.

4. Bousquet J, Van Cauwenberge PB, Khaltaev N. Allergic rhinitis and its impact on asthma: ARIA workshop report. *J Allergy Clin Immunol.* 2001;108:S147.

5. World Allergy Organization. Global resources in allergy. Allergic rhinitis and allergic conjunctivitis. www.wao.org/gloria. Updated May 1, 2006.

6. Howarth PH. Allergic and nonallergic rhinitis. In: Adkinson NF, Yuninger JW, Busse WW et al, eds. *Middleton's Allergy: Principles and Practice,* 6th ed. Mosby; 2003: 1391–1410.

7. Wilde AD, Jones AS. The nasal response to axillary pressure. *Clin Otolaryngol Allied Sci.* 2007;21:442–444.

8. Eccles R. Nasal airways. In: Busse WW, Holgate ST, eds. *Asthma and Rhinitis,* 2nd ed. London, UK: Blackwell Sciences; 2000:157.

9. Scolaro KL. Disorders related to colds and allergy. In: Berardi RR, Kroon LA, Mcdermott JH, et al. eds. *Handbook of Nonprescription Drugs.* Washington, DC: American Pharmacists Association; 2006:201–228.

10. Greiner AN, Meltzer EO. Pharmacologic rationale for treating allergic and nonallergic rhinitis. *J Allergy Clin Immunol.* 2006;118(5):985–998.

11. Kaari J. The role of intranasal corticosteroids in the management of pediatric allergic rhinitis. *Clin Pediatr (Phila).* 2006;45(8):697–704.

12. Brunton SA, Fromer LM. Treatment options for the management of perennial allergic rhinitis, with a focus on intranasal corticosteroids. *South Med J.* 2007;100(7): 701–708.

13. Nathan RA. Pharmacotherapy for allergic rhinitis: A critical review of leukotriene receptor antagonists compared with other treatments. *Ann Allergy Asthma Immunol.* 2003; 90(2):182–190.

14. Passalacqua G, Durham SR, Global allergy and asthma european network. allergic rhinitis and its impact on asthma update: Allergen immunotherapy. *J Allergy Clin Immunol.* 2007;119(4):881–891.

15. Cox L. Sublingual immunotherapy in pediatric allergic rhinitis and asthma: Efficacy, safety, and practical considerations. *Curr Allergy Asthma Rep.* 2007;7(6):410–420.

Chapter 38

Otitis Media and Sinusitis

S. Rubina Inamdar and Brookie M. Best

SEARCH STRATEGY

A systematic biomedical literature review was conducted in April 2005. The search was limited to English language articles and human subjects, and included PubMed, the Cochrane Database, and the National Guideline Clearinghouse. The current consensus documents for otitis media with effusion, and for diagnosis and management of acute otitis media can be found at the American Academy of Pediatrics website: http//www.aap.org./ Acute rhinosinusitis consensus statements can be found at the National Guideline Clearinghouse website: http//www.guideline.gov./

INTRODUCTION

Sinusitis and otitis media (OM) are two of the most common presenting conditions in primary care practice. They are frequent causes of missed school and work days, and they cost the United States health care system billions of dollars in office visits, surgeries, and medications. They have a profound impact on quality of life, work productivity, and school performance.[1–4]

Caring for patients with sinusitis and OM has changed dramatically in the past few years. The vast body of literature on sinusitis and OM suffers from widely divergent opinions regarding pathophysiology, diagnosis, and treatment. As a result of poor standardization of definitions, measures of severity, and improper clinical research design, frequently cited studies often directly contradict each other. Further, inappropriate antibiotic use leading to rising bacterial resistance to antimicrobials and growing health care costs are compelling trends that are impacting treatment approaches to these common illnesses. For these reasons, recent evidence-based reference guidelines, systematic reviews, and multidisciplinary consensus statements have been invaluable in providing guidance to clinicians.

UPPER AIRWAY ANATOMY

The upper airway is a complex system with numerous functions. It includes the nose, the sinuses and pharyngeal structures, the eustachian tubes, and the outer, middle, and inner ears (Fig. 38-1). The paranasal sinuses, consisting of the maxillary, ethmoidal, sphenoidal, and frontal sinuses are connected to the nasal passage and ultimately the pharyngeal structures. These sinuses are thought to aid the nose in providing heat and humidification to inhaled air, while also decreasing the weight of the bony skull and increasing resonance for speech. The osteomeatal complex, a narrow orifice connecting the maxillary sinuses to the nasal passage, is a critical component of sinus function. Cilia lining the walls of the sinuses provide regular clearance of mucus and debris.[5]

Healthy sinuses may produce up to 2 liters of mucus per day that goes unnoticed. Mucus thickens in response to inflammatory signals and becomes noticeable in its altered state. The infiltrate and degradation products associated with inflammation can alter the color of mucus even in the absence of true infection.

The space known as the middle ear begins at the nasopharyngeal orifice of the eustachian tube and extends to the air cells of the mastoid, petrosa, and related areas. The tympanic membrane serves as a window directly from the ear to the outer air, facilitating sound transfer and also allowing clinicians to make observations about the middle ear based on the membrane's appearance and ability to handle pressure and sound waves.

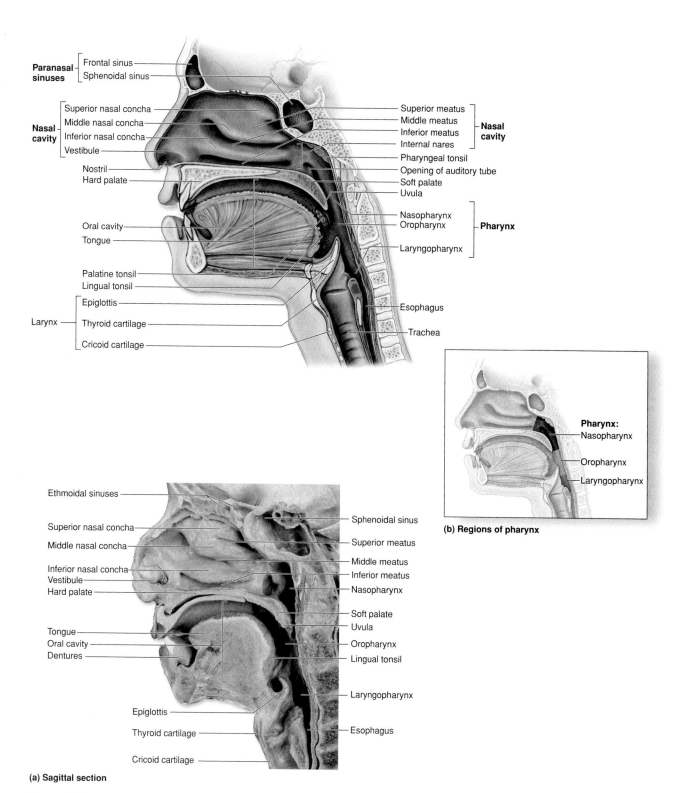

Paranasal sinuses
— Frontal sinus
— Sphenoidal sinus

Nasal cavity
— Superior nasal concha
— Middle nasal concha
— Inferior nasal concha
— Vestibule

— Nostril
— Hard palate

— Oral cavity
— Tongue

— Palatine tonsil
— Lingual tonsil

Larynx
— Epiglottis
— Thyroid cartilage
— Cricoid cartilage

— Superior meatus
— Middle meatus
— Inferior meatus
— Internal nares
Nasal cavity

— Pharyngeal tonsil
— Opening of auditory tube
— Soft palate
— Uvula

— Nasopharynx
— Oropharynx
Pharynx

— Laryngopharynx

— Esophagus

— Trachea

(b) Regions of pharynx

Pharynx:
Nasopharynx

Oropharynx

Laryngopharynx

Ethmoidal sinuses
Superior nasal concha
Middle nasal concha
Inferior nasal concha
Vestibule
Hard palate

Tongue
Oral cavity
Dentures

Epiglottis
Thyroid cartilage
Cricoid cartilage

Sphenoidal sinus
Superior meatus
Middle meatus
Inferior meatus
Nasopharynx

Soft palate
Uvula
Oropharynx
Lingual tonsil

Laryngopharynx

Esophagus

(a) Sagittal section

Figure 38-1. Anatomy of the upper airway. (Reproduced with permission from Mckinley M, O'Loughlin VD. Human Anatomy, 2nd ed. NY: McGraw-Hill; 2008:749.)

OTITIS MEDIA

OM, defined as the presence of fluid in the middle ear with signs and symptoms of inflammation, is the most common reason for an antibacterial prescription in children. In 2000, more than 13 million such antibiotic prescriptions were written, a rate of 802 per 1000 office visits for OM. Direct costs of OM were estimated at almost $2 billion in 1995, while indirect costs added more than $1 billion.[6]

The two subtypes of OM include acute otitis media (AOM) and otitis media with effusion (OME). OM with effusion is the presence of fluid in the middle ear without signs and symptoms of acute ear inflammation and infection. Unlike AOM, the fluid is usually not infected by either viruses or bacteria. The presence of a persistent effusion can result in tympanic membrane dysfunction and can have deleterious outcomes such as decreased sound conduction and superinfection with microbes. Distinguishing between these two types of OM is important, as management and outcomes differ. OME can precede or follow AOM, is associated with acute viral infections, and is more common than AOM. Thus, patients with OME and superimposed viral infection can appear to have AOM. The most important distinguishing feature is the acute onset of symptoms in AOM, whereas other features such as red tympanic membranes, decreased mobility, and air–fluid levels have poor predictive value. Sometimes, despite the best efforts of a clinician, making a definitive diagnosis is impossible and appropriate follow-up becomes paramount.

This chapter will exclude more complicated AOM associated with significant comorbid conditions such as immunodeficiencies, sensory deficits, cochlear implants, and craniofacial or neurologic abnormalities (cleft palate or Down's syndrome). Management of patients who require pressure equalization tubes will also be excluded.

EPIDEMIOLOGY AND PATHOPHYSIOLOGY

AOM is very common in pediatrics, with 70% of children having at least one episode by 3 years of age. It is most common in young children, with a peak incidence at 6 to 24 months of age; however, susceptible individuals can develop AOM well into adulthood. Patients who have persistent inflammation can progress to OME.

OME is more common than AOM, and likely affects 90% of patients before 5 years of age with approximately 2.2 million diagnosed episodes per year. More than half of children less than one year of age will develop OME. Direct and indirect costs of OME are estimated at four billion dollars.

OM may be caused by eustachian tube obstruction and secondary infection. The eustachian tube protects, aerates, and provides drainage from the middle ear. Mechanical obstruction of the eustachian tube can be caused by edema from infection or allergy, or by the presence of enlarged adenoids or nasopharyngeal tumors. This can result in poor tube function and allow entry and proliferation of pathogens in the middle ear. An alternative hypothesis for the development of OM is that the eustachian tube compliance or patency is increased, allowing easier access for pathogenic organisms. In this setting, tubal obstruction may be secondary to inappropriate function. Other contributing factors may include the adenoids as possible reservoirs for microbes, and nasopharyngeal organisms entering the middle ear as a result of reflux during swallowing.

DIAGNOSIS

Acute Otitis Media

The American Academy of Pediatrics Clinical Practice Guideline provides three main criteria for diagnosis of AOM: (1) acute onset, (2) middle ear effusion, and (3) middle ear inflammation (Table 38-1). All three components are necessary to make a definitive diagnosis of AOM. Diagnostic accuracy declines when any of the three is absent. Presence of middle ear effusion and the associated inflammation is especially important in diagnosis.

In an infant, the cardinal presenting symptom is ear pain or pulling of the ear. This symptom is often of rapid onset and associated with nonspecific symptoms such as anorexia, fever, malaise, irritability, diarrhea, and excessive crying. Symptoms can be especially subtle in neonates, and a high index of suspicion is prudent. Clinical symptoms alone are not sufficient for making the diagnosis, as most of the above symptoms are nonspecific. Symptoms such as purulent otorrhea, ear fullness, and hearing loss may be more specific but are less frequent or occur later in the course of the disease.

Examination of the patient may reveal a red tympanic membrane that may be immobile upon pneumatoscopy.

Table 38-1. Three Components of AOM Diagnosis

History of acute onset signs and symptoms
Presence of middle ear effusion
   Bulging of tympanic membranes
   Limited or absent mobility of the tympanic membrane
   Otorrhea
Signs and symptoms of middle ear inflammation.
   Distinct erythema of the tympanic membrane or
   Distinct otalgia clearly referable to the ear that interferes
     with normal activity or sleep.

The presence of full or bulging tympanic membranes associated with redness and decreased mobility is most predictive of AOM. Opacification or cloudiness of the tympanic membrane and air–fluid levels are helpful to note. Blisters on the tympanic membrane may indicate bullous myringitis, a viral infection that attacks the tympanic membranes, and can also be associated with OM. Care must be taken to differentiate the redness of inflamed tympanic membranes from the pink flush of high fever or crying. Tympanometry or acoustic reflectometry are useful when the presence of a middle ear effusion is difficult to diagnose.

OM with Effusion

The diagnosis of OME is based on the presence of fluid in the middle ear in the absence of acute symptoms. Most commonly, patients may be asymptomatic, or complain of decreased hearing, but lack the intense ear pain and nonspecific symptoms associated with acute infection. On examination, they may have pale yellow to bluish opacified tympanic membranes, with decreased motion on pneumatic otoscopy, but without significant bulging, purulent discharge, or pain. In OME the presence of air bubbles or air–fluid levels behind the tympanic membrane may indicate impending resolution.

Diagnostic Tools

The most sensitive and specific noninvasive diagnostic modality is pneumatic otoscopy when compared to myringotomy as the gold standard. In experienced hands, pneumatic otoscopy is an excellent, cost-effective, and efficient method of diagnosing effusion. In the absence of experienced otoscopists, either tympanometry or acoustic reflectometry are reliable diagnostic testing modalities. Tympanometry, also known as acoustic immittance testing, uses a sound probe to measure tympanic membrane compliance in electroacoustic terms. Tympanometry requires a tight seal and expensive calibrated equipment, but has been validated in children as young as 4 months, and with special equipment, even younger. Patients in early AOM or OME, however, may have normal tympanograms. Acoustic reflectometry is a lower cost option, with no requirement for a tight seal, but has not been validated in children below the age of two.[8]

COMORBIDITIES AND CONTRIBUTING FACTORS

A number of comorbid conditions and risk factors contribute to the development of OM (Table 38-2). The most common predisposing factor is a viral upper

Table 38-2. Risk Factors and Comorbidities Associated with Development of OM

• Bottle-feeding	• Viral upper respiratory tract infection
• Maternal smoking	
• Family history of OM	• Allergic rhinitis
• Male	• Immunodeficiencies
• Daycare	• Anatomic alterations
• Lower socioeconomic status	• Reflux
	• Barotrauma

respiratory tract infection, especially in high exposure locations such as daycare centers. Breast feeding is protective, but the benefits disappear when it is discontinued. Lower socioeconomic status is associated not only with early or recurrent AOM, but also with higher rates of hearing loss secondary to AOM. The prevalence of nasal allergy in children with OM with effusion is 35% to 50%, making allergic rhinitis (discussed in another chapter) a major predisposing factor. Anatomic alterations either from congenital defects such as cleft palate, or secondary causes such as adenoidal hypertrophy or nasotracheal intubation, can also cause functional obstruction of the eustachian tubes. Reflux can cause contamination of the middle ear space by nasopharyngeal secretions. Finally, barotrauma from air flight or diving can worsen OM.

MICROBIOLOGY OF AOM

The most common viral illnesses associated with AOM are also those most commonly associated with other upper respiratory tract infections: rhinovirus, influenzavirus, adenovirus, enterovirus, parainfluenza virus, corona virus, and respiratory syncytial virus. Viruses have been found in respiratory secretions or ear effusion fluid in 40% to 75% of patients with AOM. In 25% of cases, no pathogen is found. Bacterial causes vary by age and acuity. *Streptococcus pneumoniae* is the most prevalent cause of bacterial OM, accounting for 30% to 50% of cases. Group B *Streptococcus* is responsible for approximately 20% of neonatal and young infant disease. Nontypable *Haemophilus influenzae* cause up to 30% of OM in older children, adolescents, and adults. *Moraxella catarrhalis* is the third most common cause, responsible for up to 20% of cases. Because viruses are so commonly found in middle ear effusion, the empirical use of antimicrobials has come under some scrutiny. However, the frequency with which bacteria are isolated is high enough to require antibiotic treatment in very young infants, and in children who do not improve quickly. Immunizations against *H. influenzae* and protein

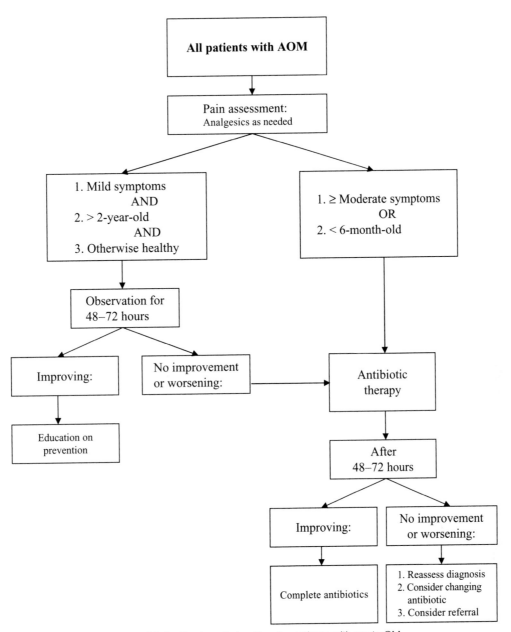

Figure 38-2. Treatment algorithm for patients with acute OM.

conjugate vaccine of *S. pneumoniae* may reduce the incidence of AOM and other infections, but these need to be confirmed in further trials.

DIFFERENTIAL DIAGNOSIS

The diagnosis most commonly confused with AOM is OME. Differentiating between these two diseases is crucial to the effective management of the patient. Other possible diagnoses associated with ear abnormalities include tympanosclerosis (a structural abnormality resulting from scarring of the tympanic membrane), cholesteatoma (a sac-like structure associated with

chronic OM), middle ear tumors, foreign bodies in the ear, and myringitis.

AOM MANAGEMENT

Proper management of AOM begins with appropriate diagnosis and includes pain management, supportive care, antibiotics in some situations, follow-up, and referral to specialists in difficult or complicated cases (Fig. 38-2). Since the complications of untreated bacterial AOM can include abscess formation, mastoiditis, hearing loss, and ultimately poor development in speech and cognition, a seemingly mild disease can have profound effects.

Table 38-3. Treatment for Acute OM

	Initial Antibiotic Regimen	
	Recommended	**Alternative**
Nonsevere illness	Amoxicillin: 80–90 mg/kg per day	Cefdinir, cefuroxime, cefpodoxime For type 1 penicillin allergy: azithromycin, clarithromycin
Severe illness	Amoxicillin–clavulanate: 90 mg/kg per day of amoxicillin, 6.4 mg/kg per day of clavulanate	Ceftriaxone, 1 or 3 days
	If Initial Antibiotic Regimen Fails	
	Recommended	**Alternative**
Nonsevere illness	Amoxicillin–clavulanate: 90 mg/kg per day of amoxicillin, 6.4 mg/kg per day of clavulanate	Ceftriaxone, 3 days For type 1 penicillin allergy: clindamycin
Severe illness	Ceftriaxone, 1 or 3 days	Tympanocentesis, clindamycin

Adapted from: Subcommittee on Management of Acute Otitis Media, American Academy of Pediatrics and American Academy of Family Physicians. Clinical practice guideline: Diagnosis and management of acute otitis media. *Pediatr.* 2004;113:1451–1465.

Most children will recover well from an episode of AOM without antibiotic therapy if the disease is not severe. For children older than 2 years of age with mild signs and symptoms, observation for 48 to 72 hours is often the most appropriate course of action. Symptomatic relief may be provided. This option should be limited to otherwise healthy children who have a caregiver who will reliably be able to observe the child, recognize symptoms of worsening illness, and have access to prompt medical care and follow-up if improvement does not occur.

Analgesics

Patients should undergo routine pain assessment, and appropriate pain-reducing treatments should be provided when needed. Various analgesics may be considered, including acetaminophen, ibuprofen, topical agents, and narcotics for severe pain. As no one agent has proven benefit over another, the product selected should incorporate patient/caregiver preference.

Antibiotics

Antibiotic treatment is recommended for infants under 6 months of age, all children with moderate to severe symptoms, and children who worsen or fail to improve over an initial observation period. For most children, amoxicillin at a dose of 80 to 90 mg/kg per day is recommended (see Table 38-3). Amoxicillin is the first-line agent because of its safety record, low cost, tolerable taste, limited antibacterial spectrum of activity, and effectiveness against susceptible and moderately resistant pneumococci. For patients with moderate to severe pain, or fever ≥39°C, initiate therapy with amoxicillin–clavulanate. Antibiotic therapy should be given for 10 days for all infants and most children, the excep-

tion being that for children older than 2 years of age who have no history of chronic or recurrent OM and intact tympanic membranes, a 5-day antibiotic treatment course can be considered.

Once antibiotic therapy is instituted, the patient's condition should improve within 48 to 72 hours. If the patient does not improve over this time frame, reassess the patient to confirm the diagnosis, and consider changing the antibacterial agent. Strong evidence supports the use of the following medications as second-line agents (see Table 38-3): amoxicillin–clavulanate, cefuroxime, ceftriaxone, cefprozil, loracarbef, cefdinir, cefixime, and cefpodoxime. Several other medications are often used for treating AOM—including trimethoprim–sulfamethoxazole, clarithromycin, erythromycin ethylsuccinate and sulfisoxazole, and azithromycin—but the evidence showing efficacy for this indication is lacking, and they should be avoided. If a patient gives a history of penicillin allergy, consider an allergy consultation, as penicillin allergy is evanescent, and proper identification of allergic individuals can increase antibiotic choice in this population.

For recurrent AOM (three or more episodes in a 6-month period, or four or more episodes in 1 year), consider antibiotic prophylaxis with amoxicillin 20 mg/kg once daily for 2 to 6 months. Prophylaxis for 12 months decreases recurrence by approximately one to two AOM episodes per child per year.[7]

Adjunct Medications

Otic antibiotic drops, such as ciprofloxacin or ofloxacin, may be added for a child with a draining middle ear. Use of nasal decongestants and corticosteroids is not supported by the literature.

Prevention

Patients/caregivers should be educated about preventing AOM. Controllable prevention measures include breastfeeding, feeding the child upright if bottle-fed, avoiding passive smoke exposure, limiting exposure to other children, encouraging correct hand-washing techniques, decreasing pacifier use after 6 months of age, and keeping immunizations up-to-date.

Referral

Patients may benefit from an otolaryngology referral if they develop mastoiditis or labyrinthitis, or if fever, agitation, or irritability persists after 48 hours despite therapy. Children with recurrent AOM of more than three times in 6 months or four to six times in 1 year can be referred to both an otolaryngologist for tympanostomy tube placement or other surgical intervention and an audiologist for hearing evaluation. Patients with recurrent AOM may benefit from an allergy and immunology evaluation to detect and treat any contributing allergic disease.

OME MANAGEMENT

The principles of management for OME include identifying patients at risk for long term sequelae with aggressive intervention when needed, and watchful waiting for children at decreased risk. In most patients, effusion will spontaneously resolve within 3 months, thereby decreasing the need for significant medical therapy. Children who are generally healthy can tolerate the brief periods associated with tinnitus, decreased hearing acuity, and possible vertigo. Children with bilateral OME of greater than 3-month duration have a 30% chance of spontaneous recovery after 6 to 12 months. Thus, after 3 months, the decision to intervene will be based on a risk/benefit analysis utilizing clinical judgment, parental preference, impact on patient health, and available medical facilities.

Hearing testing is recommended for patients with OME lasting longer than 3 months. In patients with hearing loss, testing for language delay is critical. In patients with no evidence for hearing loss or secondary structural abnormalities of the middle ear, regular observation is suggested until the effusion resolves. If evidence for structural abnormalities is seen, then patients should be referred to otolaryngology for tympanostomy tube insertion.

For patients who are already at risk for developmental delay, who have significant hearing or visual impairments, or who have cognitive or behavioral risk factors, the addition of hearing and balance abnormalities associated with OME can cause further delay. These patients require aggressive hearing, speech and language evalu-

ations, and concurrent referral to otolaryngology for possible tympanostomy tube placement. Patients should be retested after resolution of the effusion to document improvement.

A short course of antibiotics with or without steroids may result in quicker improvement. However, the long term benefits and the risk/benefit ratio have not been demonstrated, and therefore these medications are not recommended.

PROGNOSIS AND FOLLOW-UP

Most pediatric patients with AOM do well and have no residual effects in adulthood. With appropriate care and aggressive monitoring, up to 70% of patients have spontaneous resolution of their symptoms without antibiotics. In observational studies conducted in different countries, the rates of mastoiditis did not differ in places where clinicians typically treat with antibiotics earlier as compared with areas where supportive care and monitoring are used preferentially.

Most infants should have follow-up within a few days of onset of infection to detect treatment response and complications. AOM effusion often takes weeks to resolve, although symptoms may resolve quickly. For this reason, repeat antibiotics should only be used if patients appear to have continued infection and inflammation. If the effusion persists, patients should be managed for OME rather than AOM.

SINUSITIS

The definition of sinusitis is "inflammation of the paranasal sinuses." This definition is deceptive in that "sinusitis," or what is now being referred to as "rhinosinusitis," is likely a complex syndrome arising from a wide variety of causes, and therefore requires a more nuanced approach. The term rhinosinusitis is increasing in popularity as sinusitis is usually, if not always, accompanied by rhinitis. Rhinitis may occur, however, in the absence of discernable sinusitis.

Acute rhinosinusitis (ARS) is defined as symptoms of less than 4-week duration, including nasal congestion and anterior or posterior drainage, associated with facial pain or pressure with objective evidence for purulent drainage.[9] Chronic rhinosinusitis (CRS) is defined as symptoms as mentioned above that have been present for greater than 12 weeks, with objective evidence of sinus involvement such as from rhinoscopy or computed tomography (CT) imaging.

ARS is most likely infectious in origin, while CRS may be the result of multiple contributing factors including allergic inflammation, biofilms, anatomic abnormalities, fungal sensitivity, bacterial superantigens, and de novo inflammatory processes. Individuals who are diagnosed with CRS should be referred to an allergist or otolaryngologist for further evaluation and therapy. The use of recurrent surgeries to treat CRS is falling out of favor with the realization that the inflammatory processes continue after surgery, and require immunomodulation rather than mechanical clearance. Also, anatomic abnormalities, cystic fibrosis, ciliary motility disorders and immune deficiencies contributing to rhinosinusitis require unique approaches that are beyond the scope of this book. Because of the complex nature of CRS and for the sake of brevity and completeness, this chapter will focus primarily on ARS. For a more complete discussion of CRS, please refer to the Rhinosinusitis guidelines listed in the references.

EPIDEMIOLOGY AND PATHOPHYSIOLOGY

Rhinosinusitis is a highly prevalent disease affecting more than 31 million people, and is the most frequent presenting complaint to a primary care physician. It is responsible for thousands of lost workdays, school days, and decreased productivity. It significantly affects quality of life, and has well known associated comorbid conditions, such as asthma and chronic cough, that also contribute to its overall cost.

Acute viral rhinosinusitis and the common cold are likely the same entity. During an upper respiratory tract infection, nasal fluid may be forced into the sinuses, especially when a person blows their nose. This enables viral particles, cellular debris, and bacteria to be transported into the sinuses to produce a possible infection and an inflammatory response. These materials are either too thick or they become increasingly mucinous so that the normal ciliary mechanisms cannot clear them. Their persistence in sinus cavities may trigger a more exuberant inflammatory response thereby causing increased swelling, inflammation, and mucus production locally. The natural history of viral rhinosinusitis ranges from 1 to 33 days, with most patients showing improvement within 7 to 10 days, and 25% of patients having continued symptoms after 14 days.[10]

DIAGNOSIS

Inflammation of the paranasal sinuses can be the result of infectious, allergic, or irritant causes. Determining whether the cause is infectious or noninfectious is usually as simple as taking a very thorough history and physical examination. The diagnosis of allergic rhinitis is discussed in another chapter. Briefly, the hallmark of allergic disease is itching and sneezing, as compared to viral illnesses which often lack a significant pruritic component. Differentiating between the various causes

of sinus inflammation is critical to determine appropriate treatment.

The current clinical diagnostic criteria describe ARS as a cold that begins to resolve after a few days, and is better by 1 week to 10 days after onset. Acute bacterial rhinosinusitis is defined as a cold that is worse or no better after 10 to 14 days. Common symptoms include nasal congestion and anterior and/or posterior nasal drainage. Additional symptoms may include cough, sore throat, headache, facial pain or pressure, periorbital edema, earache, halitosis, tooth pain, and hyposmia. Systemic symptoms such as fatigue, increased wheeze, and fever are also possible.

Examination of the patient may reveal fever, dark shadowing under the eyes, and possible mouth breathing. Anterior nasal endoscopy can show turbinate hypertrophy and inflamed erythematous mucosa with evidence for purulent mucoid discharge. In contrast, patients with allergic rhinitis may have pale bluish mucosa. The oropharynx may be inflamed with exudates, or show evidence for post-nasal drainage in the form of mucous adherent to the posterior oropharynx or cobblestoning suggesting more chronic inflammation.

Radiographic evaluation in ARS should be undertaken if more complicated disease is suspected. The use of sinus X-rays may have some benefit, although limited CT scanning is gaining popularity. Sinus CT of both adults and children conducted at the onset of a viral respiratory tract infection reveal significant sinus abnormalities including mucosal thickening, air–fluid levels, and evidence for osteomeatal complex obstruction. While this provides evidence of inflammation in the sinuses, it does not indicate bacterial infection. CT scans are indicated in patients who have severe dramatic symptoms of unilateral facial pain and swelling associated with fever, and for patients who do not respond to initial therapy.

DIFFERENTIAL DIAGNOSIS

Most patients with symptoms that are brief and resolve spontaneously likely have the common cold. However, several other conditions can masquerade as sinus disease. Allergic rhinitis, which is a systemic illness associated with nasal congestion and purulent drainage can have many of the same signs and symptoms as ARS. Headache, even if located directly in the area of the maxillary sinuses, in the absence of significant nasal drainage, is more likely to be a migraine than rhinosinusitis. Different entities can cause symptoms similar to ARS including irritant rhinitis, rhinitis medicamentosa, intranasal cocaine use, β-blockers, head trauma, foreign bodies, tumors, and rarely, vasculitic diseases such as Wegener's granulomatosis.

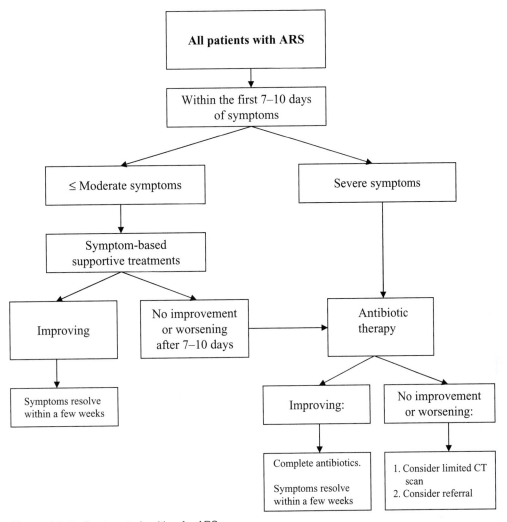

Figure 38-3. Treatment algorithm for ARS.

MICROBIOLOGY

The vast majority of ARS is viral in origin. The most common viral causes include rhinovirus (15%), influenza virus (5%) parainfluenza virus (3%) and adenovirus (2%). These viruses have numerous serotypes that impact their potency and frequency of infection. Secondary bacterial infections can occur requiring antimicrobial intervention. Several studies indicate that less than 2% of ARS in adults and up to 30% of ARS in children progress to involve a bacterial component requiring antibiotics. However, in other studies, up to 30% of patients presenting to an outpatient clinic had bacterial rhinosinusitis. The most commonly isolated bacteria in these patients are *S. pneumonia*, nontypeable *H. influenza* and *M. catarrhalis*. The organisms cultured from the sinuses vary by age of the patient, presentation, and other comorbid conditions. The *H. influenza* is often β-lactamase producing, and therefore resistant to amoxicillin. Occasionally, *S. aureus* or *S. pyogenes* may be cultured.[11]

COMORBID CONDITIONS

While patients with allergic rhinitis, OME, or asthma may not be more likely to develop ARS, complications associated with flares of these diseases may require more aggressive therapy. Acute upper respiratory viral infections can trigger asthma exacerbations and may require oral steroid supplementation during the course of the disease. Patients with concomitant allergic rhinitis and ARS may benefit from treatment with anti-histamines or an intranasal steroid to decrease persistence and severity of symptoms.[12]

MANAGEMENT

The majority of evidence-based systematic reviews and consensus documents recommend deferring antibiotic therapy for ARS until after 7 to 10 days of symptoms (for treatment algorithm of ARS, see Figure 38-3). Initial therapy should be supportive and symptom based.

Patients may utilize decongestants and mucolytics in the first few days to decrease nasal symptoms. First generation anti-histamines decrease secretions and also provide much needed sedation at night. Ibuprofen and acetaminophen may decrease pain and fever. Intranasal saline sprays and rinses can improve overall symptoms for several hours with almost minimal expense and side effects. Oxymetazoline spray, a topical decongestant, may be recommended for up to 5 days to improve nasal patency, but no longer, as tolerance will develop.

The Agency for Health Care Research and Quality published an evidence-based guideline in which they examined the cost-effectiveness of therapy. Although 69% of patients' symptoms resolved within 14 days in the absence of antibiotic therapy, patients with the most severe symptoms may benefit from the modest improvement in outcomes conferred by antimicrobial use, and may be treated earlier than 7 days.[10]

The goals of antimicrobial therapy are to reduce symptoms, decrease duration of disease, and prevent complications. The most commonly recommended antibiotics in acute uncomplicated bacterial sinusitis include amoxicillin, doxycycline, and trimethoprim/sulfamethoxazole.[13] Suggestions for the length of treatment are not uniform, although standard regimens utilize a 7-day to 10-day course. Efficacy for other more expensive antibiotics have been demonstrated, including cephalosporins, macrolides, amoxicillin–clavulanate, levofloxacin, moxifloxacin, and gatifloxacin, but cost and local resistance patterns may amend their usefulness.

Regardless of the type of antibiotic, rates of cure or clinical improvement do not differ between older and newer medications. According to the Cochrane Review, more than 80% of patients will feel better with no difference in relapse rates no matter which antibiotic is used. Patients dropped out more when treated with amoxicillin–clavulanate (4.4%) when compared with those who were treated with nonpenicillin antibiotics (1.9%).[14]

PROGNOSIS

Most patients' symptoms resolve spontaneously within a few weeks, with few residual complications. Patients who do not respond to initial therapy should be evaluated with a limited sinus CT scan to determine if other complicating factors are present, and they may benefit from referral to allergy/immunology or otolaryngology. Patients with significant comorbid illnesses such as immune deficiency, cystic fibrosis, diabetes, allergic rhinitis, asthma, or CRS would also benefit from referral. Patients with severe acute unilateral symptoms,

intense periorbital swelling, changes in vision, mental status, or with frontal or sphenoidal disease will likely require a highly aggressive approach, if not urgent evaluation by an otolaryngologist.

EVIDENCE-BASED SUMMARY

- AOM presents with acute onset symptoms, middle ear effusion and middle ear inflammation.
- Treatment for AOM in young infants is empiric antibiotics, but watchful observation may be considered in older children.
- Acute onset of illness, bulging tympanic membranes, and presence of ear pain can be used to separate AOM from OME.
- Pneumatic otoscopy is the most reliable noninvasive tool for diagnosis of AOM and OME.
- OME is likely to resolve spontaneously within 3 months.
- ARS is most likely viral in origin, and will resolve without the need for antibiotics in most patients.
- Patients with severe ARS symptoms and those whose symptoms do not resolve in 7 to 10 days, benefit from antibiotic therapy.

REFERENCES

1. Hickner JM. Acute rhinosinusitis: A diagnostic and therapeutic challenge. *J Fam Pract.* 2001;50:38-40.
2. Piccirillo JF. Clinical practice. Acute bacterial sinusitis. *N Engl J Med.* 2004;351:902-910.
3. Glasziou PP, Del Mar CB, Sanders SL, Hayem M. Antibiotics for acute otitis media in children. *Cochrane Database Syst Rev.* 2004;(1):CD000219. doi: 10.1002/14651858. CD000219.pub2.
4. Inglis AF Jr., Gates GA. Acute otitis media and otitis media with effusion. In: Cummings CW, Haughey BH, Thomas JR, Harker LA, Robbins KT, Schuller DE, et al., eds. *Otolaryngology—Head and Neck Surgery,* 4th ed. Philadelphia, PA: Elsevier Mosby; 2004:4446-4465.
5. Hulett KJ, Stankiewicz JA. Primary sinus surgery. In: Cummings CW, Haughey BH, Thomas JR, Harker LA, Robbins KT, Schuller DE et al., eds. *Otolaryngology—Head and Neck Surgery,* 4th ed. Philadelphia, PA: Elsevier Mosby; 2005: 1229-1254.
6. Institute for Clinical Systems Improvement (ICSI). Diagnosis and Treatment of Otitis Media in Children. NGC:003727. Updated May 27, 2004. Accessed May 1, 2006. http://www.icsi.org/otitis_media/diagnosis_and_ treatment_of_otitis_media_in_children_2304.html
7. Rosenfeld RM. Otitis, antibiotics, and the greater good. *Pediatrics.* 2004;114:1333-1335.

8. Paradise JL. Otitis Media. In: Behrman RE, Kliegman RE, Jenson HB, eds. *Nelson Textbook of Pediatrics.* 2004: 2138-2149.

9. Meltzer EO, Hamilos DL, Hadley JA et al. Rhinosinusitis: Establishing definitions for clinical research and patient care. *Otolaryngol Head Neck Surg.* 2004;131:S1-62.

10. Agency for Health Care Policy and Research. Diagnosis and treatment of acute bacterial rhinosinusitis: Summary, evidence report/technology assessment. www.ahrq.gov/clinic/epcsums/sinussum.htm. AHCPR publication no. 99-E015. 1999.

11. Meltzer EO, Szwarcberg J, Pill MW. Allergic rhinitis, asthma, and rhinosinusitis: Diseases of the integrated airway. *J Manag Care Pharm.* 2004;10:310-317.

12. Meltzer EO, Orgel HA, Backhaus JW et al. Intranasal flunisolide spray as an adjunct to oral antibiotic therapy for sinusitis. *J Allergy Clin Immunol.* 1993;92:812-823.

13. Snow V, Mottur-Pilson C, Hickner JM. Principles of appropriate antibiotic use for acute sinusitis in adults. *Ann Intern Med.* 2001;134:495-497.

14. Piccirillo JF. Clinical practice. Acute bacterial sinusitis. *N Engl J Med.* 2004;351:902-910.

PART 10

Hematologic Disorders

CHAPTERS

Chapter 39

Venous Thromboembolism

Rebecca Rottman and David N. Duddleston

SEARCH STRATEGY

A systematic search of the medical literature was performed on June 18, 2007. The search, limited to human subjects and journals in English language, included the National Guidelines Clearinghouse, the Cochrane database, PubMed, and UpToDate®.

INTRODUCTION

Deep vein thrombosis (DVT) and pulmonary embolus (PE) are some of the most common causes of excess morbidity and mortality in medicine today, yet it may be reduced with careful application of strategies, including increased venous circulation, early ambulation and anticoagulant medication. DVT and PE incidences are difficult to estimate since most episodes of thromboembolism are occult and recanalization occurs spontaneously. However, estimates suggest that approximately 600 000 cases occur in the United States annually with increases noted as the population ages.[1] Worldwide estimates suggest that the incidence of venous thromboembolism (VTE) ranges from 1.22 to 1.8 per 1000 person-years.[2,3] Thromboembolism is common in patients with malignancy, serious infections, serious trauma, and surgery and has a higher incidence in patients with inherited thrombophilias.[4] Mortality from pulmonary embolism has been predicted to range from 1% to 8% with an estimated mortality rate of more than 15% within the first 3 months of diagnosis.[5,6] Risk of recurrent VTE during the first year is as high as 5% to 10%, and thereafter the risk decreases to 2% to 3% annually.[7] Morbidity complications from VTE include postthrombotic syndrome, pain, leg swelling, dermatitis ulcers, hyperpigmentation, lipodermatosclerosis, and venous gangrene.[8]

Because of the burden of disease associated with DVT and PE, many risk factors have been identified (Tables 39-1 and 39-2) that are associated with thromboembolisms. Risk factor stratification and strategies to prevent thromboembolism have also been developed. This chapter will focus on evaluation and management of thromboembolism in the primary care setting.

PRESENTATION

There are several presentations of VTE, including those in peripheral veins and those in the pulmonary vasculature (see Table 39-3). In the lower extremities where most DVTs originate, there may be diffuse pain, pain localized in the affected area, or no pain at all, similarly, there may be diffuse swelling of the extremity or none, leading to a wide differential diagnosis (Table 39-4). A typical presentation would be diffuse pain and swelling in the lower extremity in someone who has recently been immobilized as a result of surgery.

Pulmonary embolism usually results from propagation of a thrombus in the pelvic region or in deep veins in the lower extremities. The clot travels up the vena cava through the right heart and terminates in the distal pulmonary vasculature.[3] PE may be occult in as many as 40% of patients found to have DVT. Pulmonary embolism can be single or multiple and can have several presentations. Symptoms range from acute dyspnea, cough, and hemoptysis to pleuritic chest pain alone or in combination with syncope or sudden death (see Table 39-5).[9] Seldom, chronically recurring PE's may result in chronic hypoxia, pulmonary hypertension or right heart failure.[10] Presenting signs and symptoms may not be specific; thus, testing is necessary for diagnosis.[11]

Table 39-1. Risk Factors for DVT and PE

Age >40	Immobilization
Long auto/plane trips	Major surgery
Malignancy	Serious infection/sepsis
Previous DVT or stroke	Acute myocardial infarction
Congestive heart failure	Nephrotic syndrome
Lower extremity fractures	Burns
Spinal cord trauma	Vasculitis
Inherited hypercoagulable states	Thrombocytosis
Pregnancy/postpartum status	Trauma
Obesity	Inflammatory bowel disease
Presence of central venous catheter	Use of oral contraceptives or hormone replacement therapy

Table 39-3. Symptoms and Signs of DVT

Symptoms	Signs
Diffuse pain in extremity	Gross swelling and edema
Pain localized along involved vein	Swelling best detected by discrepancy in measured limb circumference
Pain in knee (LE DVT) or shoulder (UE DVT)	Swelling mimicking knee effusion
Abdominal pain from pelvic thrombosis	Palpable vein tract
Symptoms referable to PE (see below)	Visible vein engorgement
No pain	Cyanotic discoloration of limb
	Homan's sign
	Warmth
	Normal findings

PHYSICAL EXAMINATION

Physical examination is often misleading, as physical signs can be subtle. Estimations are that physical findings are inaccurate in 50% of cases of DVT, and the best tool is a high index of suspicion. However, only a minority of those suspected to have DVT based on clinical criteria, actually have DVT when tested. Common findings may include disparity in limb circumference with or without pitting edema, tenderness in the extremity, positive Homan's sign (pain with active dorsiflexion of the ankle), disparity of temperature in the limb, mottled skin, palpable "cord" (vein tract) and engorged veins distal to venous obstruction. Wells and colleagues created a prediction rule for diagnosing DVT. The scoring system includes one point for various risk factors including active cancer, paralysis/paresis or recent plaster immobilization of lower extremity, recent immobilization for more than 3 days (bedridden) or major surgery within 4 weeks, localized tenderness, entire lower extremity swelling, calf swelling more than 3 cm greater than asymptomatic side, pitting edema on symptomatic leg, collateral superficial veins. If an alternative diagnosis is documented, points are subtracted from the total. A score ≥3 suggests a high probability of DVT, while a score of ≤0 suggests a low probability of DVT.[12,13] These signs may be present in the affected lower extremity or have corollary signs in the case of an upper extremity DVT. In rare cases of severe venous obstruction, skin and tissue necrosis may mimic arterial occlusion.

DIAGNOSTIC EVALUATION

Once a consideration of VTE is entered into a differential diagnosis, a diagnostic approach can be chosen. Various strategies in excluding and confirming venous thrombosis have been devised, using a combination of blood and imaging tests. A negative D-dimer test may exclude the diagnosis (i.e., level < 500 ng/mL via ELISA), although an abnormal result does not confirm it. The D-dimer test is typically used in cases with a low index of suspicion. Other blood tests are not helpful in making a diagnosis as findings such as leukocytosis are nonspecific. Imaging tests are the most helpful. Imaging tests range from noninvasive testing to contrast venography or pulmonary angiography (gold standard test). In cases of DVT of an extremity, compression ultrasonography can provide rapid and accurate diagnosis without X-ray exposure (see Fig. 39-1).[1,8,14,15]

Limitations of compression ultrasonography include cases of chronically occluded veins, inability to reveal pelvic DVT and operator variability. Normalization of ultrasound findings may take more than 1 year in 30% to 40% of cases of DVT, impedance plethysmography or MRI is more predictive of an acute DVT in the setting of prior thromboembolism in the same limb. Contrast venography is rarely indicated in light of well-validated noninvasive tests.[1,8]

Table 39-2. Inherited Hypercoagulable States

Factor V Leiden mutation	Protein C deficiency
Protein S deficiency	Anticardiolipin syndrome
Antithrombin deficiency	Dysfibrinogenemias
Prothrombin gene mutation	

Table 39-4. Differential Diagnosis for DVT

DVT	Musculoskeletal Injury
Superficial thrombophlebitis	Postthrombotic syndrome
Chronic venous insufficiency	Venous obstruction
Popliteal (Baker's) cyst	Cellulitis
Fracture	Hematoma
Hypoproteinemia	Lymphedema

Table 39-5. Symptoms and Signs of Pulmonary Embolism

Symptoms	Signs
Pleuritic chest pain	Pleuritic rub
Dyspnea	Tachypnea
Cough/hemoptysis	Tachycardia
Syncope/sudden death	Hypotension, sometimes episodic
Dyspnea on exertion	Apparent anxiety
Edema caused by right heart failure	4th heart sound
Asymptomatic	None of the above

One approach for diagnosis of PE is using helical high resolution CT scanning with a "pulmonary embolism protocol," to observe obstructions within pulmonary artery segments. Alternatively, ventilation/perfusion scanning may show a mismatch of perfusion to ventilation, indicating obstruction in a pulmonary artery. The diagnosis of pulmonary embolism may be inferred from symptoms referable to PE, along with the finding of DVT in an extremity, since the treatment of DVT parallels that of PE. Finally, in cases when there is a high clinical suspicion of PE and other techniques are unrevealing, a definitive diagnosis must be made. Pulmonary arteriography of the pulmonary tree is considered the gold standard in diagnosis but is tedious and carries risks of contrast and x-ray exposure greater than that of other techniques (see Fig. 39-2).[3,9,16]

RISK STRATIFICATION

Risk stratification allows appropriate patients to be treated as an outpatient while others must be admitted to the hospital. Some patients with simple DVT may be treated at home without admission to the hospital.[17] In cases where a diagnosis can be made expeditiously, for instance with presentation to an emergency department where immediate access to ultrasonography is available, a definitive diagnosis can be made and initial treatment begun as an outpatient. Pulmonary embolism should be addressed with questioning for near syncope, episodes of breathlessness, or pleuritic chest pain. The physical examination should focus on abnormal vital signs, splinting and a pleural rub. Oxygen saturation should be above 95% on room air. If any of these factors are abnormal, hospital admission or tests to rule out PE should be considered.

Pain should be addressed when dealing with simple DVT. Pain uncontrollable by oral medication should be treated parenterally, necessitating admission. Most DVT pain should be treatable as an outpatient.

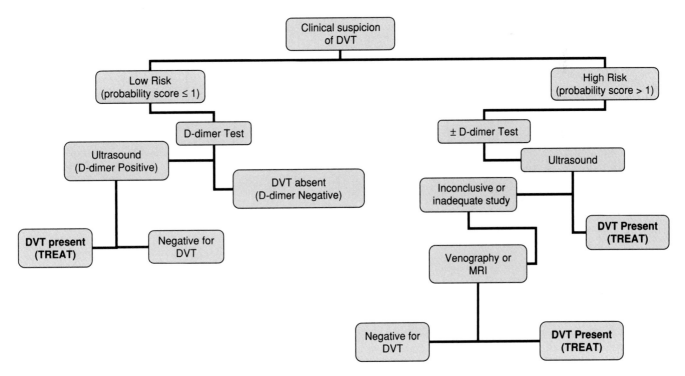

Figure 39-1. Diagnostic approach for diagnosing DVT.

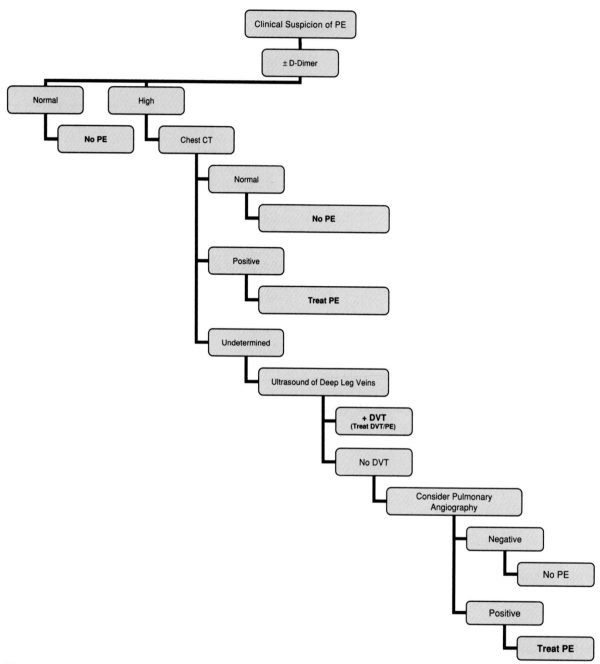

Figure 39-2. Diagnostic approach for diagnosing PE.

Lastly, since comorbid conditions frequently contribute to the development of DVT, assessment of these conditions should include the consideration of a hypercoagulable state workup for idiopathic DVT or PE. If the patient's functional capacity is significantly impaired, admission to address these issues and the DVT is warranted.

Many hospital admissions can be avoided in following the above guidelines, as long as the patient can also enter management quickly. Management has been greatly simplified with the availability of once-daily dosing of low molecular weight heparins (LMWHs). The patient should have ready access to follow-up for monitoring of the prothrombin time (PT) when warfarin therapy is begun. Complications of therapy should be assessed and managed quickly when encountered.

Table 39-6. Initial Treatment Options for DVT

Anticoagulation
Systematically administered thrombolysis
Catheter-directed thrombolysis
Catheter extraction or fragmentation and surgical thrombectomy
Vena caval interruption
Nonsteroidal anti-inflammatory agents

MANAGEMENT

PREVENTION OF VTE

Perhaps the best strategy for prevention of thromboembolism is careful evaluation of every at-risk patient and application of a guideline derived from synthesis of medical evidence. One such guideline has been published by the American College of Chest Physicians and is commonly referred to as the *Chest* guidelines.[18]

TREATMENT OF ESTABLISHED THROMBOEMBOLISM

Treatments of DVT and PE are similar. Acute PE should be managed in a hospital setting. Long-term anticoagulation therapy is the mainstay of treatment. However, other treatment options are available (see Tables 39-6 and 39-7). Most of the alternative initial treatment options are not recommended to be used routinely.[19] Complications such as post-thrombotic syndrome, chronic thromboembolic pulmonary hypertension, and superficial thrombophlebitis may occur despite appropriate management of thromboembolism.

ANTICOAGULANTS

Anticoagulants are the treatment of choice for thromboembolic disease and a good understanding of these agents is imperative. Anticoagulants are utilized to prevent thrombus extension and early and late recurrences of DVT and PE. Heparin, until recently, was the preferred initial treatment of DVT and PE. Newer agents include LMWHs that have a relatively flat dose-response curve allowing fixed dosing without intensive monitoring. Warfarin, a vitamin K antagonist (VKA), is used primarily for long-term treatment of DVT or PE and has

Table 39-7. Initial Treatment Options for PE

Anticoagulation
Systemically and locally administered thrombolytic drugs
Catheter extraction or fragmentation
Pulmonary embolectomy
Vena caval interruption

been used increasingly in prophylactic treatment after orthopedic and vascular procedures.

Unfractionated Heparin

Unfractionated heparin (UFH) is a heterogeneous mixture of polysaccharide chains ranging from 3000 to 30000 Da in size, averaging approximately 15000 Da. UFH can exert antithrombotic activity by two competing mechanisms. Pentasaccharide units scattered along the chain bind to and activate antithrombin, causing binding and subsequent inactivation of activated Factor X (Xa) in a pentasaccharide/antithrombin/Xa complex. Alternatively, by virtue of its large size, UFH can create a pentasaccharide/antithrombin/thrombin complex, essentially enveloping thrombin. This complex is the basis of measurement of the partial thromboplastin time (PTT). UFH has an equal effect on thrombin and Xa activity. UFH dosing is recommended to be given as a continuous infusion while being monitored intensively. Intermittent IV injections of UFH have been associated with a higher risk of bleeding. Over-anticoagulation with UFH can be antagonized with protamine, which binds to UFH, forming a stable salt at a ratio of 1 mg of protamine for every 100 units of UFH. When continuous UFH is used, the previous few hour's units should be included.[20]

Low Molecular Weight Heparin (Pentasaccharides)

LMWH is created by exposing heparin to enzymatic or chemical agents to fragment the large heparin molecule, making a more homogeneous mixture of shorter chains, averaging approximately 5000 Da. This exposes the pentasaccharide units along the heparin strand but leaves the chain short enough to reduce binding of thrombin. The smaller LMWH molecule confers a more predictable dose response and obviates monitoring of anticoagulation. LMWHs have a longer half-life, greater bioavailability and drug clearance, independent of dosing. LMWH has less binding to plasma proteins including those acute phase reactants in ill and injured patients. The reverse is true with UFH, which must be closely monitored to deliver the proper dose. Should measurement of anticoagulation be necessary, some laboratories can perform Factor Xa measurement. Many clinicians suggest still following hemoglobin/hematocrit, platelets and renal function (as many agents require adjustment or are not recommended in significant renal impairment). Currently three LMWHs are available in the US: enoxaparin, dalteparin, tinzaparin. Fondaparinux is a synthetic pentasaccharide heparin analog very similar to the LMWHs. To date, there is no reversal agent for LMWHs. Protamine has shown some activity for reversing effects of LMWH. Factor VII therapy has also been used in case reports to reverse anticoagulation.[20]

Table 39-8. Management of Supratherapeutic INR for DVT and PE

INR	Symptoms of Bleed or Rapid Reversal of Excessive Anticoagulant Effect Required	Risk Factors for Bleed Present *or* Increased Patient Risk of Thromboembolic Problems	Reversal Agent	Warfarin	Recheck INR (h)
Less than 5	No	Yes	None	Hold 1–3 doses/ decrease on restart	24
5–9	No	No	Vitamin K 2.5 to 5 mg po	Hold 1–3 doses/ decrease on restart	24
Greater than 9	No	No	Vitamin K 5–10 mg po with the expectation that the INR will be reduced substantially in 24–48 h. Monitor frequency and use of additional vitamin K if necessary	Hold 1–3 doses/ decrease on restart	12–24
Variable	Yes		Vitamin K 10 mg (slow IV infusion) + prothrombin complex concentrate/fresh frozen plasma/factor VIIa (repeat vitamin K (slow IV infusion) dose until INR in therapeutic range)- Every 12 h	Hold warfarin	12

Warfarin

Interestingly, warfarin initially creates a paradoxical situation of inhibiting the manufacture of procoagulant factors II, VII, IX, and X, while also inhibiting the circulating anticoagulants protein C and protein S. While the intact procoagulants are still circulating, a thrombogenic effect of warfarin may predominate, thus requiring anticoagulation by other means such as with parenteral heparin products. The homeostatic forces of coagulation and anticoagulation are balanced by procoagulants and their counterregulatory anticoagulants. The full effect of warfarin is not accomplished for several days as the intact procoagulant factors are cleared from the circulation.[21] Warfarin also crosses the placenta and therefore cannot be used in pregnancy. Its main limitation is a requirement for monitoring drug levels and dosages. Warfarin is monitored, and doses are adjusted, utilizing the international normalized ratio (INR). The INR is the ratio of a patient's PT to a control sample, raised to the power of the International Sensitivity Index value for the control sample used. Over-anticoagulation can significantly increase the risk of bleeding complications. Agents for warfarin reversal include vitamin K, fresh frozen plasma, prothrombin concentrate and factor VIIa (see Table 39-8).[21,22]

Table 39-9. UFH and LMWH Dosing Recommendations for Treatment of DVT and PE

UFH[20]	Bolus dose: 80 units/kg and 18 units/kg per hour infusion Follow hospital protocol for adjustment of dose with a PTT monitoring
Enoxaparin (Lovenox®)[23] (FDA-approved for treatment of DVT and PE)	1 mg/kg body weight SC BID for treatment 1.5 mg/kg SC daily 1 mg/kg SC daily for Creatinine Clearance < 30 mL/min
Dalteparin (Fragmin®)[24] (only FDA-approved as extended treatment of symptomatic VTE patients with cancer for up to 6 months)	200 units/kg per day SC (total body weight) for the first 30 d then 150 units/kg per day SC months 2–6 (daily dose should not exceed 18 000 units) 175 units/kg SC daily for DVT or PE treatment (caution for reduced clearance in renal insufficiency)
Tinzaparin (Innohep®)[25] (FDA-approved for treatment of DVT and PE)	7.5 mg SC daily for treatment of DVT or PE (50–100 kg patient) (caution reduced clearance in renal insufficiency, body weight less than 50 kg and the elderly)
Fondaparinux (Arixtra®)[26], a synthetic pentasaccharide (FDA approved for treatment of DVT and PE in conjunction with warfarin)	Contraindicated for Creatinine Clearance <30 mL/min

SC, subcutaneous; BID, twice daily.

Table 39-10. Initiation of Warfarin Therapy for DVT and PE

INR	Day 1	Day 2	Day 3	Day 4	Day 5
Less than 1.5	Initial dose (usually 5 mg)	No dose change	Increase dose by 0–25% of total	Increase dose by 0–25% of daily dose	Increase dose by 25% of daily dose
1.5–1.9		Decrease dose by 25–50%	No dose change or decrease by 10–25% of total	No dose change or increase by 10–25% of daily dose	Increase dose by 0–25% of daily dose
2.0–2.5		Decrease dose by 50–75%	Decrease dose by 50–75% of total	Decrease dose by 10–25% of daily dose	No change or decrease dose by 0–15% of daily dose
Greater than 2.5	Hold warfarin until INR less than 2.5 and restart at a lower dose				

INITIAL TREATMENT FOR DVT AND PE

Patients who have a high clinical suspicion or documented DVT or PE should begin anticoagulation therapy. LMWH is the treatment of choice for acute DVT and PE as a result of its predictable dose-response curve. While testing of PTT allows the clinician to judge the level of anticoagulation with intravenous UFH, maintenance of the narrow therapeutic range is fraught with complications. Inadequate dosing results in delay or lapses of treatment, and overshooting anticoagulation goals increases the risk of bleeding complications. LMWH and UFH therapy should be overlapped with VKAs for a minimum of 5 days and discontinued when the INR is stable and >2.0 (see Table 39-9).[19]

Application of clinical studies has resulted in the use of VKAs on day 1 of treatment, so as to expedite monitoring of the PT and adjustment of warfarin dosing during the customary 5-day treatment period with parenteral or subcutaneous anticoagulants. Initial dosing of warfarin is five to ten milligrams daily. Dosing with 5 mg has shown to have less excessive bleeding complications (see Table 39-10).[21] Elderly, debilitated and malnourished patients as well as those patients with congestive heart failure or liver disease should start warfarin at doses ≤5 mg daily.[22]

The Seventh ACCP Conference on Antithrombotic and Thrombolytic Therapy and the AHA/ACC Scientific Statement Guide to Warfarin Therapy have been developed to aid clinicians in the management of anticoagulation therapy.[19,21]

LONG-TERM TREATMENT FOR DVT AND PE

The safety and efficacy of long-term treatment with warfarin for DVT and PE has been extensively studied. Clinical trials have shown an increased risk for recurrent events or bleeding events when patients' INR values are maintained above or below the therapeutic range. *Chest* guideline developers looked at ideal duration of therapy as well (see Table 39-11).[19]

Table 39-11. Long-Term Treatment for DVT and PE*

Condition	INR Range	Duration of Therapy
DVT first episode (transient/reversible risk factor)	2.0–3.0	At least 3 months
DVT (first episode and idiopathic)	2.0–3.0	6–12 months (consider indefinite)
DVT (with cancer—may consider LMWH for first 3–6 months)	2.0–3.0	3–6 months (consider indefinite or until cancer resolves)
DVT (antiphospholipid antibodies or 2 or more thrombophillic conditions)	2.0–3.0	6–12 months (consider indefinite)
DVT (recurrent—2 or more episodes)	2.0–3.0	Indefinite
PE first episode (transient/reversible risk factor)	2.0–3.0	At least 3 months
PE (first episode and idiopathic)	2.0–3.0	6–12 months (consider indefinite)
PE (with cancer—may consider LMWH for first 3–6 months)	2.0–3.0	3–6 months consider indefinite or until cancer resolves)
PE (antiphospholipid antibodies or 2 or more thrombophillic conditions)	2.0–3.0	6–12 months (consider indefinite)
PE (recurrent—2 or more episodes)	2.0–3.0	Indefinite

*Risk-benefit of indefinite anticoagulation therapy must be reassessed periodically.

Table 39-12. Long-Term Management of Warfarin Therapy for DVT and PE

INR	Recommendations	Repeat INR (d)
Less than 1.5	Increase weekly dose by 10–15%	5–7
1.6–1.9	Increase weekly dose by 5–15%	7
2–3	No change in dose	*
3.1–3.5	Decrease weekly dose by 5–10%	5–7
3.6–4	Hold warfarin. Decrease weekly dose by 10–15%	5–7
4.1–9	Hold warfarin 1–2 d. Consider vitamin K 2.5–5 mg if INR close to 9 or increased bleed risk	1–2
9.1–20	Hold warfarin. Vitamin K 2.5–5 mg po. Restart warfarin when INR at goal and decreased weekly dose by at least 15–20% (may need implement other reversal recommendations)	1

*Frequency of INR testing for stable patients: (1) when INR and dose of warfarin has been stable (~2 tests), then check INR every week, (2) when INR and dose of warfarin has been stable 2 consecutive weeks, check INR every 2 weeks, (3) when INR and dose of warfarin has been stable 4 weeks, check INR every month, and (4) all patients should be checked monthly, not to exceed 4–5 weeks between laboratory draws.

Many approaches to improve anticoagulation control have been studied. Some of these approaches include therapeutic drug monitoring clinics, point of care PT testing allowing patients to adjust warfarin regimens and computer programs that aid in adjusting warfarin regimens (see Table 39-12).[19,22] Interruption of therapy may be required for patients undergoing invasive procedures. For those patients at greatest risk, including VTE within the first 3 months, bridge therapy with LMWH or UFH should be considered (see Table 39-13).[19,27]

SUMMARY

Thromboembolic disease complications may be reduced by risk assessment and appropriate pharmacologic treatment strategies. Many studies have elucidated the dosing and clinical use of anticoagulant therapy. The introduction of LMWHs has provided opportunity for outpatient treatment of DVT as well as a safe and effective alternative to heparin treatment of thromboembolic disorders. Warfarin is still the drug of choice for long-term anticoagulation by virtue of its cost. Most patients should be reevaluated periodically to assess the

Table 39-13. Prophylaxis During Interruption of Oral Anticoagulation Therapy for Invasive Procedures*

Day 10 to day 7	Stop aspirin/clopidogrel
Day 5	Stop warfarin
Day 3, day 2	Start enoxaparin 1mg/kg q12h
Day 1	Last enoxaparin dose in morning before procedure *If INR ≥ 1.8, give Vitamin K₁, 2.5 mg by mouth*
Day 0 (day of procedure)	Restart warfarin at usual dose in evening
Day +1	Restart enoxaparin at 1 mg/kg q12h
Day +4 or more	Continue enoxaparin until INR is therapeutic

*Modified from: Spyropoulos A. Bridging of oral anticoagulation therapy for invasive procedures. *Curr Hematol Rep.* 2005;4:405.

benefits of long-term anticoagulation therapy in preventing recurrent events.

REFERENCES

1. Qaseem A, Snow V, Barry P, et al. Current diagnosis of venous thromboembolism in primary care: A clinical practice guideline from the American Academy of Family Physicians and the American College of Physicians. *Ann Inter Med.* 2007;146:454.
2. Cushman M, Tsai A, White R, et al. Deep vein thrombosis and pulmonary embolism in two cohorts: The longitudinal investigation of thromboembolism etiology. *Am J Med.* 2004;117:19.
3. Goldbaher SZ. Pulmonary embolism. *Lancet.* 2004;363:1295.
4. Alikhan R, Cohen A, Combe S, et al. Risk factors for venous thromboembolism in hospitalized patients with acute medical illness: Analysis of the MEDENOX Study. *Arch Intern Med.* 2004;164:963.
5. Goldhaber SZ, Visani L, De Rosa M. Acute pulmonary embolism: Clinical outcomes in the international cooperative pulmonary embolism registry (ICOPER). *Lancet.* 1999;353:1386.
6. Hirsh J, Bates SM. Prognosis in acute pulmonary embolism. *Lancet.* 1999;353:1375.
7. Douketis JD, Kearon C, Bates S, et al. Risk of fatal pulmonary embolism in patients with treated venous thromboembolism. *JAMA.* 1998;279(6):458.
8. Tovey C, Wyatt S. Diagnosis, investigation, and management of deep vein thrombosis. *BMJ.* 2003;326:1180.
9. Stein PD, Terrin ML, Hales CA, et al. Clinical, laboratory, roentgenographic, and electrocardiographic findings in patients with acute pulmonary embolism and no preexisting cardiac or pulmonary disease. *Chest.* 1991;100(3):598.
10. Goldhaber SZ, Elliott CG. Acute Pulmonary Embolism: Part I Epidemiology, Pathophysiology, and Diagnosis. *Circulation.* 2003;108:2726.

11. Hull RD. Diagnosing pulmonary embolism with improved certainty and simplicity. *JAMA.* 2006;295(2):213.

12. Wells PS, Anderson DR, Bormanis J, et al. Value of assessment of pretest probability of deep-vein thrombosis in clinical management. *Lancet.* 1997;350:1795.

13. Wells PS, Anderson DR, Roger M, et al. Excluding pulmonary embolism at the bedside without diagnositic imaging: Management of patients with suspected pulmonary embolism presenting to the emergency department by using a simple clinical model and D-dimer. *Ann Intern Med.* 2001;135:98.

14. Scarvelis D, Wells PS. Diagnosis and treatment of deep-vein thrombosis. *CMAJ.* 2006;175(9):1087.

15. Wells PS, Owen C, Doucette S, et al. Does this patient have deep vein thrombosis? *JAMA.* 2006;295(2)199.

16. Fedullo PF, Tapson VF. The evaluation of suspected pulmonary embolism. *N Engl J Med.* 2003;349:1247.

17. Othieno R, Abu Affan M, Okpo E. Home versus in-patient treatment for deep vein thrombosis. *Cochrane Database Syst Rev.* 2007;3:CD003076.

18. Geerts WH, Pineo GF, Heit JA, et al. Prevention of venous thromboembolism: The seventh ACCP Conference on antithrombotic and thrombolytic therapy. *Chest.* 2004;126(3):338S.

19. Buller HR, Agnelli G, Hull RD, et al. Antithrombotic therapy for venous thromboembolic disease. The seventh ACCP Conference on antithrombotic and thrombolytic therapy. *Chest.* 2004;126(3):401S.

20. Hirsh J, Raschke R. Heparin and low-molecular-weight heparin. The seventh ACCP Conference on antithrombotic and thrombolytic therapy. *Chest.* 2004;126(3):188S.

21. Hirsh J, Fuster V, Ansell J, et al. American Heart Association/American College of Cardiology Foundation guide to warfarin therapy. *Circulation.* 2003;107:1692.

22. Ansell J, Hirsh J, Poller L, et al. The pharmacology and management of the vitamin K antagonists. The seventh ACCP Conference on antithrombotic and thrombolytic therapy. *Chest.* 2004;126(3):204S.

23. Lovenox [package insert]. Bridgewater, NJ: Sanofi-Aventis; 2006.

24. Fragmin [package insert]. New York, NY: Pfizer; 2007.

25. Innohep [package insert]. Boulder, CO: Pharmion Corporation; 2007.

26. Arixtra [package insert]. Research Triangle Park, NC: GlaxoSmithKline; 2005.

27. Spyropoulos A. Bridging of oral anticoagulation therapy for invasive procedures. *Curr Hematol Rep.* 2005;4:405.

Chapter 40

Anemia

R. Darryl Hamilton and Jinna Shepherd

SEARCH STRATEGY

Standard textbooks of hematology and UpToDate® were used as general reference materials. Recent advances in hematology were accessed on PubMed.

INTRODUCTION

Anemia is defined as the reduction in circulating erythrocytes as compared to age- and sex-adjusted ranges of normal. These ranges were developed since the advent of automated blood cell analysis which has allowed clinical laboratories, large and small, to screen large amounts of blood samples. However, these quantitative results must be combined with the results of an accurate history and physical examination, review of the peripheral blood smear and other, more specific, laboratory tests so that an accurate diagnosis for the cause of anemia is found. Once the diagnosis is made, then an appropriate treatment plan can be instituted so that the anemia is corrected and, ultimately, the patient's clinical condition is improved.

In both the inpatient and outpatient settings, anemia is one of the more commonly encountered clinical conditions affecting both children and adults. With respect to the ages at which anemia is encountered, differential diagnoses are often disparate. By and large, anemia in a child is generally because of congenital causes, whereas in adults, anemia is caused by an acquired etiology. In this chapter, we will evaluate some of the more common explanations of anemia, along with their treatments, as well as examine how laboratory measurements may facilitate the diagnosis and subsequent evaluation of therapies.

HISTORY AND PHYSICAL EXAMINATION

Signs and symptoms of anemia may be nonspecific, such as the noting of fatigue or dyspnea on exertion, or quite specific, such as koilonychia ("spoon nail deformity") or the presence of blood in stools. In general, all aspects of a detailed history and physical examination are important to understanding the cause of anemia. On review of systems, fatigue, shortness of breath or dyspnea on exertion, hematemesis, hemoptysis, hematochezia, and reduced mental concentration, among others, may be associated with an underlying deficiency in erythrocytes and oxygen delivery. Medical or surgical histories may point to a diagnosis (e.g., diabetes mellitus and subsequent decreased renal production of erythropoietin or a history of gastric or intestinal resection). For women who are premenopausal, noting the frequency and severity of menstruation can be helpful. Dietary factors, such as veganism or sprue, may be associated with nutritional deficiencies that lead to the development of anemia. Family history is invaluable in the evaluation of children with anemia, as congenital causes dominate the diagnoses in this age group. Occupational and recreational exposures may point to a toxin (e.g., lead) or infectious agents (e.g., mononucleosis or HIV) that result in anemia. Along with this, an accurate list of prescribed and over-the-counter medications may provide clues as well.

On physical examination, pallor of the skin or mucosal membranes is very common, although nonspecific. Likewise, tachycardia and/or systolic ejection murmurs may be present, although nondiagnostic (unless there is a history of valvular replacement). More specific findings may be related to an underlying etiology, such as koilonychia or angular cheilitis as seen in iron deficiency, or loss of vibratory or position sense as seen in

Table 40-1. Classification of Anemia Based on MCV

Decreased MCV	Normal MCV	Increased MCV
Iron deficiency	Anemia of chronic disease	B_{12} deficiency
Anemia of chronic disease	Early iron/folate/B_{12} deficiency	Folate deficiency
Thalassemia	Marrow infiltration	Liver disease
Hyperthyroidism	Combined iron/folate deficiency	Alcohol abuse
	Acute blood loss	Aplastic anemia
		Myelodysplasia
		Myeloproliferative disorder
		Hypothyroidism

chronic B_{12} deficiency. Splenomegaly in children is generally caused by production of blood elements in the spleen when there is inadequate production within the marrow spaces. Examples would include the hemoglobinopathies, such as thalassemia or sickle cell disease, or erythrocyte membrane disorders, such as hereditary spherocytosis. In adults, splenomegaly may be seen in association with autoimmune hemolytic anemia or concomitant malignancy, among other diagnoses. The history will often dictate a focused examination, such as palpation of the thyroid or examination of the urine or feces for blood, in the appropriate clinical situation.

APPROACH TO THE DIAGNOSIS OF ANEMIA

Screening for anemia is not routinely recommended as it is more frequently discovered when clinical clues suggest the need for laboratory assessment of anemia as during hospitalization, blood donation, or as part of routine annual examination. If anemia is suspected, a complete blood count with platelets, white blood cell count (WBC) with differential, and reticulocyte count should be ordered. Anemia is represented by a hemoglobin (Hgb) of <13–15 g/dL or hematocrit (Hct) <42% in men and in women a Hgb <11–13 g/dL or Hct <37%. These values vary according to ethnicity and age, but can serve as a guideline in the initial evaluation of anemia.[1] When a reduction in Hgb or Hct is found, a determination of the etiology is important.

Plasma volume may affect the measured Hgb and Hct which can be appreciated in several common scenarios. Dehydration with a decrease in plasma volume causes hemoconcentration with higher measurements of Hgb and Hct. Pregnancy results in expansion of plasma volume and lowers Hgb and Hct. An acute gastrointestinal bleed with rapid volume loss results in lower Hgb and Hct after plasma volume redistribution, which can take hours to develop.

In addition Hgb and Hct, the complete blood count provides measures of the red blood cell count and red blood cell indices. These indices include: mean corpuscular volume (MCV), mean cell hemoglobin, and mean cell hemoglobin concentration. The MCV is useful in the classification of anemia into microcytic, normocytic, or macrocytic anemias (Table 40-1). The red cell distribution width (RDW) is a statistical measurement of variation in size of the red cell.

The reticulocyte count can be useful in distinguishing types of anemia. A high reticulocyte count is consistent with rapid release of reticulocytes from the marrow into the peripheral circulation which can be seen in blood loss or hemolysis of red cells. The presence of reticulocytes in the peripheral circulation results in an elevated RDW as they are much larger than the normal RBC. A low reticulocyte count with anemia indicates ineffective erythropoiesis. Anemia caused by multiple etiologies may be associated with a low reticulocyte count, even in the presence of blood loss or hemolysis.

Additional clues to the etiology are provided by evaluation of the WBC count and differential as well as the platelet counts. A low WBC count with anemia should prompt the evaluation of abnormalities in the bone marrow. One such condition that leads to anemia and underproduction of WBC and platelets is aplastic anemia. While this can be due to specific viral infections, this condition frequently presents in young adults and is caused by an autoimmune phenomenon. Increased WBCs suggest infection or leukemia. Hypersegmented neutrophils are associated with B_{12} or folate deficiency. Platelet counts may be very high (thrombocytosis) in severe iron deficiency, inflammatory conditions, or myeloproliferative disorders. Thrombocytopenia is consistent with sepsis, infiltration of the marrow, or platelet destruction.[1]

Evaluation of the peripheral smear is essential to providing clues to determining the cause of anemia which are not readily apparent from red cell indices. Table 40-2 provides a list of abnormal characteristics of red cells and associated etiologies.

IRON METABOLISM

The most important dietary supplement to support erythrocyte formation and function is iron. Chronic daily losses of iron occur with subclinical bleeding and normal

Table 40-2. Peripheral Smear

Abnormalities of Red Cells	Common Associations
Anisocytosis (abnormal sizes)	Iron deficiency
Poikilocytosis (abnormal shapes)	Microangiopathic anemia
Hypochromia	Iron deficiency
Acanthosis (spur cells)	Liver disease
Elliptocytosis (pencil cells)	Iron deficiency
	Megaloblastic anemia
	Hereditary elliptocytosis
Macrocytosis	B$_{12}$ deficiency
Microcytosis	Iron deficiency
Rouleaux (coin stacking)	Multiple myeloma
Schistocytes (helmet cells)	Microangiopathic hemolytic anemia
	Heart valve hemolysis
Sickle cells	Sickle cell anemia
Spherocytosis	Hereditary spherocytosis
Target cells	Thalassemia
	Liver disease
	Hemoglobinopathies
Teardrop cells	Iron deficiency
	Myelofibrosis

skin exfoliation. This is balanced by absorption of iron in foods. Men and postmenopausal women absorb approximately 0.5–1.0 mg/d of dietary iron. Premenopausal women, as a result of greater blood loss with menstruation, absorb 1–2 mg/d. Dietary nonheme iron is absorbed in the proximal duodenum under acidic conditions. This iron is then complexed with ferritin, and stored in the marrow, or with transferrin and made available for immediate use to circulating RBC. Heme iron in foods, generally meats, is thought to be absorbed in a similar manner,[2] although a greater proportion of dietary heme iron is absorbed than nonheme iron. Antacids and gastric acid blockers (H2-blockers and proton pump inhibitors) decrease iron absorption, whereas vitamin C enhances iron absorption.

Red blood cell lifespans are approximately 100 to 120 days. As red blood cells age, they become less deformable, and are eventually destroyed by the cells in the reticuloendothelial system. Iron released during this process is bound to transferrin and transported to the macrophages in the bone marrow. There, iron is stored in ferritin complexes, until needed by developing erythrocyte colonies.

The gold standard for the evaluation of patients to determine the presence and availability of iron is via bone marrow aspiration. Despite its utility in this regard, it is an uncomfortable experience for patients, but carries minimal risk. Serum measurement of iron

stores is one of the most frequent laboratory studies done in the evaluation of anemia. Serum levels of iron and total iron binding capacity (TIBC) reflect the amount of iron bound to transferrin and the ability of erythrocytes to absorb iron, respectively. Iron saturation, calculated as serum iron divided by TIBC, reflects the relative availability of iron for use by circulating RBC. In general, during iron deficiency, serum measurements of iron are low whereas serum TIBC is elevated, resulting in a low iron saturation. Serum measurement of ferritin is a useful marker of storage iron, as it is produced in amounts relative to marrow stores. When ferritin is low, iron deficiency is present. However, a number of conditions can result in ferritin elevation, as ferritin is an acute phase protein. In iron deficiency associated with such disease states, ferritin will be normal to elevated, resulting in a false negative result. As discussed later, in anemia of chronic disease, serum iron and TIBC evaluation may mimic iron deficiency, but the ferritin is frequently elevated.

Erythrocytes absorb iron via membrane-bound transferrin receptors, reflected as TIBC. Circulating enzymes can cleave the extracellular domain of transferrin receptors, releasing these into the circulation. This can be measured as soluble transferrin receptors (sTFr).[3] If this value is >1.5, iron deficiency is likely present. Conditions associated with inappropriately low sTFr include chronic renal insufficiency and aplastic anemia. Both conditions are associated with decreased production of erythrocytes. Increased sTFr values are seen in conditions associated with brisk erythropoiesis, such as the chronic hemolytic states thalassemia and sickle cell disease.

IRON DEFICIENCY ANEMIA

Iron deficiency exists when the demand for iron by developing erythrocytes exceeds the supply of iron by marrow macrophages, iron stored by ferritin, or transported by transferrin. Increased requirements of iron delivery are present as a result of a number of conditions. Loss of iron via the gastrointestinal, genitourinary, and pulmonary tracts is a frequent cause of iron depletion. This is frequently visible and detectable by bedside analysis. Subclinical loss of iron via the gastrointestinal tract may occur with the ingestion of aspirin, nonsteroidal anti-inflammatory medications, or with alcohol. Genitourinary iron excretion most commonly arises in conditions that result in intravascular hemolysis. Premenopausal women, through menstruation and during pregnancy or lactation, experience large losses of iron as a result of bleeding or from incorporation into the developing fetus.

Decreased supply of iron to erythroid colonies is usually a result of ingestion of an iron-poor diet. Some patients have a decreased ability to absorb dietary iron, usually caused by concurrent use of antacids or after some gastric procedures. Patients who have undergone duodenal resection may have impaired iron absorption as well. Rare conditions exist in which iron-transporting molecules, such as transferrin, may be markedly decreased or absent.

Patients with iron deficiency may develop a range of signs of symptoms. Those generally seen with anemia, such as shortness of breath or decreased exercise tolerance, are frequent. More specific findings such as koilonychia or angular cheilitis may be present. Occasionally, patients will have a bluish tint to the sclerae, possibly because of decreased iron availability for normal collagen synthesis. Pica is a condition which may develop in patients who are iron deficient. Most commonly, this is manifested by eating ice or pagophagia. Once iron replacement therapy is begun, pica resolves fairly quickly. The other signs above may take several weeks to completely resolve. Other forms of pica include ingestion of clayish dirt or starch which decreases dietary iron absorption. Patients should be discouraged from such habits.

The bone marrow will continue to produce erythrocytes that are normocytic and normochromic despite ongoing iron losses. Once iron supply is depleted, production of microcytic, hypochromic erythrocytes ensues. Eventually the MCV decreases and then the RDW normalizes, reflecting production of similarly small erythrocytes. Once iron supplementation is begun, an increase in reticulocytosis is evident within 7 to 10 days. The Hct may normalize in 6 to 8 weeks, while the MCV may take 3 to 4 months to normalize. Several conditions exist which results in the production of microcytic, hypochromic erythrocytes other than iron deficiency. These include: anemia of chronic disease, thalassemia, hemoglobinopathies (e.g., sickle cell disease), and the rare conditions associated with decreased or absent ferritin and transferrin production. Evaluation of the bone marrow in these conditions will, in contrast to iron deficiency, show normal to increased amounts of iron.[2]

Therapy for iron deficiency is through exogenous iron. This is most easily accomplished via oral supplementation. Many preparations of elemental iron exist, and their efficacy is roughly equivalent with each other. Patients should be informed that upon beginning iron supplementation, they may experience gastrointestinal upset with nausea, diarrhea, or constipation. This generally resolves over a few days although it frequently results in patients becoming noncompliant. In patients who experience continued problems, a decrease in dose may be needed or they may take it with meals. Occasionally, changing iron preparations will alleviate some of these problems. Stools will turn dark, reflecting nonabsorbed iron. Performing an analysis for fecal occult blood will be negative, however, unless there is concomitant loss of blood via the gastrointestinal tract.

Several preparations of iron for parenteral use exist, too. There is a risk for anaphylaxis with parenteral iron, and this risk is variable with the different preparations. If the decision is made to proceed with parenteral iron, its administration must be done in a place equipped to treat anaphylaxis. Usually, stopping the infusion and administering glucocorticoids, antihistamines, or epinephrine is all that is required. However, occasionally, vasopressor support and intubation with mechanical ventilation may be needed. The risk associated with anaphylaxis far exceeds any benefit parenteral iron provides over oral supplementation, and, thus, this is done infrequently.

For patients who are iron deficient, a simple test can determine whether or not they have the capacity to absorb iron. After determination of baseline serum iron, patients take 100 mg of iron elixir on an empty stomach. Measurement of serum iron 1 and 2 hours later can identify those who can and cannot absorb iron. For those patients whose serum iron remains less than 100 mg/dL, malabsorption exists and referral for small bowel biopsy may be indicated.[4] In such cases, the administration of subcutaneous or intravenous iron preparations may be improve anemia. For patients whose iron levels rise above 100 mg/dL, iron absorption is normal absorption and the anemia is likely related to nonadherence with oral iron.

ANEMIA OF CHRONIC DISEASE

Many conditions that affect patients in the inpatient and outpatient settings can result in anemia. However, once causes such as blood loss or nutritional deficiency are excluded, the diagnosis may be difficult. Evaluation of underlying disease states may lead to the conclusion that the anemia is a result of these conditions causing either an impaired erythrocyte production or accelerated erythrocyte destruction. Therefore, the anemia is typically attributed to "chronic disease." Increasingly, a more detailed understanding of how disease states and alterations in cytokines influence erythropoiesis is being generated.[5] Chronic diseases, such as kidney disease caused by diabetes or hypertension, heart failure, autoimmune diseases such as systemic lupus erythematosus or rheumatoid arthritis, chronic infections, and malignancies may result in anemia. Endocrinopathies including hypothyroidism and hypopituitarism may cause anemia of chronic disease. Frequently, however, these conditions are often seen along with other explanations for anemia, such as blood loss or marrow infiltration by tumor or organisms. The mechanisms through which disease states influence erythrocyte production are quite varied. Abnormal iron mobilization from macrophages to developing erythrocyte colonies is influenced by inflammatory cytokines such as interleukin-1, interleukin-6, and TNF-α.[5] Renal disease may result in a suboptimal production of erythropoietin. Fever can result in physical changes in erythrocytes that result in accelerated destruction. The end result is a blunted erythrocyte production in response to decreased circulating erythrocytes.

The laboratory measurements seen in anemia of chronic disease are quite nonspecific and may exist along with other abnormalities, further clouding the diagnosis. Usually, the anemia is mild with a normal to low-normal MCV. The reticulocyte count is often low, given the degree of anemia. This may also be seen as a normal RDW value. Measurement of serum erythropoietin is useful, especially in renal disease. Low levels of erythropoietin in anemic states indicate an underproduction. Normal to high levels indicate a lack of marrow responsiveness. Serum iron levels are low, usually, however measurement of body iron stores with serum ferritin results in a normal or increased value. As ferritin is an acute phase reactant that is frequently elevated in many inflammatory conditions, a normal or elevated level does not exclude the coexistence of iron deficiency. A useful discriminating test is the serum sTFr assay. Circulating erythrocytes contain transferrin receptors that can be shed by cleavage of the extracellular domain. The circulating levels of sTFr are an accurate measure of the ability of circulating erythrocytes to bind and absorb iron. In iron replete states, the sTFr should be normal, and elevated in iron deficiency. In anemia of chronic disease, the sTFr is typically normal to slightly elevated, but much less so than seen in iron deficiency. Therefore, the usual laboratory results in anemia of chronic disease are low serum iron, low TIBC, normal sTFr, elevated ferritin, and low reticulocyte count. Table 40-3 illustrates the laboratory differences in anemia of chronic disease and iron deficiency anemia.

Therapy for anemia of chronic disease often is treatment of the underlying condition thereby increasing the ability of the marrow to produce and release erythrocytes. It may be necessary to transfuse erythrocytes, particularly in symptomatic patients. Recombinant erythropoietin administration may be helpful, especially if serum erythropoietin levels are low. Evaluation for and supplementation of other nutrients, such as iron or folic acid, may be needed. Frequently, however, these supportive measures are often not enough to correct

Table 40-3. Laboratory Characteristics of Iron Deficiency Anemia and Anemia of Chronic Disease

Laboratory Test	Iron Deficiency	Anemia of Chronic Disease
MCV	<85 fL	72–100 fL
Serum Iron	<60 ug/dL	<60 ug/dL
TIBC	>400 ug/dL	<250 ug/dL
Ferritin	<15 ng/mL	>35 ng/mL
Serum sTFr	Increased	Normal
Transferrin saturation (sFe/TIBC)	Decreased	Normal/increased
Bone marrow iron stains	Absent	Present

MCV, mean cell volume; TIBC, total iron binding capacity; sFE, serum iron.

the anemia, especially in light of the disease states that are responsible and the therapies that are undertaken to treat them.

B$_{12}$ DEFICIENCY

Vitamin B$_{12}$ is a coenzyme responsible for the normal function of methylmalonyl coenzyme A mutase and methyltetrahydrofolate-homocysteine methyl transferase. These enzymes are responsible for normal intracellular folate metabolism and nucleic acid synthesis. In the absence of B$_{12}$, purine biosynthesis is altered and nuclear function is impaired. In hematopoiesis, B$_{12}$ deficient states results in megaloblastic erythrocytes and decreased white blood cell and platelet counts.[6]

Under normal conditions, dietary B$_{12}$ is bound to "R"-binders in the low pH stomach. As food passes into the small intestine, the higher pH results in B$_{12}$ unbinding with the R-binders and binding to intrinsic factor (IF). B$_{12}$-IF then binds to cubulin in the terminal ileum where it is transported into the bloodstream. There, B$_{12}$ is bound by transcobalamin I and transcobalamin II where it is transported to tissues. Most of the measured serum B$_{12}$ amount is bound to transcobalamin I.[7]

Many conditions exist that result in impaired B$_{12}$ uptake. Strict veganism for several years will result in B$_{12}$ deficiency. Pernicious anemia, an immune-mediated destruction of gastric parietal cells (which synthesize and release IF) or of the IF itself, is the classic diagnosis for B$_{12}$ deficiency. Gastrectomy or resection of the ileum will result in B$_{12}$ deficiency either by impaired delivery of B$_{12}$-IF or the impaired uptake of B$_{12}$-IF, respectively. Pancreatic insufficiency, via decreased ability to alkalinize gastric output, will result in an inability of B$_{12}$ to bind IF.[6]

Symptoms classically associated with B$_{12}$ deficiency are related to the neurologic changes that occur. These are generally seen in distal extremity loss of vibratory or position sense. Over time, this progresses proximally to involve the entire extremities. Demyelinization of the dorsal and lateral portions of the spinal cord may result in a spastic ataxia. Cognitive difficulties, progressive dementia, and psychosis have all been attributed to B_{12} deficiency. Despite prompt replacement of B_{12}, neurologic and psychiatric abnormalities are rarely completely resolved.[8]

Erythrocytes produced during B_{12} deficiency are larger, termed macroovalocytes. Within the marrow, production of these cells is an inefficient process, and destruction within the marrow, and in the periphery, may result in elevated values of lactate dehydrogenase (LDH) and indirect bilirubin. White blood cells are similarly disrupted in B_{12} deficiency, with the most striking changes seen in the neutrophils. Normal neutrophils contain 2 to 5 nuclear lobes. In B_{12}, and folic acid, deficiency, more than 5% of the neutrophils will contain >5 lobes, so-called "hypersegmented" neutrophils. Because of the enzymes involved, deficiency of B_{12} will result in elevation of serum values for methylmalonic acid and homocysteine. In contrast, folate deficiency will result in normal methylmalonic acid levels. If a megaloblastic anemia is encountered, determination of both the methylmalonic acid and homocysteine levels is important, along with B_{12} and folic acid. Supplementation with folic acid may correct the anemia associated with B_{12} deficiency, as well as the homocysteine levels, but the methylmalonic acid levels will remain elevated.[6]

Once B_{12} deficiency is diagnosed, prompt replacement with intramuscular injections of B_{12} is undertaken at a dose of 1000 μg weekly for 8 to 10 weeks then monthly thereafter. Any B_{12} not taken up and used by the body will undergo renal clearance and urinary excretion. Once therapy has begun, prompt resolution of erythrocyte and leukocyte deficiencies will be seen, generally within several days. Within 1 or 2 months, the anemia should be completely corrected.

FOLATE DEFICIENCY

Folic acid, like B_{12}, is necessary for the normal intracellular metabolism of nucleotides and DNA/RNA synthesis. Therefore, many of the laboratory abnormalities seen in folate deficient states are also seen in B_{12} deficiency, except methylmalonic acid (see above). Unlike B_{12}, however, folate is not present in great amounts in meats and dairy products. Our daily ingestion of folate is through green, leafy vegetables and some citrus fruits. Dietary folates are polyglutamated and, through the action of intestinal enzymes, are reduced to monoglutamate-folate. This is absorbed in the duodenum or proximal jejunum and transported to the tissues.

Excess cooking of green vegetables may leach out the folate present. Excessive alcohol consumption, with concomitant poor nutritional intake, will result in decreased folate ingestion as well. Decreased dietary intake of folate is the major cause of folate deficiency, although this has lessened over time with folate fortification of bread products. Other causes of decreased folate availability may be secondary to decreased absorption (celiac disease, regional enteritis, intestinal lymphoma or amyloidosis) or increased utilization (pregnancy, end-stage renal disease, hemolytic anemia with increased marrow response).

In general, the laboratory, neurologic and psychiatric sequelae of folate deficiency are milder than that seen in B_{12} deficiency. During pregnancy, folate deficiency has been associated with neural tube defects and cognitive deficiencies in infants. Correction of folate deficiency is accomplished with oral supplementation, generally 1 mg daily. As for B_{12}, determination of serum methylmalonic acid and homocysteine levels will aid the diagnosis and evaluation of treatment. Anemia should correct itself rather quickly, and leukocyte abnormalities should promptly resolve.

SICKLE HEMOGLOBINOPATHIES

The mutation resulting in the formation of sickle hemoglobin (HbS) is found in approximately 20% of the population in equatorial Africa, Saudi Arabia, and India.[1] This region of the world is also referred to as the "malaria belt" as a result of the high presence of *Plasmodium* sp. infections. Patients with this mutation are afforded some degree of protection from malarial infection of erythrocytes. While not as prevalent in African Americans and other descendants of these regions, it comprises a large amount of nonmalignant hematology cases, particularly in urban areas. This mutation, the first abnormal hemoglobin to be discovered, results in an amino acid substitution at codon 6 in the β-globin protein from glutamic acid to valine.[8] There are now over 400 variants of hemoglobin molecules identified. These named by a letter or the place of the molecules discovery. Sickle cell hemoglobin results in a conformational change in the deoxygenated state which can allow affected Hgb molecules to polymerize, resulting in the classic sickle erythrocyte shape. Patients who are heterozygous for the sickle mutation experience no problems unless subjected to states of low oxygen tension, such as high altitudes. Homozygotes (HbSS), however, can experience a variety of systemic problems caused by the occlusion of the microvasculature in all organs.

Familial genetic variants of sickle cell disease exist, however, all forms of sickle cell disease have similar erythrocyte abnormalities that result in occlusion of the vasculature. Sickle erythrocytes are less deformable and demonstrate increased adherence to vascular endothelial cells which results in disruption of the intimal layer of vessels. Exposure of subendothelial matrix proteins activates coagulation factors thereby contributing further to vasoocclusion. Problems that are commonly seen as a result of vasoocclusion include: bone and joint pains, acute chest syndrome, splenic sequestration, stroke, retinopathy, nonhealing leg ulcers or osteonecrosis, glomerulonephritis, and priapism. The functional or anatomic asplenia from chronic infarction predisposes patients to infection from *Streptococcus pneumoniae* and possible osteomyelitis.

Sickle erythrocytes have a markedly reduced lifespan to approximately 20 days because of intra- and extravascular hemolysis. As a result, elevated levels of serum LDH and indirect bilirubin are seen, as well as increased reticulocytosis. Patients with HbSS typically have Hct values of ~25%. Occasionally patients with HbSS may present with acute decreases in Hct. This may result from folate or iron depletion or loss of erythropoietin from renal insufficiency. Parvovirus B19 infection is classically associated with aplastic crisis in patients with HbSS. The marrow may become infected with other organisms or undergo infarction, similarly resulting in aplastic crisis. Splenic sequestration, especially in patients with Hb SC disease and HbSβ$^+$ disease, can result in precipitous declines in Hct.

The diagnosis of HbSS is made via Hgb electrophoresis. Cellulose acetate electrophoresis at alkaline pH can distinguish between HbA, A2, and S. Further distinction upon citrate agar electrophoresis at acidic pH can sort out comigrating Hemoglobin, deltaHbD (from HbS) and hemoglobin C (from HbA2). Patients with sickle cell trait (HbAS) have approximately 60% HbA and 40% HbS. Concomitant α-thalassemia can have higher percentages of HbA because of the preference of α-globins binding with nonsickle β-globins. Concomitant β$^+$ thalassemia results in decreased amounts of HbA (~15%) and increased HbS (~85%). Concomitant β°thalassemia, however, has no HbA and elevated amounts of HbA2. Homozygous HbSS similarly has no HbA, but normal amounts of HbA2 and HbF.

Treatment options for sickle cell disease are a combination of prevention efforts and aggressive intervention during crises.[8] Prevention focuses on prophylactic vaccination (Pneumovax, *Haemophilus influenzae*, and Hepatitis B) and folic acid supplementation. Education of patients to avoid crisis exacerbation by proper hydration, stress reduction, and hypothermia can reduce the frequency and severity of crises. Hydroxyurea has been shown to reduce the frequency and severity of sickle crises, probably by reducing erythrocyte-endothelial adhesion and improving erythrocyte hydration. In some patients, hydroxyurea therapy results in increased levels of HbF formation, possibly decreasing sickling tendency. Hydroxyurea results in an elevated MCV, also serving as a monitor for compliance.

During a crisis, however, if interventions at home are unable to alleviate symptoms, intravenous hydration and pain control may be required. Morphine and hydromorphone are preferable to meperidine, which can lower seizure thresholds. Oxygen may be required if hypoxemia is present. In severe cases, mechanical ventilation may be required. For most cases of sickle cell crises, transfusions of blood products are not required. During splenic sequestration or aplastic crises, transfusions may bridge recovery from these events. For acute chest syndrome, cerebrovascular accidents, or ocular vasoocclusion, exchange transfusions to keep HbA >70% is necessary. Recent trials examining patients who have experienced cerebrovascular accidents have shown that continued exchange transfusion has beneficial effects in reducing subsequent events.[8]

THALASSEMIA

Adult hemoglobin (HbA) is a tetramer, composed of two α-globin proteins and two β-globin proteins. The genes for α-globin are located on chromosome 16, with each chromosome containing two alleles for α-globin, for a total of four. The genes for β-globin are located on chromosome 11 within a cluster of genes capable of producing ε, γ-, δ-, and β-globin.[2] Each chromosome 11 contains one gene cluster each. During fetal development, production is restricted to γ-globin, with the resultant production of fetal Hgb, $α_2γ_2$, or HbF. After birth, gene switching results in primarily β-globin production, although there is some δ-globin ($α_2δ_2$ or HbA2) and HbF being produced. Patients with normal α-globin and β-globin production will have, on Hgb electrophoresis, 90% to 95% HbA, and 5% to 10% HbA2 and HbF.

Thalassemia is a condition in which there is deficient production of α-globin (α-thalassemia) and/or β-globin (β-thalassemia). The end result is the production of a decreased amount of HbA, with increased amounts of other globin tetramers. Depending on the type and severity of the respective deficiencies, the erythrocytes produced may exhibit decreased MCV, "target-cell" conformation, and/or globin tetramer inclusions. Because of their size and shape, they may undergo destruction in the periphery or within the marrow, causing a picture of hemolytic anemia. This is seen on the peripheral smear as microspherocytes or schistocytes and on serum chemistries with increased LDH and increased indirect bilirubin. With hemolysis of any origin, Hgb is released into the plasma and degraded, with the heme moiety bound by haptoglobin. Once haptoglobin has been depleted, excess heme is cleared by the kidneys and taken up by urothelial cells. This can be seen on urinary cytology as hemosiderin-laden urothelial cells are sloughed.

α-THALASSEMIA

The deficient production of α-globin is primarily seen in patients with African, Middle Eastern, Southeast Asian, or Mediterranean ancestries. This deficiency is primarily accomplished by allele deletion or the production of a truncated form of the protein.[8] Functionally, however, it results in a decreased amount of α-globin production. Hgb electrophoresis measures the relative percentages of each type of Hgb in the circulation. The majority of α-thalassemic patients will have relatively normal amounts of HbA, HbA2, and HbF, as all of these contain two α-globins each. With increasing deletion of α alleles, the Hgb electrophoresis may become abnormal, as it isolates more amounts of HbH (β_4). To make an accurate diagnosis of α-thalassemia, DNA-sequencing of α alleles is required, although rarely clinically indicated. As there are four globin alleles, there are actually six possible genotypes (Table 40-4). For zero, one, or two allele deletions, the Hgb electrophoresis will be essentially normal. The erythrocytes may display variable amounts of microcytosis, "target"-shapes, and anemia. By and large, however, these patients are asymptomatic, despite the size and shape of the erythrocytes as well as the increased extravascular hemolysis that is present. This hemolysis is generally very well compensated by chronic, increased marrow production of erythrocytes. As long as adequate iron and folate are present, severe anemia should not be present.

For three allele deletion, HbH disease, the Hgb electrophoresis displays increased amounts of β_4 and HbF and decreased amounts of HbA. The erythrocytes demonstrate severe microcytosis and evidence of hemol-

ysis. Despite this, no therapy is required, unless there is severe anemia. In these instances, to compensate for the degree of anemia, the spleen begins to produce blood cells (extramedullary hematopoiesis). The resultant splenomegaly may become massive, causing intra-abdominal compression of other organs. Splenectomy alleviates this problem, although does not correct the underlying anemic picture.

Hydrops fetalis, or four allele deletion, is usually lethal in utero or soon after birth. As there is no α-globin production, there is primarily Hb Bart (γ_4) in erythrocytes. These globin molecules have very high O_2-affinities, preventing off-loading of oxygen to the developing tissues, producing lactic acidosis and tissue edema.

β-THALASSEMIA

Defects in β-globin production can be quite varied. Mutations may result in the absent expression of a β gene and no β-globin production (β°-thalassemia) or the production of a truncated or defective β-globin (β⁺-thalassemia).[8] Seen primarily in populations of Mediterranean, Middle Eastern, Southeast Asian, and Indian descent, the degree of ineffective erythropoiesis is generally more severe than is seen with α-thalassemia. Proportionate to the degree of anemia, the microcytosis is more severe, as is the degree of extravascular hemolysis and destruction within the marrow spaces. As there are two possible defects within each β-globin gene, there are six possible genotypes (Table 40-5).

With decreased amounts of normal β-globin being produced, the cell will increase, to some degree, the amounts of δ-globin and γ-globin. The result of this can be seen on Hgb electrophoresis, with decreased amounts of HbA and increased amounts of HbA2 and HbF. If patients contain one functional β-globin gene, there will still be >50% HbA as the α-globin will preferentially associate with β-globin rather than the δ- and γ-globins.

In β-thalassemia minor, patients generally have a mild microcytic anemia with frequent target cells. The MCV is <70 fL and there are increased amounts of reticulocytes and, occasionally, nucleated red blood cells. On Hgb electrophoresis, there is increased amounts of HbA2 (>3.5%) and HbF. As patients are

Table 40-4. α-Thalassemia Genotypes

αα/αα	Normal production of α-globin
A-/αα	α⁺ thalassemia; seen in ~1/3 of African Americans
−/αα	α-thalassemia 1 (α°-thalassemia); seen primarily in Asian populations
A-/α-	α-thalassemia 2; seen in African and Mediterranean populations
A-/−	HbH disease (β_4)
−/−	hydrops fetalis; Hb Bart (γ_4) production

Table 40-5. β-Thalassemia Genotypes

B/β	Normal
B/β⁺ or β/β°	β-thalassemia minor
B°/β⁺ or β⁺/β⁺	β-thalassemia intermedia
B8/b8	b-thalassemia major; Cooley's anemia

minimally symptomatic, no therapy or transfusions are required.

In β-thalassemia intermedia, the microcytosis and anemia are more severe than seen in β-thalassemia minor. Significant splenomegaly and marrow expansion can develop to accommodate the increase in erythropoiesis. If splenomegaly becomes symptomatic, splenectomy can achieve symptom relief, without an impact on hematopoiesis. With splenectomy, there can be a marked increase in the amount of nucleated red blood cells in the circulation. With the significant anemia and the amount of hemolysis present, there is marked increase in iron absorption and availability. Eventually, patients may require iron chelation therapy with deferoxamine to prevent hepatic damage from iron overload.[2]

Patients who have Cooley's anemia, or β-thalassemia major, marrow expansion occurs in all the bones, particularly the skull and long bones. Children with this disorder frequently have growth and developmental delays as a result. These children require an aggressive transfusion program with concurrent iron chelation therapy. There is functional asplenia despite the massive splenomegaly, and recurrent bacterial infections, classically *Yersinia enterocolitica*, develop. In many centers throughout the world, allogeneic bone marrow transplantation for affected children offers the potential for cure of this disease.[2]

MICROANGIOPATHIC ANEMIA

Microangiopathic hemolytic anemia is a syndrome which results in intravascular hemolysis of red blood cells caused by a variety of underlying disorders. Mechanical heart valves may cause sheer stress and resulting lysis of cells. Disseminated intravascular hemolysis, thrombotic thrombocytopenic purpura, hemolytic-uremic syndrome, accelerated hypertension, vasculitis, or eclampsia may be associated with this anemia. Examination of the peripheral smear shows a normocytic anemia with thrombocytopenia and anisocytosis, poikilocytosis, or the presence of schistocytes. An elevated reticulocyte count is the result of rapid bone marrow response to hemolysis and anemia. An elevated LDH and bilirubin and decreased haptoglobin result from hemolysis.

The treatment of the syndrome is to address the underlying abnormalities which may include sepsis, autoimmune disorders, pregnancy, or severe hypertension.

CONCLUSION

Patients in the primary care setting often present with anemia. Through a careful history and physical examination and judicious use of appropriate laboratory tests, clues to the etiology will often present themselves. Initiation of appropriate treatment depends upon the correct diagnosis, and treatment of concomitant medical illnesses. In those situations in which the diagnosis is unclear or outside the scope of a primary care setting, referral to a hematologist should be considered.

EVIDENCE-BASED SUMMARY

- The diagnosis of anemia requires a search for the underlying etiology.
- Adults with anemia of chronic disease may benefit from administration of erythropoietin supplementation.
- Iron replacement is not necessary for anemia of chronic disease.
- Ferritin is a useful measure of iron stores.
- The sTFr assay is elevated in iron deficiency and normal to increased in anemia of chronic disease.
- B$_{12}$ and folate deficiency can result in megaloblastic anemia and hypersegmented neutrophils. Patients may develop neurologic changes.
- Sickle cell anemia is associated with many life-threatening consequences.
- Hgb electrophoresis is used to evaluate abnormalities of Hgb in variants of sickle cell anemia and thalassemias.

REFERENCES

1. Schrier SL. Approach to the adult patient with anemia. www.uptodate.com. Accessed March 13, 2007.
2. Hoffman R, Benz E, Shattil S, et al. *Hematology: Basic Principles and Practice,* 4th ed. Philadelphia, PA: Elsevier; 2005.
3. Punnonen K, Irjala K, Rajamaki A. Serum transferrin receptor and its ratio to ferritin in the diagnosis of iron deficiency. *Blood.* 1997;89:1052.
4. Cook JD. Iron Deficiency Anemia. *Curr Ther Hematol Oncol.* 1987;3:9.
5. Jongen-Lavrencic M, Peeters HR, Wognum A, et al. Elevated levels of inflammatory cytokines in the bone marrow of patients with rheumaloid arthritis and anemia of chronic disease. *J Rheumatol.* 1997;24:1504.
6. Carmel R. Current concepts in cobalamin deficiency. *Annu Rev Med* 2000;51:357.
7. George J, Williams M, et al. *American Society of Hematology Self-Assessment Program.* Washington, DC: Blackwell; 2003.
8. Steinberg MH. Management of sickle cell disease. *N Engl J Med.* 1999;340:1021.

PART 11

Infectious Diseases

CHAPTERS

Chapter 41

Lower Respiratory Tract Infections

Kelly Echevarria and Kathryn Sabol

SEARCH STRATEGY

A systematic search of the medical literature was performed on November 15, 2007. The search included relevant articles from UpToDate®, Ovid, Guidelines from the Infectious Diseases Society of America (IDSA), the American Thoracic Society (ATS), and Centers for the Disease Control and Prevention (CDC).

INTRODUCTION

Lower respiratory tract infections are a significant cause of morbidity and mortality in the United States and one of the major reasons for unscheduled physician office visits. In 1997, there were more than 10 million office visits by adults for acute bronchitis in the United States.[1] Although bronchitis and pneumonia are often felt to be a spectrum of the same disease by patients and health care providers, they are in fact distinct, and require different treatment approaches. This chapter will discuss the epidemiology and evidence-based management of acute uncomplicated bronchitis and community-acquired pneumonia (CAP). Bronchitis occurring in patients with underlying lung disease, often termed acute exacerbations of chronic bronchitis, will not be addressed here.

ACUTE BRONCHITIS

EPIDEMIOLOGY AND MICROBIOLOGY

Acute uncomplicated bronchitis is a common inflammatory condition of the tracheobronchial tree that affects as many as 5% of adults each year.[2] In contrast to more nonspecific respiratory syndromes, a majority of patients with bronchitis seek medical care from a physician. This is a result of the prevailing belief that bron-

chitis is a bacterial infection that requires antibiotic therapy to hasten resolution. In fact, literature supports the vast majority of cases of uncomplicated acute bronchitis that have a nonbacterial cause.[2] Viruses, including influenza A and B, parainfluenza, respiratory syncytial virus (RSV), rhinoviruses, adenoviruses and coronaviruses are among the more common etiologic agents. RSV seems to be of concern especially in older adults, where a significant percentage of cases will be associated with pneumonia. The only nonviral causes that have been convincingly implicated in acute uncomplicated bronchitis are *Bordetella pertussis*, *Mycoplasma pneumoniae* and *Chlamydophila pneumoniae*, and are thought to account for 5% to 10% of cases of acute bronchitis.[2] *B. pertussis* may be a particularly common cause of prolonged cough, but antibiotic therapy is not of clinical benefit, unless begun early in the illness.[3] Pathogens common to other respiratory tract infections like otitis media and pneumonia, including *Streptococcus pneumoniae*, *Haemophilus influenza* and *Moraxella catarrhalis* have not been convincingly shown to be etiologic agents in acute bronchitis in patients without underlying lung disease.

CLINICAL PRESENTATION AND DIAGNOSTIC EVALUATION

The hallmark of acute bronchitis is a cough, which may be purulent or nonpurulent, and is often prolonged in duration. Many patients begin with symptoms typical of a viral upper respiratory tract infection, but progress to persistent cough. Pulmonary function tests have been shown to be abnormal in nearly half of these patients. Bronchial hyperresponsiveness is typically evident for 2 to 3 weeks, although it may persist for up to 2 months.[3] The main focus in the evaluation of patients is in differentiating uncomplicated bronchitis from pneumonia, which requires antibiotic therapy. Although no one symptom can reliably distinguish these conditions, recent guidelines suggest the absence of vital sign abnormalities (heart rate $\geq$100 beats/min, respiratory rate $\geq$24 breaths/min, or temperature $\geq$38°C) and absence of focal physical findings on chest examination (rales, egophony, or fremitus) reduce the likelihood of pneumonia to the point where further diagnostic testing is usually unnecessary. One caveat to this is that older patients with pneumonia often present with atypical symptoms. A higher index of suspicion and diagnostic workup is indicted in these patients even in the absence of vital sign abnormalities.[3] Also, in patients with a cough persisting for longer than 3 weeks, evaluation of other causes of chronic cough such as postnasal drip, asthma and gastroesophageal reflux may be useful.

MANAGEMENT

Reviewing the etiologies should make it obvious that antimicrobial therapy is unlikely to benefit patients with acute uncomplicated bronchitis. Numerous clinical trials and meta-analyses support this claim, showing no or minimal benefit of antibiotics over placebo on duration of illness, limitation of activity or loss of work.[2,4] Although older studies were criticized for design flaws, a recent well-designed study of azithromycin versus a vitamin C control found no benefit of antibiotics on health-related quality of life or return to work.[5] Other trials have shown a benefit of albuterol over antibiotics, possibly because of the decreasing bronchial hyperresponsiveness.[6] The usefulness in patients without airway obstruction, however, is controversial. A recent meta-analysis did not find benefit in the routine use of β-agonists for acute bronchitis.[7] Despite the fact that antibiotics provide minimal benefit, a recent survey found over 60% of patients who visited a physician for bronchitis were given a prescription for an antibiotic, and over half of those were for broad-spectrum antibiotics.[8] This is in the face of a public health crisis, where few antibiotics are in the developmental pipeline and antibiotic resistance both in and out of hospitals is soaring. As a result, in 2001 the CDC partnered with the American Academy of Family Physicians, the American College of Physicians-American Society of Internal Medicine, and the IDSA to issue a joint statement on the management of uncomplicated acute bronchitis.[2] The guideline focuses on ruling out pneumonia (see Subsection "Clinical Presentation and Diagnostic Evaluation" above), and educating patients on the lack of benefit of antimicrobial therapy for acute bronchitis. Antibiotics are not recommended for patients with acute uncomplicated bronchitis, regardless of cough duration. Education is critical as physicians cite patient expectations a major reason for prescribing antibiotics despite the lack of benefit. Clinicians should employ tactics such as referring to bronchitis as a "chest cold," explaining the dangers of resistance and antibiotic adverse effects, and counseling patients about appropriate symptomatic management and realistic estimates of cough duration. The societal and financial harm of antibiotic misuse cannot be overstated. Antibiotic use predicts antibiotic resistance both in a society as well as individual patients, and is associated with worse patient outcomes. Finally, the cost of unnecessary prescriptions for respiratory tract infections has been estimated at over $700 million each year in the United States alone.[3] It is encouraging that interventions designed to reduce unnecessary antibiotic use have found significant reduction in the prescription of antibiotics without increasing adverse outcomes or return physician visits.

EVIDENCE-BASED TREATMENT OF ACUTE BRONCHITIS

- The vast majority of acute bronchitis in adults without underlying lung disease is viral in origin and requires no treatment other than supportive care.
- Older patients may not manifest classic symptoms of pneumonia and providers should have a lower threshold for obtaining a chest radiograph in patients with symptoms of bronchitis and wheezing.
- β-Agonists may provide some relief in patients with symptoms of acute bronchitis, especially in the setting of chronic cough.
- Indiscriminate use of antibiotics leads to increased cost and resistance, and may not improve patient satisfaction with their providers.

COMMUNITY-ACQUIRED PNEUMONIA

EPIDEMIOLOGY AND MICROBIOLOGY

CAP is an acute infection of the pulmonary parenchyma. It is associated with symptoms of acute infection accompanied by an infiltrate on chest radiograph in patients who have not been recently hospitalized or resided in a long-term care facility.[9] Approximately 4 million cases of CAP are diagnosed each year, resulting in an estimated 10 million physician visits, 600 000 hospitalizations, and 45 000 deaths in the United States.[10] Nearly 80% of these patients are treated in the outpatient setting, with a consequent mortality of less than 1%.

The etiologic agent of CAP remains elusive in up to half of the patients, even with extensive diagnostic testing. *S. pneumoniae* is consistently the most common pathogen isolated in nearly every prospective series of CAP. Other pathogens commonly isolated include

H. influenzae, and *M. catarrhalis,* and the atypical organisms—*M. pneumoniae, C. pneumoniae,* and *Legionella pneumophila.* Respiratory viruses have also been implicated, especially Influenza A and B, parainfluenza, and RSV.[9-11] Some patients may have more than one etiologic agent responsible for CAP, such as a mixture of typical and atypical organisms.

CLINICAL PRESENTATION AND DIAGNOSTIC EVALUATION

Symptoms of CAP include fever, productive or nonproductive cough, pleuritic chest pain and dyspnea. Older patients may present with atypical symptoms such as confusion or failure to thrive.[11] Unfortunately, physical examination is neither sensitive nor specific in diagnosing CAP.[9] Guidelines endorsed by the IDSA and the ATS strongly recommend chest radiographs in all patients when the diagnosis of CAP is considered.[11] Providers should avoid feeding the problem of antibiotic overuse and resistance by treating suspected patients with antibiotics. A sputum gram stain and culture is also useful, but may not be possible, particularly in the outpatient setting.[11] In hospitalized patients, additional diagnostic testing should include a complete blood count and differential, chemistry testing, and a measure of oxygenation (oximetry or arterial blood gas). Blood cultures are optional in most cases, but should be performed in patients with severe CAP, chronic liver disease, and alcohol abuse or in those failing therapy. If the chest radiograph shows evidence of pleural effusion or cavitary pneumonia, blood and sputum cultures should be obtained.[11] Newer diagnostic tests such as the pneumococcal urinary antigen may also prove useful in some situations.

MANAGEMENT

Impact of Initial Site of Treatment

The decision to treat a patient with CAP as an outpatient or an inpatient may be the single most important clinical decision throughout the course of illness.[9,11] Overall mortality for patients with CAP is approximately 14%. However, it is less than 1% for outpatients and nearly 30% in patients treated in the hospital. Determination of initial treatment site should be based on several factors, including age, severity of illness, other comorbid conditions and social support issues. A number of factors have been shown to be associated with an increased risk of mortality (Table 41-1).

Applying these risk factors is difficult. It has been suggested physicians often overestimate a patient's risk of death, with a resultant increase in hospitalization rates. Considering that the average cost of care for inpatient management of CAP is $7500 versus $150-350

Table 41-1. Criteria for Severe CAP

Respiratory rate $\geq$ 30 breaths/min
PaO$_2$/FiO$_2$ $\leq$ 250
Multilobar infiltrates
Confusion/disorientation
Uremia (BUN $\geq$ 20 mg/dL)
Leukopenia (WBC count < 4000 cells/mm^2)
Thrombocytopenia (platelet count < 100 000 cells/mm^2)
Hypothermia (core temperature < 36°C)
Hypotension requiring aggressive fluid resuscitation
Need for invasive mechanical ventilation
Need for vasopressors for septic shock

Adapted from Ref. 11.

for outpatient care, considerable energy has been expended to identify patients at low risk of death who may benefit from outpatient therapy.[12] One method to accomplish this is through the use of prognostic scoring systems such as the Pneumonia Severity Index (PSI) and the CURB-65.[13,14] The PSI is a tool to predict short-term mortality with CAP and divides patients into five risk classes. Patients are categorized as class I if they are younger than 50 years of age, have normal mental status, relatively normal vital signs and do not possess any of the five comorbid conditions—neoplastic disease, liver disease, congestive heart failure, cerebrovascular disease, or renal disease. Classes II to V are based on points assigned for demographic factors, comorbid conditions, physical findings, and laboratory and radiographic findings. Investigators found that patients in class I or II are at lower risk for mortality (<1%) and can generally be treated as outpatients. Patients in class III have slightly higher mortality (1%–3%) and may require brief observation in an inpatient unit. Finally, patients in class IV or V are at the highest risk (10%–30% mortality) and require hospitalization. Although the PSI is useful, it is complicated to calculate, is heavily weighted by age, and does not account for social issues such as substance abuse, noncompliance, and poor family support. More recently, a modification of the British Thoracic Society criteria, known as CURB-65 has been correlated with risk for mortality.[14] Patients are assigned a point for confusion, BUN > 20 mg/dL, respiratory rate $\geq$30 breaths/minute, low blood pressure (SBP <90 or DBP $\leq$60 mm Hg) and age $\geq$ 65 years. The number of points correlates well with mortality, with rates of 0.7%, 2%, 9%, 14%, 40%, and 57%, respectively, for those patients with 0, 1, 2, 3, 4, or 5 factors. As a result, patients with a score of 0 to 1 could be treated as outpatients, while those with higher scores should be hospitalized. The use of either scoring system can decrease the number of patients hospitalized with CAP, but it is unclear which is superior. The ease of the CURB-65 makes it a quick and useful tool to assist in the

Table 41-2. Empiric Antibiotic Therapy for CAP in Outpatients

Population	Drug Therapy
Previously healthy adults No recent antibiotic therapy	Macrolide* or doxycycline
Recent antibiotic therapy or comorbidities present	Respiratory fluoroquinolone[†] β-lactam[‡] plus a macrolide or doxycycline

*Azithromycin or clarithromycin.
[†]Levofloxacin 750 mg, moxifloxacin, gemifloxacin.
[‡]High-dose amoxicillin (1g three times daily), high-dose amoxicillin/ clavulanate (2g twice daily), ceftriaxone, cefpodoxime, or cefuroxime.
Adapted from Ref. 11.

decision to hospitalize. Whichever scoring system the physician chooses should be supplemented with clinical judgment, and recognition of social factors that may compromise the safety of outpatient treatment.

Antibiotic Treatment

Antibiotics are the mainstay of therapy for CAP. As described above, pneumonia is caused by a variety of pathogens. Given the difficulty in establishing an etiologic diagnosis, treatment is largely empiric. Initial antibiotic therapy for outpatients with CAP is based on two factors. These include the presence or absence of recent antibiotic therapy and the presence of comorbidities, such as cardiopulmonary disease, diabetes, renal or liver disease, asplenia, and malignancy. Patients should also be assessed for risk of infection with multidrug-resistant pathogens, including recent hospitalization or nursing home residence. These patients should be treated as healthcare-associated pneumonia, rather than CAP.[15] Initial suggested empiric antibiotic regimens are listed in Table 41-2.

Outpatients who are otherwise healthy with no recent antibiotic use or comorbidities can be given a macrolide antibiotic or doxycycline. Each demonstrates adequate coverage of the likely organisms (*S. pneumoniae, H. influenzae, M. pneumoniae* and *C. pneumoniae*). In patients with recent antibiotic use or co morbid conditions, coverage for penicillin nonsusceptible *S. pneumoniae* should be considered (see Subsection "Drug-Resistant *S. pneumoniae*" below). If aspiration is suspected coverage of oral anaerobes with either amoxicillin-clavulanate or clindamycin is indicated.

Drug-Resistant *S. pneumoniae*

Drug-resistant *S. pneumoniae* (DRSP) (penicillin MIC ≥4 mcg/mL) has been a problem in recent years. Risk factors for DRSP include age >65 years, β-lactam use within the previous 3 months, alcoholism, immunosuppressive illness, and exposure to a child in daycare.[11] Resistance to penicillin in *S. pneumoniae* often results in resistance to other classes of drugs, such as tetracyclines and macrolides. If DRSP is suspected, several β-lactam

antibiotics can still successfully be used. Ideal choices include high-dose amoxicillin (1 g three times daily) or amoxicillin/clavulanate (2 g twice daily). Other suitable agents to consider include cefuroxime or cefpodoxime.[11] Respiratory fluoroquinolones are active against the majority of strains of DRSP.

Appropriate duration of treatment remains an area of uncertainty. Few controlled trials have been conducted assessing length of treatment for CAP. Physicians should consider the offending pathogen, response to treatment, and complications. A reasonable course of therapy is 7 to 10 days for most patients. Recent studies have found durations of as short as 5 days to be successful in a large percentage of patients, although further study is needed.[11]

Initial response to therapy is often seen within the first 3 days of antibiotic therapy, although defervescence may not occur until several days later. Radiographic findings are much slower to resolve and can be abnormal for several months. Several considerations should be taken into account in patients who fail to respond to initial therapy. These include incorrect diagnosis, host failure, incorrect antibiotic or dose, unusual pathogen, adverse drug reactions, or complications such as empyema.

Viral Causes of Pneumonia

As discussed earlier many viruses cause pneumonia and may account for up to half of patients hospitalized for an acute respiratory condition.[11] Influenza also predisposes patients to bacterial superinfection. Patients with cardiopulmonary conditions and those older than 65 years of age are at increased risk for complications and death from influenza.[11] Rapid antigen tests for influenza A and B are available and are recommended for early identification and treatment initiation. Treatment with antiviral agents within 48 hours of symptom onset will reduce the duration of illness by 1 to 2 days.[11] Preliminary data also suggest early use of antivirals may decrease the incidence of lower respiratory tract complications.[16] The neuraminidase inhibitors, zanamivir and oseltamivir, are active against both influenza A and B. Oseltamivir is given orally while zanamivir is administered through inhalation; oseltamivir is recommended in patients with concurrent asthma or COPD due to the risk of bronchospasm with zanamivir. Amantadine and rimantadine currently have a very limited role in the treatment and prophylaxis of influenza due to an increased rate of resistance in circulating influenza viruses.[17]

Prevention

Considering the morbidity and mortality associated with CAP, prevention is an important goal. The best data on prevention of CAP comes from the influenza vaccine, where meta-analysis demonstrates the administration of the influenza vaccine in elderly adults decreases the overall incidence of pneumonia by 53%, hospitalization by 50% and death by 68%.[18] The CDC currently recommends that all patients 6 to 59 months or ≥50 years of age, pregnant women and patients with chronic medical conditions be administered the influenza vaccine yearly.[17] Vaccination is also recommendation for health care workers to prevent transmission to high-risk patients. In 2003, the U.S. Food and Drug Administration (FDA) approved a live, attenuated influenza vaccine that is administered intranasally, and is recommended for healthy persons aged 5 to 49 years. Because it is a live vaccine, it should be avoided in children younger than 5 years of age and individuals older than 50 years of age, patients with chronic pulmonary, cardiac or metabolic conditions, and those with underlying immunosuppressive conditions. Health care workers, family members, and those with close contact to immunosuppressed individuals should also be excluded from receiving the intranasal vaccine. High-risk patients exposed to influenza should be considered for chemoprophylaxis with antivirals.

Studies demonstrating overall effectiveness of the 23-valent pneumococcal vaccine for prevention of pneumonia are less conclusive. The pneumococcal vaccine is recommended for all adults older than 65 years of age, and younger patients with chronic diseases such as diabetes, cardiovascular or lung diseases, alcoholism, renal failure, and immune system disorders.[11] Revaccination is recommended 5 years after the first.

EVIDENCE-BASED TREATMENT OF CAP

- The decision whether or not to hospitalize a patient with CAP may be the most important treatment decision and there are several scoring systems which can aid providers.
- Treatment decisions should be based on risk factors for drug-resistant organisms, such as recent antibiotic use and comorbidities.
- Coverage for atypical organisms should always be included in empiric treatment regimens.
- Prevention of pneumonia in high-risk patients through the use of influenza and pneumococcal vaccine is extremely important.

REFERENCES

1. Schappert SM. Ambulatory care visits to physician offices, hospital outpatient departments and emergency departments: United States 1997. *Vital and Health Statistics*. Series 13, No. 143. Hyattsville, MD: U.S. Department of Health and Human Services, Centers for Disease Control and Prevention, National Center for Health Statistics; 1999. DHHS publication no. 2000-1714.

2. Gonzales R, Bartlett JG, Besser RE, et al. Principles of appropriate antibiotic use for treatment of uncomplicated acute bronchitis: Background. *Ann Intern Med.* 2001;134:521-529.

3. Aagaard E, Gonzales R. Management of acute bronchitis in healthy adults. *Infect Dis Clinics of North America.* 2004;18: 919-937.

4. Bent S, Saint S, Vittinghoff E, et al. Antibiotics in acute bronchitis: A meta-analysis. *Am J Med.* 1999;107:62-67.

5. Evans A, Husain S, Durairaj L, et al. Azithromycin for acute bronchitis: A randomized, double-blind controlled trial. *Lancet.* 2002;359:1648-1654.

6. Hueston WJ. A comparison of albuterol and erythromycin for the treatment of acute bronchitis. *J Fam Pract.* 1991;33:476-480.

7. Smucny JJ, Flynn CA, Becker LA, et al. Are Beta-2-agonists effective treatment for acute bronchitis or acute cough in patients without underlying pulmonary disease? A systematic review. *J Fam Pract.* 2001;50:945.

8. Steinman M., Landefeld CS, Gonzales R. Predictors of broad-spectrum antibiotic prescribing for acute respiratory tract infections in adult primary care. *JAMA.* 2003;289:719-725.

9. Bartlett JG, Dowell SF, Mandell LA, et al. Practice guidelines for the management of community-acquired pneumonia in adults. *Clin Infect Dis.* 2000;31:347.

10. Mandell L. Epidemiology and etiology of community-acquired pneumonia. *Infect Dis Clinics.* 2004;18:761-776.

11. Mandell LA, Bartlett JG, Dowell SF, et al. Infectious Diseases Society of America/American Thoracic Society consensus guidelines on the management of community-acquired pneumonia in adults. *Clin Infect Dis.* 2007;44:527–572

12. Lave JR, Lin CC, Fine MJ. The cost of treating patients with community-acquired pneumonia. *Semin Respir Crit Care Med.* 1999;20:189-198.

13. Fine MJ, Auble TE, Yealy DM, et al. A prediction rule to identify low-risk patients with community-acquired pneumonia. *N Engl J Med.* 1997;336(4):243.

14. Lim WS, van der Eerden MM, Laing R, et al. Defining community acquired pneumonia severity on presentation to the hospital: An international derivation and validation study. *Thorax.* 2003;58:377-382.

15. Guidelines for the management of adults with hospital-acquired, ventilator-associated and healthcare-associated pneumonia. *Am J Resp Crit Care Med.* 2005;171:388-416.

16. Kaiser L, Wat C, Mills T, et al. Impact of oseltamivir treatment on influenza-related lower respiratory tract complications and hospitalizations. *Arch Intern Med.* 2003;163: 1667-1672.

17. Prevention and Control of Influenza. Recommendations of the Advisory Committee on Immunization Practices (ACIP). *MMWR.* 2007;56/RR-6.

18. Gross PA, Hermogenes AW, Sacks HS, et al. The efficacy of influenza vaccine in elderly persons: A meta-analysis and review of the literature. *Ann Intern Med.* 1995;123: 518-527.

Chapter 42

Skin and Soft Tissue Infections

Douglas N. Fish

SEARCH STRATEGY

A systematic search of the medical literature was performed in January, 2008. The search, limited to human subjects and English language journals, included MEDLINE®, PubMed, the Cochrane Database of Systematic Reviews, and UpToDate®. The current Infectious Disease Society of America practice guidelines for management of skin and soft tissue infections and those for diabetic foot infections can be found at www.idsociety.org.

The skin serves as a barrier between humans and their environment and therefore functions as a primary defense mechanism against infections. The skin consists of the following layers and structures: (1) the epidermis, the outermost nonvascular layer of the skin, (2) the dermis, the layer of skin directly beneath the epidermis which consists of connective tissue containing blood vessels and lymphatics, sensory nerve endings, sweat and sebaceous glands, hair follicles, and smooth-muscle fibers, and (3) the subcutaneous fat, a layer of loose connective tissue beneath the dermis which primarily consists of fat cells. Beneath the subcutaneous fat lies the fascia, which separates the skin from underlying muscle. Skin and soft tissue infections (SSTIs) may involve any or all layers of the skin, fascia, and muscle. They may also spread far from the initial site of infection and lead to more severe complications, such as endocarditis, sepsis, or streptococcal glomerulonephritis. The treatment of SSTIs may at times necessitate both medical and surgical management. Various infections of the skin are a common reason for patients seeking attention from primary care providers; cellulitis was listed as the primary reason for office visits in approximately 2% of members of one health plan.[1] It is therefore imperative that primary care providers have adequate knowledge of the appropriate evaluation and management of common SSTIs.

Bacterial infections of the skin can broadly be classified as primary or secondary (see Table 42-1).[2] Primary bacterial infections usually involve areas of previously healthy skin and are typically caused by a single pathogen. In contrast, secondary infections occur in areas of previously damaged skin and are frequently polymicrobic. SSTIs are also classified as complicated or uncomplicated. Infections are considered complicated when they involve deeper skin structures (fascia, muscle layers, etc.), require significant surgical intervention, or occur in patients with compromised immune function (diabetes mellitus, human immunodeficiency virus [HIV], etc.).[3]

The skin and subcutaneous tissues are normally extremely resistant to infection but may become susceptible under certain conditions. Even when high concentrations of bacteria are applied topically or injected into the soft tissue, resultant infections are rare. The majority of SSTIs result from the disruption of normal host defenses by processes such as skin puncture, abrasion, or underlying diseases (e.g., diabetes). The nature and severity of the infection depends on both the type of microorganism present and the site of inoculation.[2,3]

IMPETIGO

Impetigo is a superficial skin infection that is seen most commonly in children of age 2 to 5 years, and is easily transmitted from person to person. The infection is generally classified as bullous or nonbullous based on clinical presentation. Impetigo is most common during hot, humid weather, which facilitates microbial colonization of the skin. Minor trauma, such as scratches or insect bites, then allows entry of organisms into the superficial layers of skin and infection ensues. Impetigo

Table 42-1. Classification of Skin and Soft Tissue Infections Encountered in Primary Care[2,5]

Primary infections
    Impetigo
    Erysipelas
    Folliculitis
    Furuncles and carbuncles
    Cellulitis
Secondary infections
    Infected bite wounds
        Animal bites
        Human bites
    Diabetic Foot infections

Table 42-2. Bacterial Etiology of Skin and Soft Tissue Infections

Infection	Pathogens
Impetigo	*S. aureus*, Group A streptococci (*S. pyogenes*)
Erysipelas	Group A streptococci, rarely *S. aureus*
Folliculitis	*S. aureus*
Furuncles and carbuncles	*S. aureus*
Cellulitis	*S. aureus*, group A streptococci; MRSA becoming more common; enteric Gram-negative bacilli and/or anaerobes occur in diabetics, injection drug users
Infected bite wounds Animal bites	*P. multocida*, streptococci, staphylococci, *Moraxella, Neisseria, Bacteroides*, other anaerobes
Human bites	Streptococci, *S. aureus, Haemophilus, E. corrodens*, anaerobes
Diabetic foot infections	*S. aureus*, streptococci, enteric Gram-negative bacilli, *P. aeruginosa; Bacteroides, Peptostreptococcus*, other anaerobes

MRSA, methicillin-resistant *S. aureus*

is highly communicable and readily spreads through close contact, especially among siblings, day care centers, and schools.[2,4]

ETIOLOGY[2,4,5]

Traditionally, nearly all cases of impetigo were caused by group A streptococci (i.e., *Streptococcus pyogenes*) (refer to Table 42-2). However, *Staphylococcus aureus*, either alone or in combination with *S. pyogenes*, has more recently emerged as the principal cause of impetigo. The bullous form is caused by strains of *S. aureus* capable of producing exfoliative toxins. The bullous form most frequently affects neonates and accounts for approximately 10% of all cases of impetigo.

CLINICAL PRESENTATION[1,2,4,5]

Nonbullous impetigo manifests initially as small, painless vesicular lesions on the skin. These vesicles usually occur on exposed areas of the skin such as the face and extremities. The vesicles then rapidly become pustules. These pustules usually then rupture within 4 to 6 days and form characteristic thick, golden-yellow crusts. Itching is common and scratching spreads the infection. Most lesions heal without scars and systemic manifestations of the infection are minimal.

Bullous impetigo is characterized by skin lesions which are superficial, thin-walled, fluid-filled with clear or amber-colored liquid, ranging in size from 0.5 to 3 cm in diameter, and surrounded by an erythematous margin. The bullae may be flaccid or tense, and they also eventually rupture to release fluid and form a shiny film over the denuded area.

DIAGNOSTIC EVALUATION[2,4]

Diagnosis of impetigo is usually made by history and examination. This infection most commonly occurs in children, and soliciting a careful history from the child

or parents will often reveal the presence of some sort of minor trauma prior to appearance of the lesions. The presence of new vesicular and older pustular lesions, the latter associated with the characteristic honey-yellow crusts, are usually sufficient to make the diagnosis. Microbiological diagnosis is usually not required, but may be made by culturing the base of lesions that have had the crusts removed. In bullous impetigo, microbiological diagnosis may be made by culturing fluid aspirated from the lesions. However, cultures are usually not necessary since this infection is caused almost exclusively by *S. aureus*.

MANAGEMENT[1,2,4,5]

Although impetigo may resolve spontaneously, antimicrobial treatment is indicated to relieve symptoms, prevent formation of new lesions, and prevent complications such as a secondary cellulitis. Antibiotic selection for management of impetigo is summarized in Table 42-3. Penicillinase-resistant penicillins, for example, dicloxacillin, are preferred for treatment because of the increased incidence of infections caused by *S. aureus*. Amoxicillin/ clavulanic acid and first-generation cephalosporins such as cephalexin are also effective. Although penicillin is effective for infections known to be caused by *S. pyogenes*, impetigo is usually treated empirically without microbiological diagnosis and antistaphylococcal agents are initially recommended. Penicillin-allergic patients can be treated with clindamycin or erythromycin; however, resistance to erythromycin among *S. aureus* and *S. pyogenes* is increasing in some geographical areas and this drug should be used cautiously. Mupirocin 2% ointment (applied topically 3 times daily) is as effective as erythromycin and provides a useful alternative to systemic antibiotic therapy in some patients.[6] Retapamulin 1% ointment (applied topically twice daily) may also be considered as an alternative to systemic therapy for the treatment of mild impetigo. The usual duration of antibiotic therapy is 7 to 10 days. In addition to antibiotics, removal of the crusts by soaking with soap and warm water is helpful in the healing of the ruptured lesions and providing symptomatic relief, particularly for itching often associated with the thick crusts. With proper treatment, healing of skin lesions is generally rapid and occurs without residual scarring.

ERYSIPELAS

Erysipelas is a superficial cellulitis of the skin with prominent lymphatic involvement. Infections are most common in infants, young children, and older people. Predisposing factors include venous stasis, diabetes mellitus, alcohol abuse, and nephrotic syndrome. Erysipelas also commonly occurs in areas of preexisting lymphatic obstruction or edema.[2,7]

ETIOLOGY

Organisms which cause erysipelas gain access to underlying tissues through small breaks in the skin. The infection is almost always caused by group A β-hemolytic streptococci (*S. pyogenes*). Very rarely these infections are caused by *S. aureus*.[2,4,7]

CLINICAL PRESENTATION[2,4,7]

Approximately 70% to 80% of erysipelas infections are found on the lower extremities, the remainder involving the face. Erysipelas is characterized by a painful lesion with a bright red, edematous, indurated appearance and an advancing, raised border that is sharply demarcated from adjacent normal skin. The intense red color and burning pain associated with this skin infection has led to the common name of St. Anthony's fire. The sharply demarcated border and lesions which are raised above the level of the surrounding skin are the two clinical features that differentiate erysipelas from cellulitis. Fever and malaise are prominent clinical features of erysipelas and leukocytosis is common. Because erysipelas itself can cause lymphatic obstruction, a risk factor for this type of infection, it tends to recur in areas of previous infection. Approximately 30% of patients will have a recurrent infection within 3 years of a previous episode of erysipelas.

DIAGNOSTIC EVALUATION

Diagnosis is nearly always made based on the characteristic lesion. Cultures obtained by aspiration of the advancing edges of the lesion or by punch biopsy may yield causative organisms, but the overall presentation of the infection is distinctive enough that cultures are not routinely recommended.

MANAGEMENT[1,2,5,7]

The goal of treatment of erysipelas is rapid eradication of the infection. Most cases of erysipelas are relatively mild and can be treated in the outpatient setting with oral antibiotics, although more extensive lesions may require hospitalization and parenteral antibiotics. Mild-to-moderate cases of erysipelas in both adults and children may be treated with penicillin V potassium (VK) (Table 42-3). A penicillinase-resistant penicillin or first-generation cephalosporin are also acceptable treatments. Mild-to-moderate erysipelas in penicillin-allergic patients may be treated with clindamycin or erythromycin.

Erysipelas generally responds quickly to appropriate antimicrobial therapy with marked improvement usually seen within 48 hours. Temperature and white blood cell count should return to normal within 48 to 72 hours. Erythema, edema, and pain should also gradually resolve.

FOLLICULITIS

Folliculitis is inflammation of the hair follicle. Infection occurring at the base of the eyelid is referred to as a stye. Folliculitis can be caused by physical injury, chemical irritation, or infection. Inadequate chlorine levels in whirlpools, hot tubs, and swimming pools which lead to the presence of large numbers of bacterial organisms may cause outbreaks of folliculitis.[1,2,4]

ETIOLOGY

S. aureus is the most common cause of folliculitis. Folliculitis associated with contaminated whirlpools and hot tubs are often caused by *Pseudomonas aeruginosa*. This organism, as well as other Gram-negative bacilli, has also been associated with folliculitis as a complication in patients with acne. Most cases seen by primary care practitioners will, however, be caused by *S. aureus*.[1,2,4]

CLINICAL PRESENTATION AND DIAGNOSTIC EVALUATION

Folliculitis is associated with small (2–5 mm), erythematous, sometimes pruritic papular lesions. These lesions

Table 42-3. Recommended Drugs and Dosing Regimens for Initial Outpatient Treatment of Skin and Soft Tissue Infections

Type of Infection	Drug and Oral Adult Dose	Drug and Daily Oral Pediatric Dose
Impetigo	Dicloxacillin 250–500 mg every 6 h Amoxicillin/clavulanic acid 875 mg/125 mg every 12 h Cephalexin 250–500 mg every 6 h Clindamycin 300–600 mg every 6–8 h[*] Mupirocin ointment every 8 h[*] Retapamulin ointment every 12 hours[*]	Dicloxacillin 25–50 mg/kg in four divided doses Amoxicillin/clavulanic acid 40 mg/kg (of the amoxicillin component) in two divided doses Cephalexin 25–50 mg/kg in four divided doses Clindamycin 10–30 mg/kg per day in 3–4 divided doses[*] Mupirocin ointment every 8 h[*] Retapamulin ointment every 12 hours[*]
Erysipelas	Penicillin VK 250–500 mg every 6 h Dicloxacillin 250–500 mg every 6 h Cephalexin 250–500 mg every 6 h Erythromycin 250–500 mg every 6 h[*]	Penicillin VK 40,000–90,000 units/kg in four divided doses Dicloxacillin 25–50 mg/kg in four divided doses Cephalexin 25–50 mg/kg in four divided doses Erythromycin 30–50 mg/kg in four divided doses[*]
Folliculitis	None; warm saline compresses usually sufficient	
Furuncles and carbuncles	Dicloxacillin 250–500 mg every 6 h Clindamycin 300–600 mg every 6–8 h[*]	Dicloxacillin 25–50 mg/kg in four divided doses Clindamycin 10–30 mg/kg/d in 3–4 divided doses[*]
Cellulitis	Dicloxacillin 250–500 mg every 6 h Amoxicillin/clavulanic acid 875 mg/125 mg every 12 h Cephalexin 250–500 mg every 6 h Cefadroxil 500–1000 mg every 12 h Fluoroquinolone (levofloxacin 500–750 mg every 24 h or moxifloxacin 400 mg every 24 h)[*] TMP/SMX 160 mg/800 mg every 12 h[*] Doxycycline 100–200 mg every 12 h[*]	Dicloxacillin 25–50 mg/kg in four divided doses Amoxicillin/clavulanic acid 40 mg/kg (of the amoxicillin component) in two divided doses Cephalexin 25–50 mg/kg in four divided doses Cefadroxil 30 mg/kg in two divided doses Clindamycin 10–30 mg/kg/d in 3–4 divided doses[*] TMP/SMX 4–6 mg/kg (of the trimethoprim component) every 12 h[*]
Animal bite	Amoxicillin/clavulanic acid 875 mg/125 mg every 12 h Doxycycline 100–200 mg every 12 h[*] Dicloxacillin 250–500 mg every 6 h + Penicillin VK 250–500 mg every 6 h Cefuroxime axetil 500 mg every 12 h + metronidazole 250–500 mg every 8 h or clindamycin 300–600 mg every 6–8 h Fluoroquinolone (levofloxacin 500–750 mg every 24 h or moxifloxacin 400 mg every 24 h) + metronidazole 250–500 mg every 8 h or clindamycin 300–600 mg every 6–8 h[*]	Amoxicillin/clavulanic acid 40 mg/kg (of the amoxicillin component) in two divided doses Dicloxacillin 25–50 mg/kg in four divided doses + Penicillin VK 40,000–90,000 units/kg in four divided doses Cefuroxime axetil 20–30 mg/kg in two divided doses + metronidazole 30 mg/kg in 3–4 divided doses or clindamycin 10–30 mg/kg/d in 3–4 divided doses TMP/SMX 4–6 mg/kg (of the trimethoprim component) every 12 h + metronidazole 30 mg/kg in 3–4 divided doses or clindamycin 10–30 mg/kg/d in 3–4 divided doses[*]
Human bite	Amoxicillin/clavulanic acid 875 mg/125 mg every 12 h Doxycycline 100–200 mg every 12 h[*] Dicloxacillin 250–500 mg every 6 h + Penicillin VK 250–500 mg every 6 h Cefuroxime axetil 500 mg every 12 h + metronidazole 250–500 mg every 8 h or clindamycin 300–600 mg every 6–8 h Fluoroquinolone (levofloxacin 500–750 mg every 24 h or moxifloxacin 400 mg every 24 h) + metronidazole 250–500 mg every 8 h or clindamycin 300–600 mg every 6–8 h[*]	Amoxicillin/clavulanic acid 40 mg/kg (of the amoxicillin component) in two divided doses Dicloxacillin 25–50 mg/kg in four divided doses + Penicillin VK 40,000–90,000 units/kg in four divided doses Cefuroxime axetil 20–30 mg/kg in two divided doses + metronidazole 30 mg/kg in 3–4 divided doses or clindamycin 10–30 mg/kg/d in 3–4 divided doses TMP/SMX 4–6 mg/kg (of the trimethoprim component) every 12 h + metronidazole 30 mg/kg in 3–4 divided doses or clindamycin 10–30 mg/kg/d in 3–4 divided doses[*]
Diabetic foot infections	Amoxicillin/clavulanic acid 875 mg/125 mg every 12 h Fluoroquinolone (levofloxacin 750 mg every 24 h or moxifloxacin 400 mg every 24 h) + metronidazole 250–500 mg every 8 h or clindamycin 300–600 mg every 6–8 h[*]	

[*] Recommended for patients with penicillin allergy.
TMP/SMX, trimethoprim/sulfamethoxazole.

are often topped by a central pustule. Systemic signs of infection such as fever and malaise are uncommon, although they have been reported in cases caused by *P. aeruginosa*.[1,2,4] Folliculitis associated with contaminated whirlpools and hot tubs generally appears within 48 hours after exposure to the contaminated water.[2]

The pruritic lesions are usually found on the buttocks, hips, and axillae and are typically limited to the trunk below the upper part of the chest or neck, corresponding to the water level. Diagnosis is usually made by the characteristic clinical findings and cultures or more extensive work-up are seldom performed.

MANAGEMENT[1,2,4]

Treatment of folliculitis generally requires only local measures, such as warm saline compresses, or topical antibiotic therapy with clindamycin, erythromycin, mupirocin, or benzoyl peroxide (Table 42-3).[6] Topical agents are generally applied 2 to 4 times daily for 7 days. Many follicular infections resolve spontaneously without medical or surgical intervention, generally within 5 days. Lesions may need to be incised if they do not respond to a few days of moist heat and over-the-counter topical agents. Following drainage, most lesions begin to heal within several days. Scarring or more serious complications rarely develop from mild cases of folliculitis. Folliculitis associated with whirlpools or hot tubs which does not spontaneously resolve, or which appears to be worsening, may be treated with oral ciprofloxacin or levofloxacin.[2]

FURUNCLES AND CARBUNCLES

Furuncles and carbuncles occur when a follicular infection extends from around the hair shaft to involve the deeper areas of the skin. A furuncle, commonly known as an abscess or boil, is a walled-off mass of purulent material arising from a hair follicle. Furuncles differ from folliculitis in that furuncles affect the dermis and subcutaneous tissue rather than only the superficial epidermis. The lesions are called carbuncles when they coalesce to form large, deep masses which extend to the subcutaneous tissue, often in areas covered with thick or inelastic skin. Risk factors for furuncles and carbuncles include obesity, treatment with corticosteroids, immune defects, and diabetes mellitus.[1,2,4]

ETIOLOGY

S. aureus is nearly always the causative pathogen of furuncles and carbuncles.

CLINICAL PRESENTATION[1,2,4]

Furuncles can occur anywhere on hairy skin, but generally develop in areas subject to friction and perspiration. These infections commonly occur on the face, neck, axillae, and buttocks. Furuncles begin as firm, tender, red nodules that then become painful and fluctuant. The lesions are usually discrete and occur as single nodules, although multiple nodules also occur. Spontaneous drainage of pus is common, after which the lesions subside.

Carbuncles are usually located at the base of the neck, on the back, or on the thighs. The lesions are large, deep, and indurated with obvious swelling of the surrounding tissues. Fever, chills, and malaise are frequent complaints, and some patients may appear acutely ill or "toxic." The lesions usually eventually open and drain externally through multiple sinus tracts along the hair follicles. Areas of undrained pus are frequent, and cellulitis or bacteremia may occur as complications of severe carbuncles. Leukocytosis may be present in patients with large or severe carbuncular lesions or in those with secondary complications. Endocarditis and osteomyelitis occur rarely.

DIAGNOSTIC EVALUATION

Diagnosis of a furuncle or a carbuncle is usually made based on the characteristic appearances of the lesions. Drainage fluids may be sent for culture, but this is not usually done since the infection is invariably caused by *S. aureus*.

MANAGEMENT[1,2,4]

Small furuncles can generally be treated with moist heat, which promotes localization and drainage of pus. Large and/or multiple furuncles and carbuncles are generally treated with a penicillinase-resistant penicillin such as dicloxacillin for 7 to 10 days (Table 42-3). An alternative agent for penicillin-allergic patients is clindamycin. Surgical incision and drainage is indicated for large furuncles that do not spontaneously drain and/or are fluctuant in nature; most carbuncles also require incision and drainage.

CELLULITIS

Cellulitis is defined as an acute, spreading infection of the skin and subcutaneous tissue. Cellulitis is considered a serious disease because of the propensity of the infection to spread through lymphatic tissue and to the bloodstream. Although cellulitis may affect patients of all ages, more than one-half of patients who develop cellulitis have an underlying condition such as drug or alcohol abuse, obesity, diabetes mellitus, peripheral vascular disease, or preexisting edema.[2,4,5] The presence of a foreign body, such as an intravenous catheter, also increases the risk of developing cellulitis. Cellulitis may occur when the skin barrier is broken, as with a cut, bite, or abrasion. In older patients, cellulitis of the lower extremities may be complicated by thrombophlebitis. Other complications of cellulitis include local abscess formation, osteomyelitis, septic arthritis, and sepsis in more severe cases.[2,4,5]

ETIOLOGY

Although any organism may cause cellulitis, the most common bacterial causes are group A streptococci and

Staphylococcus species.[1,2,4,5] In certain populations, other organisms may be prevalent. For example, patients with diabetes may develop cellulitis caused by multiple pathogens including Gram-negative and anaerobic organisms. *Haemophilus influenzae* was considered a common pathogen in children before the *H. influenzae* type b vaccine was introduced.[2] The rising incidence of infections caused by community-acquired methicillin-resistant *S. aureus* (CA-MRSA) is a major concern in the outpatient setting.[5,8]

Acute cellulitis with mixed aerobic and anaerobic flora generally occurs in diabetics, where the skin is adjacent to some site of trauma, at sites of surgical incisions to the abdomen or perineum, or where host defenses have been otherwise compromised (e.g., vascular insufficiency). Injection drug users are also predisposed to polymicrobic cellulitis and abscess formation at the site of injection. Infecting organisms are believed to originate from the skin and/or oropharynx, as well as from contaminated needles, syringes, and diluents. *S. aureus* and streptococci are the most common organisms isolated from these infections, but anaerobic bacteria (especially oropharyngeal anaerobes) are also commonly found as part of polymicrobic infections.[2,4,5]

CLINICAL PRESENTATION[2,4,5]

Cellulitis most commonly affects the head, neck, and upper and lower extremities. The most common signs and symptoms associated with cellulitis include pain, tenderness, nonpruritic erythema, swelling, and warmth at the site of infection. The borders of the infected tissues may appear demarcated compared to the adjoining tissue that is not affected, but the borders of the infection are often poorly defined. Vesicles and bullae filled with clear fluid are common, although pustular lesions are also occasionally present. Some patients may experience a prodrome, which may include chills, malaise, anorexia, nausea, and vomiting. Fever and white blood cell count elevation may occur in some patients but are not present in all.

DIAGNOSTIC EVALUATION[2,4,5]

Needle aspiration of the infected area may identify the pathogenic organism in up to 60% of patients, but the yield of such cultures is often much lower in routine practice. In general, needle aspiration and cultures of the infected area are unnecessary in uncomplicated cases because empiric antibiotic therapy is effective in the majority of cases. Cultures should be considered if the infection is complex; if there is an increased risk of complications, as in very young patients or older adults and in patients with diabetes, peripheral vascular disease, or immunosuppression; or if a standard course of antibiotics has failed. Blood cultures are positive in <5% of patients and are not routinely performed in mild-to-moderate infections.

Most patients with cellulitis of mild-to-moderate severity may be successfully managed with oral antibiotics in the outpatient setting. However, more severe cases or infections in patients with significant comorbidities may necessitate the need for hospitalization and treatment with parenteral antibiotics. The decision to hospitalize a patient will be based on the location of the cellulitis (particularly face or head), presence of severe systemic symptoms, presence of complications such as abscess or osteomyelitis, underlying diseases such as poorly controlled diabetes mellitus or drug- or disease state-induced immunosuppression, the patient's ability to be adherent with drug therapy or return to the clinic if problems develop, and the clinicians' subjective overall assessment of the severity of the infection.[1,2,4,5,9] As a general guideline, patients who are afebrile, not toxic-appearing, and who are otherwise healthy or with no unstable comorbid conditions are usually suitable for outpatient therapy with oral antibiotics.[5] Conversely, patients having a toxic appearance, unstable comorbidities, a limb-threatening infection, or other life-threatening infection such as gangrenous infection or necrotizing fasciitis will require initial hospitalization, parenteral antimicrobial therapy, and often some type of surgical intervention. Periorbital cellulitis (infection of the tissues surrounding the eye) should always be initially treated with parenteral antibiotics.[10]

MANAGEMENT[1,2,4,5,9,11]

The goal of therapy of acute bacterial cellulitis is rapid eradication of the infection and prevention of further complications. Optimal cellulitis treatment is based on a number of factors, including the most likely causative organisms, penetration of the antibiotic to the site of infection, concurrent medications, medication allergies, patient compliance issues, and cost. Antimicrobial therapy of bacterial cellulitis is directed against the type of bacteria either documented, or suspected to be present based on the clinical presentation. The most likely organism may vary depending on patient age and concomitant diseases such as diabetes mellitus or HIV infection. In general, although, empiric therapy of uncomplicated cellulitis should be effective against streptococci and *S. aureus*.

Local care of cellulitis includes elevation and immobilization of the involved area to decrease swelling. Initial application of cool sterile saline dressings may help to decrease pain and inflammation. These should be followed, when tolerated, by moist heat to aid in localization of the infection, promote drainage and remove exudates, and decrease edema. Surgical intervention (incision and drainage or debridement) may often be required for severe cellulitis but is not usually required for the treatment of cellulitis in patients appropriately treated in the primary care setting. Abscesses may also be associated with infections caused by CA-MRSA; these lesions should likewise be incised and drained when present.

Commonly used antibiotics for outpatient management of cellulitis are shown in Table 42-3. Because staphylococcal and streptococcal cellulitis are usually indistinguishable, and because >90% of all *S. aureus* strains produce penicillinase enzymes, administration of an oral penicillinase-resistant penicillin (dicloxacillin or cloxacillin) is usually recommended. Amoxicillin/clavulanic acid and first-generation cephalosporins such as cefadroxil or cephalexin are also commonly used for mild-to-moderate infections. Other oral cephalosporins, such as cefaclor, cefprozil, and cefpodoxime proxetil, are also effective in the treatment of cellulitis but are considerably more expensive. In patients allergic to β-lactam antibiotics, clindamycin is an appropriate choice. If documented to be a mild cellulitis secondary to streptococci, oral Penicillin VK may be administered.

The increasing incidence of infections caused by CA-MRSA is of great concern as a result of the inadequacy of standard recommended therapy for cellulitis (traditionally consisting of a β-lactam agent). Although the most optimal treatment for CA-MRSA infections is not known, initial therapy with trimethoprim/sulfamethoxazole (TMP/SMX) or a tetracycline (i.e., doxycycline or minocycline) should be considered in geographic areas in which CA-MRSA infections are commonly encountered.[2,8,12] Because TMP/SMX may not provide adequate activity against group A streptococci, the empiric addition of a β-lactam agent to TMP/SMX has also been advocated; however, whether such initial combination therapy improves clinical outcomes is not clear. Patients begun on β-lactam antibiotic regimens should be closely monitored for appropriate response to therapy. Empiric therapy with agents which are highly active against multidrug-resistant Gram-positive cocci, for example, linezolid, is not routinely recommended as a result of the significantly higher cost of these drugs and usually adequate response to TMP/SMX or a tetracycline.[8,12]

Amoxicillin/clavulanic acid and cephalosporins may be preferred in the setting of diabetes because of their broader spectrum of antibacterial activity and the potential for infection with Gram-negative bacilli as well as Gram-positive pathogens. Fluoroquinolones (levofloxacin or moxifloxacin) may also be recommended for adult diabetic patients because of their expanded spectrum of activity. Although these fluoroquinolones have been shown to be effective for uncomplicated SSTIs including cellulitis, they are considered to be alternative rather than first-line agents because of increasing reports of resistance among both Gram-positive and Gram-negative bacteria as well as increased treatment costs compared to other therapies.[2,4,9] Because patients with diabetes are at higher risk for CA-MRSA, clinicians must be alert to the potential for infection with this pathogen and patient response to therapy must be monitored very closely.[5]

Infections in injection drug users are generally treated similarly to those in other types of patients. It is also important that blood cultures be obtained, as 25% to 35% of patients may be bacteremic. Also, patients should be assessed for the presence of abscesses; incision, drainage, and culture of these lesions are of extreme importance. Initial antimicrobial therapy should include coverage for anaerobic organisms, in addition to *S. aureus* and streptococci. In areas where methicillin-resistant *S. aureus* (MRSA) is prevalent, hospitalization for treatment with parenteral antibiotics should be considered.[2,5,9]

The usual duration of therapy for cellulitis is 10 to 14 days. However, patients with peripheral vascular disease, chronic venous stasis, alcoholic cirrhosis, or diabetes may have significantly delayed response to therapy and may require a total of 3 to 4 weeks of therapy.

BITE WOUNDS

GENERAL CONSIDERATIONS[2,5]

Infections associated with bite wounds, either from animals or humans, are considered to be serious illnesses as they can manifest 4 to 24 hours after the injury, cause extensive skin and subcutaneous tissue injury, and are potentially limb threatening, requiring extensive surgical debridement. Most bite wounds will be initially evaluated in the primary care setting, either in offices and clinics or through emergency departments. Knowledge of appropriate evaluation and management is therefore very important for primary care clinicians.

The initial care of the patient with a bite wound should include a detailed history including time lapse from injury to clinic or emergency department visit. Inspection of the wound with attention to deepness, whether tendons and ligaments are affected, and presence of foul odor are necessary to determine whether treatment may be attempted in the outpatient setting with oral antibiotics alone or whether hospitalization and surgical interventions may potentially be required. Cultures (aerobic and anaerobic) and a complete blood count are important for evaluating treatment options, and a surgical consult should be obtained for wounds which are deep, obviously infected, and/or associated with extensive injury to tissues, ligaments, or tendons. Time is essential to prevent permanent damage, particularly if the hand is involved.

Treatment of bite wounds with antibiotic therapy is appropriate for an established infection. If the wound does not adequately respond within 24 hours, a return visit to the clinic or emergency department may be necessary for reevaluation. Finally, appropriate measures for rabies and tetanus vaccination should be considered in all patients.

ANIMAL BITES[2,5]

Dog bites account for approximately 80% of all animal bite wounds requiring medical attention. Dog bites most commonly occur in males less than 20 years of age. More than 70% of these bites are to the extremities. Bites to the face occur less commonly and are mostly seen in children younger than 15 years of age. Patients at greatest risk of acquiring an infection after a bite have had a puncture wound (usually the hand), have not sought medical attention within 12 hours of the injury, and are older than 50 years of age.

Cat bites account for approximately 5% to 15% of all reported animal bites and are the second most common cause of animal bite wounds in the United States. Bites and scratches caused by cats most commonly occur on the upper extremities and, in contrast to dog bites, most cat-related injuries are reported in women. Infections associated with cat bites are estimated to occur in 30% to 50% of injuries and happen at a rate more than double that seen with dog bites.

Etiology

Infections from dog bite wounds are caused predominantly by organisms of the dog's oral flora. Most infections are polymicrobial and involve an average of five bacterial pathogens (Table 42-2). *Pasteurella* species are most frequently isolated; other common aerobes include streptococci, staphylococci, *Moraxella,* and *Neisseria.* The most common anaerobes are *Fusobacterium, Bacteroides, Porphyromonas,* and *Prevotella.* Cultures of both infected and noninfected bite wounds have similar bacteria present, with aerobic organisms isolated from 74% to 90% and anaerobic organisms isolated from 41% to 49% of wounds.[2,5]

Infections associated with cat bites or scratches are caused by *Pasteurella multocida* in approximately 75% of cases; this bacteria is part of the normal flora of 50% to 70% of healthy cats. Mixed aerobic and anaerobic infections have been reported in the majority of cat bite wounds.[2,5] Both tularemia (*Pasteurella tularensis*) and rabies have also been transmitted by cat bites.

Clinical Presentation

Primary care providers see two distinct groups of patients seeking medical attention for animal bites.[2,5] The first group presents within 8 to 12 hours of the injury and has not yet developed infection; these patients require only general wound care, repair of tear wounds, or rabies and/or tetanus treatment. The second group of patients presents more than 8 to 12 hours after the injury has occurred and is usually seeking medical attention for infection-related complaints. Such complaints include pain, erythema, purulent discharge, and swelling. Localized cellulitis is generally present with pain at the site of injury. The cellulitis usually spreads proximally from the initial site of injury and a gray malodorous discharge may be encountered. If *P. multocida* is present, a rapidly progressing cellulitis may be observed with pain and swelling developing within 24 to 48 hours after the initial injury. Infections developing within the first 24 hours of a bite are most often caused by *P. multocida,* while infections developing more than 36 to 48 hours after the bite are more likely to be infected with staphylococci or streptococci. In contrast to some other SSTIs, fever is uncommon and fewer than 20% of patients have concomitant adenopathy or lymphangitis.

Diagnostic Evaluation

Documentation of the mechanism of injury is important. Because the rabies virus can be transmitted via saliva, rabies may be a potential complication of a bite. Capture of the animal for determination of rabies immunization history is essential. It is also important for the patient's tetanus immune status to be determined.

Cultures obtained from early and/or noninfected bite wounds are not of great value in predicting the subsequent development of infection.[2,5] Cultures are therefore not recommended for wounds that are seen within 8 hours or more than 24 hours after the bite injury when the incidence of infection is low. In the case of bite wounds with clinical signs of established infection, samples for both aerobic and anaerobic cultures should be obtained. Purulent discharge is a common finding in infected bite wounds and is easily sent for culture. Radiographic evaluation of the affected part should be considered when infection is documented in proximity to a bone or joint.

Management

Wounds should be thoroughly irrigated with a large volume (>150 mL) of sterile normal saline. Proper irrigation will reduce the bacterial count in the wound; prompt, thorough irrigation of the wound with soap or iodine solution may also reduce the development of rabies. Antibiotic solutions do not offer any advantage over saline. In addition to irrigation, when possible, the injured area should be immobilized and elevated. It is important to stress to patients that the affected area should be elevated for several days or until edema has resolved.[2]

Tetanus does not commonly occur after animal bites. However, immunization history in regard to the tetanus vaccine should be reviewed with each patient. Administration of tetanus–diphtheria toxoids and/or tetanus immune globulin should be considered if immunization histories are incomplete and/or tetanus vaccinations have been inadequate, particularly in patients with more extensive wounds or if soil contamination has occurred.[2,5]

The role of prophylactic antimicrobial therapy for the early, noninfected bite wound remains controversial.[2,5,13] Controlled studies, retrospective evaluations, and meta-analyses have not definitively shown benefits with prophylactic antibiotics for noninfected bites.[13] Because up to 20% of bite wounds may become infected, a 3- to 5-day course of antimicrobial therapy is generally recommended, especially for patients at greater risk for infection (patients >50 years of age, deep puncture wounds, wounds to the hands, and wounds in immunocompromised hosts).[2,5,13] Prophylactic treatment should be directed at the typical aerobic and anaerobic oral flora of the animal as well as the skin flora of the bite victim. Antibiotic regimens suggested for empiric oral therapy of bite wounds from dogs and cats usually consist of either amoxicillin/clavulanic acid or doxycycline.[5] Alternative regimens include a first- or second-generation cephalosporin plus clindamycin, or penicillin in combination with a first-generation cephalosporin or clindamycin. Although these latter combination regimens are effective, they are also more expensive and more difficult for good patient adherence. Doxycycline has good activity against *P. multocida*, is less expensive than amoxicillin/clavulanic acid, and is also suitable for patients who are allergic to penicillins. Although conclusive clinical data are lacking, fluoroquinolones may also be considered in β-lactam allergic patients. Doxycycline should not be used in children and/or pregnant women.

Patients who present with established infections should be evaluated regarding whether therapy is best accomplished with oral antibiotics or parenteral therapy. More severe infections for which initial parenteral antibiotic therapy may be more appropriate include those involving the head or hands, those accompanied by extensive cellulitis or lymphangitis, significant systemic signs and symptoms, wounds in which bones or joints may be involved, and wounds in which pain is disproportionate to the apparent severity of the injury.[2,5]

The recommended treatment of infected animal bites is amoxicillin/clavulanic acid.[5] Doxycycline is an effective alternative agent, particularly in penicillin-allergic, nonpregnant adults. Dicloxacillin plus penicillin VK has also been recommended. Second-generation cephalosporins such as cefuroxime axetil, fluoroquinolones, and TMP/SMX may also be effective options but should be combined with metronidazole or clindamycin to provide adequate antianaerobic activity. The duration of antibiotic treatment is usually 7 to 10 days.

Results of any available Gram stains or cultures should be used to confirm the appropriateness of antibiotic therapy. Surgical evaluation and/or wound debridement may be needed if signs and symptoms of infection have not substantially improved, or the wound has become worse, within 24 to 48 hours after beginning therapy.

HUMAN BITES

Human bites are the third most frequent type of bite (after dogs and cats). Infected human bites usually occur secondary to bites inflicted by another individual, or from clenched-fist injuries resulting from one person hitting another in the mouth. Bites by others can occur to any part of the body, but most often involve the hands. The areas most commonly affected by clenched-fist injuries are the third and fourth metacarpophalangeal joints.[2,5]

Human bites are generally more serious than animal bites and carry a higher likelihood of infection than do most animal bites; infectious complications occur in 10% to 50% of cases. Bites to the hand are most serious and more frequently become infected. Clenched-fist injuries are particularly prone to infection because the force of a punch may carry bacteria into deep tissue spaces. The injury also often causes a breach in the capsule of the metacarpophalangeal joint and leads to direct inoculation of bacteria into the joint or bone. Clenched-fist injuries may also be associated with severing of tendons or nerves, or breaking of bones.[2,5]

Etiology

Infections of human bite wounds are most often caused by the normal oral flora but may also involve normal flora of the skin. These are typically polymicrobial infections which include both aerobic and anaerobic microorganisms.[2,5] *Streptococcus* species (especially *S. anginosus*) are the most common isolates, followed by *Staphylococcus* species (predominately *S. aureus*). *Haemophilus* species and *Eikenella corrodens* are also commonly isolated from human bite wounds. Anaerobic pathogens are involved in approximately 40% of human bites, with a slightly higher incidence in clenched-fist injuries. Anaerobes recovered from human bite infections commonly include *Prevotella*, *Fusobacterium*, *Veillonella*, and *Peptostreptococcus* species.

Clinical Presentation

Most clenched-fist injuries are already infected by the time patients seek medical care. Patients with infected bites to the hand may develop a painful, throbbing, swollen extremity. Wounds often have a purulent discharge, and patients often complain of a decreased range of motion. Signs of infection include erythema, swelling, and clear or purulent discharge. Adjacent lymph nodes may be enlarged. In clenched-fist injuries, edema may cause substantial limitation to a joint's range of motion.

Diagnostic Evaluation

Surgical assessment of wounds should be considered if it appears that deeper tissues may have been injured or if accumulations of pus have occurred. Surgical exploration, debridement, or excision and drainage may be required in many cases. Clenched-fist injuries in particular should also be evaluated for evidence of damage to tendons, joints, and nerves because of the potential for more extensive and/or severe damage to the hand and resultant loss of function.[2,5]

Samples for bacterial cultures (both aerobic and anaerobic), usually from purulent drainage fluids, should be collected in all patients with established infection. Peripheral leukocytosis of 15 000 to 30 000 cells/mm^3 may be seen in many infections, therefore the white blood cell count should be monitored for resolution of infection. If damage to a bone or joint is suspected, radiographic evaluation should be undertaken.

Management

Similar to animal bites, management of human bite wounds consists of aggressive irrigation, surgical debridement if necessary, and immobilization of the affected area. Tetanus toxoid and antitoxin may be indicated. If the biter is known to be HIV-positive or may have important risk factors, the victim should have a baseline blood specimen drawn to determine preexposure HIV status and then be retested in 3 months and 6 months. Bite wounds should also be thoroughly and vigorously irrigated with a virucidal agent such as povidone-iodine. Bite victims exposed to blood-tainted saliva from a person known to have HIV infection should be offered antiretroviral chemoprophylaxis.

All patients with noninfected hand bite injuries should be given prophylactic antibiotic therapy.[5] Initial therapy should consist of amoxicillin/clavulanic acid or doxycycline. A penicillinase-resistant penicillin such as dicloxacillin in combination with Penicillin VK may also be administered. Prophylactic therapy should be given for 3 to 5 days as for animal bites. First-generation cephalosporins or macrolides are not recommended since sensitivity of *E. corrodens* to these agents is variable.

Patients with infected bite wounds should be carefully evaluated to determine the most appropriate route of antibiotic administration. Hospitalization for minor wounds is not necessary if surgical repair of vital structures has not been performed or is not necessary. Patients in whom parenteral antibiotic therapy may be most appropriate include those with wounds characterized by the following: large in area; evidence of involvement of deeper tissues, joints, or bones; accumulations of pus, particularly in or around joint spaces; any evidence of damage to tendons, joints, or nerves; or those wounds subjectively felt to be severe in nature on the basis of clinical assessment.[2,5] Patients suffering clenched-fist injuries are often most appropriately treated with parenteral antibiotics. Immunocompromised patients and those who are unlikely to be adherent to antibiotic regimens should also receive parenteral therapy.[2,5]

Patients who are suitable candidates for oral antibiotic therapy should be empirically started on amoxicillin/clavulanic acid or doxycycline pending results of cultures.[5] Penicillin plus a penicillinase-resistant penicillin would be a suitable alternative regimen. A combination of clindamycin plus a fluoroquinolone or TMP/SMX may also be used as an alternative therapy for the penicillin-allergic patient. Duration of therapy for infected bite injuries should be 7 to 14 days.

Results of any available Gram stains or cultures should be used to confirm the appropriateness of antibiotic therapy. Surgical evaluation and/or wound debridement may be needed if signs and symptoms of infection have not substantially improved, or the wound has become worse, within 24 to 48 hours after beginning therapy.

DIABETIC FOOT INFECTIONS

Disorders of the foot are among the most common complications of diabetes. The three major types of foot infections seen in diabetic patients include deep abscesses of the central plantar space (arch); cellulitis of the dorsum, often arising from infections in the toes; and mal perforans ulcers, that is, chronic ulcers of the sole of the foot. Osteomyelitis is one of the most serious complications of foot problems in diabetic patients and may occur in 30% to 40% of infections. It is estimated that 25% of diabetic patients experience significant soft tissue infection at some time during the course of their lifetime; these infections are the cause of lower extremity amputations in approximately 15% to 20% of patients.[5,14] Of these patients, approximately 10% to 20% will undergo additional surgery or amputation of a second limb within 12 months of the initial amputation. Foot infections are clearly associated with significant morbidity, cost, and decreased functionality and quality of life in diabetic patients.[2,5,14]

Three key factors involved in the development of diabetic foot problems are neuropathy, angiopathy and ischemia, and immunologic defects.[5,14] Any of these disorders can occur in isolation; however, they frequently occur together. Neuropathies may cause muscular imbalance, abnormal stresses on tissues and bone, and repetitive injuries. Also, decreased pain sensation may cause an absence of pain and unawareness of minor injuries and ulceration. Atherosclerosis in diabetic patients causes problems with both small vessels (microangiopathy) and large vessels (macroangiopathy) that can result in varying degrees of ischemia, ultimately leading to skin breakdown and infection. Finally, diabetic patients typically have impaired phagocytosis and intracellular microbicidal function as compared to non-diabetics, possibly related to angiopathies and tissue ischemia. These defects in cell-mediated immunity make patients with diabetes more susceptible to certain types of infection and also impair wound healing.

Etiology

Diabetic foot infections typically involve a number of different bacterial pathogens. Diabetic foot infections are usually polymicrobic in nature and involve an average of 4 to 6 isolates per culture. Table 42-4 lists the bacterial etiology in 346 diabetic patients with microbiologically documented infections who were enrolled in three recent comparative studies.[15–17] Staphylococci (especially *S. aureus*) and streptococci are the most

Table 42-4. Frequency of Bacterial Isolates from Diabetic Foot Infections[15–17]

Organisms	Percent of Infections (%)
Aerobes	69–79
Gram-positive	45–66
S. aureus	13–46
Streptococcus spp.	10–14
Enterococcus spp.	8–20
Coagulase-negative staphylococci	7–12
Gram-negative	24–37
Proteus spp.	5
Enterobacter spp.	2–3
E. coli	3–5
Klebsiella spp.	2
P. aeruginosa	2–7
Other Gram-negative bacilli	3–7
Anaerobes	25–44
Peptostreptococcus spp.	8–27
B. fragilis group	5–11
Other *Bacteroides* spp.	3–4
Clostridium spp.	0–2
Other anaerobes	5–7

common pathogens, although Gram-negative bacilli and/or anaerobes occur in approximately 30% to 50% of cases. Common Gram-negative bacteria involved in diabetic foot infections include *Escherichia coli, Klebsiella* species, and *Proteus* species. *P. aeruginosa* is found in usually 2% to 10% of infections. *Bacteroides fragilis* and *Peptostreptococcus* species are among the most common anaerobes isolated. Hospitalization, surgical procedures, and prolonged or broad-spectrum antibiotic therapy increases the risk of infection with antibiotic-resistant pathogens such as MRSA.[14] Similar to cellulitis, infection with CA-MRSA is becoming more common in diabetic foot wounds.[5,14]

Clinical Presentation[5,14]

Infections are often much more extensive and much deeper than they initially appear. Patients with peripheral neuropathy often seek medical care for swelling or erythema in the foot with the absence of pain. Typical clinical signs of infection as seen with other types of SSTIs may not be present in the diabetic foot as a result of angiopathy and neuropathy. When present, infected lesions vary in size and in clinical features. Erythema, edema, warmth, presence of pus, draining sinuses, pain, and tenderness are common clinical features of infected wounds; however, some of these signs and symptoms may be absent in some patients. Fever may also be absent in many patients. It has been noted that 50% of patients with limb-threatening infection have no systemic signs or symptoms.

Diagnostic Evaluation

Specimens for culture and sensitivities should be routinely collected. However, routine swab cultures of ulcerative lesions are difficult to interpret because non-pathogenic organisms often colonize the surface of the wounds. Cultures of material from sinus tracts are also unreliable. Cultures and sensitivity tests should therefore be done with specimens obtained from a deep culture obtained after surgical debridement whenever possible.[16] Before culturing, the wound should be vigorously scrubbed with saline-moistened sterile gauze to remove any overlying necrotic debris. Cultures then can be obtained from the wound base, preferably from expressed pus. Because of the complex microbiology of these infections, wounds must be cultured for both aerobic and anaerobic organisms.[5,14–17] The presence of osteomyelitis must also be assessed via radiograph, bone scan, and/or bone culture, as appropriate.

Management

The goal of therapy of diabetic foot infections is preservation of as much normal limb function as possible while preventing additional infectious complications. Up to

Table 42-5. Classification of Infection in Diabetic Patients with Foot Wounds[14]

Wound Characteristics	Severity; Treatment Recommendation
No purulence, no signs/symptoms of inflammation (e.g., purulence, erythema, pain, tenderness, warmth, or induration)	Uninfected; no antibiotic therapy indicated
Presence of ≥2 signs/symptoms of inflammation (as listed above), cellulitis or erythema extend ≤2 cm around ulcer and limited to skin or superficial subcutaneous tissues, no complications or systemic findings	Mild infection; most cases appropriate to treat as outpatient with oral antibiotics
Presence of inflammation (as with mild infection), patient clinically stable but with ≥1 of the following: Cellulitis/erythema >2 cm around ulcer, lymphangitis, spread through deeper tissues, deep-tissue abscess, gangrene, or involvement of muscle, tendon, bone or joint	Moderate infection; most cases appropriate to treat as outpatient with oral antibiotics
Presence of infection with systemic involvement and/or clinical instability (e.g., fever, chills, tachycardia, hypotension, mental status changes, vomiting, leukocytosis, metabolic acidosis, severe hyperglycemia, acute renal dysfunction)	Severe infection; requires hospitalization and treatment with parenteral antibiotics

90% of these infections can be successfully treated with a comprehensive treatment approach that includes both wound care and antimicrobial therapy. However, one of the most important initial tasks in the management of diabetic foot infections is to recognize which patients require immediate hospitalization rather than treatment as an outpatient. Determination of the most appropriate treatment setting is often very difficult and somewhat controversial. One system for classifying the severity of diabetic foot wounds has recently been published by the International Consensus on the Diabetic Foot (Table 42-5). Infections categorized as mild-to-moderate in severity can usually be treated with oral antibiotics in the outpatient setting. Complicating factors which make oral antibiotics less appropriate for these infections include the need for urgent diagnostic testing, likely inability to adhere to antibiotic therapy, or factors that may affect the ability to provide good wound care. Patients with severe infections should be hospitalized for treatment with parenteral antibiotics. Patients with wounds classified as uninfected should of course not receive any antibiotic therapy.

After carefully assessing the extent of the lesion and obtaining necessary cultures, necrotic tissue must be thoroughly debrided and wounds drained as required. Wounds must be kept clean and dressings changed frequently (two to three times daily). Glycemic control must be maximized in all patients to ensure optimal wound healing. Bedrest for leg elevation and control of any edema is another important component of comprehensive wound management. Finally, appropriate antimicrobials must be initiated.

The optimal antimicrobial therapy for diabetic foot infections has yet to be defined. Many different agents have been studied and generally provide clinical cure rates of 60% to 85% in published studies.[5,14] Many clinicians consider amoxicillin/clavulanic acid to be the preferred agent because of its broad spectrum of activity which includes staphylococci, streptococci, enterococci, and many Enterobacteriaceae and anaerobes. Although amoxicillin/clavulanic acid does not have activity against *P. aeruginosa*, most mild-to-moderate infections are not likely to involve *P. aeruginosa* and activity against this organism has not been proven to lead to better outcomes. Fluoroquinolones such as ciprofloxacin and levofloxacin, which provide coverage against *P. aeruginosa*, have been extensively studied as monotherapy but are perhaps most appropriately used in combination with metronidazole or clindamycin to provide anaerobic activity.[14] Oral moxifloxacin has enhanced anaerobic activity and is a suitable fluoroquinolone for oral monotherapy of mild-to-moderate infections in which *P. aeruginosa* is less likely. Although MRSA is becoming more common in diabetic foot infections, use of agents such as linezolid is not recommended for initial therapy unless properly obtained cultures document the presence of this pathogen.[5,8,12,14]

Mild-to-moderate infections should generally be treated for at least 10 to 14 days, although regimens of 21 days or more are often required. In cases of underlying osteomyelitis, treatment should continue for 6 to 12 weeks. After healing of the infection has occurred, a well-designed program for prevention of further infections should be instituted.

Therapy should be carefully reevaluated after 48 to 72 hours to assess favorable response. Change in therapy (or route of administration, if oral) should be considered if clinical improvement is not observed during this time. For optimal results, drug therapy should be appropriately modified according to information from deep tissue culture and the clinical condition of the patient.

EVIDENCE-BASED SUMMARY

- Impetigo is a superficial skin infection that is most commonly seen in young children and usually caused by group A streptococci (i.e., *S. pyogenes*), or occasionally *S. aureus*. Impetigo usually manifests as small, painless vesicular lesions and pustules on the face and extremities and is associated with thick, golden-yellow crusts. Appropriate antibiotics for impetigo include dicloxacillin, amoxicillin/clavulanate, and first-generation cephalosporins (e.g., cephalexin). Mild cases may also be treated with topical mupirocin or retapamulin ointments rather than with systemic antibiotics.

- Erysipelas is a superficial infection of the skin that is most common in infants, young children, and older people. Erysipelas is characterized by a painful lesion with a bright red, edematous appearance and is differentiated from cellulitis by the presence of raised lesions with a sharply demarcated border. Most cases are caused by group A streptococci and can be successfully treated with Penicillin VK, a penicillinase-resistant penicillin, or a first-generation cephalosporin.

- Folliculitis is inflammation of the hair follicle and is most commonly caused by *S. aureus*. This infection is associated with small, erythematous, sometimes pruritic papular lesions which are often topped by a central pustule. Folliculitis is usually treated with local measures such as warm saline compresses, or topical antibiotic therapy with clindamycin, erythromycin, mupirocin, or benzoyl peroxide.

- Furuncles and carbuncles occur when a folliculitis extends from the hair shaft to involve the deeper areas of the skin; these infections are also usually caused by *S. aureus*. Furuncles are commonly known as an abscesses or boils, while carbuncles coalesce to form large, deep masses which extend to subcutaneous tissues. Small furuncles are generally treated with moist heat, while large and/or multiple furuncles and carbuncles are usually treated with a penicillinase-resistant penicillin plus surgical incision and drainage.

- Cellulitis is an acute, spreading infection of the skin and subcutaneous tissue and is considered a serious infection with many potential complications. Group A streptococci and staphylococci are most commonly seen, although mixed infections involving Gram-negative bacilli and anaerobes may occur in diabetics, traumatic wounds, injection drug users, surgical incisions sites in the abdomen or perineum, or where host defenses have been otherwise compromised (e.g., vascular insufficiency). The increasing incidence of infection caused by CA-MRSA is also a major concern in the outpatient setting. Patients who are afebrile, not toxic appearing, and who are otherwise healthy or with no unstable comorbid conditions are usually appropriate for outpatient therapy with oral antibiotics such as dicloxacillin, amoxicillin/clavulanate, or first-generation cephalosporins. Fluoroquinolones or amoxicillin/clavulanate are most appropriate when the presence of Gram-negative pathogens is suspected. Initial therapy with TMP/SMX or a tetracycline (i.e., doxycycline or minocycline) should be considered in geographic areas in which CA-MRSA infections are commonly seen. Appropriate wound care including incision and drainage or debridement, if required, is also important in the proper management of cellulitis.

- Bite wounds, either from animals or humans, are considered to be serious infections because they can cause extensive skin and subcutaneous tissue injury, and are potentially limb threatening with the need for extensive surgical debridement. Surgical assessment of human bite wounds to the hand should be considered if deeper tissues are involved or accumulations of pus have occurred. Surgical exploration, debridement, or excision and drainage may be required in bite wounds to the hand, particularly with clenched-fist injuries; these infections may also require parenteral rather than outpatient-based therapy. Infected animal or human bites may be treated with amoxicillin/clavulanate or doxycycline. A 3- to 5-day course of prophylactic antibiotics may also be considered in patients in whom an established infection has not yet developed.

- Diabetic foot infections are typically polymicrobial in nature and require careful assessment to determine the extent and severity of tissue involvement. Many mild-to-moderate infections can be successfully treated with a comprehensive treatment approach that includes both wound care and oral antimicrobial therapy in the outpatient setting. Wounds must be thoroughly debrided, drained, and kept clean with frequent dressing changes. Glycemic control must be maximized in all patients to ensure optimal wound healing. Amoxicillin/clavulanate, or a fluoroquinolone with or without metronidazole or clindamycin are considered appropriate antibiotics for initial therapy of mild-to-moderate infections.

REFERENCES

1. Stulberg DL, Penrod MA, Blatny RA. Common bacterial skin infections. *Am Fam Physician.* 2002;66:119–124.
2. Swartz MN. Cellulitis and subcutaneous tissue infections, In: Mandell GL, Bennett JE, Dolin R, eds. *Principles and Practice of Infectious Diseases,* 5th ed. New York, NY: Churchill Livingstone; 2000:1037–1057.
3. DiNubile MJ, Lipsky BA. Complicated infections of skin and skin structures: When the infection is more than skin deep. *J Antimicrob Chemother.* 2004;53(Suppl S2): ii37–ii50.
4. Bhumbra NA, McCullough SG. Skin and subcutaneous infections. *Prim Care Clin Office Pract.* 2003;30:1–24.
5. Stevens DL, Bisno AL, Chambers HF, et al. Practice guidelines for the diagnosis and management of skin and soft-tissue infections. *Clin Infect Dis.* 2005;41:1373–1406.
6. Lio PA, Kaye ET. Topical antibacterial agents. *Infect Dis Clin North Am.* 2004;18:717–733.
7. Eriksson B, Jorup-Roenstroem C, Karkkonen K, et al. Erysipelas: Clinical and bacteriologic spectrum and serological aspects. *Clin Infect Dis.* 1996;23:1091–1098.
8. Eady EA, Cove JH. Staphylococcal resistance revisited: Community-acquired methicillin resistant Staphylococcus aureus—an emerging problem for the management of skin and soft tissue infections. *Curr Opin Infect Dis.* 2003;16:103–124.
9. Nichols RL. Optimal treatment of complicated skin and skin structure infections. *J Antimicrob Chemother.* 1999;44:19–23.
10. Tovilla-Canales JL, Nava A, Tovilla y Pomar JL. Orbital and periorbital infections. *Curr Opin Ophthalmol.* 2001;12: 335–341.
11. Hutchison LC. Antimicrobial therapy and resistance in dermatologic pathogens of the elderly. *Dermatol Clin.* 2004;22:63–71.
12. Raghavan M, Linden PK. Newer treatment options for skin and soft tissue infections. *Drugs.* 2004;64:1621–1642.
13. Medeiros I, Saconato H. Antibiotic prophylaxis for mammalian bites. *Cochrane Database Syst Rev.* 2001;CD001738.
14. Lipsky BA, Berendt AR, Deery HG, et al Diagnosis and treatment of diabetic foot infections. *Clin Infect Dis.* 2004;39:885–910.
15. Nichols RL, Smith JW, Gentry LO, et al. Multicenter randomized study comparing levofloxacin and ciprofloxacin for uncomplicated skin and skin structure infections. *South Med J.* 1997;90:1193–1200.
16. Pellizzer G, Strazzabosco M, Presi S, et al. Deep tissue biopsy vs. superficial swab culture monitoring in the microbiological assessment of limb-threatening diabetic foot infection. *Diabet Med.* 2001;18:822–827.
17. Lipsky BA, Armstrong DG, Citron DM, et al. Ertapenem versus piperacillin/tazobactam for diabetic foot infections (SIDESTEP): Prospective, randomized, controlled, double-blinded, multicentre trial. *Lancet.* 2005;366:1695–1703.

Chapter 43

Tuberculosis

Rocsanna Namdar and Charles A. Peloquin

SEARCH STRATEGY

This chapter reflects current recommendations from the American Thoracic Society/Centers for Disease Control (CDC)/Infectious Disease Society of America on the treatment of tuberculosis; diagnostic standards and classification of tuberculosis in adults and children; targeted tuberculin skin testing; treatment of latent tuberculosis infection (LTBI); and prevention and treatment of tuberculosis among patients infected with human immunodeficiency virus (HIV). It also includes the most recently published data addressing the diagnosis and treatment of tuberculosis, plus the authors' three decades of experience.

INTRODUCTION

Tuberculosis (TB) remains a leading infectious killer globally. TB is caused by *Mycobacterium tuberculosis*, which can produce either a silent, latent infection, or a progressive active disease.[1] If left untreated, or improperly treated, TB causes progressive tissue destruction and eventually death. TB remains out of control in many developing countries. One-third of the world's population currently is infected, and drug resistance is increasing in many areas.[1]

EPIDEMIOLOGY

Approximately, 2 billion people are infected by *M. tuberculosis* worldwide, and roughly 2 million to 3 million people die from active TB each year, despite the fact that it is curable.[1-3] In the United States, about 13 million people are latently infected with *M. tuberculosis*, meaning that they are not currently sick, but they could fall ill with TB any time. The United States had over 14 000 new cases of active TB in 2005, and about 1500 deaths[4] (for detailed data analysis visit the CDC website at http://www.cdc.gov/nchstp/tb).

RISK FACTORS FOR INFECTION

Location and Place of Birth

California, Florida, Illinois, New York, and Texas accounted for over 50% of all TB cases in 2005.[4] Within these states, TB is most prevalent in large urban areas.[3] The percentage of foreign-born TB patients in the United States has increased annually since 1986, reaching 54% in 2005.[4] Two-thirds of these patients came from Mexico, the Philippines, Vietnam, India, China, Haiti, and South Korea.[4] Close contacts of pulmonary TB patients are most likely to become infected.[2-3] These include family members, coworkers, or coresidents in places such as prisons, shelters, or nursing homes.

Race, Ethnicity, Age, and Gender

In the United States, in 2005, non-Hispanic blacks accounted for 27.9% of all TB cases, and Hispanics accounted for 28.4%.[5] Asians and Pacific Islanders accounted for about 22%, while non-Hispanic whites accounted for only 21% of the new TB cases.[5] TB is most common among people aged 25 to 44 years, followed by those aged 45 to 64 years (28%) and more than 65 years (21%).

Coinfection with HIV

HIV is the most important risk factor for active TB, especially among people aged 25 to 44 years.[2,3,5,6] Roughly 10% of US TB patients are coinfected with HIV, while approximately 20% of TB patients aged 25 to

44 years are coinfected with HIV.[4,5] HIV coinfection may not increase the risk of acquiring *M. tuberculosis* infection, but it does increase the likelihood of progression to active disease.[1,6] Further, TB and HIV patients share a number of behavioral risk factors that contribute to the high rates of coinfection.[2,7,8]

Risk Factors for Disease

Once infected with *M. tuberculosis*, a persons' lifetime risk of active TB is about 10%.[2,3,6] The greatest risk for active disease occurs during the first 2 years after infection. Children younger than 2 years, adults older 65 years, and immunocompromised patients have greater risks. HIV-infected patients with *M. tuberculosis* infection are 100 times more likely to develop active TB than normal hosts.[3,9]

ETIOLOGY

After staining, microscopic examination ("smear") detects about 8000 to 10 000 organisms/mL of specimen. A patient can be "smear negative" but still show a growth of *M. tuberculosis* on culture. Microscopic examination also cannot determine species. On culture, *M. tuberculosis* grows slowly, doubling about every 20 hours. This is very slow compared to gram-positive and gram-negative bacteria, which double about every 30 minutes.

CULTURE AND SUSCEPTIBILITY TESTING

Direct susceptibility testing involves inoculating specialized media with organisms taken directly from a concentrated, smear-positive specimen, producing susceptibility results in 2 to 3 weeks.[1,10,11] Indirect susceptibility, obtained from a pure culture of the organisms, takes several more weeks. The most common agar method, known as the proportion method, also takes many weeks to produce results. The Bactec system uses liquid media and detects live mycobacteria in 9 to 14 days.[1,10,11] Rapid-identification tests include nucleic acid probes and DNA fingerprinting using restriction fragment length polymorphism analysis, and polymerase chain reaction.[1,6,10,12–14]

TRANSMISSION

M. tuberculosis is transmitted from person to person by coughing or sneezing.[2,6,15] This produces "droplet nuclei" that are dispersed in the air. Each droplet nuclei contains 1 to 3 organisms. About 30% of individuals who experience prolonged contact with an infectious TB patient become infected.

PATHOPHYSIOLOGY

PRIMARY INFECTION

Primary infection usually results from inhaling droplet nuclei that contain *M. tuberculosis*.[2,6,16]

The progression to clinical disease depends on three factors: (1) the number of *M. tuberculosis* organisms inhaled (infecting dose), (2) the virulence of these organisms, and (3) the host's cell-mediated immune response.[2,4,6,12,15,17] If pulmonary macrophages inhibit or kill the bacilli, the infection is aborted.[15] If the macrophages do not do this, the organisms continue to multiply, and *M. tuberculosis* eventually can spread throughout the body through the bloodstream.[2,6,15] *M. tuberculosis* most commonly infects the posterior apical region of the lungs.

After about 3 weeks, T lymphocytes become activated, and begin to secrete Interferon-gamma and the other cytokines. These stimulate macrophages to become bactericidal and to form granulomas.[15] Over 1 to 3 months, tissue hypersensitivity occurs, resulting in a positive tuberculin skin test.[2,6,16] About 5% of patients (usually children, the older adults, or the immunocompromised) experience "progressive primary" disease prior to skin test conversion.[18,19] This presents as a progressive pneumonia, and frequently spreads, leading to meningitis and other severe forms of TB.[18]

REACTIVATION DISEASE

Roughly 10% of infected patients develop reactivation disease; and nearly half of these cases occur within 2 years of infection.[2,6,12] The apices of the lungs are the most common sites for reactivation (in 85% of cases).[2] The inflammatory response produces caseating granulomas, which will eventually liquefy and spread locally, leading to the formation of a hole (cavity) in the lungs. Bacterial counts in the cavities can be as high as 10^8/mL of cavitary fluid.[2,15] If left untreated, pulmonary TB continues to destroy the lungs, resulting in hypoxia, respiratory acidosis, and eventually death.

EXTRAPULMONARY AND MILIARY TB

Caseating granulomas at extrapulmonary sites can undergo liquefaction, releasing tubercle bacilli and causing symptomatic disease.[2,6] Extrapulmonary TB without concurrent pulmonary disease is more common in HIV-infected patients. The diagnosis of TB is difficult and often delayed in immunocompromised hosts.[2,3,6] Occasionally, a massive inoculum of organisms enters the bloodstream, causing a widely disseminated form of the disease known as miliary TB. It is named for the millet seed appearance of the small granulomas seen on chest radiograph, and it can become fatal rapidly.[16] Miliary TB is a medical emergency, requiring immediate treatment.

INFLUENCE OF HIV INFECTION ON PATHOGENESIS

HIV infection is the largest risk factor for active TB.[2,6,16] As CD4+ lymphocytes multiply in response to the mycobacterial infection, HIV multiplies within these cells and selectively destroys them. In turn, the TB-fighting lymphocytes are depleted.[16] HIV-infected patients infected with TB deteriorate more rapidly unless they receive antimycobacterial chemotherapy.[20,21] Most physicians elect to begin TB treatment first, and once this is under control, begin HIV treatment as well. Starting both treatments at the same time can lead to paradoxical worsening of the TB.[12,22]

CLINICAL PRESENTATION

TB classically presents with symptoms such as weight loss, fatigue, a productive cough, fever, and night sweats.[1,2,6,17] The onset of TB may be gradual, and the diagnosis may not be considered until a chest radiograph is performed.[2,6,17] As the infection progresses, cavitation is often seen on the radiograph. Physical examination is nonspecific, but suggestive of progressive pulmonary disease. Dullness to chest percussion, rales, and increased vocal fremitus are frequently observed on auscultation. Abnormal laboratory data usually are limited to moderate elevations in the white blood cell count with a lymphocyte predominance.

Patients coinfected with HIV may have atypical presentations.[1,2,6,16,23] As their CD4+ counts decline, HIV-positive patients are less likely to have positive skin tests, cavitary lesions, or fever. Pulmonary radiographic findings may be minimal or absent. Extrapulmonary TB typically presents as a slowly progressive decline in organ function.[2,6,16,17] Abnormal behavior, headaches, or convulsions suggest tuberculous meningitis.[6,16]

THE OLDER ADULTS

TB in the older adults is easily confused with other respiratory diseases. Many clinical findings are muted, or absent altogether. TB in the older adults is far less likely to present with positive skin tests, fevers, night sweats, sputum production, or hemoptysis.[2,16,24,25] In contrast, mental status changes are twice as common in the older adults, and mortality is 6 times higher.[2,16,24]

CHILDREN

TB in children, especially those younger than 12 years, may present as a typical bacterial pneumonia, called progressive primary TB.[17–19] Unlike adults, pulmonary TB in children often involves the lower and middle lobes.[17–19] Dissemination to the lymph nodes, gastrointestinal and genitourinary tracts, bone marrow, and meninges is fairly common. Because cavitary lesions are uncommon, children do not spread TB readily. However, TB can be rapidly fatal in a child, and it requires prompt chemotherapy.

DIAGNOSIS

SKIN TESTING

The Mantoux test is the preferred TB skin test. Tubersol 5 TU brand of the purified protein derivative appears to be the preferred product.[2,17,20] Injection should produce a small, raised, blanched wheal to be read by an experienced professional in 48 to 72 hours. Criteria for interpretation are listed in Table 43-1.[1,2,6,17,20] The CDC does not recommend the routine use of anergy panels.[20,26] The "booster effect" occurs in patients who do not respond to an initial skin test, but show a positive reaction if retested about a week later.[17,26]

ADDITIONAL TESTS

Sputum collected in the morning usually has the highest yield of organisms.[2,10,17] Daily sputum collections over 3 consecutive days are recommended. Sputum induction with aerosolized hypertonic saline may produce a diagnostic sample. Bronchoscopy, or aspiration of gastric fluid via a nasogastric tube, may be attempted in selected patients.[17] For patients with suspected extrapulmonary TB, samples of draining fluid, biopsies of the infected site, or both may be attempted. Blood cultures are positive occasionally, especially in AIDS patients.[17,23,27]

TREATMENT OF TB

GENERAL APPROACHES TO TREATMENT

Monotherapy can be used only for infected patients who do not have active TB (LTBI as shown by positive skin test). Once active disease is present, a minimum of two drugs and generally three or four drugs must be used simultaneously.[2,6,12,28] The shortest duration of treatment generally is 6 months, and 2 to 3 years of treatment may be necessary for cases of multidrug-resistant TB (MDR-TB).[2,6,12,28] Directly observed therapy (DOT) by a health care worker is a cost-effective way to ensure the completion of treatment.[2,6,12,28–30]

Table 43-1. Criteria for Tuberculin Positivity by Risk Group

Reaction ≥5 mm of Induration	Reaction ≥10 mm of Induration	Reaction ≥15 mm of Induration
HIV-positive persons	Recent immigrants (i.e., within the last 5 y) from high-prevalence countries	Persons with no risk factors for TB
Persons with recent contacts with TB patients	Injection drug users	
Fibrotic changes on chest radiograph consistent with prior TB	Residents and employees[†] of the following high-risk congregate settings: prisons and jails, nursing homes and other long-term facilities for the older asults, hospitals and other health care facilities, residential facilities for patients with AIDS, and homeless shelters	
Patients with organ transplants and other immunosuppressed patients (receiving the equivalent of ≥15 mg/d of prednisone for 1 mo or more)[*]	Mycobacteriology laboratory personnel	
	Persons with the following clinical conditions that place them at high risk: silicosis, diabetes mellitus, chronic renal failure, some hematologic disorders (e.g., leukemias and lymphomas), other specific malignancies (e.g., carcinoma of the head or neck and lung), weight loss of ≥10% of ideal body weight, gastrectomy, and jejunoileal bypass	
	Children younger than 4 y of age or infants, children, and adolescents exposed to adults at high risk	

[*]Risk of TB in patients treated with corticosteroids increases with higher dose and longer duration.
[†]For persons who are otherwise at low risk and are tested at the start of employment, a reaction of ≥15 mm induration is considered positive.
HIV, human immunodeficiency virus; TB, tuberculosis; AIDS, acquired immunodeficiency syndrome.
Source: Adapted from Centers for Disease Control and Prevention. Screening for tuberculosis and tuberculosis infection in high-risk populations: Recommendations of the Advisory Council for the Elimination of Tuberculosis. *MMWR.* 1995;44(No. RR-11):19–34.

NONPHARMACOLOGIC THERAPY

Nonpharmacologic interventions aim to (1) prevent the spread of TB, (2) find where TB has already spread, using contact investigation, and (3) replenish the weakened (consumptive) patient to a state of normal weight and well-being. Public health departments perform functions (1) and (2). Clinicians involved in the treatment of TB should verify that the local health department has been notified of all new cases of TB. Surgery may be needed to remove destroyed lung tissue, space-occupying infected lesions ("tuberculomas"), and certain extrapulmonary lesions.[2,12,28]

PHARMACOLOGIC THERAPY

Treating LTBI

Isoniazid is the preferred drug for treating LTBI.[2,6,12,28] Generally, isoniazid, 300 mg daily (5–10 mg/kg of body weight), is given alone for 9 months. Lower doses are less effective.[2,31] The treatment of LTBI reduces a person's lifetime risk of active TB from about 10% to about 1% (Table 43-2).[20] Rifampin, 600 mg daily for 4 months, can be used when isoniazid resistance is suspected, or when the patient cannot tolerate isoniazid.[2,19,32,33] Rifabutin, 300 mg daily, might be substituted for rifampin for patients at high risk of drug interactions. The combination of pyrazinamide plus rifampin is no longer recommended because of higher than expected rates of hepatotoxicity.[34] When resistance to isoniazid and rifampin is suspected in the isolate causing infection, there is no regimen proven to be effective.[2,28]

Treating Active Disease

Combination chemotherapy is required for treating active TB disease. The patient should receive at least two drugs to which the isolate is susceptible, and generally four drugs are given at the onset of treatment. Isoniazid and rifampin should be used together whenever possible, as they are the best drugs for preventing drug resistance.[2,6,28,35,36] Drug susceptibility testing should be done on the initial isolate for all patients with active TB. These data should guide the selection of drugs over the course of treatment.[2,6,12,28]

The standard TB treatment regimen is isoniazid, rifampin, pyrazinamide, and ethambutol for 2 months, followed by isoniazid and rifampin for 4 months, for a total of 6 months of treatment.[2,12,28] A total of 9 months of isoniazid and rifampin treatment is required for patients with cavitation on initial chest radiograph, positive cultures at the completion of 2 months initial-phase treatment, and in patients initially treated without pyrazinamide. Treatment should be continued for at least 6 months from the time they convert to smear and culture negative.[2,6,12,28] Some authors recommend therapeutic drug monitoring for such patients.[2,28,36,37] Table 43-3 shows the recommended treatment regimens for TB. When isoniazid and rifampin cannot be used, treatment durations become 2 years or more,

Table 43-2. Recommended Drug Regimens for Treatment of Latent Tuberculosis Infection in Adults

Drug	Interval and Duration	Comments	Rating* HIV−	Evidence† HIV+
Isoniazid	Daily for 9 mo[‡][§]	In HIV-infected patients, isoniazid maybe administered concurrently with NRTIs, protease inhibitors, or NNRTIs	A (II)	A (II)
	Twice weekly for 9 mo[‡][§]	DOT must be used with twice-weekly dosing	B (II)	B (II)
Isoniazid	Daily for 6 mo[§]	Not indicated for HIV-infected persons, those with fibrotic lesions on chest radiographs, or children	B (I)	C (I)
	Twice weekly for 6 mo[§]	DOT must be used with twice-weekly dosing	B (II)	C (I)
Rifampin	Daily for 4 mo	For persons who are contacts of patients with isoniazid-resistant, rifampin-susceptible TB.		
		In HIV-infected patients, protease inhibitors or NNRTIs should generally not be administered concurrently with rifampin; rifabutin can be used as an alternative for patients treated with indinavir, nelfinavir, amprenivir, ritonavir, or efavirenz, and possibly with nevirapine or soft-gel saquinavir[¶]	B(II)	B(III)

*Strength of recommendation: A = preferred; B = acceptable alternative; C = offer when A and B cannot be given.
†Quality of evidence: I = randomized clinical trial data; II = data from clinical trials that are not randomized or were conducted in other populations; III = expert opinion.
‡Recommended regimen for children younger than 18 years of age.
§Recommended regimens for pregnant women. Some experts would use rifampin and pyrazinamide for 2 months as an alternative regimen in HIV-infected pregnant women, although pyrazinamide should be avoided during the first trimester.
¶Rifabutin should not be used with hard-gel saquinavir or delavirdine. When used with other protease inhibitors or NNRTIs, dose adjustment of rifabutin may be required.
HIV, human immunodeficiency virus; NRTI, nucleoside reverse transcriptase inhibitor; NNRTI, non-nucleoside reverse transcriptase inhibitor; DOT, directly observed therapy; TB, tuberculosis.
Source: Adapted from Centers for Disease Control and Prevention. Targeted tuberculin testing and treatment of latent tuberculosis infection. *MMWR.* 2000;49(RR-6):31.

regardless of immune status.[2,12,28,36] When intermittent therapy is used, DOT is essential. Doses missed during an intermittent TB regimen decrease its efficacy and increase the relapse rate. When the patients' sputum smear results convert to negative, the risk of infecting others is greatly reduced, but it is not zero.[2,15,28] Such patients can be removed from respiratory isolation, but they must be careful not to cough on others, and should meet people only in well-ventilated places.

Adjustments to the regimen should be made once the susceptibility data are available.[2,12,28] Drug resistance should be expected in patients presenting for the retreatment of TB. Two or more drugs not previously used before, with in vitro activity against the patient's isolate, should be added to the regimen, as needed.[2,12,28] TB specialists should be consulted regarding cases of drug-resistant TB.[2,12,28] *It is critical to avoid monotherapy, and it is critical to avoid adding a single drug to a failing regimen.*[2,12,28]

SPECIAL POPULATIONS

Patients with central nervous system TB usually are treated for longer periods (9–12 months instead of 6 months,).[2,12,28] Extrapulmonary TB of the soft tissues can be treated with conventional regimens.[2,12,28] TB of the bone is typically treated for 9 months, occasionally with surgical debridement.[2,12,28] TB in children may be treated with regimens similar to those used in adults, although some physicians extend treatment to 9 months.[2,12,17,18,28,32,38] Pediatric doses of isoniazid and

rifampin on a milligram per kilogram basis are higher than those used in adults (see Table 43-4).[28]

Pregnant women receive the usual treatment of isoniazid, rifampin, and ethambutol for 9 months.[2,28,32,36,38] Pyrazinamide has not been studied in a large number of pregnant women, but anecdotal data suggest that it may be safe.[28] Vitamin B_6 should be provided. Streptomycin, other aminoglycosides, capreomycin, and ethionamide are generally avoided.[28,39] Para-aminosalicylic and cycloserine are used sparingly.[39] Quinolones generally are avoided in pregnancy.[28,39] Although most anti-TB drugs are excreted in breast milk, the amount of drug received by the infant through nursing is insufficient to cause toxicity. Quinolones should be avoided in nursing mothers, if possible.

HUMAN IMMUNODEFICIENCY VIRUS

Patients with AIDS or other immunocompromising conditions may be managed with chemotherapeutic regimens similar to those used in immunocompetent individuals, although treatment is often extended to 9 months (Table 43-3).[2,12,28] The precise duration of treatment remains a matter of debate. Highly intermittent regimens (twice or once weekly) are not recommended for HIV-positive TB patients.[28] Prognosis has been particularly poor for HIV-infected patients infected with MDR-TB. Some patients with AIDS malabsorb their oral medications, and drug interactions are common.[2,28,36,37] For these reasons, serum drug concentration monitoring should be strongly considered in this population.

Table 43-3. Drug Regimens for Culture-Positive Pulmonary Tuberculosis Caused by Drug-Susceptible Organisms

Initial Phase			Continuation Phase				Rating* (Evidence)[†]	
Regimen	Drugs	Interval and Doses[‡] (Minimal Duration)	Regimen	Drugs	Interval and Doses[‡§] (Minimal Duration)	Range of Total Doses (Minimal Duration)	HIV–	HIV+
1	INH RIF PZA EMB	7 d/wk for 56 doses (8 wk) or 5 d/wk for 40 doses (8 wk)[¶]	1a	INH/RIF	7 d/wk for 126 doses (18 wk) or 5 d/wk for 90 doses (18 wk)[¶]	182–130 (26 wk)	A (I)	A (II)
			1b	INH/RIF	Twice weekly for 36 doses (18 wk)	92–76 (26 wk)	A (I)	A (II)**
			1c[††]	INH/RPT	Once weekly for 18 doses (18 wk)	74–58 (26 wk)	B (I)	E (I)
2	INH RIF PZA EMB	7 d/wk for 14 doses (2 wk)[¶], then twice weekly for 12 doses (6 wk) or 5 d/wk for 10 doses (2 wk), then twice weekly for 12 doses (6 wk)	2a	INH/RIF	Twice weekly for 36 doses (18 wk)	62–58 (26 wk)	A (II)	B (II)**
			2b[††]	INH/RPT	Once weekly for 18 doses (18 wk)	44–40 (26 wk)	B (I)	E (I)
3	INH RIF PZA EMB	3 times weekly for 24 doses (8 wk)	3a	INH/RIF	3 times weekly for 54 doses (18 wk)	78 (26 wk)	B (I)	B (II)
4	INH RIF EMB	7 d/wk for 56 doses (8 wk) or 5 d/wk for 40 doses (8 wk)[¶]	4a	INH/RIF	7 d/wk for 217 doses (31 wk) or 5 d/wk for 155 doses (31 wk)[¶]	273–195 (39 wk)	C (I)	C (II)
			4b	INH/RIF	Twice weekly for 62 doses (31 wk)	118–102 (39 wk)	C (I)	C (II)

*Definitions of evidence ratings: A = preferred; B = acceptable alternative; C = offer when A and B cannot be given; E = should never be given.

[†]Definitions of evidence ratings: I = randomized clinical trial; II = data from clinical trials that were not randomized or were conducted in other populations; III = expert opinion.

[‡]When DOT is used, drugs may be given 5 d/wk and the necessary number of doses adjusted accordingly. Although there are no studies that compare five with seven daily doses, extensive experience indicates this would be an effective practice.

[§]Patients with cavitation on initial chest radiograph and positive cultures at completion of 2 months of therapy should receive a 7-month (31-week; either 217 doses [daily] or 62 doses [twice weekly]) continuation phase.

[¶]The 5 d/wk administration is always given by DOT. Rating for 5 d/wk regimens is A (III).

**Not recommended for HIV-infected patients with CD4+ cell counts <100 cells/mL.

[††]Options 1c and 2b should be used only in HIV-negative patients who have negative sputum smears at the time of completion of 2 months of therapy and who do not have cavitation on the initial chest radiograph. For patients started on this regimen and found to have a positive culture from the 2-month specimen, treatment should be extended for an extra 3 months.

HIV, human immunodeficiency virus; EMB: ethambutol; INH: isoniazid; PZA: pyrazinamide; RIF: rifampin; RPT: rifapentine.

Source: Adapted from Centers for Disease Control and Prevention. Treatment of tuberculosis. *MMWR.* 2003;52 (RR-11).

Table 43-4. Antituberculosis Drugs for Adults and Children*

Drug	Daily Doses†	Adverse Effects	Monitoring
Isoniazid	Adults: 5 mg/kg (300 mg). Children: 10–15 mg/kg (300 mg).	Asymptomatic elevation of aminotransferases, clinical hepatitis, fatal hepatitis, peripheral neurotoxicity, CNS effects, lupus-like syndrome, hypersensitivity, monoamine poisoning, diarrhea.	• LFT monthly in patients who have preexisting liver disease or who develop abnormal liver function that does not require discontinuation of drug. • Dosage adjustments may be necessary in patients receiving anticonvulsants or warfarin.
Rifampin	Adults‡: 10 mg/kg (600 mg). Children: 10–20 mg/kg. (600 mg)	Cutaneous reactions, gastrointestinal reactions (nausea, anorexia, abdominal pain), flu-like syndrome, hepatotoxicity, severe immunologic reactions, orange discoloration of bodily fluids (sputum, urine, sweat, tears), drug interactions caused by induction of hepatic microsomal enzymes.	• Rifampin causes many drug interactions. For a complete list of drug interactions and effects refer to CDC website: http://www.cdc.gov/tb/TB_HIV_Drugs/Table2.htm
Rifabutin	Adults‡: 5 mg/kg (300 mg). Children: Appropriate dosing unknown.	Hematologic toxicity, uveitis, gastrointestinal symptoms, polyarthralgias, hepatotoxicity, pseudojaundice (skin discoloration with normal bilirubin), rash, flu-like syndrome, orange discoloration of bodily fluids (sputum, urine, sweat, tears).	• Drug interactions of rifabutin are less problematic than rifampin.
Rifapentine	Adults: 10 mg/kg (continuation phase) (600 mg) Dosed weekly. Children: The drug is not approved for use in children.	Similar to those associated with rifampin.	• Drug interactions are being investigated and are likely similar to rifampin.
Pyrazinamide	Adults: Based on IBW. 40–55 kg, 1000 mg; 56–75 kg, 1500 mg; 76–90 kg, 2000 mg. Children: 15–30 mg/kg.	Hepatotoxicity, gastrointestinal symptoms (nausea, vomiting), nongouty polyarthralgia, asymptomatic hyperuricemia, acute gouty arthritis, transient morbilliform rash, dermatitis.	• Serum uric acid can serve as a surrogate marker for compliance. • LFTs in patients with underlying liver disease.
Ethambutol§	Adults: Based on IBW. 40–55 kg, 800 mg; 56–75 kg, 1200 mg; 76–90 kg, 1600 mg. Children‡: 15–20 mg/kg daily.	Retrobulbar neuritis, peripheral neuritis, cutaneous reactions.	• Baseline visual acuity testing and testing of color discrimination. • Monthly testing of visual acuity and color discrimination in patients taking >15–20 mg/kg, renal insufficiency, or receiving the drug for >2 mo
Cycloserine	Adults¶: 10–15 mg/kg per day, usually 500–750 mg/d in 2 doses. Children: 10–15 mg/kg per day.	CNS effects	• Monthly assessments of neuropsychiatric status. • Serum concentrations may be necessary until appropriate dose is established.
Ethionamide	Adults**: 15–20 mg/kg per day, usually 500–750 mg/d in a single daily dose or 2 divided doses. Children: 15–20 mg/kg per day.	Gastrointestinal effects, hepatotoxicity, neurotoxicity, endocrine effects.	• Baseline LFTs. • Monthly LFTs, if underlying liver disease is present. • TSH at baseline and monthly intervals.
Streptomycin	Adults: See footnote.†† Children: 20–40 mg/kg per day.	Ototoxicity, neurotoxicity, nephrotoxicity.	• Baseline audiogram, vestibular testing, Romberg testing, and Scr. • Monthly assessments of renal function and auditory or vestibular symptoms.

(continued)

Table 43-4. Antituberculosis Drugs for Adults and Children* (*Continued*)

Drug	Daily Doses[†]	Adverse Effects	Monitoring
Amikacin/ kanamycin	Adults: See footnote.[††] Children: 15–30 mg/kg per day, intravenously or intramuscularly as a single daily dose.	Ototoxicity, nephrotoxicity.	• Baseline audiogram, vestibular testing, Romberg testing, and Scr. • Monthly assessments of renal function and auditory or vestibular symptoms.
Capreomycin	Adults: See footnote.[††] Children: 15–30 mg/kg per day, intravenously or intramuscularly as a single daily dose.	Nephrotoxicity, ototoxicity.	• Baseline audiogram, vestibular testing, Romberg testing, and Scr. • Monthly assessments of renal function and auditory or vestibular symptoms. • Baseline and monthly serum K^+ and Mg^{++}.
p-Aminosalicylic acid	Adults: 8–12 g/d in 2 or 3 doses. Children: 200–300 mg/kg per day in 2–4 divided doses.	Hepatotoxicity, gastrointestinal distress, malabsorption syndrome, hypothyroidism, coagulopathy.	• Baseline LFTs and TSH. • TSH every 3 mo.
Levofloxacin	Adults: 500–1000 mg daily. Children: See footnote.[‡‡]	Gastrointestinal disturbance, neurologic effects, cutaneous reactions.	• No specific monitoring recommended.
Moxifloxacin	Adults: 400 mg daily. Children: See footnote.[§§]		
Gatifloxacin	Adults: 400 mg daily. Children: See footnote.[¶¶]		

*For purposes of this document, adult dosing begins at the age of 15 years.
[†]Dose per weight is based on ideal body weight. Children weighing more than 40 kg should be dosed as adults.
[‡]Dose may need to be adjusted when there is concomitant use of protease inhibitors or nonnucleoside reverse transcriptase inhibitors.
[§]The drug can likely be used safely in older children but should be used with caution in children younger than 5 years, in whom visual acuity cannot be monitored. In younger children, ethambutol (at the dose of 15 mg/kg per day) can be used if there is suspected or proven resistance to isoniazid or rifampin.
[¶]It should be noted that although this is the dose recommended generally, most physicians with experience using cycloserine indicate that it is unusual for patients to be able to tolerate this amount. Serum concentration measurements are often useful in determining the optimal dose for a given patient.
**The single daily dose can be given at bedtime or with the main meal.
[††]Dose: 15 mg/kg per day (1 g), and 10 mg/kg in persons more than 50 years of age (750 mg). Usual dose: 750–1000 mg administered intramuscularly or intravenously, given as a single dose 5–7 d/wk and reduced to 2 or 3 times per week after the first 2–4 months or after culture conversion, depending on the efficacy of the other drugs in the regimen.
[‡‡]The long-term (more than several weeks) use of levofloxacin in children and adolescents has not been approved because of concerns about effects on bone and cartilage growth. However, most experts agree that the drug should be considered for children with tuberculosis caused by organisms resistant to both isoniazid and rifampin. The optimal dose is not known.
[§§]The long-term (more than several weeks) use of moxifloxacin in children and adolescents has not been approved because of concerns about effects on bone and cartilage growth. The optimal dose is not known.
[¶¶]The long-term (more than several weeks) use of gatifloxacin in children and adolescents has not been approved because of concerns about effects on bone and cartilage growth. The optimal dose is not known.
CNS, central nervous system; LFT, liver function tests; IBW, ideal body weight; TSH, thyroid stimulating hormone.
Source: From Centers for Disease Control and Prevention. Treatment of tuberculosis. *MMWR.* 2003;52 (RR-11).

RENAL FAILURE

Isoniazid and rifampin do not require dose modification in renal failure.[31,36,39] Pyrazinamide and ethambutol typically are reduced to 3 times weekly.[28,31] Renally cleared TB drugs include the aminoglycosides (amikacin, kanamycin, and streptomycin), capreomycin, ethambutol, cycloserine, and levofloxacin.[28,31,33,39] Dosing intervals need to be extended for these drugs. Serum concentration monitoring must be performed for cycloserine to avoid dose-related toxicities in renal failure patients.[33,36,37]

HEPATIC FAILURE

Anti-TB drugs that rely on hepatic clearance for elimination include isoniazid, rifampin, pyrazinamide, ethionamide, and p-aminosalicylic acid.[39] About 50% of the ciprofloxacin is cleared by the liver. Elevations of serum transaminase concentrations generally are not correlated with the residual capacity of the liver to metabolize drugs, so these markers cannot be used as guides for drug dosing. Further, isoniazid, rifampin, pyrazinamide, and to a lesser degree, ethionamide, p-aminosalicylic acid, and rarely ethambutol, may cause hepatotoxicity.[28,36,39] These patients require close monitoring and may benefit from serum concentration monitoring.

THE TB DRUGS

The interested reader is referred to several other publications for more detailed information regarding these drugs.[2,11,28,34–37,39–42] A summary of daily doses, adverse effects, and monitoring parameters of first-line and second-line anti-TB drugs is provided in Table 43-4.[28]

EVALUATION OF THERAPEUTIC OUTCOMES

The most serious problem with TB therapy is patient's nonadherence to the prescribed regimens.[43,44] Unfortunately, there is no reliable way to identify such patients a priori. The most effective way to achieve this end is with DOT.[2,11,28] The use of DOT in nearly all patients with TB may be of benefit.[45] For patients who are acid fast bacillus smear positive, sputum samples should be sent for AFB stains every 1 to 2 weeks until two consecutive smears are negative. This provides early evidence of a response to treatment.[28] Once on maintenance therapy, sputum cultures can be performed monthly until two consecutive cultures are negative, which generally occurs over 2 to 3 months. If sputum cultures continue to be positive after 2 months, drug susceptibility testing should be repeated, and serum concentrations of the drugs should be checked.

Serum chemistries, including blood urea nitrogen, creatinine, aspartate transaminase, alanine transaminase, and a complete blood count with platelets should be performed at baseline and periodically thereafter, depending on the presence of other factors that may increase the likelihood of toxicity (advanced age, alcohol abuse, pregnancy).[2,28] Hepatotoxicity should be suspected in patients whose transaminases exceed 5 times the upper limit of normal or whose total bilirubin exceeds 3 mg/dL, and in patients with symptoms such as nausea, vomiting, or jaundice. At this point, the offending agent(s) should be discontinued. Sequential reintroduction of the drugs with frequent testing of liver enzymes is often successful in identifying the offending agent; other agents may be continued (Table 43-4).[28]

THERAPEUTIC DRUG MONITORING

Therapeutic drug monitoring (TDM) or applied pharmacokinetics is the use of serum drug concentrations to optimize therapy.[28,36,37] Non-AIDS patients with drug-susceptible TB generally do well, and TDM may be used if they are failing appropriate DOT (no clinical improvement after 2 to 4 weeks or smear positive after 4 to 6 weeks). On the other hand, patients with AIDS, diabetes, cystic fibrosis, and various gastrointestinal disorders often fail to absorb these drugs properly and are candidates for TDM. In addition, patients with hepatic or renal disease should be monitored, given their potential for overdoses. In the treatment of MDR-TB, TDM may be particularly useful.[39,41] Finally, TDM of the TB and HIV

drugs is perhaps the most logical way to untangle the complex drug interactions that take place. For a complete list of drug interactions visit the CDC website at http://www.cdc.gov/nchstp/tb/tb_hiv_drugs/toc.htm.[46]

EVIDENCE-BASED SUMMARY

- In the United States, TB disproportionately affects ethnic minorities as compared to whites, reflecting greater ongoing transmission in ethnic minority communities. Additional TB surveillance and preventive treatment is required within these communities.
- Coinfection with HIV and TB accelerates the progression of both diseases, thus requiring rapid diagnosis and treatment of both diseases.
- Mycobacteria are slow-growing organisms; in the laboratory, they require special stains, special growth media, and long periods of incubation to be isolated and identified.
- TB can produce atypical signs and symptoms in infants, the older adults, and immunocompromised hosts, and it can progress rapidly in these patients.
- LTBI can lead to reactivation disease years after the primary infection occurred.
- The patient suspected of having active TB disease must be isolated until the diagnosis is confirmed and they are no longer contagious. Often, isolation takes place in specialized "negative pressure" hospital rooms to prevent the spread of TB.
- Isoniazid and rifampin are the two most important TB drugs; organisms resistant to both of these drugs (MDR-TB) are much more difficult to treat.
- Never add a single drug to a failing regimen!
- DOT should be used whenever possible to reduce treatment failures and the selection of drug-resistant isolates.

REFERENCES

1. *Report on the Global Tuberculosis Epidemic.* World Health Organization, Geneva, Switzerland; 1998.
2. Iseman MD. *A Clinician's Guide to Tuberculosis.* Philadelphia, PA: Lippincott Williams & Wilkins; 2000.
3. McCray E, Weinbaum CM, Braden CR, et al. The epidemiology of tuberculosis in the United States. *Clin Chest Med.* 1997;18:99–113.

4. Centers for Disease Control and Prevention. Trends in Tuberculosis Morbidity—United States, 1992–2002. *MMWR.* 2003;52:222–224.

5. Centers for Disease Control and Prevention. Trends in tuberculosis morbidity—United States, 2005. *MMWR.* 2006, 55;305–308.

6. Haas DW. Mycobacterium tuberculosis. In: Mandell GL, Bennett JE, Dolin R, eds. *Principles and Practice of Infectious Diseases.* 5th ed. New York, NY: Churchill Livingstone; 2000:2576–2607.

7. Small PM, Shafer RW, Hopewell PC, et al. Exogenous reinfection with multidrug-resistant *Mycobacterium tuberculosis* in patients with advanced HIV infection. *N Engl J Med.* 1993;328:1137–1144.

8. Beck-Sague C, Dooley SW, Hutton MD, et al. Hospital outbreak of multidrug-resistant *Mycobacterium tuberculosis* infections: Factors in transmission to staff and HIV-infected patients. *JAMA.* 1992;268:1280–1286.

9. Centers for Disease Control and Prevention. Meeting the challenge of multidrug-resistant tuberculosis: Summary of a conference. *MMWR.* 1992;41(R-11):51–71.

10. Heifets L. Mycobacteriology laboratory. *Clin Chest Med* 1997;18:35–53.

11. Heifets LB. Drug susceptibility tests in the management of chemotherapy of tuberculosis. In: Heifets LB, ed. *Drug Susceptibility in the Chemotherapy of Mycobacterial Infections.* Boca Raton, FL: CRC Press; 1991:89–122.

12. Daley CL, Chambers HF. Mycobacterium tuberculosis complex. In Yu VL, Weber R, Raoult D, eds. *Antimicrobial therapy and vaccines.* Volume I, Microbes, 2nd ed. New York, NY: Apple Trees Productions; 2002:841–865.

13. Roberts GD, Böttger EC, Stockman L. Methods for the rapid identification of mycobacterial species. *Clin Lab Med.* 1996;16:603–615.

14. Sandin RL. Polymerase chain reaction and other amplification techniques in mycobacteriology. *Clin Lab Med.* 1996;16:617–639.

15. Piessens WF, Nardell EA. Pathogenesis of tuberculosis. In: Reichman LB, Hershfield ES, eds. *Tuberculosis. A Comprehensive International Approach.* 2nd ed. New York, NY: Marcel Dekker; 2000:241–260.

16. Daniel TM, Boom WH, Ellner JJ. Immunology of tuberculosis. In: Reichman LB, Hershfield ES, eds. *Tuberculosis. A Comprehensive International Approach.* 2nd ed. New York, NY: Marcel Dekker; 2000:157–185.

17. American Thoracic Society/Centers for Disease Control and Prevention. Diagnostic standards and classification of tuberculosis in adults and children. *Am J Respir Crit Care Med.* 2000;161:1376–1395.

18. Peloquin CA, Berning SE. Tuberculosis and multi-drug resistant tuberculosis in children. *Pediatr Nurs.* 1995;21:566–572.

19. Correa AG. Unique aspects of tuberculosis in the pediatric population. *Clin Chest Med.* 1997;18:89–98.

20. American Thoracic Society/Centers for Disease Control and Prevention. Targeted tuberculin skin testing and treatment of latent tuberculosis infection. *Am J Respir Crit Care Med.* 2000;161:S221–S247.

21. Pape JW, Jean SS, Ho JL, et al. Effect of isoniazid prophylaxis on incidence of active tuberculosis and progression of HIV infection. *Lancet.* 1993;342:268–272.

22. Narita M, Ashkin D, Hollender ES, Pitchenik AE. Paradoxical worsening of tuberculosis following antiretroviral therapy in patients with AIDS. *Am J Respir Crit Care Med.* 1998;158:157–161.

23. Barnes PF, Bloch AB, Davidson PT, Snider DE. Tuberculosis in patients with human immunodeficiency virus infection. *N Engl J Med.* 1991;324:1644–1650.

24. Alvarez S, Shell C, Berk SL. Pulmonary tuberculosis in elderly men. *Am J Med.* 1987;82:602–606.

25. Umeki S. Comparison of younger and elderly patients with pulmonary tuberculosis. *Respiration.* 1989;55:75–83.

26. Centers for Disease Control and Prevention. Anergy skin testing and preventive therapy for HIV-infected persons: revised recommendations. *MMWR.* 1997;46(RR-15):1–10.

27. Bouza E, Diaz-Lopez MD, Moreno S, et al. Mycobacterium tuberculosis bacteremia in patients with and without human immunodeficiency virus infection. *Arch Intern Med.* 1993;153:496–500.

28. American Thoracic Society/Centers for Disease Control/Infectious Disease Society of America. Treatment of tuberculosis. *Am J Respir Crit Care Med.* 2003;167:603–662.

29. Fujiwara PI, Larkin C, Frieden TR. Directly observed therapy in New York City. *Clin Chest Med.* 1997;18:135–148.

30. Weis SE. Universal directly observed therapy. *Clin Chest Med.* 1997;18:155–163.

31. Malone RS, Fish DN, Spiegel DM, Childs JM, Peloquin CA. The effect of hemodialysis on isoniazid, rifampin, pyrazinamide, and ethambutol. *Am J Respir Crit Care Med.* 1999;159:1580–1584.

32. Vallejo JG, Starke JR. Tuberculosis and pregnancy. *Clin Chest Med.* 1992;13:693–707.

33. Malone RS, Fish DN, Spiegel DM, Childs JM, Peloquin CA. The effect of hemodialysis on cycloserine, ethionamide, para-aminosalicylate, and clofazimine. *Chest.* 1999;116:984–990.

34. Centers for Disease Control and Prevention. Update. fatal and severe liver injuries associated with rifampin and pyrazinamide for latent tuberculosis infection, and revisions in the American Thoracic Society/CDC recommendations. *MMWR.* 2001;50(34):733–735.

35. Mitchison DA. Basic mechanisms of chemotherapy. *Chest.* 1979;76(Suppl 6):771–781.

36. Peloquin CA. Pharmacological Issues in the Treatment of Tuberculosis. *Ann NY Acad Sci.* 2001;953:157–164.

37. Peloquin CA. Therapeutic drug monitoring in the treatment of tuberculosis. *Drugs.* 2002;62:2169–2183.

38. Hamadeh MA, Glassroth J. Tuberculosis and pregnancy. *Chest.* 1992;101:1114–1120.

39. Peloquin CA. Antituberculosis drugs: Pharmacokinetics. In: Heifets LB, ed. *Drug Susceptibility in the Chemotherapy of Mycobacterial Infections.* Boca Raton, FL: CRC Press; 1991:59–88.

40. McEvoy GK, ed. *AHFS Drug Information*. Bethesda, MD: American Soc Health-Systems Pharmacists; 2003.

41. Holdiness MR. Clinical pharmacokinetics of the antituberculosis drugs. *Clin Pharmacokinet*. 1984;9:511–544.

42. Girling DJ. Adverse effects of antituberculous drugs. *Drugs*. 1982;23:56–74.

43. Brudney K, Dobkin J. Resurgent tuberculosis in New York City: Human immunodeficiency virus, homelessness, and the decline of tuberculosis control programs. *Am Rev Resp Dis*. 1991;144:745–749.

44. Mahmoudi A, Iseman MD. Pitfalls in the care of patients with tuberculosis: Common errors and their association with the acquisition of drug resistance. *JAMA*. 1993;270:65–68.

45. Chaulk CP, Bartlett JG, Chaisson RE. *15 Years of Directly Observed Therapy for TB*. Program and Abstracts. 32nd Annual Meeting. Infectious Diseases Society of America. Orlando, FL. October 7–9, 1994. Abstract 181.

46. Peloquin CA. Agents for tuberculosis. In: Piscitelli SC, Rodvold KA, eds. *Drug Interactions in Infectious Diseases*. Totowa, NJ: Humana Press; 2001:109–120.

Chapter 44

Urinary Tract Infections and Prostatitis

Elizabeth A. Coyle and Randall A. Prince

SEARCH STRATEGY

A systematic search of the medical literature was performed on November 2006. The search included relevant articles from PubMed, Ovid, and guidelines from the Infectious Diseases Society of America.

INTRODUCTION

Urinary tract infections (UTIs) are one of the most commonly occurring bacterial infections, accounting for millions of patient visits annually.[1–3] Approximately one in three females will have had a UTI by their mid-twenties. In the older adults, infection rates in men and women are similar.

A UTI is defined as the presence of microorganisms in the urinary tract that cannot be accounted for by contamination. UTIs are classified by several methods. Commonly, describing them by anatomic site or as uncomplicated or complicated is most typical. The main classification method used in this chapter will be the categorization of UTIs as uncomplicated or complicated. Tables 44-1 to 44-3 present summary lists on clinical presentation, diagnostic criteria, and empiric therapy.

UNCOMPLICATED UTI

EPIDEMIOLOGY AND MICROBIOLOGY

Uncomplicated infections occur in individuals who lack structural or functional abnormalities of the urinary tract that may interfere with the normal flow of urine or voiding mechanism. Normal healthy females of child-bearing age are the individuals who fit this category almost exclusively. Males are excluded from this UTI classification because their infections most often represent a structural or neurologic abnormality.

Approximately 20% of the females will suffer from a symptomatic UTI during their lifetime. A marked increase in the UTI after puberty is thought to be associated with sexual activity as the percentage of nonpregnant females having significant bacteriuria increases to as much as 4% compared to 1% before puberty. Unfortunately, a significant percentage (20%) of women will have recurrent infections as either uncomplicated or complicated. The women still classified as uncomplicated, but experiencing recurrent UTIs, have less than three UTIs within a year. Most physicians would classify a more frequent UTI presentation, regardless of clinical presentation or anatomical site, as complicated UTI.

The microbiology of uncomplicated UTIs by the definition stated shows *Escherichia coli* to be the causative bacterium in approximately 80% of cases.[4,5] Other organisms that are less frequently encountered include *Staphylococcus saprophyticus*, *Proteus mirabilis*, and *Klebsiella pneumoniae*. The surveillance data demonstrating the predominance of *E. coli* in uncomplicated UTI has major implications for the empiric management of uncomplicated UTI.

CLINICAL PRESENTATION AND DIAGNOSTIC EVALUATION

Typical symptoms in the primary care setting are frequency, dysuria, and urgency (see Table 44-1).[4,6] A

Table 44-1. Diagnostic Criteria for Significant Bacteriuria

$\geq 10^2$ CFU coliforms/mL or $\geq 10^5$ CFU noncoliforms/mL in a symptomatic female
$\geq 10^3$ CFU bacteria/mL in a symptomatic male
$\geq 10^5$ CFU bacteria/mL in asymptomatic individuals on two consecutive specimens
Any growth of bacteria on suprapubic catheterization in a symptomatic patient
$\geq 10^2$ CFU bacteria/mL in a catheterized patient

CFU, colony forming units.

Table 44-2. Clinical Presentation of Urinary Tract Infections in Adults

Signs and symptoms
Lower UTI: dysuria, urgency, frequency, nocturia, suprapubic heaviness
Gross hematuria
Upper UTI: Flank pain, fever, nausea, vomiting, malaise
Physical examination
Upper UTI: costovertebral tenderness
Laboratory tests
Bacteriuria
Pyuria (white blood cell count $>10/mm^3$)
Nitrite-positive urine (with nitrite reducers)
Leukocyte esterase–positive urine
Antibody-coated bacteria (upper UTI)

significant number of patients will have hematuria. Systemic presentation such as fever, malaise, and nausea are not to be expected. The finding of dysuria requires careful consideration of non-UTI diseases, particularly sexually transmitted diseases. Utilizing the patient history with a urinalysis is quite often sufficient for the diagnosis of uncomplicated UTI. Dipstick methods for the determination of pyuria and the presence of bacteriuria are quite helpful in the outpatient setting. When used together, their specificity is usually about 90% and their sensitivity at least 60%.[7] Negative dipstick results with a high suspicion of UTI will require a microscopic examination for better detection confidence. Urine culture is not necessary in uncomplicated UTI unless treatment failure is an issue.[1]

MANAGEMENT

Our desired goals are to eradicate the organism(s), prevent recurrence, and prevent or treat the consequences of the infection. Utilizing appropriate pharmacological intervention is most often effective in treating or preventing infection consequences and eradicating the organism(s). However, preventing recurrence may not follow appropriate management for a variety of reasons. Use of a nonantimicrobial in uncomplicated UTIs is common, but often without evidence-based data. For example, the dysuria associated with UTI is a result of the infection and the appropriate antimicrobial therapy

Table 44-3. Empiric Treatment of Urinary Tract Infections and Prostatitis

Infectious Disease	Causative Organisms	Treatments
Uncomplicated UTI	*E. coli, S. saprophyticus*	Trimethoprim–sulfamethoxazole × 3–5 d Quinolone × 3–5 d
Complicated UTI		
Pregnancy	*E. coli, S. saprophyticus*	Amoxicillin–clavulanate × 7 d Cephalosporin × 7 d Trimethoprim–sulfamethoxazole × 7 d (avoid during third trimester)

Pyelonephritis	*E. coli, Proteus* spp.,
	  K. pneumoniae, P. aeruginosa,
	  S. fecalis
		Quinolone × 14 d
		  (oral for mild to moderate)
		Trimethoprim–sulfamethoxazole × 14 days
		  (oral for mild to moderate)
		Extended spectrum penicillin plus aminoglycoside × 14 days
		  (oral therapy may complete a total of 2 weeks of therapy)

Recurrent UTI		Trimethoprim–sulfamethoxazole, 1/2 single-strength tablet
		  daily × 6 mo
		Nitrofurantoin 50 mg daily × 6 mo
		  (Suppressive therapy for >3 UTIs/yr)

Prostatitis		
Acute	*E. coli, K. pneumoniae*	Trimethoprim–sulfamethoxazole × 4–6 wk Quinolone × 4–6 wk (IV therapy may be needed initially)
Chronic	*E. coli, K. pneumoniae,* *Proteus* spp.; *P. aeruginosa*	Trimethoprim–sulfamethoxazole × 6 wk or longer Quinolone × 6 wk or longer

will eliminate this symptom. Therefore, the practice of using urinary analgesics for dysuria is not usually warranted. Encouraging fluids, however, is prudent as a natural means of eliminating bacteria from the urinary tract.[2]

Therapy is directed against *E. coli* as it is the predominant causative organism.[1,5] Unfortunately, this organism, like many others, has developed an increasing resistance to many antimicrobial agents. Of particular note is the ever-increasing resistance of *E. coli* to ampicillin and many cephalosprins. Some areas of the United States have been experiencing an increase in resistance by *E. coli* to the product trimethoprim–sulfamethoxazole.[8,9] It is, therefore, incumbent upon the physician to know the local susceptibility patterns of antimicrobial agents to potential urinary pathogens.

The length of therapy for uncomplicated UTI has been debated for several years. Current data suggest short-course therapy to be the most appropriate approach. The use of single-dose therapy should be discouraged as lower cure rates and high recurrence has been documented. Short-course therapy (3 or 5 days) still has the advantages of increased patient adherence, decreased cost, fewer side effects, and reduced recurrence rates as compared with single-dose therapy.[4,10–13] Using 1 or 2 weeks of therapy for uncomplicated UTI is not recommended owing to increased side effects, increased cost, and no marked increase in efficacy. The data suggest that either fluorinated quinolone or trimethoprim–sulfamethoxazole be used empirically in uncomplicated UTI. Other agents, such as nitrofurantoin may be effective. In the case of nitrofurantoin, short-course therapy is not as efficacious as for fluorinated quinolones or trimethoprim–sulfamethoxazole; therefore, a treatment course of at least 7 days should be used.

COMPLICATED UTI

Basically, complicated UTIs are those that do not meet the definition of uncomplicated UTI. For example, all UTIs in males are complicated, as males will have some predisposing factor(s) for acquiring a UTI. Regardless of gender, complicated UTI occurs due to predisposing factor(s) such as a congenital abnormality or distortion of the urinary tract, a stone, indwelling catheter, prostatic hypertrophy, obstruction, and/or neurologic deficit that interferes with the normal flow of urine and urinary tract defenses.[14,15] Additionally, upper tract infection, that is, pyelonephritis, will be considered as a complicated UTI because its treatment usually is prolonged and directed by laboratory testing. For clarity, the various types of complicated UTIs will be discussed individually rather than attempt to discuss complicated UTI as a homogenous topic.

GENERAL EPIDEMIOLOGY AND MICROBIOLOGY

No specific figures are available on the number of cases of complicated UTIs per year, but it is safe to estimate there occur thousands of complicated UTIs annually in the United States. Pyelonephritis alone accounts for several hundred thousand cases annually, with about half of them, requiring hospitalization.[16] At particular risk are pregnant women since complicated UTI is associated with premature labor and low-birth-weight infants.[17] Older adults, both men and women, experience a significant incidence of complicated UTI and are susceptible to urosepsis.[18] General risk factors associated with complicated UTIs are listed in Table 44-1.

As compared to uncomplicated UTI, *E. coli* causes less than 50% of complicated UTIs. As a subset, acute pyelonephritis in an otherwise normal, healthy individual is caused by *E. coli* in 80% of cases. Enterococci, *Pseudomonas aeruginosa*, *K. pneumoniae*, *Proteus* spp., staphylococci, and *Enterobacter* spp. are often isolated in complicated UTI with *E. coli* and enterococci being the most commonly isolated organisms.[10,19]

OVERALL CLINICAL PRESENTATION AND DIAGNOSTIC EVALUATION

The clinical signs and symptoms are quite diverse. Fever, flank pain, costovertebral angle tenderness and other systemic signs and symptoms generally lead one to an initial suggestion of upper tract infection (see Table 44-1). However, dysuria, frequency, and urgency may also be present. There are a multitude of presenting signs and symptoms for complicated UTI and no one constellation fits perfectly. Older adults, the immunocompromised host, the catheterized patient, and so on, all have potential differing presentations. Therefore, any clinical presentation of signs and symptoms suggestive of urinary tract invasion warrants further diagnostic testing.

Urine culture and urinalysis are required for the confirmation of complicated UTI. Usually obtaining a midstream clean-catch urine specimen showing at least 10^2 organisms/mL with suggestive symptoms is confirmatory. If noncoliform organisms are noted, then at least 10^5 organisms/mL would be confirmatory. Counts less than 10^2/mL do not rule out UTI, particularly in men and pregnant women. Pyuria and hematuria are commonly noted in complicated UTI. Table 44-2 lists the criteria of significant bacteriuria for differing conditions.[20]

UTIs IN MALES

Except for the age extremes, the incidence of infection in males is less than females. In very young males, structural anomalies are usually responsible for UTI but as the male ages into adulthood, UTI often occurs as the result of urinary tract instrumentation. In the older male, both structural (prostatic hypertrophy) and instrumentation factors may cause UTI. Recurrence of infection is seen in the older male because of the prostate being the site of continued bacterial seeding of the urinary tract. Urinalysis and urine culture should be obtained before therapy initiation as infections in the male are not as predictable as in women.

Most physicians will treat male UTI with a course of therapy directed by laboratory analysis for 10–14 days. Short-term therapy should not be used. Initial therapy usually involves the use of fluoroquinolone or trimethoprim–sulfamethoxazole.[21] If recurrent infections exist, treatment periods of at least 6 weeks may be used.[22] Long-term therapy courses have demonstrated more successful cure rates than the 2-week therapy. Even with long-term therapy, recurrent infections are difficult to cure and success is related to factors such as prostatic involvement, obstruction, and more than one causative organism. Alterations in treatment due to unsuccessful treatment are directed by further urine culture testing and diagnostic workup where appropriate.

RECURRENT INFECTIONS

Recurrent infections are quite common and the majority are caused by reinfection of a new organism different from the organism causing the preceding infection. The patient is typically female with a history of lower tract infections.

For patients experiencing less than three infections per year, each new infection should be treated as a separate acute process. Short-term therapy for each infection would be prudent. In addition, self-administration of antimicrobials at the onset of symptoms has been successful and convenient for some women.[23] The physician may choose from several treatment strategies based upon the predisposing factors, number of episodes per year, and patient's preference. A couple of common factors associated with recurrence are sexual intercourse and diaphragm or spermicide use for birth control. Additional management choices include self-administered therapy, postcoital therapy, and continuous low-dose prophylaxis.

Patients with more than three infections per year and not having any apparent reason for the recurrences are treated with long-term prophylactic therapy. After a conventional course of therapy for a given UTI, prophylaxis is instituted. Older men, women, and children have benefited from long-term prophylaxis by having a marked reduction in their symptomatic UTIs. For example, women have had recurrence rates drop to less than one infection per patient-year from an initial rate of three per patient-year.[24] Trimethoprim–sulfamethoxazole (one-half of a single-strength tablet), trimethoprim (100 mg daily), fluoroquinolone (one tablet daily), and nitrofurantoin (50 or 100 mg daily) all reduce the rate of reinfection when used in single-agent therapy.[24] During prophylactic therapy (usually 6 months in length), urine cultures are obtained monthly, so that a conventional course of therapy can be instituted based on the last culture results in case the patient develops a UTI on the prophylaxis therapy.

Women experiencing symptomatic reinfection after sexual intercourse may be treated with postcoital single-dose prophylactic therapy.[25] Postintercourse voiding should also be encouraged. A lack of estrogen may be responsible for recurrence in postmenopausal women owing to an increase in *E. coli* vaginal colonization. Topically applied estrogen cream may be helpful in this setting.

If recurrence is due to relapse, that is, persistence of infection with the same organism after therapy for an isolated UTI, then the therapeutic approach focuses on assessing the patient for structural anomalies, prostatitis (for males), and infection of the renal tissue. If short-course therapy was used for the initial UTI, then a 2-week course is now prudent. Failing a conventional course would require a few weeks of therapy; therapy should then be continued for another 2 to 4 weeks. Urological investigation will be necessary in those not having success with the aforementioned therapies, and very prolonged therapy may be needed, particularly when no apparent cause for relapse is found.

ACUTE PYELONEPHRITIS

When signs and symptoms of upper tract infection are present as stated earlier, aggressive management is usually warranted. Depending on the overall presentation, hospitalization may be necessary. The initial workup should be a Gram stain of the urine, urinalysis, and culture and sensitivity tests. The therapeutic objections in this setting should be to achieve not only therapeutic urine concentrations of an appropriate antimicrobial, but also effective plasma concentration of it, as well. Additionally, an agent that will provide suitable renal tissue effectiveness seems prudent for full eradication of the invading organism.

Again, fluoroquinolone or trimethoprim–sulfamethoxazole for a 2-week course of oral therapy is effective in mild or moderate cases.[1,26] If the Gram stain shows a gram-positive coccus, *Streptococcus faecalis* should be considered, and therapy with ampicillin should be used. The seriously ill patient will require hospitalization and parenteral therapy at least initially. A number of antimicrobial agents are effective in these patients such as combination therapy of an aminoglycoside and ampicillin or an extended-spectrum beta-lactam antimicrobial, a fluoroquinolone, or a carbapenem.[1,26] Therapy should stabilize the patient within 24 hours and a significant reduction in the bacteriology should be demonstrated within a couple of days. If an appropriate response is not seen in few days, further investigation along with a switch in antimicrobial therapy, based on recent blood and/or urine culture reports, is needed. Follow-up urine cultures should be performed 2 weeks after completion of therapy to ensure an appropriate outcome and to check for possible relapse.

UTI IN PREGNANCY

A variety of factors contribute to the development of bacteriuria and UTI in the pregnant patient via physiological or urine component changes promoting bacterial growth. Up to 40% of bacteriuric pregnant patients will develop pyelonephritis. If untreated, asymptomatic bacteriuria has the potential to cause significant adverse effects, including prematurity, low birth weight, and stillbirth.[27,28] Therapy is a particular challenge for the physician, as the therapy needs to be effective and safe for the patient as well as the unborn child. The use of a sulfonamide, cephalosporin, or penicillin agent for a week of therapy is very effective. Follow-up urine cultures posttherapy are recommended.

UTI IN CATHETERIZED PATIENTS

In the hospital or nursing home setting, it is the use of an indwelling catheter that is frequently associated with infection of the urinary tract. The risk of infection from a single catheterization in a healthy patient is quite low; however, bacteriuria is going to occur in the patient with an indwelling catheter, regardless of therapeutic approaches.[29–31] One may delay the appearance of bacteria in the urine, but with sufficient time, all catheterized patients will suffer from bacteriuria. The use of aseptic techniques for catheterization, a closed drainage system, and prophylactic antimicrobials may have improved the overall incidence of UTIs in the catheterized patient by a few weeks, but these methods do not eliminate the finding.[30,32] The presence of a foreign body in the urinary system for a sufficient period of time will lead to bacteriuria and potentially UTI. Unfortunately, UTI symptoms in catheterized patient are not clearly defined and may not be of predictive value. When bacteriuria occurs in the asymptomatic, short-term catheterized patient (<30 days), the use of systemic antibiotics should be withheld and the catheter removed as soon as possible. If the patient becomes symptomatic, the catheter should be removed

and systemic treatment be used for a couple of weeks. As bacteriuria will occur in the long-term catheterized patients, urine cultures should be done periodically and if the patient becomes symptomatic, therapy should be instituted as per the last urine culture results.

PROSTATITIS

INTRODUCTION

Bacterial prostatitis, an inflammation of the prostate gland and surrounding tissue as a result of infection, is classified as either acute or chronic. Pathogens and significant inflammatory cells must be present in prostatic secretions and urine to make the diagnosis of bacterial prostatitis. Up to 50% of males develop some form of prostatitis during their lifetime.[33,34] The acute form typically is an acute infectious disease characterized by a sudden onset of fever, tenderness, and urinary and constitutional symptoms while chronic prostatitis presents with the following symptoms: urinating difficulty, low back pain, perineal pressure or a combination of these symptoms.

It would appear that intraprostatic reflux of infected urine plays a significant role in the development of prostatitis.[33,34] Indwelling urethral catheterization, urethral instrumentation, and transurethral prostatectomy in patients with infected urine can cause prostatitis. In addition, the activity of prostatic antibacterial factor and its dependency on zinc concentrations is of undetermined significance in the development of prostatitis.[35]

MICROBIOLOGY

E. coli is the predominant organism in acute prostatitis and occurs in 75% of cases. Other gram-negative organisms frequently isolated include *K. pneumoniae*, *P. mirabilis*, and less frequently, *P. aeruginosa*, *Enterobacter* spp., and *Serratia* spp.[33,34] *E. coli* most commonly causes chronic bacterial prostatitis with other gram-negative organisms isolated less frequently. The importance of gram-positive organisms in chronic bacterial prostatitis remains controversial.

CLINICAL PRESENTATION

The clinical presentation of acute and chronic prostatitis is presented in Table 44-4. The diagnosis of acute bacterial prostatitis can be made from the patient's clinical presentation and the presence of significant bacteriuria. In contrast, chronic bacterial prostatitis is more difficult to diagnose and treat. Chronic bacterial prostatitis is typically characterized by recurrent UTIs with the same pathogen, is the most common cause of recurrent UTI

Table 44-4. Clinical Presentation of Bacterial Prostatitis

Signs and symptoms
    Acute bacterial prostatitis: high fever, chills, malaise, myalgia, localized pain (perineal, rectal, sacrococcygeal), frequency, urgency, dysuria, nocturia, and retention
    Chronic bacterial prostatitis: voiding difficulties (frequency, urgency, dysuria), low back pain, and perineal and suprapubic discomfort
Physical examination
    Acute bacterial prostatitis: swollen, tender, tense, or indurated gland
    Chronic bacterial prostatitis: boggy, indurated (enlarged) prostate in most patients
Laboratory tests
    Bacteriuria
    Bacteria in expressed prostatic secretions

in males, and remains asymptomatic in many patients. Because physical examination of the prostate is often normal, urinary tract localization studies are critical to the diagnosis of chronic bacterial prostatitis.[36]

MANAGEMENT

The therapeutic objectives for bacterial prostatitis are similar to that of UTI. Generally speaking, acute prostatitis responds nicely to pharmacologic intervention. Prostatic penetration of antimicrobials occurs because the acute inflammatory reaction alters the cellular membrane barrier between the bloodstream and the prostate. Most patients can be managed with oral antimicrobial agents, such as trimethoprim–sulfamethoxazole and the fluoroquinolones, with intravenous therapy rarely necessary. The length of therapy is kept to be 4 weeks to minimize the risk of chronic prostatitis development. Some physicians may use suppressive therapy for recurrent infections (see Table 44-4).[37]

Chronic bacterial prostatitis rarely results in cure, despite the achievement of appropriate systemic concentrations of a suitable antimicrobial. It seems that despite these systemic concentrations, prostatic fluid/tissue concentrations are not appropriate. Several factors that determine antibiotic diffusion into prostatic secretions include lipid solubility, amount of unionized drug, and pH gradient from plasma to prostatic tissue.

Appropriate antimicrobial choices considering the potential infecting organisms and desirable antimicrobial characteristics for prostatic activity include fluoroquinolones and trimethoprim–sulfamethoxazole (the sulfa component probably adds little for efficacy). Therapy should be continued for 4 to 6 weeks initially with long treatments necessary in select cases. Suppressive therapy can be an option for regimen failures.

EVIDENCE-BASED SUMMARY

Uncomplicated urinary tract infections
- Uncomplicated UTIs are most common in an otherwise healthy female who lacks structural or functional abnormalities of the urinary tract.
- Eighty-five percent of uncomplicated UTIs are caused by *E. coli*, and the remainder are caused primarily by *S. saprophyticus*, *Proteus* spp., and *Klebsiella* spp.
- Symptoms of lower UTIs include dysuria, urgency, frequency, nocturia, and suprapubic heaviness.
- The goals of treatment of UTIs are to prevent or treat systemic consequences of infections, eradicate the invading organism(s), and prevent the recurrence of infection.
- Uncomplicated UTIs can be managed most effectively with short-course (3 days) therapy with either trimethoprim–sulfamethoxazole or fluoroquinolone.
- In choosing appropriate antibiotic therapy, physicians need to be cognizant of antibiotic resistance patterns, particularly to *E. coli*. Recently, trimethoprim–sulfamethoxazole has demonstrated diminished activity against *E. coli* in some areas of the country, with reported resistance up to 20%.

Complicated urinary tract infections
- Most often complicated infections are associated with a predisposing lesion of the urinary tract; however, the term may be used to refer to all other infections, except for those in the otherwise healthy adult female.
- Complicated UTIs can involve more systemic symptoms such as fever, nausea, vomiting, and flank pain.
- Enterococci, *P. aeruginosa*, *K. pneumoniae*, *Proteus* spp., staphylococci, and *Enterobacter* spp. are often isolated in complicated UTI with *E. coli* and enterococci being the most commonly isolated organisms.
- Complicated infections require longer treatment periods (2 weeks) usually with one of these agents.

Prostatitis
- Acute bacterial prostatitis can be managed with many agents that have activity against the causative organism.
- Therapy with trimethoprim–sulfamethoxazole or fluoroquinolone is preferred for 4 to 6 weeks.
- Chronic prostatitis requires an agent that is not only active against the causative organism but also concentrates in the prostatic secretions.

REFERENCES

1. Warren JW, Abrutyn E, Hebel JR, et al. Guidelines for antimicrobial treatment of uncomplicated acute bacterial cystitis and acute pyelonephritis. *Clin Infect Dis.* 1999;29: 745–758.
2. Fihn SD. Acute uncomplicated urinary tract infection in women. *N Engl J Med.* 2003;349:259–266.
3. Foxman B. Epidemiology of urinary tract infections: Incidence, morbidity, and economic considerations. *Am J Med.* 2002;113(1A):5S–13S.
4. Stamm WE, Hooton TM. Management of urinary tract infections in adults. *N Engl J Med.* 1993; 329:1328–1334.
5. Gordon KA, Jones RN, et al. Susceptibility patterns of orally administered antimicrobials among urinary tract infection pathogens from hospitalized patients in North America: Comparison report to Europe and Latin America. Results from the SENTRY Antimicrobial Surveillance Program (2000). *Diagn Microbiol Infect Dis.* 2003;45: 295–301.
6. Bent S, Nallamothu BK, Simel DL, Fihn SD, Saint S. Does this woman have an acute, uncomplicated urinary tract infection? *JAMA.* 2002;287(20):2701–2710.
7. Wallach J. *Interpretation of Diagnostic Tests.* 7th ed. Philadelphia, PA: Lippincott, Williams and Wilkins; 2000.
8. Steinke DT, Seaton RA, Phillips G, et al. Factors associated with trimethoprim-resistant bacteria isolated from urine samples. *J Antimicrob Chemother.* 1999;43:841–843.
9. Ti TY, Kumarasinghe G, Taylor MB, et al. What is true community-acquired urinary tract infection? Comparison of pathogens identified in urine from routine outpatient specimens and from community clinics in a prospective study. *Eur J Clin Microbiol Infect Dis.* 2003;22:242–245.
10. Stamm WE, Hooton TM. Management of urinary tract infections in adults. *N Engl J Med.* 1993; 329:1328–1334.
11. Tice AD. Short-course therapy of acute cystitis: A brief review of therapeutic strategies. *J Antimicrob Chemother.* 1999;43(A):85–93.
12. Irvani A, Klimberg I, Briefer C, et al. A trial comparing low-dose, short-course ciprofloxacin and standard 7-day therapy with co-trimoxazole or nitrofurantoin in the treatment of uncomplicated urinary tract infections. *J Antimicrob Chemother.* 1999;43(A):67–75.
13. McCarty JM, Richard G, Huck W, et al. A randomized trial of short-course ciprofloxacin, ofloxacin, or trimethoprim–sulfamethoxazole for treatment of acute urinary tract infections in women. *Am J Med.* 1999;106:292–299.
14. Alper BS, Curry SH. Urinary tract infection in children. *Am Fam Physician.* 2005;72(12):2483–2488.
15. Shand DG, Nimmon CC, O'Grady F, et al. Relation between residual urine volume and response to treatment of urinary infection. *Lancet.* 1970;1:1305–1306.
16. Hooton TM, Stamm WE. Diagnosis and treatment of uncomplicated urinary tract infection. *Infect Dis Clin North Am.* 1997;11:551–581.

17. Gilstrap LC, Ramin SM. Urinary tract infection during pregnancy. *Obstet Gynecol Clin North Am.* 2001;28:581–591.
18. Shortliffe LM, McCue JD. Urinary tract infections at the age extremes: pediatrics and geriatrics. *Am J Med.* 2002; 113(1A):55S–66S.
19. Ramakrishnan K, Scheid DC. Diagnosis and management of acute pyelonephritis in adults. *Am Fam Physician.* 2005;71: 933–944.
20. Platt R. Quantitative definition of bacteriuria. *Am J Med.* 1983;75:44–52.
21. Lipsky BA. Prostatitis and urinary tract infection in men: What's new; what's true? *Am J Med.* 1999;106:327–334.
22. Gleckman R, Crowley M, Natsios GA. Therapy of recurrent invasive urinary tract infection in men. *N Engl J Med.* 1979;301:878–880.
23. Wong ES, McKevitt M, Running K, et al. Management of recurrent urinary tract infections with patient-administered single-dose therapy. *Ann Intern Med.* 1985;102:302–307.
24. Hooton TM. Recurrent urinary tract infection in women. *Int J Antimicrob Agents.* 2001;17:259–268.
25. Stapleton A, Latham RH, Johnson C, et al. Post-coital antimicrobial prophylaxis for recurrent urinary tract infection. *JAMA.* 1990;264:703–706.
26. Melekos MD, Naber KG. Complicated urinary tract infections. *Int J Antimicrob Agents.* 2000;15:247–256.
27. Christensen B. Which antibiotics are appropriate for treating bacteriuria in pregnancy? *J Antimicrob Chemother.* 2000;46(S1):29–34.
28. McDermott S, Dagiuse V, Mann H, et al. Perinatal risk for mortality and mental retardation associated with maternal urinary tract infections. *J Fam Pract.* 2001;50:433–437.
29. Trautner BW, Darouiche RO. Catheter-associated infections; pathogenesis affects prevention. *Arch Intern Med.* 2004; 164(8): 842–850.
30. Tambyah PA, Maki DG. Catheter-associated urinary tract infection is rarely symptomatic. *Arch Intern Med.* 2000; 160:678–682.
31. Ohkawa M, Sugata T, Sawaki M, et al. Bacterial and crystal adherence to the surfaces of indwelling urethral catheters. *J Urol.* 1990;143:717–721.
32. Johnson JR, Duskowski MA, Wilt TJ. Systemic review: antimicrobial urinary catheters prevent catheter-associated urinary tract infections in hospital patients. *Arch Intern Med.* 2006;144(2):116–126.
33. Schaefer AJ. Urinary tract infection in men: State of the art. *Infection.* 1994;22(1):S19–S21.
34. Drieger JN, Nyberg L, Nickel JC. NIH concensus definition and classification of prostatitis. *JAMA.* 1999;282: 236–237.
35. Fair WR, Couch J, Wehner M. Prostatic antibacterial factor: Identity and significance. *Urology.* 1976;7:169–177.
36. Meares EM. Prostatitis. *Med Clin North Am.* 1991;75:405–424.
37. Wagenlehner FM, Naber KG. Current challenges in the treatment of complicated urinary tract infections and prostatitis. *Clin Microbiol Infect.* 2006;12(3):67–80.

Chapter 45
Sexually Transmitted Diseases

Laurajo Ryan

SEARCH STRATEGY

A search and evaluation of the medical literature was performed on January 22, 2008. This search was limited to studies published in English concerning human trials. An Ovid search was performed, as was a search of the Centers for Disease Control and Prevention website and the National Guideline Clearinghouse.

Sexually transmitted diseases (STDs) are a heterogeneous group of infections with a wide variety of causative agents. The pathogens associated with STDs run the range from bacterial, viral, and fungal sources to parasitic organisms. The common link between the infecting agents and the diseases they cause, is their propensity to be spread through sexual contact.

Primary care providers are in the unique position to not only diagnose and treat current STD infections, but they also have the opportunity to reduce STD transmission through risk reduction counseling. Screening for STD risk factors should occur at each health care contact and education on safer sexual practices is appropriate for all at-risk patients. Counseling measures aimed at preventing transmission of STDs must be delivered in a nonjudgmental manner and should address each patient's particular risk factors. Patients who seek testing for one STD should also be offered testing for all STDs, including HIV.

Risk factors for acquiring STDs include young age, socioeconomic factors, immune status, sexual orientation and sexual behaviors among others. Specific behaviors associated with increased risk of infection with a STD (regardless of other risk factors) include multiple sexual partners, male with male sex, and sexual contact with those people known to be infected with STDs.

Short of abstinence, the best protection against contracting a STD is participation in a mutually monogamous relationship with an uninfected partner. Consistent and proper usage of latex condoms offers the next best protection against STDs.

Although STDs occur more commonly in males than females, the complications associated with STDs tend to be more severe in women. These complications can include damage to the reproductive system, increased risk of cervical cancer and disease transmission to the neonate during pregnancy or childbirth.

This chapter will focus on the most commonly encountered STDs (Table 45-1). The recommendations contained in this chapter are derived from the Centers for Disease Control and Prevention (CDC) treatment guidelines.[1]

In general, patients who actively seek treatment and evaluation of STDs complain of genital ulcers, urethritis, cervicitis, or copious vaginal discharge and itching. The signs and symptoms of many STDs are similar which makes testing for specific etiology paramount, since prompt treatment can limit further disease spread. All patients who are evaluated for STDs should also be screened for HIV.[1]

VIRAL INFECTIONS

STDs that are caused by viral agents produce lifelong infections. The course of the specific disease is variable, and is dependent upon both viral and host factors. Treatment is aimed at transmission prevention, symptom suppression and decreasing morbidity and mortality. Hepatitis A (HAV), hepatitis B (HBV) and hepatitis C can be transmitted sexually, unfortunately, HAV and HBV and human papillomavirus (HPV) are the only STDs for which approved vaccines are available.

Table 45-1. Sexually Transmitted and Sexually Transmissible Microorganisms

Bacteria	Viruses	Other*
Transmitted in adults predominantly by sexual intercourse		
Neisseria gonorrhoeae	HIV (types 1 and 2)	*Trichomonas vaginalis*
Chlamydia trachomatis	Human T-cell lymphotropic virus type I	*Phthirus pubis*
Treponema pallidum	Herpes simplex virus type 2	
Haemophilus ducreyi	HPV (multiple genotypes)	
Calymmatobacterium granulomatis	HBV†	
Ureaplasma urealyticum	Molluscum contagiosum virus	
Sexual transmission repeatedly described but not well defined or not the predominant mode		
Mycoplasma hominis	Cytomegalovirus	*Candida albicans*
M. genitalium	Human T-cell lymphotropic virus type II	*Sarcoptes scabiei*
Gardnerella vaginalis and other vaginal bacteria	(?) Hepatitis C, D viruses	
Group B *Streptococcus*	HSV-1	
Mobiluncus spp.	(?) Epstein–Barr virus	
Helicobacter cinaedi	Kaposi's sarcoma-associated herpesvirus‡	
Sporothrix fennelliae	Transfusion-transmitted virus	
Transmitted by sexual contact involving oral-fecal exposure; of declining importance in homosexual men		
Shigella spp.	HAV	*Giardia lamblia*
Campylobacter spp.		*Entamoeba histolytica*

*Includes protozoa, ectoparasites, and fungi.
†Among the US patients for whom a risk factor can be ascertained, most HBV infections are transmitted sexually or by injection drug use.
‡Human herpesvirus type 8.

GENITAL HERPES

Genital herpes lesions are caused by two separate virion, herpes simplex virus type 1 (HSV-1) and herpes simplex virus type 2 (HSV-2). HSV-1 is typically associated with perioral lesions, these lesions are commonly termed "fever blisters." HSV-2 is the more common cause of genital lesions, although it should be kept in mind that either virus can cause infection in either region. It is estimated that at least 45 million persons in the United States are infected with genital herpes.[2] Infections with HSV-1 and HSV-2 are, as with other viral infections, lifelong.

Clinical Presentation

The initial manifestation of genital herpes usually presents as blisters in the genital and/or perianal area, which later burst and form painful ulcers (Table 45-2). These ulcers characteristically last weeks to months, and occasionally are so severe as to require hospitalization. Subsequent outbreaks tend to be less severe, both in intensity and in duration than the initial outbreak, and many infected persons never experience another symptomatic episode after the initial flare.[3] Viral transmission can occur even when there are no visible

Table 45-2. Clinical Features of Genital Ulcers

Disease	Clinical Diagnosis	Painful Ulcers	Inguinal Adenopathy	Comment
Syphilis	Indurated, relatively clean base; heals spontaneously	No	Firm, rubbery nodes; tender	Primary (chancre); secondary (rash, mucocutaneous lesions, lymphadenopathy); tertiary (cardiac, ophthalmic, auditory, CNS lesions)
Herpes simplex infection	Multiple, small, grouped vesicles coalesce and form shallow ulcers; vulvovaginitis	Yes	Tender bilateral adenopathy	Cytologic detection insensitive; false-negative culture common; type-specific serologic test
Chancroid	Multiple, painful, irregular, purulent ulcers	Yes	Painful, suppurative, inguinal lymph nodes	Cofactor for HIV transmission; 10% have HSV or syphilis

Source: Adapted from Centers for Disease Control and Prevention: STDs treatment guidelines-2002. *MMWR.* 2002;51(RR-6).

lesions, in fact, many of those who are infected are completely asymptomatic and unaware they carry the disease. Asymptomatic viral shedding is more typical with HSV-2 than it is with HSV-1, and is also more common during the first year of infection.[2,4] Herpes viruses are transmitted when infected bodily secretions come in contact of with mucosal or abraded tissue. Women are more susceptible to infection than are men, probably because of the more extensive contact of mucosal surfaces during sexual activity. Herpes virus may also be transmitted neonatally during vaginal birth; the risk for transmission is exceptionally high if the mother contracts the virus near the time of delivery.[5] Current recommendations state that women with active herpetic lesions at the time of onset of labor should deliver via cesarean section to protect against herpes transmission. However, even those women who are asymptomatic at time of delivery can pass the virus; cesarean delivery has not been proven 100% protective against vertical transmission.[6,7]

DIAGNOSTIC EVALUATION

Genital herpes may be diagnosed clinically by history, physical presentation, and visual inspection, although this method is not optimal as many infected patients are asymptomatic. Several modes of laboratory testing have been employed, but none has proven fully satisfactory. Virological testing to isolate HSV within cell cultures is the preferred detection method in those who present with genital lesions. When testing mucocutaneous lesions, the sensitivity is highest for HSV early in the course of the outbreak, and rapidly declines as the ulcers heal.[7]

Sensitivity also declines when testing recurrent outbreaks as opposed to testing the initial disease presentation.[6] Polymerase chain reaction assays to amplify HSV DNA are sensitive, but very expensive, and their role in testing has not been fully defined. Since cytological Tzanck testing which stains cells obtained from lesions is both nonspecific and insensitive, it is only helpful when positive.[2]

Treatment

Antiviral therapy combined with disease counseling and transmission prevention is the mainstay of treatment for genital herpes. Systemic antiviral drugs are used for symptomatic treatment. Daily suppressive therapy with systemic antiviral drugs can reduce both the severity and frequency of outbreaks.[8] These drugs may also be used upon symptom recurrence to reduce the severity and length of the outbreak, but intermittent therapy does not decrease the frequency of outbreaks. Sustained oral antiviral treatment cannot eliminate the virus from the body, but it can decrease viral shedding, possibly reducing, but not eliminating, the risk of transmitting the virus to a sexual partner.[8] Topical antiviral treatments have shown little efficacy in the treatment of genital herpes and are not recommended. Acyclovir, valacyclovir and famcyclovir have all been shown in randomized clinical trials to provide benefit in the treatment of genital herpes.[9–12]

Treatment of initial symptomatic episode (Table 45-3) is usually prescribed for 7 to 10 days, but if healing is not complete on day 10, therapy will usually be extended. The decision to treat episodically only during outbreaks or to administer daily suppressive therapy is ultimately driven by the severity and frequency of outbreaks the patient experiences.

GENITAL WARTS

Condyloma acuminatum, commonly know as genital warts, are caused by HPV. It is estimated that approximately 50% of sexually active people are infected with HPV, and a high percentage of persons are unaware of their infection. HPV encompasses a large group of viruses, more than 30 strains of which have been shown to be sexually transmitted. The most serious consequence of HPV is cervical cancer.[13] Approximately 90% of all cervical cancers are associated with HPV infection. In June 2006, the FDA approved the HPV vaccine Gardasil for use in females 9 to 26 years of age. The vaccine is protective against four of the most common strains of HPV which together account for more than 90% of cases of genital warts.[14]

Clinical presentation

Genital warts typically appear externally as painless, pink or flesh colored swellings of the skin of the genital region, perineum, and perianal region. These warts can appear singly or in clusters and may occasionally be found on the face. Genital warts can also manifest internally on the cervix, vaginal walls, and anus or within the urethra, in which case the patient is unlikely to be aware of the infection. After infection with HPV, signs of infection may take months to appear, or the infected person may never develop symptoms. Visible signs need not be present to transmit the virus.

Diagnostic Evaluation

Diagnosis of genital warts is by visual identification. Many asymptomatic women are presumptively diagnosed with HPV on the basis of an abnormal Papanicolaou test (Pap smear). Biopsy and DNA identification of HPV is also available for women who present with mild cervical dysplasia, although tests are not normally warranted in routine management of genital warts.

Table 45-3. Antimicrobial Therapy for STDs

Disease	First-Line Treatment	Alternate(s)
Chlamydia	Azithromycin 1 g po single dose Doxycycline 100 mg po bid × 7 d	Erythromycin 500 mg po qid × 7 d Ofloxacin 300 mg po bid × 7 d Levofloxacin 500 mg po qd × 7 d
Gonorrhea	Cefixime 400 mg po single dose Ceftriaxone 125 mg IM single dose Ciprofloxacin 500 mg po single dose Ofloxacin 400 mg po single dose Levofloxacin 250 mg po single dose	Spectinomycin 2 g IM single dose Spectinomycin 2 g IM single dose Gatifloxacin 400 mg po single dose
Trichomoniasis	Metronidazole 2 g po single dose	Metronidazole 500 mg po bid × 7 d
Bacterial vaginosis	Metronidazole 500 mg po bid × 7 d Metronidazole vaginal gel 0.75% qd for 5 d	Clindamycin 2% cream intravaginally qhs × 7 d
Syphilis (primary, secondary, early tertiary)	Benzathine penicillin G 2.4 million units IM d in a single dose	Doxycycline 100 mg po bid × 14
Syphilis (latent, tertiary)	Benzathine penicillin G 2.4 million units IM weekly × 3 weeks	
HSV (primary)	Acyclovir 400 mg po tid × 7-10 d Famciclovir 250 mg po tid × 7-10 d Valacyclovir 1 g po bid × 7-10 d	Acyclovir 200 mg po 5 times a day × 7-10 d
HSV (recurrent)	Acyclovir 400 mg po tid × 5 d Famciclovir 125 mg po bid × 5 d Valacyclovir 500 mg po bid × 5 d	Acyclovir 800 mg po 5 times a day × 7-10 d Valacyclovir 1 g po qd × 5 days
Chancroid	Azithromycin 1 g po single dose Ceftriaxone 250 mg IM single dose Ciprofloxacin 500 mg po bid × 3 d	Erythromycin base 500 mg po qid × 7

Source: Adapted from the Centers for Disease Control and Prevention: STDs treatment guidelines-2002. *MMWR.* 51(RR-6), 2002.

Treatment

No specific treatment for genital warts has proven to be more effective than any other treatment. This includes watchful waiting, as symptoms can resolve without treatment. If active therapy is desired, the regimen is based on wart location (moist or dry area), amount of skin area involved and preference of the patient and provider.[13] Three main avenues of treatment are available: surgical, laser therapy or topical treatment. Treatment can take place in the provider's office or topical therapy can be administered at home by the patient. Common office treatments include cryotherapy with liquid nitrogen, surgical removal of individual warts or application of a caustic agent such as trichloroacetic acid. Common at-home topical therapies are podofilox 0.5% applied to affected area in cycles of twice daily application for 3 days, alternating with no therapy for 4 days, repeated over a 4-week period, or imiquimod 5% applied before bed, 3 nights each week for 16 weeks.

BACTERIAL INFECTIONS

A great number of different organisms including spirochetes and both gram-negative and gram-positive bacteria cause sexually transmitted bacterial infections.

SYPHILIS

Syphilis is an STD that is considered a reportable disease in every state. It is caused by the spirochete *Treponema pallidum.* Transmission is through direct mucous membrane contact or through an abrasion in nonmucous tissue with a syphilis lesion of an infected sexual partner. Exposure can also occur in the womb. After initial infection, syphilis has an incubation period that normally lasts approximately 3 weeks, but it can last up to 3 months. If left untreated, syphilis progresses through several different phases: primary, secondary, latent, and tertiary. Neurosyphilis can occur at any point in the disease. Each stage of syphilis presents with its own specific set of symptoms.

Clinical Presentation

Primary Syphilis. After the dormant period, primary syphilis presents with painless genital ulcers or chancres at the site of infection (Table 45-2). The lesion or lesions (more than one chancre may occur if more than one spirochete penetrated at initial exposure) can arise on the external genitals or perianal area where they are visible, but they can also occur in the vagina, rectum or in the mouth where they are not as evident. The chancres are round in shape, indurated, and usually painless. This primary lesion can last up to two months, but may disappear as quickly as one week even without treatment.

Secondary Syphilis. Secondary syphilis manifests as skin rash 14 to 42 days after appearance of the primary chancre if the primary stage is left untreated. The rash typically occurs on the palms of the hands and the soles of the feet. The rash is often accompanied by general malaise, fever, and lymphadenopathy. Independent of treatment, the rash usually disappears in 4 to 6 weeks.

Latent Syphilis. During latent syphilis, the infected person shows no symptoms of the disease, but will have positive infection upon serological testing. The early latent period is defined as up to 1 year from infection by the U.S. Public Health Service. Late latent syphilis is the period of asymptomatic infection greater than 1 year post infection. The late latent stage is generally considered to be noninfectious, except during pregnancy, but the disease may still progress to the tertiary stage.

Tertiary Syphilis. Tertiary or late syphilis can develop anywhere from 1 to 30 years after initial infection in untreated persons. Tertiary syphilis is characterized by organ damage; particularly cardiovascular damage, neurological damage and the presence of benign gumma that can involve any organ.

Diagnostic Evaluation

Microscopic inspection of fluid from chancres or enlarged lymph nodes can identify *T. pallidum* on darkfield examination; the spirochete can also be identified through direct fluorescent antibody tests. Two types of serological examinations are useful for diagnosis when fluid samples are not available and syphilis is suspected. Nontreponemal tests such as the Venereal Disease Research Laboratory (VDRL) and Rapid Plasma Reagin (RPR) test for antibodies. Both VDRL and RPR can yield false-positive results and alone are not appropriate for diagnosis. Positive nontreponemal serology tests should be confirmed by treponemal serological testing such as fluorescent treponemal antibody absorbed (FTA-ABS) or *T. pallidum* particle agglutination (TP-PA). Serial nontreponemal antibody testing correlates to disease activity, and can be used to track disease progression. After successful treatment of primary or secondary syphilis, the patient almost invariably becomes seronegative, while patients treated for tertiary or late latent syphilis tend to remain seropositive.

Treatment

Parenteral penicillin G is the mainstay of syphilis treatment in all stages of the disease. Penicillin G is used preferentially for treatment of syphilis over other penicillin preparations because of the drug's long half-life. Differences in the growth patterns of *T. pallidum* depend on the length of infection; for this reason, the specific disease stage determines the appropriate treatment regimen. Since *T. pallidum* resistance to penicillin has not developed, alternative drug regimens that do not contain penicillins are only appropriate treatment in those who are truly penicillin allergic. Penicillin G is the only drug shown to be safe and effective for syphilis treatment during pregnancy. Pregnant women who report a penicillin allergy should undergo skin testing for confirmation; penicillin desensitization should be conducted if an allergy is confirmed. Specific treatment regimens recommended by the CDC are listed in Table 45-3.

GONORRHEA

It is estimated that infection with *Neisseria gonorrhoeae* causes more than half a million new cases of gonorrhea each year in the United States alone.[1] In many men, quickly developing symptoms of urethral infection cause them to seek prompt treatment, but often women (and some men) will remain asymptomatic. Additionally, many of those infected with gonorrhea are coinfected with *Chlamydia trachomatis*. Most authorities recommend an agent that is effective against both *N. gonorrhoeae* and *C. trachomatis* be added to primary gonorrhea therapy. Presumptive therapy is often cheaper than actually testing for chlamydial infection in those with gonorrhea.[1]

Clinical Presentation

Patients who are infected with gonorrhea display a highly variable clinical picture. Within 2 to 8 days of infection, most men will develop symptoms of urethritis including dysuria, increased urinary frequency and purulent discharge from the penis. These disturbing symptoms usually cause infected men to seek treatment. Women, on the other hand, may experience symptoms that are nonspecific such as dysuria, increased urinary frequency, and increased vaginal discharge if symptoms are present at all. Unfortunately, gonorrhea is often not diagnosed in women until disease complications such as pelvic inflammatory disease (PID) have developed. PID is a common cause of female infertility. The most common site of gonorrheal infection in women is the endocervical canal, but also occurs in the cervix itself. Both men and women can also contract infection of the oropharynx, rectum, or eyes. Left untreated, gonorrhea infection can disseminate in the blood (bacteremia), and ultimately cause skin lesions and septic arthritis.

Diagnostic Evaluation

Diagnosis in women is problematic since they are so often asymptomatic; therefore screening of at-risk persons is paramount. Diagnosis in men is more straightforward given that they typically present shortly after onset of symptoms. Clinically, the Gram stain is the most useful initial technique for identification of the *N. gonorrhoeae* bacterium in urethral or vaginal discharge. *N. gonorrhoeae* is a gram-negative intracellular diplococcus. Ambiguous Gram stain smears require that a culture be performed. Most people are colonized with neisseria in the oropharynx, so Gram stain is not useful for diagnosis of suspected pharyngeal gonorrhea.

Treatment

Gonorrheal resistance to antibiotic treatment is increasing worldwide. Gonorrheal resistance may be either plasmid-mediated (penicillins, tetracycline) or chromosomally mediated (penicillins, tetracycline and fluoroquinolones).[15] Resistance to fluoroquinolones has spread to the point that the CDC recommends against using this class of drugs to treat gonorrhea in the United States.[16] Local resistance patterns should be used to guide choice of treatment from within the CDC recommended regimens (Table 45-3).[17]

If chlamydial coinfection cannot be ruled out, the patient should receive a concomitant course of doxycycline or azithromycin.

CHLAMYDIA INFECTIONS

Chlamydia infections are the most common bacterial STDs in the United States. The causative bacterium is *C. trachomatis*. *Chlamydia* infections are particularly dangerous, because even when signs/symptoms are mild, the patient is still contagious and an untreated infection may cause irreparable harm. In women, PID, ectopic pregnancy, and irreversible infertility can result from chlamydial infection. As stated in the section on gonorrhea, coinfection with both *N. gonorrhea* and *C. trachomatis* is quite common and many authorities recommend treatment for both infections if either bacterium is detected.

Clinical Presentation

In patients who display symptoms (75% of women and 50% of men are asymptomatic), mucopurulent vaginal or penile discharge, accompanied by a burning sensation during urination are the most common findings. Symptoms typically appear 1 to 3 weeks after

Table 45-4. Treatment of Infectious Urethritis and/or Cervicitis

Syndrome/Microorganism	First-Line Therapy	Alternative Therapy
Empiric therapy (treat for both *N. gonorrhoeae* and *C. trachomatis*)	Combination therapy for both organisms (see below)	
Gonococcal urethritis (*N. gonorrhoeae*)	Ceftriaxone, 125 mg IM ×1 Ciprofloxacin,* 500 mg orally × 1 Cefixime, 400 mg orally × 1	Spectinomycin,† 2 g IM × 1 Ceftizoxime,‡ 250–500 mg IM × 1 Cefuroxime axetil,‡ 1 g orally × 1
Nongonococcal urethritis (*C. trachomatis* or *U. urealyticum*)	Doxycycline,§ 100 mg orally twice daily × 7 d Azithromycin, 1 g orally × 1	Erythromycin base, 500 mg orally four times daily × 7 d Erythromycin ethylsuccinate, 800 mg orally four times daily × 7 d Ofloxacin, 300 mg orally twice daily × 7 d Amoxicillin, 500 mg orally twice daily × 7 d
Recurrent/persistent urethritis	Ensure patient is compliant with therapy Evaluate for possible reexposure to untreated infected sexual partner Wet mount +/− culture for *Trichomonas vaginalis*	Retreat Retreat Metronidazole,¶ 2 g orally × 1 plus erythromycin base, 500 mg orally four times daily × 7 d OR Erythromycin ethylsuccinate, 800 mg orally four times daily × 7 d

*The fluoroquinolones should not be used during pregnancy or in patients less than 18 years of age. The CDC no longer recommends use of fluroquinolones for patients in the U.S.
†Spectinomycin, once widely used for the treatment of gonorrhea, has the disadvantages of higher cost, requirement for injection, and lack of sustained high-serum bactericidal levels.
‡Ceftizoxime and cefuroxime are well tolerated but less active.
§Doxycycline should not be used during pregnancy.
¶Metronidazole should not be given during the first trimester of pregnancy. Metronidazole may cause a disulfiram-like reaction with alcohol.

infection. Infection may also be present in the throat of those who have oral sex and the anus and rectum of those who receive anal sex.

Diagnostic Evaluation

Diagnosis of chlamydial infection is made by detection of *C. trachomatis* by either culture or nucleic acid amplification tests. If the patient is in a risk group with a particularly high prevalence of *Chlamydia* and gonorrhea, and the disease is clinically suspected, the CDC recommends empiric treatment, especially in those unlikely to return for treatment.

Treatment

Therapy for chlamydial infections (Table 45-4) commonly includes treatment with either azithromycin or doxycycline. Both regimens have proven efficacious in clinical trials. In some patient groups the azithromycin may be preferred because it can be given as directly observed single-dose therapy.

CHANCROID

Chancroid infection is caused by *Haemophilus ducreyi*, a gram-negative bacillus, and is an important cofactor for the transmission of HIV infection. Infection with chancroid is not commonly detected in the Unites States, but has been associated with periodic regional outbreaks. All patients diagnosed with chancroid should be tested for HIV since infections with *H. ducreyi* increases transmission rates of HIV.

Clinical Presentation

Chancroid presents as highly painful genital ulcers 3 to 5 days after sexual exposure to an infected partner. The ulcer itself is not indurated, but typically appears necrotic with purulent discharge and may be accompanied by inguinal lymphadenopathy. Untreated, the enlarged lymph (bubo) may form an abscess.

Diagnostic Evaluation

H. ducreyi is the causative agent in chancroid infections, but the culture media used to make specific diagnosis has a low sensitivity. Polymerase chain reaction testing is available commercially, although there are no FDA approved assays. Presumptive diagnosis is made based on the presence of painful genital ulcers only when syphilis and herpes simplex virus have been ruled out by examination of the exudative fluid from the ulcer. The presence of painful genital ulcers when associated with regional lymphadenopathy is also highly suggestive of chancroid infection.

Treatment

Chancroid is treated with a macrolide antibiotic (erythromycin, azithromycin), or ceftriaxone or ciprofloxacin (Table 45-3). Treatment results in clinical cure in approximately one week, although resistance to ciprofloxacin and erythromycin is increasing worldwide and treatment should be based on local resistance patterns.

In the primary care setting, detecting and preventing transmission of STDs is of paramount importance. STD risks should be discussed openly and honestly with patients, and CDC guidelines should serve as the basis for treatment recommendations.

EVIDENCE-BASED SUMMARY

- STDs include a wide variety of infections including bacterial, viral and fungal pathogens
- Risk factors for STDs include young age, socioeconomic factors, immune status, sexual orientation, and sexual behaviors such as sexual contact with those known to be infected, and multiple sexual partners
- The spread of STDs can be limited by participating in a mutually monogamous relationship and by consistent, proper use of a latex condom
- HAV, HBV, and HPV are the only STDs for which approved vaccinations are available
- The presentation of many STDs are very similar, which makes laboratory testing to determine the specific pathogen mandatory
- Infections with the herpes-virus are lifelong, and although symptoms may not be present, the disease is still transmissible

REFERENCES

1. Centers for Disease Control and Prevention. Sexually transmitted diseases treatment guidelines 2002. 2002; 51(No. RR-6):1–79.
2. Leone P. Reducing the risk of transmitting genital herpes: Advances in understanding and therapy. *Curr Med Res Opin.* 2005;21(10):1577–1582.
3. Kimberlin DW, Rouse DJ. Clinical practice. Genital herpes. *N Engl J Med.* 2004;350:1970.
4. Brock BV, Selke S, Benedetti J, et al. Frequency of asymptomatic shedding of herpes simplex virus in women with genital herpes. *JAMA.* 1990;263:418.
5. Brown ZA, Gardella C, Wald A, et al. Genital herpes complicating pregnancy. *Obstet Gynecol.* 2005;106(4): 845–856.

6. Leung DT, Sacks SL. Current recommendations for the treatment of genital herpes. *Drugs*. 2000;60:1329–1352.

7. ACOG Committee on Practice Bulletins—Gynecology. ACOG practice bulletin: Clinical management guidelines for obstetrician–gynecologists, number 57, November 2004. Gynecologic herpes simplex virus infections. *Obstet Gynecol*. 2004;104 (5 Pt 1):1111–1118.

8. Wald A. New therapies and prevention strategies for genital herpes. *Clin Infect Dis*. 1999;28(Suppl):S4.

9. Diaz-Mitoma F, Sibbald RG, Shafran SD, Boon R, Saltzman RL. Oral famciclovir for the suppression of recurrent genital herpes: a randomized controlled trial. *JAMA*. 1998;280:887–892.

10. Chosidow O, Drouault Y, Lecontae-Veyriac F, et al. Famciclovir vs. aciclovir in immunocompetent patients with recurrent genital herpes infections: A parallel-groups, randomized, double-blind clinical trial. *Br J Dermatol*. 2001;144:818–824.

11. Fife KH, Barbarash RA, Rudolph T, Degregorio B, Roth RE. Valaciclovir versus acyclovir in the treatment of first-episode genital herpes infection: results of an international, multicenter, double-blind randomized clinical trial. *Sex Transm Dis*. 1997;24:481–486.

12. Patel R, Bodsworth NJ, Wooley P, et al. Valacyclovir for the suppression of recurrent genital HSV infection: A placebo controlled study of once-daily therapy. *Genitourin Med*. 1997;73:105–109.

13. Kurman RJ, Henson DE, Herbst AL, Noller KL, Schiffman MH, National Cancer Institute Workshop. Interim guidelines for management of abnormal cervical cytology. *JAMA*. 1994;1994(271):1866–1869.

14. Gardisil [package insert]. Whitehouse Station, NJ: Merck & Co; 2006.

15. O'Brien JP, Goldenberg DL, Rice PA. Disseminated gonococcal infection: a prospective analysis of 49 patients and a review of pathophysiology and immune mechanisms. *Medicine (Baltimore)*. 1983;62(6):395–406.

16. Centers for Disease Control and Prevention (CDC). Update to CDC's sexually transmitted diseases treatment guidelines, 2006: Fluoroquinolones no longer reccommended for treatment of gonococcal infections. *MMWR*. 2007;56:332–336.

17. Emmert DH, Kirchner JT. Sexually transmitted diseases in women: Gonorrhea and syphilis. *Postgrad Med*. 2000;107(2):181–197.

INDEX

Page numbers followed by *f* and *t* indicate figures and tables, respectively.